PHARMACOLOGY
An Introduction
to Drugs

second edition

PHARMACOLOGY
An Introduction
to Drugs

Michael C. Gerald
Professor
Division of Pharmacology
College of Pharmacy
The Ohio State University

PRENTICE-HALL, INC., ENGLEWOOD CLIFFS, NEW JERSEY 07632

Library of Congress Cataloging in Publication Data

Gerald, Michael C., (date)
  Pharmacology, an introduction to drugs.

  Includes bibliographies and index.
  1. Pharmacology. 2. Drugs. I. Title. [DNLM:
1. Drugs. 2. Pharmacology. QV 38 G354p]
RM300.G47 1981   615'.1   81-1540
ISBN 0-13-662098-1   AACR2

Editorial/production supervision
  and interior design by Kathleen M. Lafferty
Cover design by Edsal Enterprises
Manufacturing buyer: John B. Hall

Printed in the United States of America

10 9 8 7 6 5 4 3 2 1

Prentice-Hall International, Inc., *London*
Prentice-Hall of Australia Pty. Limited, *Sydney*
Prentice-Hall of Canada, Ltd., *Toronto*
Prentice-Hall of India Private Limited, *New Delhi*
Prentice-Hall of Japan, Inc., *Tokyo*
Prentice-Hall of Southeast Asia Pte. Ltd., *Singapore*
Whitehall Books Limited, *Wellington, New Zealand*

To my loving wife, Gloria,
and to Melissa and Marc

Contents

section three —————————————

DRUGS AFFECTING
THE CENTRAL NERVOUS SYSTEM   **163**

section four —————————————

DRUGS AFFECTING THE CARDIOVASCULAR
SYSTEM AND KIDNEYS   **389**

section five —————————————

DRUGS AFFECTING THE ENDOCRINE SYSTEM   **439**

Preface

Since the appearance of the first edition of *Pharmacology: An Introduction to Drugs,* drug-related news stories have continued to favorably compete for headlines in newspapers or for prominent segments on evening news broadcasts with the economy, the energy crisis, foreign affairs, and even revelations of political scandals. While interest in drugs has remained high, the focus appears to have shifted. I share the impression of many of my colleagues across the continent that interest in drug (substance) abuse is somewhat less intense than it was a decade ago and has now stabilized; fascination in the mystical and metaphysical effects of mind-altering substances, as espoused in the writings of Aldous Huxley, Havelock Ellis, Timothy Leary, and others, and as warmly embraced as gospel by students on campuses across the land some years ago, is less in vogue at present.

Students now seem to be seeking a more scientific, biomedical, and toxicological orientation to the study of drugs and other biologically active substances and now appear less interested in the social and legal aspects of drug usage. The sphere of general interest in drugs has been expanded to include the role of endorphins and the prostaglandins in health and disease and their involvement in the actions of drugs; the therapeutic utility of interferon and laetrile as anticancer agents; the benefits versus risks associated with the chronic use of oral contraceptives and oral antidiabetic agents; the potential dangers associated with the use of saccharin, phencyclidine (PCP), and marijuana; and the possible hazards to the developing fetus caused by the maternal use of alcohol or aspirin. The brisk sales enjoyed by guides to self-medications bear adequate testimony to the rise of the health-conscious consumer seeking to play an active role in the selection of his or her drugs. This edition reflects and emphasizes many of these areas of interest and concern.

While five new chapters have been prepared for this edition and sixteen chapters have undergone major revision or the extensive addition of significant new topics or sections, and all chapters have been updated and refined for clarity, the basic objectives, approach, and style of this text have been retained. The very kind formal book reviews and the informal compliments conveyed to me by mouth and mail from instructors and students in North America and abroad reinforce my desire to retain this well-received format.

Drugs will continue to be defined broadly to include medicines used for the treatment of disease as well as other biologically active chemicals, with the exception of foods. This text is designed to be read with enjoyment by students at several levels. First, it is written for the student who possesses minimal formal scientific preparation but who desires or requires a basic understanding of the actions and biological effects of drugs, their therapeutic uses, if any, and their potential dangers. Every effort has been made to provide such a reader with the technical vocabulary and the scientific and health-related background required to appreciate and comprehend drug-induced effects. Conversely, although the book is simply written, it does not, therefore, assume that the reader seeks a grossly oversimplified treatment of basic concepts. In this regard, the text presents an intellectual challenge for the scientifically well-versed student who seeks a distillation of the contemporary concepts underlying the basic and applied principles of pharmacology.

The text continues to provide the instructor with considerable flexibility concerning the choice of subject material and the order in which the eight major sections and the 32 chapters are presented or assigned for independent reading. The scope of subjects is sufficiently broad enough to facilitate the selection of materials that will best complement and supplement the many possible diverse objectives of a contemporary one semester-quarter course. The contents of this text, and the most significant revisions incorporated in this revision, are summarized as follows:

Section One, in particular Chapters 1 through 3, introduces the fundamental principles that serve as the foundation of pharmacology and the remainder of the book. This revision places considerable emphasis on the relationship between the dose and the biological response (Chapter 2) and expands the discussion of the influence of old age, placebos, and drug-drug interactions on the response to drugs. Section Two, "Drugs Affecting the Peripheral Nervous System," has been updated to include our better understanding of autonomic receptor concepts, and Chapter 8 more extensively examines the effects of toxins and venoms on the nervous system.

Many changes appear in Section Three (Chapters 9 through 18), "Drugs Affecting the Central Nervous System," which occupies about one-third of the entire text. Since various aspects of the nonmedical use of drugs and the concept of drug dependence appear throughout this section, the chapter "Drug Abuse in Today's Society" has been moved to an earlier position (Chapter 10) and greater muscle has been placed on drug use in athletic competition. To better reflect advances in knowledge and reader concern, new or greatly expanded sections have been devoted to the fetal alcohol syndrome, alcohol–drug interactions, and medical hazards of chronic alcoholism (Chapter 12); the opiate receptor and endogenous (natural) opiates called endorphins (Chapter 13); the pharmacology of the prostaglandins and their relationship to the actions of aspirin-like drugs (Chapter 14); cocaine (Chapter 15); mania and the benzodiazepine (Valium-like) antianxiety agents (Chapter 16); phencyclidine (Chapter 17); and the potential dangers and possible therapeutic uses of marijuana (Chapter 18). Appetite suppressants and the use of amphetamine-like drugs for the treatment of hyperkinetic disorders have been moved to Chapter 15 from Section Two.

Section Four contains greater stress on cardiac arrhythmias and their drug treatment (Chapter 21) and an almost completely rewritten chapter (22) on antihypertensive agents, which now also includes an extensive treatment of kidney physiology and diuretic agents. The control of fertility, a comparison of alternative contraceptive methods, the potential dangers of oral contraceptives (Chapter 23), and a gaze into possible future treatment approaches to diabetes mellitus (Chapter 24) appear in Section Five (endocrine drugs).

Section Six, dealing with the treatment of common gastrointestinal and respiratory disorders, is an addition in this revision. The use of antacids and other drugs for the management of peptic ulcer disease appears in Chapter 25, while the following chapter considers the properties and therapeutic uses of laxatives and antidiarrheal agents. Chapter 27 evaluates contemporary treatments used for the symptomatic relief of the common cold and the treatment of allergic disorders and asthma. The scope of the antimicrobial agents has been broadened in Chapter 29 of Section Seven (chemotherapy), while prominent consideration of the cell cycle and cancer chemotherapy, interferon, and laetrile have been added to Chapter 30.

In the intervening years since the appearance of the first edition, probably no single area of pharmacology has attracted increasingly greater attention than toxicology. This interest is mirrored in Section Eight of the revised text. Chapter 31 presents a broad overview of the many facets of the field, including environmental, economic, and forensic toxicology; the nature of the adverse effects of drugs and other chemicals; chemical mutagenesis, carcinogenesis, and teratogenesis; and acute poisoning and its emergency treatment. After examining the pharmacology of nicotine in Chapter 32, the nature of tobacco dependence and the health hazards associated with smoking are evaluated.

In Section Five we discuss the critical importance of feedback systems in maintaining homeostasis, which is essential for the survival of living organisms. Similarly, feedback from an author's readers is essential for the continued viability of his or her literary works, and, in this regard, your comments and suggestions will be sincerely appreciated. Many thanks are extended to Dr. Ralf G. Rahwan for providing me with very extensive feedback and to the staff of Prentice-Hall for expediting the production of this book.

Michael C. Gerald

General Concepts
of Pharmacology

1

Drugs
and Society

*A desire to take medicine is, perhaps, the great feature which distinguishes
man from other animals.*

—Sir William Osler (1891)

Ever since the arrival of humans on earth millions of years ago, first among
their most fundamental quests has been the search for foodstuffs for sustenance.
In an attempt to subserve this end, our forebears no doubt randomly sampled
the plants, animals, and minerals of their environment. Careful observation of
their animal neighbors, and emulation of them, helped prehistoric people select
their dinner.

Whereas ofttimes this sampling procedure proved fruitful, it could also be a
dangerous one—when, for example, by chance the seeds of *Strychnos nux vomica*
(which contain the deadly alkaloid strychnine) were chosen or the ovaries of the
pufferfish (an excellent source of tetrodotoxin, one of the most powerful poisons
known to man). Conversely, imagine the surprise of the first Peruvian Indian to
chew coca leaves. The resulting physical and mental "high" (euphoria, a feeling
of well-being) with diminished sensations of hunger can be attributed to cocaine.
If pain and hunger coexisted at the time our ancestors first imbibed the juices of
the opium poppy, perhaps upon awakening many hours later without pain, they
associated these effects with the plant.

Thus, primitive people observed that while some natural products could be
utilized as nutrients, and others were capable of relieving the symptoms of disease, still others induced harmful or even lethal effects. The branch of science
known as pharmacology is concerned with all of these types of effects.

More specifically, **pharmacology** *is the scientific study of the interaction of
chemical agents with living organisms.* Note that this definition does not attempt
to distinguish between a *desirable* interaction (for example, the cure of life-
threatening pneumonia with penicillin) and an *undesirable* interaction (such as

3

lead poisoning in children resulting from an ingestion of paint chips). We observe that both the interactions promoting the welfare of the organism enabling it to better survive and the interactions producing detrimental effects leading to its discomfiture, injury, or death are of interest to the pharmacologist. Whereas the distinction between "undesirable" and "desirable" interactions is usually rather obvious, we shall shortly observe that the particular disease and the individual patient must also be considered prior to arriving at such a judgment.

In this book we shall not restrict our discussions exclusively to human "living organisms," but, where germane, shall at times refer to the effects of drugs on other animals and on plants. Although foods are chemical agents that interact with living organisms to induce effects, they will not be considered in this work. Let us now depart from tradition and consider a **drug** to be *any chemical agent that is capable of interacting with living organisms to produce biological effects.*

STAGES IN THE DEVELOPMENT OF THERAPEUTICS

Humanity's crude awareness of disease is as old as its cognizance of hunger. Although cause and effect relationships were not understood, primitive people still knew when they were ill. Thus, as we observed, the use of drugs in the treatment of disease **(therapeutics)** is very ancient, no doubt long predating recorded history. The selection of drugs was at first fortuitous, and their continued use was based upon empirical considerations. **Empirical therapeutics** is based on *clinical evidence that a drug is effective, although the mechanism by which it acts is unknown.* For example, while colchicine has been used for thousands of years and continues to be employed for the treatment of acute attacks of gout, only in recent years has the basis for its beneficial effects been uncovered. Aspirin had been employed for approximately seven decades for the treatment of arthritis and rheumatism before the mechanism of its anti-inflammatory effects was ascertained in the early 1970s.

It should be observed that the sampling and use of drugs on an empirical basis is not merely a point of historical interest. This testing procedure is employed today by young amateur pharmacologists who sample a variety of medicine-chest products in an attempt to uncover a previously unidentified pleasurable psychic effect.

In contrast to the empirical use of drugs, modern therapeutics is primarily based upon more rational principles where the mechanism of drug action is basically understood.

We are unable to assign fixed dates to the stages in the development of therapeutics because the progression to each succeeding stage was dependent upon the specific level of development (scientific and religious) of the countries or even villages in which such development took place. Generally, however, *the development of therapeutics* may be arbitrarily divided into three stages: mystical, empirical, and specific.

Mystical Stage

The mystical stage, by far the oldest, still exists today in more primitive cultures. Strongly influenced by religion, this stage employed three major vehicles of therapy: prayers, surgery, and drugs.

God (or gods) were invoked with *prayers* to protect our ancestors against black magic, evil spirits, and demons, at a time when belief in astrology was even more widespread than in this "age of Aquarius." While some aspects of mysticism are still with us, it might be suggested that the sacrifice of a virgin has been discontinued because of scarcity of subjects with such qualifications.[1]

This same spirit of mysticism existed in colonial Salem, Massachusetts, where in 1692 nineteen persons were hanged in keeping with the words of the Bible commanding that "Thou shalt not suffer a witch to live" (Exodus 22:18). Even until the beginning of the eighteenth century, mentally ill patients were believed to be possessed by Satan and, hence, part of the therapeutic regimen was to "beat the devil out of them," in a very literal sense.

The second type of mystical therapy was *surgery*. This was exemplified in first-century Peru by trephining. In this procedure, a hole was bored through the skull in an attempt to relieve headaches or cure mental disease and epilepsy by enabling devils and demons to depart from the body of the possessed. We may be skeptical about the effectiveness of trephining in the treatment of disease, but there is little doubt that many of these ancient Peruvian surgeons possessed great skill. One exhumed skull had five such holes, with evidence that the patient survived the operations.

As might be expected, the use of *drugs* in the mystical stages was almost exclusively based upon superstition. The supposition that one could transfer innate attributes, for example, led to the use of tiger's blood as a beverage to endow the imbiber with strength. In the southwestern part of our country, the ingestion of "mescal buttons" (from the peyote cactus) is still practiced by members of the Native American Church of North America as an integral part of their religious ceremony in order to transport their souls up to God. For hundreds of years, the Christian missionaries sought to prevent the Indians from obtaining peyote. The Indians considered this plant to be "the flesh of the gods," while the missionaries contended that its use was a sure path to hell. In 1962, three Navajo members of the Church were convicted of using peyote in violation of California law. This conviction was reversed by a higher court which deemed this plant a sacramental symbol, since it was used by a Christian church in place of bread and wine, and was the "theological heart" of the religion.

[1] A.C. Kinsey, *Sexual Behavior in the Human Female* (Philadelphia: Saunders, 1953).

Empirical Stage

After many years of experience and astute clinical observations, the *empirical stage* of therapeutics rose to prominence. The first recorded compilations of drugs useful in the treatment of disease are found in the Egyptian medical papyri, so called because they were written on sheets prepared from the papyrus plant. The most famous of these was the *Ebers papyrus* (1550 B.C.) which recommends castor oil and aloe (laxatives), opium (analgesic or "pain killer"), colchicine (antigout), and many other drugs currently employed as therapeutic agents. These ancient Egyptian writings also suggested that moldy bread be applied to skin bruises, thus predating Alexander Fleming's discovery of penicillin from these molds by 3500 years.

Dioscorides, a first-century contemporary of the well-known violinist Nero, prepared a formulary arranged according to the source of the drug (plant, animal, or mineral) rather than the disease entity. In addition to a description of the source, for purposes of identification and field collection, information was provided concerning the preparation of the drug, methods of administration, and therapeutic indications for its use. Foremost in the empirical stage was the great Greek scientist and physician *Galen* (A.D. 131–201) whose dogmatic, and sometimes erroneous, teachings were to dominate medicine for 1500 years. His formulations, termed "galenicals," popularized the principle of *polypharmacy,* a term used to denote a prescription containing dozens of ingredients. The rationale for the inclusion of many of these ingredients can be traced to the medical theories and superstitions of the period.

Specific Stage

The practice of polypharmacy continued uninterrupted until the Middle Ages, when rebellious individuals such as *Paracelsus* (1493–1541) attacked the traditional prescribing philosophies of Galen. This Swiss physician-scientist vociferously advocated the use of simple, yet specific, compounds for the treatment of disease. Moreover, he declared that the alchemists of the time would better utilize their energies in developing drugs rather than in the eternal search for the philosopher's stone to transform lead into gold. This marked the beginning of the *specific stage* in the development of therapeutics, a phase dependent upon parallel advances in pharmacology, physiology, medicine, pathology, chemistry, and biochemistry.

To illustrate this evolutionary process, let us briefly consider morphine, a very widely used pain killer. During the Middle Ages when *polypharmacy* was still in vogue, prescriptions generally contained mixtures of several plants with a variety of extraneous substances added. A very simple preparation was Paracelsus's laudanum, which contained opium, gold, and pearls. (Note that even Paracelsus retained vestiges of polypharmaceutical formulation.) Perhaps in response to the outrageous cost of this prescription, *crude preparations* were introduced which contained a single drug or at least a preparation derived from a single plant, such as opium. Morphine was isolated from opium by the German apothecary Sertürner (1806), and this marked the introduction of *chemically pure active constituents* into modern therapeutics. Among morphine's many actions is that of stimulating vomiting, but because of the relative nonspecificity of this effect, morphine is not so employed in therapeutics. However, when treated with concentrated hydrochloric acid, morphine forms apomorphine, a highly specific and potent emetic used for the treatment of poisonings. Thus, we are now in the age of *synthetic drugs*, an age in which drugs are developed with the aim of greater specificity of action and enhanced potency and with fewer undesirable effects. In the mid-1970s several peptides (amino acid–containing compounds) were isolated from animal brains and found to possess morphine-like pharmacological activity; these substances have been termed *endorphins* or *enkephalins.* Scientists in many parts of the world are now actively seeking to identify other such natural compounds as well as to synthesize synthetic derivatives. It is hoped that this research will provide a better understanding of the mechanisms by which the body responds to pain and other emotional behaviors as well as provide leads for the development of safer morphine-like pain-relieving drugs lacking potential for abuse.

THE EVOLUTION OF PHARMACOLOGY

The science of **pharmacology** evolved primarily from *physiology,* a discipline concerned with the function of living organisms. In fact, nineteenth-century pharmacologists were often physiologists who turned their attention to the effects of drugs on living systems. Whereas these early scientists studied the gross effects of drugs, interest was later focused upon the specific effects of such chemicals on particular organ systems, with the desire to ascertain the basic mechanism responsible for these effects. In more recent years, many pharmacological studies have employed *biochemical* techniques in their research. The biochemical or molecular pharmacologist wishes to explain drug action on the basis of changes in the chemistry of the cell. In the final analysis, we find that drug molecules are interacting with the molecules of the cells of the body to produce an effect that may profoundly influence the entire body or even large segments of society.

In the last few decades we have seen tremendous advances in pharmacology. Many familiar drugs that we now take for granted were unknown in the last generation. Of the 25 single-ingredient drugs most frequently prescribed in the United States in 1979, 80 percent were introduced after 1950 and over one-half after 1960. Not only are individual drugs new, but more significantly, entire classes of drugs are of recent vintage. Antihistamines, antibiotics, and glucocorticoidal (cortisone-like) hormones were developed in the 1940s. The polio vaccine, oral contraceptives, and effective drugs for the management of high blood pressure and the treatment of mental disorders appeared in the following decade. Antiviral agents and levodopa (a unique breakthrough in the management of Parkinson's disease) arrived in the 1960s. The 1970s witnessed the development of improved drugs for the treatment of cancer, bacterial, viral, and fungal diseases, high blood pressure, asthma, and ulcers of the gastrointestinal tract, as well as many synthetic derivatives of the naturally occurring prostaglandins which possess great potential as therapeutic agents for the treatment of a wide range of diseases. We are optimistic that in the future pharmacological advances will be made in the treatment of cancer and parasitic diseases that ravage large proportions of the developing tropical nations and that more effective drugs will become available for the management of cardiovascular diseases and to prevent the rejection of organ transplants.

Unfortunately a large percentage of the currently available drugs, with the exception of antibiotics, merely relieve the symptoms of disease without effecting a cure. Drugs used for the treatment of schizophrenia and depression bear testimony to this shortcoming. A major ultimate objective of pharmacology and therapeutics is the development of drugs capable of *curing disease.*

WHAT IS PHARMACOLOGY?

Pharmacology is generally considered to be concerned with the *study of drugs*.[2] Prior to 1955, a **drug** could be characterized as *a chemical used in the diagnosis, prevention, treatment, or cure of disease.* In 1955 this time-honored definition was found to be inadequate after the introduction of oral contraceptives. Assuming that pregnancy is not a disease, "the pill" does not fall into any of the above categories.

A revision of our definition of drugs to include *all chemicals that affect living processes* is in order, and this definition is sufficiently general to encompass *all* chemicals affecting *all* living organisms. Thus, a study of useful therapeutic agents such as aspirin, a pesticide such as DDT, mercury poisoning in fish, and hydrogen sulfide polluting our air does not lie outside our broad scope of interest. We shall not, however, include foods, notwithstanding the fact that they fall within our broad definition.

Pharmacology is a basic medical science and its development and progress is based on the accomplishments and triumphs of other scientific disciplines. A person standing on the shoulders of a giant may see farther than the giant himself. Upon whose shoulders is pharmacology perched? Our "giant" is not one, but rather the accumulative knowledge from such sciences as biology,

---

[2] Although pharmacology deals with the study of all drug-induced effects in all animal species, **clinical pharmacology** concerns itself with an examination of the therapeutic effects and uses of drugs in the management of disease in humans and domesticated animals.

physiology, biochemistry, pathology, microbiology, psychology, and medicinal chemistry. At the same time, pharmacology supplies one of the essential building blocks in the edifice of scientific knowledge (Figure 1-1). Advances in pharmacology and the use of drugs as specific chemical tools have enhanced our basic understanding of each of these sciences.

- *Physiology* is the study of the function of the systems of living organisms.
- *Biochemistry* is concerned with the chemical reactions responsible for the maintenance of life.
- *Pathology* is an investigation of the morphologic, functional, and chemical changes responsible for disease; if we are attempting to learn about the use of drugs in the treatment of disease, a fundamental knowledge of the disease state is essential.
- *Microbiology* is the study of microorganisms (bacteria, protozoa, viruses, fungi) that are responsible for infectious and parasitic diseases.
- *Psychology* is concerned with the study of human and animal behavior. We are interested in how drugs alter normal behavior and correct abnormal behavior.
- *Medicinal chemistry* is the study of the relationship between the chemical structure of a drug and its biological activity.

This list of credits is not intended to be exhaustive, and omissions should not be interpreted as demeaning a particular discipline.

The study of pharmacology may be subdivided into its basic components, which may be considered to have both basic science and applied science elements; these are pharmacodynamics, therapeutics, and toxicology.

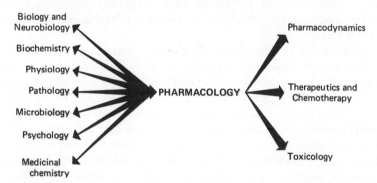

FIGURE 1-1. Pharmacology: Its Roots and Branches. Our contemporary knowledge of pharmacology is based to a large extent upon discoveries made in other scientific disciplines. Conversely, the use of drugs and other research methodologies developed by pharmacologists have led to a better understanding of the fundamental principles underlying these disciplines. This symbiotic relationship is denoted by the double arrows on the left half of the figure. The basic science and applied science applications of pharmacology appear on the right.

Pharmacodynamics, a basic experimental science, is a study of *where a drug acts in the body* (on which system, at which organ, tissue, organelle) and *how it acts* (what is the mechanism of action in physiological and/or biochemical terms). Pharmacodynamics also deals with the *absorption, distribution, metabolism (biotransformation), and elimination of drugs.*

Therapeutics (or pharmacotherapy) is a general term describing the *use of drugs in the treatment of disease.*[3] **Chemotherapy** is a specific type of therapeutics in which drugs are employed to *kill or weaken invading cells or organisms* (microbes, worm parasites, and so forth). Implicit in this definition is the prerequisite that the drug will be far more toxic to the invader (the microbe) than to the host (you)—this is the principle of *selective toxicity.*

As will be introduced shortly, and discussed throughout the remainder of this book, *all drugs are potential poisons when given in sufficient doses.* With this thought in mind, it is easy to comprehend why **toxicology,** *the study of poisons and the treatment of poisoning,* cannot be cleanly pared from pharmacology.

RELEVANCY OF PHARMACOLOGY TO SOCIETY

In the past decade, drug-related news stories have favorably competed with foreign affairs, the economy, the energy crisis, and even revelations of political scandals for headlines in newspapers or for prominent segments on evening news broadcasts. Informed citizens are encouraged by reports from laboratories describing new breakthroughs in the war against cancer or viral diseases, while horrified by claims that commonly used drugs, artificial sweeteners and other food additives, and environmental chemicals cause cancer or birth defects.

When viewed as "chemicals affecting life processes," drugs touch upon many diverse and apparently unrelated avenues of life—from algae "feeding" happily on phosphate detergents, to DDT affecting the normal development of eagles in their shells, to the alcoholic mother giving birth to a baby with severe physical abnormalities, to a national intelligence agency administering LSD to unsuspecting subjects, to anxious parents insisting that pediatricians give their children antibiotics for the common cold. The lowest common denominator in these examples is the **misuse** or **abuse of drugs** to the detriment of humankind. Obviously, a good starting place is to consider the *rational use of drugs* by readers and their families. This means employing drugs only when there is a sound medical justification for their use and in the doses prescribed.

At a very early age children begin to think of drugs as a cure for all their pains and suffering. They observe their parents consuming vitamins, weight-reducing capsules, tranquilizers, aspirins, antacids, and laxatives. Television

---

[3] Voltaire's definition of therapeutics and physicians is somewhat less charitable: "Doctors are men who prescribe medicine of which they know little to cure diseases of which they know less in human beings of whom they know nothing."

portrays the immediate drug-induced transformation of wretched souls into joyfully happy people with the mere swallow of a small tablet. It might be argued that these conditioning processes strongly contribute to later experimentation with drugs in an attempt to escape from the normal frustrations of life.

Many adults believe that a direct linear relationship exists between the dose of the drug taken and the amount of benefit received—if one tablet is good, two tablets should provide twice the beneficial effects. We shall attempt to disprove this common illusion.

We shall now consider the relevancy of *pharmacological knowledge to different segments of society.* This discussion will include the health professions, public health, social problems, agriculture and agronomy, chemical warfare, toxicology, criminology and criminalistics, and industrial and household solvents and detergents.

Health Professions

As might be anticipated, the greatest interest in drugs, and the only area in which they are formally studied, is in the health science professions. These include medicine, veterinary medicine, dentistry, nursing, allied health professions, pharmacy, health education, and nutrition.

Medicine and Veterinary Medicine

Medicinal agents are employed by these professions for the diagnosis, prevention, treatment, and cure of disease, for alleviation of the symptoms of disease, and for contraception. In addition to treating disease in domesticated and farm animals, *veterinary medicine* is also interested in promoting the growth rate and fertility of poultry and pigs and cattle. The Food and Drug Administration has banned the use of antibiotics in poultry and pigs and the use of diethylstilbestrol (a female sex hormone) in cattle feed. In both instances, concern exists regarding the presence of drug residues in animals who will eventually find their way to our dinner platter.

Dentistry

Dentists employ a limited number of drugs consisting mainly of minor tranquilizers to allay apprehension prior to their operative procedures, local anesthetics to depress pain in the specific area to be operated upon, analgesic agents to reduce postoperative pain, and, often, antibiotics to prevent infection before and after the procedures.

Nursing

The nurse is responsible for the proper administration of drugs in the hospital ward and, therefore, is very concerned with such factors as dose, route, time, and frequency of administration. Often the nurse is the first to recognize undesirable effects induced by the drug. Moreover, the nurse is playing an increasingly important role in the drug education of the patient and family.

Allied Health Professions

During the course of their daily activities, the occupational therapist, physical therapist, medical technologist, medical dietitian, and other health professionals all interact with hospitalized patients who are receiving medication. This is not at all surprising because the average patient, during a normal period of hospitalization, receives nine different drugs. Some of these drugs may modify the patient's activity or emotional behavior, while other drugs may alter accurate interpretation of laboratory results.[4] Moreover, the diet of the patient should be carefully selected so that it does not include foods capable of interfering with the desired therapeutic effects of the medication.[5] The study of pharmacology thus provides allied health professionals with a better understanding of an important and often essential component of the total medical treatment of the patient.

Pharmacy

Of all the health professions, pharmacy[6] has the broadest interest in drugs, since it is concerned with the identification, standardization, storage, compounding, and dispensing of drugs. Pharmacists employ their knowledge of drug uses, doses, side effects, and contraindications to advise both the prescriber and patient.

Health Education

In recent years, society has recognized that drug abuse is no longer solely the problem of adult addicts or the residents of ghetto communities. We now realize that the illicit use of drugs has entered middle-class and wealthy communities and is a problem in primary and secondary schools. While several years ago our health education teacher was concerned with the dangers of tobacco and alcohol, drug abuse information concerning narcotics (heroin), stimulants (amphetamine), depressants (barbiturates), and marijuana is currently taking precedence. Education concerning the dangers of these drugs is now mandatory in the primary and secondary schools of many states. Millions

---

[4] N.V. Constantino and H.F. Kabat, "Drug-Induced Modifications of Laboratory Test Values—Revised 1973," *American Journal of Hospital Pharmacy* **30**: 24–71 (1973).

[5] E. A. Hartshorn, "Food and Drug Interactions," *Journal of the American Dietetic Association* **70**: 15–19 (1977).

[6] The terms *pharmacy* and *pharmacology* are commonly but erroneously used interchangeably.

of Americans, representing a broad cross-section of the nation, use marijuana on a regular basis.

Nutrition

The inclusion of nutrition in this discussion is warranted primarily because foods and, more particularly, vitamins can prevent as well as successfully treat malnutrition and vitamin deficiencies. In a country as affluent as the United States these diseases should be, but are not yet, only of historical interest.

Public Health

There exists a great overlap of mutual interests between the health professionals and the public health investigators. The consequences of environmental pollution or smoking and the potential hazards of the indiscriminate use of food additives, as well as the benefits of water fluoridation and mass polio immunizations, are of equal concern to both groups.

Environmental Pollution

A causal relationship between air pollution and respiratory diseases was recognized even in fourteenth- and fifteenth-century England, when Kings Richard II and Henry V initiated steps to regulate the use of coal. Could they have predicted 4000 deaths in the London smog of 1952? Among the most important chemical air pollutants are sulfur dioxide and carbon monoxide (end products of fuel combustion) and nitrogen oxides (from automotive exhausts and tobacco smoke). No less important is the pollution of our water with pesticides, mercury, and other toxic chemicals.

Food Additives

Saccharin, an artificial sweetener, is currently in a state of limbo. While some studies in animals suggest that it causes cancer, the United States Congress has enacted legislation permitting it to remain on the market until its carcinogenic potential in humans is more fully assessed.

Fluoridation

Notwithstanding the medical and political fears of some members of our communities, fluoridation of water has proved to be a safe, inexpensive, and effective method of substantially reducing the incidence of dental caries, especially when children drink this water during the first eight years of life. We shall not attempt to resolve the question of whether fluoridation of an entire city's drinking water impinges upon the private rights of individuals who are opposed to mass medication.

Smoking

There appears to be a high correlation between the incidence of smoking and cancer of the lung and upper respiratory tract, chronic bronchitis, and coronary heart disease. Tobacco smoke contains a variety of substances that could account for this carcinogenicity (the ability to produce cancer), the most important of which are the coal tar hydrocarbons. Nicotine, although not a carcinogen, is a very toxic compound employed as an insecticide spray. The nausea, vomiting, headache, and dizziness experienced by the neophyte smoker can be attributed to nicotine.

Social Problems

For all of us, the social problems associated with drugs are probably of greatest relevance, interest, and concern. These problems include drug abuse and misuse, population control, mercy killing, and modification of innate intelligence.

Drug Abuse

Foremost among these social dilemmas is drug abuse, a topic of casual interest decades ago when it was mainly a problem of the ghetto poor. With the realization that the "speed freak," "acid head," and "dope addict" also reside in "good, middle-class homes," the public, largely encouraged by the news media, has become intensely concerned.

Students seeking the truth about drugs have been torn between two apparently irreconcilable philosophies. On the one hand, they have been enticed by "notes from the underground" exalting the wonders of "acid" and "Acapulco gold"; simultaneously, they have often been subjected to, and insulted by, the lies and half-truths of the well-meaning establishment. The full disclosure of the facts in an objective manner, regardless of whether or not they turn the drug user on or off, is the new emerging philosophy.

Birth and Death

Drugs are now capable of controlling life and death, even in the absence of disease. Ten million women in the United States today are preventing the creation of life by chemical means, namely, "the pill." Learned physicians and scientists are grappling with an evaluation of the benefits versus the risks inherent in the use of oral contraceptives. Control of the population explosion hangs in the balance, but the possible long-term effects of these drugs on our children and grandchildren are as yet unknown. Relatively safe and highly effective drugs are now available to terminate undesired pregnancies, thus fueling the debate over one of the most emotionally charged issues that has recently confronted Americans—the legalization of abortion.

What about the other end of the spectrum, that is, permitting life to cease? Here, the use of drugs is less within the medical realm but rather a moral question. Is the practice of euthanasia (mercy killing) justified in order to terminate a life filled with pain and suffering associated with an incurable disease? Should life be prolonged in the unconscious, vegetative patient, when by the mere discontinuation of artificial respiration or drugs vitality will cease?

Enhancement of Intelligence

Drugs can improve our existence in many ways. However, will too much good have a possible unfavorable end result? The movie "Charley" asks a question that may have to be answered within the next decades: Would society as a whole benefit from a drug capable of markedly enhancing intelligence? Who then would eagerly embark upon the less glamorous, more menial tasks required by the community? These social and moral issues cannot and should not be answered exclusively by the scientists responsible for the development of these drugs, but rather by the people who will inherit the consequences.

Agriculture and Agronomy

The application of pesticides such as DDT to the soil has greatly increased the quantity and quality of crops harvested. However, surrounding waters have become contaminated with these persistent compounds, directly resulting in large fish kills, as well as in interference with other forms of marine and wildlife. DDT and chemically related pesticides have been banned based upon the argument that disruptions in the ecological balance of nature and possible long-term dangers to humans from ingestion of pesticide residues in the diet far outweigh the agricultural advantages.

Chemicals are also being utilized to enhance the growth rate of plants. The faster maturation of plants for use as foods delights the farmer, while the horticulturist is perhaps equally pleased by the eradication of weeds.

Chemical Warfare

Among the most controversial applications of drugs are their use in chemical warfare, where a variety of diverse compounds have been employed for their toxic effects to plants and humans. Defoliants and crop-destroying agents[7] were used in Vietnam to eliminate natural camouflage as well as enemy food supplies. It should be appreciated that these agents are not selectively destructive, and their use has resulted in the widespread devastation of

---

[7] Compounds such as 2,4-D ([2,4-dichlorophenoxy] acetic acid) are plant hormones that act as herbicides by very markedly increasing the rate of growth of weeds to a level where they eventually "burn themselves out."

mangrove forests (used for building homes and as a source of firewood and cover for wildlife), hardwood forests (timber industry), as well as the crops for civilian populations.

There are several categories of chemical agents that have already been used or are potentially available for use in combat. Among these are irritating agents (tear gas, Mace), vesicant or blistering agents ("mustard gas" of World War I infamy), agents producing lung damage (phosgene), and nerve gases (GB). This last class is the newest and most lethal. In the late 1970s the American public was startled by disclosures that the CIA had been conducting covert studies with potent mind-altering chemicals such as LSD.

Toxicology, Criminology, and Criminalistics

In many instances where death has occurred in a mysterious or suspicious fashion, an autopsy is ordered and an attempt is made to uncover a possible drug-induced cause of suicide or homicide. The forensic toxicologist is frequently asked to analyze the body fluids of poisoned but living patients for positive identification of the offending chemical so that specific treatment can be instituted. Similarly, blood or exhaled air is assayed in persons suspected of driving under the influence of alcohol.

At present, drugs are available that are capable of temporarily *modifying antisocial behavior,* but the next decade may see the development of compounds that have very long-lasting effects. Although this seems to be a laudable objective, the far reaching consequences of altering human behavior and thought processes may be a serious threat to our individuality. Placed in the hands of a dictator, such a drug could easily transform a democratic society into a monolithic Oceania, as depicted in *1984.*

Industrial and Household Solvents and Detergents

A wide variety of familiar household products are capable of producing serious injury if used in the absence of adequate precautions. After long exposure to a variety of common solvents used as paint thinners, dry cleaners, and furniture polishes (petroleum ether, kerosene, gasoline, and carbon tetrachloride), lung, liver, and kidney damage may occur as well as signs of central nervous system depression. These latter signs include the slowing of activity, dizziness, mental confusion, and coma. Soaps and detergents containing "enzymes" that produce dazzling white washes have been reported to produce respiratory difficulties and allergic skin reactions in workers responsible for their manufacture.

In this section we have attempted to show that interest in pharmacology is not the exclusive domain of the health professionals and stodgy scientists working on esoteric research problems in ivy-covered, cloistered laboratories.

Rather, drugs and chemicals can be considered potent forces whose use and misuse have dynamic medical, legal, social, and moral consequences to society as a whole.

SUMMARY

The human quest to successfully treat the diseases that have plagued people over the ages evolved progressively from the chance observation that ingestion of a selected part of a plant, animal, or mineral alleviated suffering to regular use of that natural product when common disease symptoms were present. Often, the use of such drugs was strongly colored by mystical beliefs. At a later age, and still with us until this century, was the empirical use of drugs. Advancements in pharmacology and related biomedical sciences have fostered the rational use of specific drugs for the more effective treatment of disease.

The pharmacologist attempts to gain information about the fundamental nature of drug action (pharmacodynamics), as well as the clinical application of these facts for the treatment of disease (therapeutics). All too often, the public has been very well aware of the benefits derived from drugs, but grossly unenlightened about the dangers associated with the abuse or misuse of these potent chemicals.

Drugs cease to remain the exclusive domain of the health professional and scientist. Because their use has spread to all segments of society, it is important that we all acquire a better understanding of their value and limitations. With this knowledge, we must impose the responsibility to ensure their proper usage.

Health professionals (medicine, veterinary medicine, dentistry, nursing, allied health professions, pharmacy, health education, and nutrition) employ drugs on a daily basis in the course of their normal activities. Public health and social problems—air and water pollution, drug abuse, smoking and disease, prevention of life, and the termination of life—are issues of concern to all individuals. All of us must participate in deciding whether chemical warfare or the modification of antisocial behavior are ever morally justified.

Whereas mere pharmacological knowledge will not resolve these problems, the informed member of society will be in a better position to arrive at a more objective, less emotional verdict when called upon to decide.

SUPPLEMENTARY READINGS

General References and Textbooks

DiPalma, J. R. ed., *Drill's Pharmacology in Medicine.* 4th ed. New York: McGraw-Hill, 1971.

Doull, J., C. D. Klassen, and M. O. Amdur, eds., *Casarett and Doull's Toxicology: The Basic Science of Poisonings.* 2nd ed. New York: Macmillan, 1980.

Gilman, A. G., L. S. Goodman, and A. Gilman, eds., *Goodman and Gilman's The Pharmacological Basis of Therapeutics.* 6th ed. New York: Macmillan, 1980.

Goldstein, A., L. Aronow, and S. M. Kalman, *Principles of Drug Action: The Basis of Pharmacology.* 2nd ed. New York: John Wiley, 1974.

Sources of In-Depth Sophisticated Reviews

Advances in Pharmacology.

Annual Review of Pharmacology and Toxicology.

Annual Review of Physiology.

Handbook of Experimental Pharmacology. New York: Springer-Verlag.

International Encyclopedia of Pharmacology and Therapeutics. Oxford, England: Pergamon Press.

Pharmacological Reviews.

Physiological Reviews.

Historical and Educational Perspectives

Gerald, M., and J. P. Long, eds., *Instruction in Pharmacology: New Approaches and New Faces.* Basel: S. Karger, 1979.

Holmstedt, B., and G. Liljestrand, eds., *Readings in Pharmacology.* New York: Macmillan, 1963.

Leake, C. D., "The Scientific Status of Pharmacology," *Science* **134:** 2069–79 (1961).

2

The Nature
of Drug Action

Such considerations raise the obvious question as to whether it is worthwhile attempting physico-chemical interpretations of cell-drug reactions. The author believes that such attempts are worthwhile, even in our present incomplete state of knowledge, because the formulation of provisional hypotheses provides an object for further research. The only danger is when such provisional hypotheses are mistaken for definitely established laws, and as a result inhibit rather than stimulate further investigation.

—A.J. Clark (1937)

It is relatively simple to observe the gross effects of drugs. We know that amphetamine stimulates mental and physical activity, while barbiturates, such as phenobarbital, depress such activities; that chlorpromazine (Thorazine) reduces the mental aberrations of schizophrenia; and that antihistamines relieve symptoms of allergies. How do these effects occur? If all these drug effects could be attributed to a simple, all-encompassing mode of action, uncovering the mysteries associated with the mechanisms responsible for the actions of these drugs would be greatly simplified, but not very intellectually challenging. However, scientists have long given up attempting to find such a unifying theory that would be applicable for all drugs.

This chapter will introduce some general concepts concerning the mechanisms by which drugs are able to produce their effects. After considering the distinction between drug actions and effects, we shall discuss the nature of a drug's interaction with enzymes, membranes, and pharmacological receptors. The kinds of actions drugs are capable or incapable of producing, the quantification of the resulting effects, and the therapeutic applications of drugs for the treatment of disease will also be examined.

GENERAL CONCEPTS CONCERNING DRUG EFFECTS

Actions and Effects

At the outset, it will be useful for us to distinguish between the actions of drugs and their effects. *Actions* of drugs are the underlying biochemical and/or physiological mechanisms by which these chemicals produce responses in living organisms. The observed consequences of these actions are called the drugs' *effects*. Two examples will illustrate this distinction. Penicillin interferes with the incorporation of essential compounds into the cell wall of certain bacteria. This action has the effect of preventing the manufacture of cell walls and results in the death of the microbe. When fever exists, aspirin is able to reduce body temperature to normal. This effect is thought to result from the action of this drug on heat-regulating centers located in the hypothalamus. This center, located in the brain, stimulates the widening of the small blood vessels of the skin, thus permitting the dissipation of heat from the body.

Primary and Secondary Drug Effects

One of the most basic principles in pharmacology is that *no drug produces a single effect*. Because drugs are not uniquely selective, it is useful to differentiate between the primary and secondary effects of drugs.

The *primary effect* of a drug is the desired therapeutic effect; it is the basic reason the physician prescribes the drug. *Secondary effects* are all other effects produced in addition to the primary one, and these may be desirable or undesirable, depending upon the patient's individual medical problem and the therapeutic objective sought by the physician or drug user.

For the purposes of illustrating the distinction between primary and secondary drug effects, only two effects of dextroamphetamine (Dexedrine) will be considered: (1) its appetite-suppressing effects and (2) its ability to stimulate the central nervous system, which produces a feeling of well-being, elevated mental spirits, and enhanced mental alertness and physical activity. If dextroamphetamine is prescribed as an appetite suppressant, appetite suppression is the primary effect; central nervous system stimulation must necessarily be a secondary effect. These stimulatory effects may or may not be viewed as being undesirable. By brightening the mental outlook of a patient who might otherwise be depressed by restrictions in the diet, these activating effects are highly desirable. However, when the drug is taken too close to bedtime, insomnia often results. This is obviously undesirable. During World War II, amphetamine was used by military combatants on both sides for its mental and physical stimulating properties. In this instance, appetite suppression was a secondary effect.

Diphenhydramine (Benadryl) is widely used for the treatment of allergies. Unfortunately, this drug produces (as do virtually all other members of the antihistamine class) a high incidence of drowsiness resulting from central nervous system depression. This secondary effect is very undesirable for automobile drivers, operators of farm equipment, or students cramming on the night prior to their final examination. On the other hand, diphenhydramine is a relatively safe drug and has been employed as a mild sedative for children. Nonprescription (over-the-counter, OTC) sleep-facilitating products, such as Compoz and Sominex, have capitalized on the drowsiness induced by antihistamines which are usually incorporated as the active ingredient of this proprietary class of drugs.

A drug may produce many effects that result from a single action, or many different actions may cause a single effect. After consideration of drug-receptor interactions in the next section, we shall return to a discussion of why drugs are neither specific nor selective in their effects.

MECHANISMS OF DRUG ACTION

The biological effects observed after a drug has been administered are the result of an interaction between that chemical and some part of the organism. In some cases, this interaction is highly specific, whereas in other instances, some nonspecific chemical or physical properties of the drug account for the observed effects. We have chosen to divide these mechanisms into two major categories: those involving a drug-receptor interaction and those in which a receptor interaction is not directly involved.

DRUG-RECEPTOR INTERACTIONS

A **receptor** is a term used to refer to *those chemical constituents of the cell with which a drug interacts to produce its pharmacological effects.* Whereas some of these constituents have been identified as being a part of macromolecules such as enzymes and nucleic acids, in most cases their chemical nature remains obscure.

A friendly word of caution should be offered to inquisitive students wishing to maintain a favorable rapport with their professor. Do not request that he or she pass a receptor around the room neatly preserved in a specimen jar. Moreover, it would be imprudent to ask your professor to draw the precise chemical structure of a receptor site. At present, with few exceptions, the receptor is merely a conceptual device utilized by the pharmacologist to describe the nature of the interaction of drugs with living organisms to produce a biological effect. When the exact chemical structure of these cellular target sites is isolated and identified, the pharmacologist will be very eager to discard the vague term, "receptor," and substitute for it the name of the precise molecule in question. However, for the time being, the term receptor will continue to be employed.

Concepts and Theories of Drug-Receptor Interactions

After attachment to a receptor site, a drug may either initiate a response or prevent a response from occurring (Figure 2–1). An **agonist** is a drug capable of interacting with a receptor to produce a response. When an **antagonist** attaches to the receptor, no response is produced, and, moreover, in the presence of an antagonist, the response normally elicited by its agonist is reduced or totally prevented. In most instances, a rather specific chemical structure is required for a drug to act as an agonist or antagonist.

The terms *affinity* and *intrinsic activity* are often used to describe the nature of the drug-receptor interaction. *Affinity* refers to the relative tendency of a drug to combine with its receptor. *Intrinsic activity* or *efficacy* refers to the capacity of a drug to produce a pharmacological response after it has interacted with its receptor. An *agonist* possesses both efficacy and intrinsic activity, while an *antagonist* has efficacy but lacks intrinsic activity.

Two agonists interacting at a common receptor site may produce an equivalent pharmacological response at markedly different doses. While many plausible reasons may be offered to explain this difference, it is possible that the more *potent* drug (the drug producing its effects at the lower dose) may have greater intrinsic activity for the receptor site. The significance of potency differences will be explored in a later section of this chapter. The highlights of three theories attempting to explain the nature of drug-receptor interactions will be briefly presented. These are the occupation theory, the rate theory, and theories involving drug-induced protein changes.

The occupation theory states that the magnitude of the response produced by a drug is directly proportional to the number of receptor sites occupied. A maximum drug-induced effect occurs when all sites are occupied. The theory argues that both agonists and antagonists are able to form drug-receptor complexes, but whereas the agonist possesses activity to produce stimulation, the antagonist lacks this activity.

The rate theory contends that it is the rate of drug-receptor complexes that is crucial, and not the number of these complexes. The theory postulates that the rate of complex formation and breakdown is very rapid, and this complex formation creates many stimulatory impulses in a finite period of time. By contrast, the antagonist is envisioned as forming a stable complex with the receptor that does not readily break down, thus preventing the interaction of an agonist with that receptor.

Several theories have been advanced, which, in very general terms, suggest that an agonist exerts its actions by inducing *temporary structural changes in the protein constituents of the receptor site.* Such structural alterations might promote an activating effect, such as an increase in the permeability of a cell membrane to nutrients and other essential compounds. If the alteration in protein structure results in a less stable drug-receptor complex, the prerequisites for the rate theory would be satisfied. Antagonists might produce struc-

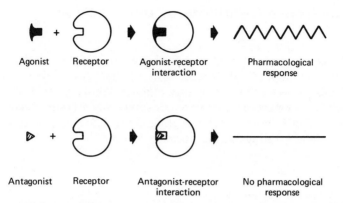

Agonist — Receptor — Agonist-receptor interaction — Pharmacological response

Antagonist — Receptor — Antagonist-receptor interaction — No pharmacological response

FIGURE 2–1. Drug-Receptor Interactions. The agonist is theorized to be capable of neatly fitting and interacting with the receptor site to produce a pharmacological response. On the other hand, the antagonist only partially fits the receptor site; its structure is such that it is unable to cause an effect. By preventing the agonist from combining with the receptor, it prevents the agonist-induced effects.

tural changes that would preclude the formation of a suitable agonist-receptor complex.

A comprehensive exposition of these theories is clearly beyond the scope of this text. The interested reader should consult the references cited at the end of this chapter for an intensive treatment of these concepts.

Lack of Drug Selectivity and Specificity

After its administration a drug may be widely distributed to many parts of the body. The mere observation that a drug has its primary effects on one organ does not justify the assumption that the drug is concentrated at this site. Whereas some drugs possess greater specificity of action than others, *all drugs are capable of producing more than one effect.* These multiple effects may be explained as follows. First, a single type of pharmacological receptor, located in different parts of the body, is responsible for the initiation of a variety of responses, depending upon the anatomical site at which it is situated. Stimulation of the cholinergic receptor results in a reduction in heart rate, a drop in blood pressure, constriction of the pupils, marked salivation, enhanced gastric acid secretion in the stomach, and constriction of the bronchioles. Chapter 7 will discuss the basis for these effects. Second, we should recognize that, although a drug may preferentially interact with a single receptor site, it often interacts with other receptors, although less effectively. Chlorpromazine (Thorazine), a tranquilizer widely used for the treatment of psychosis, acts at the norepinephrine, dopamine, serotonin, acetylcholine, and histamine receptor sites. This drug's very diverse pharmacological effects can be attributed to its lack of receptor selectivity.

NONRECEPTOR MECHANISMS OF DRUG ACTION

Although drug-receptor interactions have attracted the greatest amount of interest and work input by pharmacologists, mechanisms not directly involving receptors are just as worthy of our consideration. We shall classify nonreceptor mechanisms of drug action into five major subdivisions: (1) drug actions on enzymes; (2) antimetabolites; (3) chelating agents; (4) drugs acting on cell membranes; and (5) drugs acting nonspecifically.

Drug Actions on Enzymes

Long before birth and until the time of death, our cells are actively engaged in building up and tearing apart the constituents in our bodies. Collectively, we refer to these processes as *metabolism*, a term derived from the Greek meaning "a turning about." The buildup of body constituents is called anabolism; the breakdown process is catabolism. These dynamic events are the result of chemical reactions occurring within our bodies. Biochemistry concerns itself with these so-called reactions of intermediary metabolism.

Enzymes

You may recall from your experiments in the chemistry laboratory that when you sought to make or synthesize a compound it was often necessary to heat the chemicals in reaction vessels to relatively high temperatures, or to add acids or bases to adjust the pH in order to improve upon the reaction conditions, or to let the reactants mix for many hours or days before you could triumphantly recover the products of your labor. Unlike the test tube, your body cannot withstand high temperatures or marked changes in pH, nor can it patiently wait for many hours or days until some essential body constituents are formed. To facilitate and control the reactions of intermediary metabolism, the body requires catalysts. These substances are present in very small amounts and are capable of hastening the rate at which a reaction occurs, without themselves undergoing a permanent change in structure.

In biological systems, these catalysts are the enzymes, which are an absolute requisite for all life—from the simplest unicellular microorganism to the complex human body. More than 1000 enzymes are known to exist, *each* of which is a very specific protein substance, composed of different combinations of simple amino acids. Generally, one enzyme is capable of catalyzing only one of the body's many ongoing chemical reactions. In the absence of a particular enzyme, which may be the result of a genetic defect, a specific chemical reaction in the body will fail to occur. Phenylketonuria (PKU) is a genetically transmitted disease, resulting in marked mental deficiency that has been attributed to the absence of an essential enzyme termed phenylalanine hydroxylase.

While some enzymes can function as catalysts very adequately by themselves, others require a nonprotein substance called a *cofactor* to be active. This cofactor is often a simple metallic ion of an element such as magnesium (Mg^{2+}), zinc (Zn^{2+}), manganese (Mn^{2+}), iron (Fe^{3+}), copper (Cu^{+}, Cu^{2+}), or sodium (Na^{+}). In other instances, the cofactor is an organic molecule called a *coenzyme*. Sometimes both the metallic ion and the coenzyme must be present for enzyme activity.[1]

Drugs

Because of the cardinal role enzymes play in making these essential reactions of intermediary metabolism possible, it should be readily appreciated that drug-induced changes in the activity of enzymes are likely to have profound effects on the body as a whole.

A large number of drugs have been shown to *stimulate* the activity of enzymes responsible for the inactivation of normal body steroids. The steroids are a class of compounds grouped together because of similarities in chemical structure; they include the male and female hormones, cortisone-like hormones, and bilirubin, a pigment responsible for jaundice. At present, we do not know whether these drug-induced effects are harmful or not. Preliminary studies suggest that certain diseases, such as jaundice in newborns, may be treated successfully by stimulating the enzymes responsible for the breakdown (catabolism) of body constituents that are present in excessive quantities.

In addition to the very specific enzymes that take part in intermediary metabolism, relatively nonspecific enzymes are present in the liver and are responsible for the breakdown of drugs. As will be discussed in detail in Chapter 3, over 200 compounds are able to stimulate the activity of these so-called liver microsomal drug-metabolizing enzymes. Many of these are commonly used drugs or other compounds frequently encountered in our day-to-day living.

In subsequent chapters, we shall encounter examples of drugs whose mechanism of action may be attributed to an ability to inhibit enzymes. Cholinesterase inhibitors prevent the breakdown of acetylcholine and are used as insecticides and potential nerve gases, as well as for the treatment of glaucoma and myasthenia gravis. Monoamine oxidase inhibitors prevent the inactivation of norepinephrine; many investigators contend that, by elevating norepinephrine concentrations in the brain, these drugs are able to reverse depression. Certain diuretics are able to remove excessive body fluids by increasing the output of urine as a result of the inhibition of the enzyme carbonic anhydrase.

[1] The student seeking greater in-depth appreciation of enzymes should consult any modern textbook of biochemistry.

Antimetabolites

By a series of specific biochemical reactions, living organisms are capable of converting simple starting materials to end products (metabolites) that are essential for their survival. *Antimetabolites* are a group of drugs that chemically resemble natural intermediate products required for the ultimate biosynthesis of essential metabolites. These drugs compete with the intermediate product for a common enzyme system. The "counterfeit incorporation" of the drug into the biosynthetic pathway in preference to the natural intermediate biochemical results in the formation of an abnormal end product that the living organism is incapable of utilizing to sustain life. Examples of commonly employed antimetabolites include the anticancer drug methotrexate and the sulfonamides ("sulfa drugs") used to combat bacterial infections.

Chelating Agents

A drug may exert its action because it is able to participate in a specific interaction with a metallic ion. This ion may be a natural constituent of the body, present in either normal or abnormally elevated concentrations, or it may be a foreign toxic metal. *Chelating agents*[2] are capable of specifically or preferentially combining with metals to form a drug-metal complex that is nontoxic and readily eliminated from the body. Such drugs have been found to be particularly useful as antidotes in the treatment of poisoning by heavy metals. Commonly employed chelating agents include dimercaprol (for antimony, arsenic, and mercury poisoning), dimercaprol and edetate (lead poisoning), and deferoxamine (iron poisoning).

Drugs Acting on Cell Membranes

Our interest in drugs affecting the *permeability of the cell membrane* is of obvious importance in view of the fundamental role the membrane plays in the selective passage of certain ions, nutrients, and other essential compounds into the cell. The selective admittance of some substances, with the simultaneous exclusion of others, is essential for the maintenance of normal cellular function (Chapter 3).

Drugs interfering with the movement of the positively charged cations sodium and/or potassium are capable of stabilizing the membrane of nerves thereby preventing their normal excitation. Membrane stabilization is thought

---

[2] The term *chelate* is derived from the Greek word *chele* ("crab's claw"), pictorially describing how the drug surrounds the metal to form a complex.

to be responsible for the ability of ether and other general anesthetics to cause loss of consciousness and for phenytoin (Dilantin) to reduce the incidence of seizures in epileptic patients.

Many hormones and drugs have been shown to produce effects on their target cells by stimulating the activity of *adenylate cyclase,* an enzyme system located in the membrane of the target cell. Activation of this enzyme promotes the formation of cyclic AMP which produces effects characteristic of that hormone (Chapter 22). The hormone insulin promotes the movement of the sugar glucose from the plasma into the cell; this increase in cell membrane permeability results from the interaction of insulin with adenylate cyclase. In juvenile diabetes mellitus there is an absence or deficiency of insulin leading to inadequate amounts of glucose entering the cell.

Drugs Acting Nonspecifically

The pharmacological effects of some drugs may be a *nonspecific consequence of their chemical or physical properties.* Among the best sources of these drugs is your medicine chest. If you were to mentally inventory its contents, undoubtedly you would find such items as powders for after shave or bath or for diaper rash, a styptic pencil, suntan lotions, mouthwashes, and antiseptic agents.

An *antiseptic* is a drug that kills or retards the growth of microbes on the skin, thus reducing the possibility of infection developing in wounds. Drugs in this class are termed *protoplasmic poisons* because they nonspecifically act on all cells (bacterial and human) with which they come in contact. Phenol (carbolic acid), introduced in 1867 by Lister [3] as a germicide, is a classical example. This compound kills a wide variety of microorganisms within minutes after contact and acts by general precipitation and inactivation of protoplasmic proteins. An unfortunate consequence is the destruction of healthy tissues and a retardation of the normal healing processes. Less irritating antiseptics commonly used in the home today include tincture (alcoholic solution) of iodine, thimerosal (Merthiolate), and merbromin (Mercurochrome).[4]

---

[3]Lord Lister did not invent the mouthwash Listerine, although undoubtedly this product was named in his honor. Listerine contains boric acid, aromatic oils, and 25 percent alcohol, but, notwithstanding Lister's great contribution to medical science, no phenol.

[4]Until 1972, *hexachlorophene* was a common antiseptic ingredient found in 300–400 products widely used as soaps, shampoos, toothpastes, mouthwashes, anti-acne products, and vaginal deodorants. Surgeons used this antibacterial agent to reduce the bacteria on their hands prior to operations. It had been a routine practice at many hospitals to wash newborn infants with hexachlorophene as a prophylactic measure against nursery epidemics of staphylococcal skin infections. In 1972 the Food and Drug Administration established strict limitations on its use after studies in animals revealed that its application to skin was associated with a risk of systemic toxicity and, in particular, brain damage in infants.

SITES OF DRUG ACTION

In the previous sections, we examined some very fundamental concepts regarding drug-receptor interactions, as well as drug-induced effects not involving receptor sites. **Pharmacodynamics** is concerned with the *sites at which drugs act and the mechanism by which this action occurs.* Applying the previously presented material, let us now view mechanisms of drug action from a somewhat different perspective, namely, the *site* and the *general nature* of the drug-cell interaction. Based upon these criteria drugs may be classified as (1) those acting exclusively by physical means outside cells, (2) those acting outside the cell via chemical interactions, (3) those acting on the cell membrane by a physical and/or chemical interaction, and (4) those acting by modifying biochemical reactions within the cell (Figure 2–2).

Drugs Acting Outside Cells by Physical Means

Outside sites of action include the external surfaces of the skin and the cavities of the gastrointestinal tract. Common examples of drugs that act on these sites include ointments, sprays, and dusting powders, which act to alleviate pain from sunburn, repel insects, or relieve itching of the feet, respectively. In addition, some orally administered drugs act solely by physical means. For example, one group of appetite suppressants is composed of undigestible gums that swell when they come into contact with the stomach's fluids; by supplying bulk, they provide a feeling of fullness. Another example is mineral oil, which facilitates bowel movements and relieves constipation by coating and softening the fecal contents of the colon.

Drugs Acting Outside Cell Membranes by Chemical Interactions

We have previously considered that chelating agents form a chemical complex with metallic ions by this mechanism. Antacids are alkaline substances that chemically neutralize excessive gastric acid (hydrochloric acid) in the stomach. This is a biological example of a simple acid-based neutralization reaction familiar to all students of chemistry.

Drugs Acting on the Cell Membrane by Physical and/or Chemical Interactions

To add to our earlier discussion of drug interactions at or on cell membranes, we should emphasize that some drug receptor sites are known to be located on the membrane. Hence, it is rather reasonable to assume that drug agonists and antagonists act at this same receptor site. Polymyxin B

(Aerosporin) and amphotericin B (Fungizone) are clinically employed for the treatment of bacterial and fungal infections, respectively. Each of these antibiotics interacts with different specific chemical constituents on the microbial cell membrane, damaging and thereby impairing its function as a selective barrier, and resulting in the death of these microbes.

Drugs Acting within the Cell by Modifying Normal Biochemical Reactions

Dicumarol and warfarin, two very commonly used anticoagulants ("blood thinners") effective after administration by mouth, inhibit blood clotting mechanisms by interfering with the synthesis of vitamin K–dependent clotting factors by the liver. Certain drugs employed for the treatment of cancer act by inhibiting the synthesis of essential proteins or nucleic acids by tumor cells. Interference with the patient's ability to synthesize these biochemicals is largely responsible for the wide range of adverse effects produced by these anticancer agents.

Cells require oxygen and energy to survive, and this energy is supplied by metabolic reactions occurring in the mitochondria. Administration of thyroid hormone markedly stimulates the rate of these metabolic reactions. Cytochromes are iron-containing proteins concerned with cellular oxidation. Hydrocyanic (HCN, prussic) acid, is an extremely poisonous substance used in "gas chambers," and was formerly employed in Nazi genocide mass murder extermination camps. Cyanide (CN^-) attacks and inactivates the cytochrome system preventing tissues from taking up and utilizing the oxygen in oxyhemoglobin.

At this point, the inquisitive reader may ask why some drugs only act *outside* or on the cell membrane, whereas others are able to act *inside* the cell. This very fundamental question can be answered by looking at the physical and

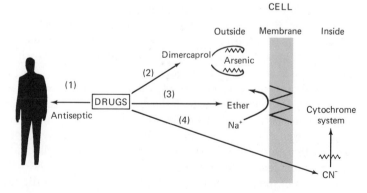

FIGURE 2–2. Sites and Mechanisms of Drug Action. Drugs act (1) by physical means outside the cell, (2) by chemical interactions outside the cell, (3) on cell membranes by physical and/or chemical interactions, and (4) inside the cell to alter biochemical reactions.

chemical characteristics of the drug in question. These properties will determine whether or not a drug is able to cross the cell membrane and act within the cell. We shall specifically come to grips with this problem when we discuss "Drug Passage across Cell Membranes" in Chapter 3.

CATEGORIZATION OF DRUG ACTIONS

The previous section discussed the sites at which drugs act and the basic mechanisms responsible for these actions. Let us now examine the types of actions that drugs produce in the cells, tissues, or organs of living organisms.

All drugs act by stimulating or depressing cellular activity, replacing deficient substances, killing or weakening invading foreign organisms, or causing irritation. These distinctions are not as definitive as we might expect and desire, and we find that some compounds fit into more than one category. These actions should not be confused with the therapeutic uses of drugs, which are the ultimate applications of these actions for the treatment of disease.

Stimulation and Depression

Drugs may act by stimulating or depressing the normal physiological function of specific organs. *Stimulation* is an increase in the rate of functional activity of a cell or in the amount of secretion from a gland. *Depression* denotes a reduction in such activity. Amphetamine and caffeine stimulate the central nervous system, whereas alcohol and phenobarbital depress the brain.

At this juncture, it is appropriate to state that *drugs cannot endow a tissue or cell with properties they do not inherently possess.* Thus, no drug is capable of stimulating an epithelial cell located in the mouth to release insulin. Similarly, a drug cannot transform a muscle fiber in such a manner that it functions as a nerve cell. However, drugs can stimulate or depress the *normal* activity of a nerve or muscle cell. In addition, stimulants such as amphetamine possess a biphasic activity. That is, at moderate doses, amphetamine causes stimulation, whereas at high doses it causes depression.

Let us examine another fundamental principle of drug action with the following example. In congestive heart failure, the heart is incapable of effectively pumping blood throughout the body. This situation is not unlike that of a pump handle of a well that is being very rapidly, but incompletely, depressed at each stroke, so that very little water is pumped from the well, and with a considerable but inefficient expenditure of energy. Digitalis stimulates the force of each contraction of the heart, while simultaneously depressing the rate, thus enabling the heart to serve as a more effective pump.

This example illustrates a second fundamental limitation on the properties of drugs: *They are unable to restore diseased organ or tissue function to normal by a direct action.* Rather, drugs act indirectly by providing more favorable conditions for the body's normal repair mechanisms to come into play. Phenobarbital does not correct the underlying defect that is responsible for epilepsy, but it does depress the excessive activity of nerve cells in the cerebral cortex, and thereby reduces the incidence of seizures. Antihistamines such as tripelennamine (Pyribenzamine) do not cure allergies, but they do prevent the agonist, histamine, from initiating an allergic response. By blocking the histamine receptor site, the antihistamine antagonist is, in effect, depressing the ability of histamine to exert its actions.

In theory, at least, can drugs be developed that will enhance intelligence? If we consider intelligence to be manifested by the ability to learn and retain information, it would appear to be clearly within the realm of possibility that a drug, "Smarts," might stimulate RNA or DNA synthesis in the brain. It has been suggested that these nucleic acids play a role in short- and long-term memory and memory storage.

Replacement

Drugs may *replace* essential body compounds that are either absent or present in less than optimal concentrations. A common example of such replacement therapy is the administration of insulin to a diabetic. In geographic areas where seafood is not generally a regular part of the diet, endemic goiter is frequently observed. The addition of very small amounts of iodine to table salt (0.1 g of potassium iodide per 1000 g of salt, or 0.01%) prevents this swelling of the thyroid gland.

Killing Foreign Organisms

Chemotherapeutic agents act by killing or preventing the multiplication of invading foreign organisms such as worms or bacteria. Penicillin exerts its bactericidal effects by blocking the synthesis or manufacture of the bacterial cell wall. Chloroquine inactivates DNA in *Plasmodium,* thus preventing replication of the protozoan responsible for malaria.

Antibiotics do not cure infectious diseases exclusively by virtue of their direct lethal effects on bacteria but require the cooperation of the body's normal immune defense mechanisms. Heart transplant recipients receive immunosuppressive drugs to prevent rejection of the foreign heart; however, an unfortunate consequence of this depression of immune mechanisms is that it renders the patient defenseless against invading bacteria.

Irritation

A group of drugs acts by the relatively nonspecific mechanism of irritation. Liniments are irritants that relieve muscular pain by stimulating blood flow to a localized area. In some laxatives, such as Ex-Lax and Feen-A-Mint, the active ingredient is phenolphthalein. This compound is thought to act in part by causing irritation of the inner wall of the colon, which initiates peristalsis and eventual defecation. In addition to its properties as a laxative, phenolphthalein is frequently employed in laboratories as a chemical indicator for the neutralization of acids with bases.

QUANTITATIVE CHARACTERIZATION OF DRUG EFFECTS

> *When you cannot measure it, when you cannot express it in numbers—you have scarcely, in your thoughts, advanced to the stage of Science, whatever the matter may be.*
>
> —Lord Kelvin (1824–1907)

Thus far, our discussions of drug-induced effects have been qualitative in nature; that is, drugs were merely said to stimulate or depress. If, however, as Kelvin indicates, pharmacology is a science, we should be able to ascribe numbers to our observations and to indicate by how much a biological response is increased or decreased. This *quantitative characterization of drug effects* is not only of interest when pursuing the experimental aspects of pharmacology but also of obvious significance to the clinician employing drugs as therapeutic agents in human or animal patients.

The **dose** administered influences the concentration of that chemical available at its site of action in the biological system at a given time. As we shall discuss in Chapter 3, the processes of absorption and distribution determine what proportion of the drug molecules administered will reach their site(s) of action, and what period of time must elapse before a drug-induced effect is perceived. Moreover, just as drugs do not elicit an effect at the precise instant of their administration, their biological effects do not persist for an infinite period of time. The processes of redistribution, metabolism (biotransformation), and elimination are responsible for removing drug molecules from their sites of action.

Thus the *concentration* of a drug at its site of action determines the *intensity* of its effects (or response). The concentration is influenced by the dose administered and by that instant of time at which the drug response is evaluated (Figure 2–3). **Pharmacokinetics** is that branch of pharmacology concerned with the interrelationships of dose, time. and biological response.

We shall now consider the concepts of dose-response and time-response relationships which are of fundamental importance for all students of pharmacology and therapeutics.

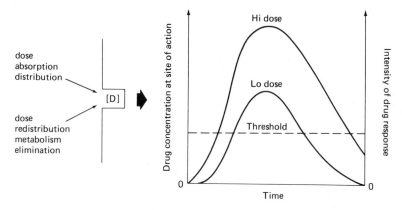

FIGURE 2–3. Interrelationships of Dose, Time, and Pharmacological Response. The concentration of drug at its site of action [D], determined by the dose administered and the rate and degree of absorption and distribution, influences the intensity of the drug response. This drug concentration must exceed a minimal (threshold) level to produce a perceptible response. The duration of the drug response is influenced by the dose administered and processes that remove the drug from its site of action, namely, redistribution, metabolism (biotransformation), and elimination.

Dose-Response Relationships

The relationship between the dose of the drug administered and the intensity of the resulting response is commonly depicted by a dose-response curve. Dose-response relationships may be graded or quantal (Figures 2–4 and 2–5, respectively).

Graded Dose-Response Relationships

As the dose of a given drug administered is increased, the magnitude (intensity) of the drug-induced response generally increases in a smooth and gradual manner; this is termed a *graded* or *quantitative* dose-response relationship (Figure 2–4). The dependent variable (the response) is commonly plotted on the ordinate (*y*-axis) employing an arithmetic scale, while the independent variable (the dose) is plotted on the abscissa (*x*-axis).[5]

A *threshold dose* is the lowest dose capable of producing a barely perceivable response; less than this critical concentration, a *subthreshold dose,* fails to elicit a detectable response. The threshold dose of a given drug may differ depending upon the specific response we choose to study. For example, the threshold dose of a barbiturate required to kill an individual is approximately ten times higher than that dose required to produce sleep. Sodium

[5] While the dose may be plotted using an arithmetic scale, doses are commonly transformed to a logarithmic equivalent. The use of a log-dose response curve permits the display of a wider dosage range on a single scale and often converts the dose-response relationship from a hyperbolic curve to a line segment which is more useful when comparing drugs.

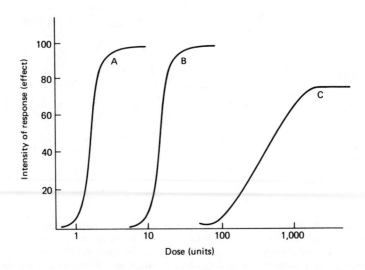

FIGURE 2-4. Hypothetical Graded Log Dose-Response Curves. Drug A is more potent than B which is more potent than C. Drugs A and B have equivalent efficacy which is greater than C; drug C cannot produce a greater effect regardless of the dose administered. Doses less than 1, 10, and 100 units are subthreshold for drugs A, B, and C, respectively.

fluoride is a potent rat poison; at considerably lower doses, however, it has been shown to be highly effective in preventing dental caries in children. From this example a general principle of pharmacology emerges—namely, *even the most deadly poisons, when administered at sufficiently low (subthreshold) doses, are nontoxic.*

The *maximum effect* or *efficacy* is the greatest response produced by a specific drug regardless of the dose administered. Some drugs, by virtue of their inherent properties, are only capable of producing a certain maximum effect (for example, only 50 or 75 percent) and are incapable of producing a theoretical 100 percent effect (Figure 2-4). Nitrous oxide ("laughing gas") is incapable of producing the same level of general anesthesia as either ether or halothane (Fluothane) and, therefore, cannot be used alone in certain types of major operations.

For many drugs, an attempt to enhance efficacy by increasing the dosage may result in a proportionately greater incidence of side effects which often sets a maximum limit on the amount of drug that can be safely tolerated. When treating advanced cases of rheumatoid arthritis with aspirin, the physician does not realistically anticipate being capable of totally eliminating all symptoms associated with this chronic, debilitating, inflammatory disease; rather an attempt is made to reduce the symptoms to a tolerable level without eliciting undue drug-induced discomfort. While relatively small doses of dextro-amphetamine (Dexedrine) enhance athletic performance, high doses of this stimulant impair such performance as the result of adverse side effects.

Dose-response curves are frequently used to evaluate and compare the potency and therapeutic index of related drugs.

Potency refers to the absolute amount of drug (that is, the *dose*) required to produce a specified pharmacological effect (Figure 2–4). The fact that drug A is more potent than drug B (that is, less of A is required to produce an equivalent pharmacological effect), does not denote that A is necessarily a superior therapeutic agent. Knowledge of drug potency alone does not enable us to predict whether the more potent drug is more or less toxic. A far more valid indicator is the therapeutic index (see below). The following hallucinogenic agents produce equivalent behavioral effects in humans, notwithstanding a 1000-fold difference in potency:

	mg	Relative Potency
Mescaline	200	X
Psilocybin	2	100X
LSD-25	0.2	1000X

Quantal Dose-Response Relationships

Whereas the graded dose-response relationship depicts a progressive increase in the magnitude of the pharmacological response with increasing doses, many pharmacological effects are *all-or-none* in nature. For example, is the woman pregnant or not pregnant after employing a contraceptive drug at a dose of X? Does the mosquito survive after exposure to Y concentration of DDT? Does Z dose of alcohol impair a specified simulated driving activity? (See Figure 2-5.)

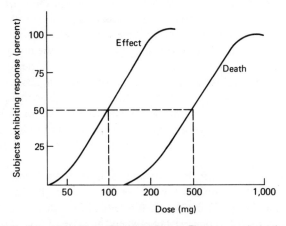

FIGURE 2–5. Quantal Log Dose-Response Curves. These curves depict those doses of a test compound required to produce the desired pharmacological effect (left) and death (right). Groups of ten mice were injected with different doses of the compound, and the percentage of animals exhibiting each of these responses was noted. The median effective dose (ED50) and median lethal dose (LD50) of this test compound were determined to be 100 mg and 500 mg, respectively, and, therefore, its therapeutic index (LD50/ED50) is 5.

The quantal dose-response curve generally assumes the shape of a normal distribution (Gaussian or bell-shaped) curve (Figure 3–6). From this curve or from the curves depicted in Figure 2–5, we can calculate the dose required to produce a specified response in 50 percent of our test subjects. This is referred to as the *median effective dose,* commonly abbreviated ED50; if death of the test animal was selected as the end point, an analogous curve could be used to determine the median lethal dose or LD50.

As noted above, mere knowledge of drug potency provides us with little insight as to the relative safety of that compound. Ideally, we want drugs whose toxic or lethal effects are only manifested at doses far in excess of those doses required to produce the desired therapeutic effect(s). The **therapeutic index** (T.I.; therapeutic ratio) is used to express the *relative margin of safety* of a drug, and in the experimental laboratory is calculated as the median lethal dose/median effective dose or LD50/ED50.[6]

In a clinical setting, a more meaningful and realistic formula for calculation of the therapeutic index is LD1/ED99. The reason for the distinction between the laboratory and clinic should be self-evident. When drugs are to be employed as therapeutic agents, we would like to compare ratios of drug safety based upon doses that are effective in virtually all patients (ED99) while lethal to none (LD1). A ratio calculated on the basis of LD0/ED100 would, of course, be far more desirable but marked variation in drug sensitivity among test subjects makes this theoretically ideal ratio extremely difficult to determine.

How large must the therapeutic index be? Obviously, it must be greater than 1 if the drug is to possess any clinical utility; the greater this ratio, the safer the drug. A single therapeutic index cannot be established for all classes of drugs. Compare the relative safety of digitalis (T.I. = 1.5–2.0) with penicillin (T.I. > 100). The normal therapeutic dose of digitalis is about one-half the lethal dose, whereas penicillin is extremely nontoxic for the nonallergic patient. Thus, evaluation of whether one drug is therapeutically superior to another is not based upon the absolute dose required to produce the desired effect or toxicity. Rather it is the ratio of these two values that must be considered. Drugs A and B have a LD50 of 10 and 1000 mg, respectively, and an ED50 of 0.1 and 10 mg. Since both drugs have an equivalent therapeutic index of 100, on the basis of the available evidence, one would conclude that they are equally desirable therapeutically.

If a drug is employed for the treatment of more than one medical disorder, and different doses are required for the treatment of each condition, the drug will have multiple therapeutic indexes. While the lethal dose of codeine remains constant, a fourfold difference exists between the dose of this narcotic required to suppress cough (its antitussive effects) and the dose used to relieve pain (its analgesic effect).

---

[6] Based upon statistical considerations, it is more reliable for us to compute the therapeutic index and compare drugs at the median (50%) dose rather than at extreme ends of the dose-response curve, for example, the ED10 or ED90.

Time-Response Relationships

Some drugs act very rapidly after administration, whereas others manifest their activity hours or even days later. Television advertisements promoting aspirin-containing, headache-relieving products attempt to capitalize on such differences. The length of time a drug continues to exert its effects is also of importance. That is, will victims of peptic ulcers be obliged to take their antacid every one to two hours, or can they take a product that will provide relief for four hours after a single dose?

Evaluation of time-response relationships involves three basic parameters: latency, maximal effect, and duration of action. *Latency or onset of action* denotes the length of time it takes for a drug to produce an observable effect after it has been administered. *Maximal effect* is the time required for a drug to exert its peak or greatest effects. *Duration of action* is the period of time a drug continues to produce a response after a single dose. A general time-response curve is illustrated in Figure 2–3. Differences in the time-response effects of different insulin preparations are illustrated in Figure 24–1.

These time-response parameters are influenced by a variety of factors, some of which include: (1) the route of drug administration, for example, oral versus intravenous; (2) the solubility of the drug, which modifies the rate at which the drug is absorbed into the blood from its site of administration; (3) the speed with which the drug is distributed to its site of action; and (4) the time required for the drug to be chemically inactivated (metabolized or biotransformed) and excreted or otherwise removed from the body. Chapter 3 will discuss each of these factors in detail.

THERAPEUTIC USES OF DRUGS

The sites of drug action, the mechanisms responsible for these actions, and the resulting effects comprise those aspects of pharmacology called *pharmacodynamics.* The ultimate practical application of this knowledge for the *treatment of disease* is termed **therapeutics.** In classical terms, drugs are generally thought of as being synonymous with therapeutic agents. There are four basic therapeutic uses of drugs: the diagnosis, prevention, cure, and alleviation of the symptoms of disease. Drugs are also used to prevent and terminate pregnancy (contraception and abortion, respectively).

Diagnosis of Disease

Drugs may be used as tools to diagnose the presence of disease which is often detected by impaired or abnormal functions of organs. Frequently employed diagnostic agents include: sodium iodide (131_I) for the identification of thyroid abnormalities or cancer, sulfobromophthalein for liver function tests, and glucose tolerance tests for the diagnosis of diabetes. Barium sulfate is used to uncover abnormalities of the upper gastrointestinal tract, while organic iodine compounds are employed as contrast agents to visualize the gall bladder and the presence of stones therein.

Prevention of Disease

The ultimate objective of medicine is the prevention of disease. In this regard, drugs have played a significant role. Vitamins are an integral part of many American breakfasts in order to prevent deficiency diseases. A substantial reduction in the incidence of caries has been observed in children living in communities having fluoridated drinking water. The most dramatic prevention of diseases has occurred as a direct result of mass immunizations employing vaccines that prevent smallpox, diptheria, poliomyelitis, and measles. A vaccine to prevent the common cold has been extremely difficult to develop because of the many different types of viruses that cause colds.

Cure of Disease

With the exception of the chemotherapeutic agents, most classes of drugs only relieve the symptoms of disease rather than produce a cure or completely eradicate a disease. Even chemotherapeutic agents are not uniformly effective; the relative ineffectiveness of most anticancer drugs dramatically emphasizes these shortcomings. On the positive side, penicillin, piperazine (Antepar), and chloroquine (Aralen) have been quite effective in the cure of pneumonia caused by bacteria, pinworm, and malaria, respectively.

Alleviation of the Symptoms of Disease

As indicated in the previous paragraph, most commonly employed therapeutic agents merely relieve the symptoms of disease without producing a cure. The body must then bear the burden of making the required physiological, biochemical, and psychological adjustments to effect a cure of the disease. Drugs in this class do not alter the underlying cause of the disease process, but merely relieve the symptoms in a relatively nonspecific fashion.

Aspirin is extremely effective in reducing fever (antipyretic agent), regardless of whether the fever is of bacterial or viral origin. This drug does not influence the cause of the symptoms, but only the resulting fever. Similarly, morphine relieves the severe pain caused by terminal cancer or a bone fracture. Chlorpromazine (Thorazine) permits schizophrenics to return to the "real world," regardless of the nature of their biochemical or psychological aberrations.

Contraception and Abortion

Since we assume that pregnancy is not a disease, contraceptive agents have added a completely new dimension to the classical definition of what constitutes a drug. Prior to 1955, all drugs fit into one of the previously discussed four categories. That is, they all were used for the treatment of disease. "The pill," currently used monthly by ten million women in the United States, has clearly established a place for itself in therapeutics not withstanding a number of potentially dangerous adverse effects. More recently, prostaglandin derivatives have become clinically available that are capable of terminating undesired pregnancies more safely and effectively than previously employed chemical agents or surgical procedures.

SUMMARY ————————————————————————

This chapter has considered the nature of the interaction of chemical substances, broadly termed *drugs*, with living organisms. A drug does not produce one and only one effect as a result of this interaction. Rather a drug is not unlike a master key capable of opening several, but not all, locks. Some master keys can open a great number of locks, while others, only two or three. Some drug-induced effects may be highly desirable and serve as the basis for the drug's therapeutic use, while other effects are undesirable and limit the clinical application of the drug.

Drug effects are frequently attributed to an interaction with a receptor site. Both agonists and antagonists are thought to bind to macromolecular receptors, but antagonists are unable to initiate a response, and prevent the agonist from so acting. Theories regarding the drug-receptor interaction suggest that the effects may depend upon (1) the number of receptors occupied, (2) the rate at which a drug-receptor complex is formed and broken, or (3) drug-induced changes in the structure of the proteins comprising the receptor site. A drug's relative lack of specificity may be explained by considering that drugs are capable of interacting with more than one receptor site. Moreover, receptor sites responsive to the same drug serve dissimilar functions in different parts of the body.

Drug actions not mediated by attachment to receptor sites may produce their effects as a result of nonspecific chemical or physical interactions, specific chemical reactions with ions or molecules, or by counterfeit incorporation into biochemical reactions (antimetabolites).

We have observed that drugs may have several sites of action and mechanisms by which they interact with living organisms. These include: (1) actions outside the cell by physical means, (2) actions outside the cell by chemical interactions, (3) actions on cell membranes by physical and/or chemical mechanisms, and (4) actions within the cell that modify chemical reactions. The end result of these actions may be stimulation or depression of cellular activity, replacement of deficient essential compounds to the body, lethal effects to invading foreign organisms, or irritation. In no instance does the drug confer the tissue or cell with properties it does not inherently possess. Furthermore, the drug is incapable of directly repairing a diseased tissue; this can only be accomplished by the normal body repair mechanisms.

The magnitude of a drug-induced effect may be evaluated with respect to the dosage employed or the time period that has elapsed after drug administration; these interrelationships of dose, time, and pharmacological response are examined in the science of pharmacokinetics. Dose-response relationships, which may be graded or quantal (all-or-none), are used to evaluate threshold doses and efficacy or the maximum effect that the drug is capable of producing; potency or the absolute amount of drug (dose) required to produce a given pharmacological response; and the therapeutic index, which expresses the ratio of the lethal dose and the effective dose. Time-response relationships seek to evaluate the latency or onset of drug effects, the time required before the maximum effect is achieved, and the duration of drug effects.

Therapeutics consists of the diagnosis, prevention, cure, and alleviation of the symptoms of disease. Additional categories include drugs used for the prevention and termination of pregnancy (contraception and abortion, respectively), nondisease entities.

SUPPLEMENTARY READINGS

Albert, A., *Selective Toxicity*. 6th ed. New York: John Wiley, 1979.

Clark, A. J., *The Mode of Action of Drugs on Cells*. London: Arnold, 1933.

Dikstein, S., ed., *Fundamentals of Cell Pharmacology*. Springfield, Ill.: Charles C Thomas, 1973.

Goldstein, A., L. Aronow, and S. M. Kalman, *Principles of Drug Action*. 2nd ed. New York: John Wiley, 1974.

Featherstone, R.M., ed., *A Guide to Molecular Pharmacology–Toxicology*, Parts I-II. New York: Marcel Dekker, 1973.

Rang, H.P., ed., *Drug Receptors*. Baltimore: University Park Press, 1973.

Smythies, J. R., and R. J. Bradley, eds., *Receptors in Pharmacology*. New York: Marcel Dekker, 1978.

Tallarida, R. J., and L. S. Jacob, *The Dose-Response Relation in Pharmacology*. New York: Springer-Verlag, 1979.

3

Factors Modifying
the Response to Drugs

One cannot possibly practice good medicine and not understand the fundamentals underlying therapy.

—Fuller Albright (1900–)

In our discussions thus far, we have tacitly assumed that after a drug is administered, it somehow reaches its site of action, interacts with a receptor or acts through a nonreceptor mediated mechanism, and after a finite period of time ceases to elicit a pharmacological effect. This chapter is concerned with the events that occur between the time the drug is introduced into the body and the time it is finally eliminated. These intermediate steps are termed absorption, distribution, biotransformation or metabolism, and excretion. In the second major section of this chapter this fundamental information will be directly applied when we consider the factors that modify the response to drugs.

Some drugs are apparently equipped with "seven league boots" that enable these chemicals to enter all parts of the body; others are restricted in their access to selected sites in the body. A study of drug **absorption** and **distribution** will attempt to account for some of these differences. Since drugs do not have an infinitely long duration of action in the body, biological mechanisms must be present for terminating their actions and removing these chemicals from the body. **Biotransformation** or **metabolism** of drugs is responsible for chemical changes in the parent drug molecule causing inactivation after chemical alteration of the drug molecule has occurred; the resulting metabolite is **excreted** or **eliminated** from the body. These interrelationships are depicted in Figure 3–1 and will be discussed in detail on the succeeding pages of this chapter.

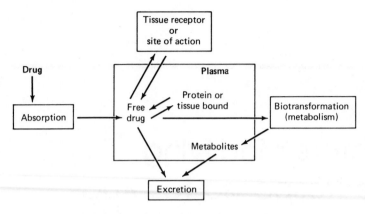

FIGURE 3-1. Fate of a Drug after Absorption.

DRUG PASSAGE ACROSS CELL MEMBRANES

Each of the factors to be subsequently considered, that is, absorption, distribution, biotransformation, and excretion, requires the *passage of the drug across a cell membrane.* These membranes consist of a bimolecular layer of lipid or fat-like molecules coated with a protein layer on each surface. The ability of a drug to cross this membrane depends upon its chemical and physical properties.

Physical-Chemical Considerations

Let us briefly consider some selected basic background information concerning the chemistry of drugs that will improve our understanding of the modes by which these compounds cross cell membranes. The chemical structure of a drug determines whether a drug will be more fat-soluble or water-soluble. In addition, certain reactive portions of the molecule, or functional groups, are responsible for the interaction of the drug with the tissue receptors.

Most drugs are weak *organic acids or bases,* and, therefore, at the physiological pH[1] of body fluids, drug molecules exist as a mixture of the non-ionized or uncharged molecular form and the ionized or charged form. The relative proportion of each form is dependent upon the pH of the body fluid in which the drug is present and the ionization or dissociation constant of the drug. Weak organic acids (such as aspirin and other salicylates, barbiturates,

---

[1] The term pH refers to the negative logarithm of the hydrogen ion concentration. This term signifies the relative degree of acidity or basicity (alkalinity) of a solution on a scale of 0–14. A value of 7 denotes neutrality, less than 7 indicates acidity, and greater than 7, basicity. The pH of blood and most body fluids normally ranges from 7.35 to 7.45.

and sulfonamides) are predominantly nonionized in acidic body fluids, such as the urine, whereas they become ionized in the slightly alkaline environment of the plasma and small intestines. The converse is true for weak organic bases (morphine and other opiates, amphetamines, and antihistamines). (See Table 3–1.)

TABLE 3-1. INFLUENCE OF pH ON IONIZATION AND THE PASSAGE OF DRUGS ACROSS LIPID (CELL) MEMBRANES

Drug Type	Acidic (low pH) Environment		Alkaline (high pH) Environment	
	Predominant Form	Passage Across Lipid Membranes	Predominant Form	Passage Across Lipid Membranes
Weak acid	$R-COOH$	High	$R-COO^{\ominus} + H^{\oplus}$	Low
e.g., aspirin	OCOCH$_3$ / COOH (benzene ring) — Nonionized (uncharged)		OCOCH$_3$ / COO$^-$ + H$^+$ (benzene ring) — Ionized (charged)	
Weak base	$R-NH_3^+$	Low	$R-NH_2$	High
e.g., amphetamine	CH$_3$ group, benzene ring, $-CH_2CH-NH_3^{\oplus}$ — Ionized (charged)		CH$_3$ group, benzene ring, $-CH_2CH-NH_2$ — Nonionized (uncharged)	

When we examine the properties of a drug molecule that influence its passage across cell membranes, one factor continually reappears, namely, the relative lipid solubility of the compound. As a general rule, we observe that drugs are more lipid-soluble (fat-soluble) and less water-soluble when they are nonionized or uncharged; conversely, ionized or charged molecules are less lipid-soluble and more water-soluble. Relatively strong bases are occasionally used as drugs. These compounds are almost completely ionized at the physiological pH of the body, and are, therefore, virtually lipid-insoluble.

Thus, at any time we find that a drug is present in the body as a mixture of ionized and nonionized molecules. It is the relative lipid solubility of the nonionized molecule that determines whether or not a drug (1) will be absorbed, (2) will be distributed to all parts of the body (such as the brain), (3) will cross cell membranes and act within the cells, or (4) will be readily excreted in the urine. To a lesser extent the molecular size of the drug is of importance.

Drugs are able to traverse cell membranes by one or more of the following modes: filtration, diffusion, and active transport. Most drugs cross cell membranes by either diffusion or active transport, while other compounds utilize both these processes.

Filtration

Cell membranes have channels or pores that permit small water-soluble molecules and ions (sodium, potassium, chloride) to pass through by simple filtration. The size of these pores differs with particular cell membranes. For example, the pores found in capillary membranes are relatively large (40 Å)[2] and permit the filtration of most molecules, with the exception of large molecular proteins. However, most other cell membranes have a pore size diameter of only 4 Å, thus enabling only water and small drugs having a molecular weight of 100–200 to cross. We shall soon see that some large lipid-insoluble compounds are capable of crossing cell membranes by an active transport process.

Diffusion

Larger lipid-soluble molecules and most drugs are able to cross cell membranes by *passive diffusion.* This transfer process results from the dissolution of a lipid-soluble drug in the lipid portion of the cell membrane and thereafter diffusing across this barrier. This is in agreement with the familiar chemical axiom stating that "like dissolves like." Thus, the ability of a molecule to diffuse across a membrane is directly related to its lipid solubility. Studies correlating the relationship between the relative lipid solubility and the potency of general anesthetic agents (ether, chloroform, nitrous oxide) or the antibacterial activity of alcohols are classic.

The *concentration gradient* across the cell membrane strongly influences the rate of diffusion. Drug molecules tend to move toward the side of the membrane where there are fewer molecules. As a consequence, we see that drugs flow "downhill" from a region of higher concentration to an area of lower drug concentration. When an equal concentration is attained on each side of the membrane, such as inside and outside a cell, a steady-state is said to exist, and there is no additional net transfer of drug molecules.

Active Transport

Many lipid-insoluble molecules that are, in addition, too large to pass through pores by filtration (that is, have a molecular weight greater than 100–200) are nevertheless capable of crossing cell membranes. This phe-

---

[2] Å = angstrom: 100,000,000 Å = 1 centimeter = 0.39 in.

nomenon may be explained on the basis of an *active transport carrier* mechanism with which the drug is able to combine temporarily to form a complex.

This carrier system is analogous to a shuttle bus traveling from a hotel to a nearby convention hall. The bus deposits its passengers at the hall and then returns to the hotel for additional passengers. To get aboard this bus, a special pass is required, designating the individual as a bona fide conventioneer. Although the bus has a limited capacity, perhaps for only 25 passengers, for practical purposes the capacity of the convention hall is unlimited, holding several thousand persons.

Let us now examine the *active transport system,* which is depicted in Figure 3-2. Consider a drug that is outside the cell membrane and that does not have the required chemical and physical properties that would enable it to cross the membrane unassisted. The drug loosely combines with a carrier that is able to transport it across the membrane and deposit it inside the cell. The carrier then returns to the outside of the membrane to pick up additional drug molecules.

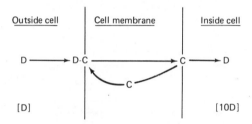

FIGURE 3-2. Schematic Representation of Proposed Active Transport Drug-Carrier System. D is a drug that is too lipid-insoluble to diffuse across the membrane and is too large to pass by filtration through the pores. C is a carrier that is able to freely diffuse across the membrane. D-C is the drug-carrier complex. In an active transport system, drugs can be transported against a concentration gradient. [D] and [10D] are the relative drug concentrations outside and inside the cell, respectively.

The required characteristics for such an **active transport carrier system** include: (1) there must be a source of *energy;* (2) there must be *substrate specificity*—that is, only molecules with certain chemical characteristics can be actively transported; (3) only a finite number of molecules can be transported at any one time, indicating that the carrier can be *saturated;* and (4) drugs can be transported from areas of low concentration to those of higher concentration. Thus, drugs can be transported against a *concentration gradient,* which differs from passive diffusion. The characteristics associated with filtration, diffusion, and active transport are summarized in Table 3-2 and Figure 3-3.

TABLE 3-2. SUMMARY OF MODES BY WHICH DRUGS CROSS CELL MEMBRANES

	Filtration	Diffusion	Active Transport
Size of drug	Small (molecular weight <100-200)	Small or large	Small or large
Solubility	Lipid or water	Lipid	Lipid or water
Chemical specificity	No	No	Yes
Energy requirements	No	No	Yes
Passage against a concentration gradient	No	No	Yes
Rate of passage determined by	Size of drug molecule Concentration gradient	Lipid solubility Concentration gradient	Energy Carrier saturation Structural specificity

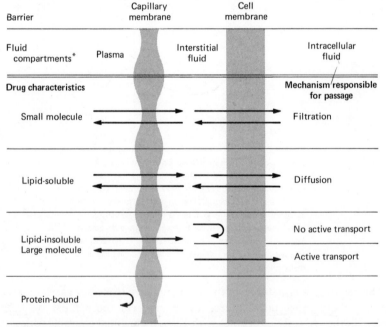

*The average 70 kg (154 lb) man is made up of 40 liters (40 quarts) of water, or about 57% of his total weight. Of these 40 liters, 25 liters are within the 100 trillion cells of the body (intracellular fluid); the remaining 15 liters of water, termed extra-cellular water, are subdivided into several compartments. Two of these are the plasma (noncellular part of the blood—3 liters) and the interstitial fluid (water lying in the spaces between the cells—12 liters).

FIGURE 3-3. Passage of Drugs across Membrane Barriers. Drug transfer is influenced by the size of the molecule, lipid solubility, presence of an active transport system, and protein binding. With the exception of protein-bound drugs, almost all commonly used drugs are able to cross readily the walls of the capillary membranes. This affects the transfer of these compounds from the plasma to the interstitial fluid. Small molecules enter the cell by filtration across the cell membrane; lipid-soluble drugs pass through the membrane by diffusion. Lipid-insoluble drugs of larger dimensions require an active transport carrier mechanism to cross the cell membrane. Protein-bound drugs do not leave the plasma in the bound state.

ABSORPTION

Drugs may act at the site of drug administration or, more commonly, at some distant part of the body. Anti-acne creams, dandruff shampoos, and powders for athlete's foot all act on the skin at the site of administration; antacids act in the stomach and do not require absorption into the bloodstream to exert their pharmacological effects. It is far more common for the target site to be inaccessible to direct application of the drug. Diuretics act on the kidneys, barbiturate sedative-hypnotics depress brain activity, and digitalis influences the function of the heart. In most cases, drugs must enter the blood and be carried by this fluid to the appropriate locus of action. *Absorption* may be defined as the transfer of a drug from its site of administration to the blood.

The speed of drug absorption, and the extent to which it occurs, is dependent upon the route of drug administration selected, the physical-chemical properties of the drug, and the surface area available for the drug to penetrate.

Route of Administration

The physical-chemical properties of the drug, the intended site of drug action, and time-response factors influence which route of administration is selected (Table 3–3). When the ultimate locus of drug action is remote from this site of administration, the drug must be delivered in a manner that will insure its entry into the blood. Most commonly, this is accomplished by giving the drug by mouth (orally) or injection (parenterally). A dermatologist treating facial acne would not be expected to prescribe a suppository. Conversely, a glycerin suppository for a constipated infant would be more rational than an ointment of the same compound applied to the skin of the buttock.

The onset of action after the oral administration of a drug generally occurs within one hour. When an immediate effect is imperative in a life-threatening situation, the problem of absorption after oral administration may be totally obviated by giving the drug intravenously or intraarterially. These routes deliver the drug directly into the bloodstream and make it immediately available for distribution to the appropriate site of drug action.

Physical-Chemical Properties

Absorption into the bloodstream from the site of administration is strongly dependent upon the *solubility* of the compound. When a drug is in solution, it is more rapidly absorbed than when the same compound is taken as a solid. Insoluble drugs are very poorly absorbed into the blood after oral administration of the solid drug, and in some instances such compounds are virtually unabsorbed. This can be highly advantageous, for example, when the antibiotic neomycin is used to sterilize the gastrointestinal tract prior to abdominal surgery.

TABLE 3-3. ROUTES OF ADMINISTRATION OF DRUGS

Route	Where Administered	Advantages	Possible Disadvantages	Examples
Topical	On skin or mucous membrane	Drug at site of action	Possible absorption, sensitization and allergy	Ointments, creams, eye and nose drops, vaginal jellies
Systemic 1. Oral	Distributed in the body to a location distant from the site of administration; given by mouth and absorbed from stomach or intestines Sublingual: placed under the tongue	Safest Most convenient Most economical	Irritating: nausea and vomiting Destruction by intestinal enzymes Food interferes with absorption Uncooperative patient	Penicillin tablets Quinine capsules Ipecac syrup
2. Rectal	Placed into lower rectum as a suppository	Useful when patient is vomiting or unconscious Drug does not pass through liver before entering systemic circulation (not metabolized as rapidly)	Irregular and incomplete absorption Irritation to rectal mucosa Inconvenient	Trimethobenzamide (Tigan) suppositories (antiemetic) Aspirin suppositories
3. Inhalation	Gaseous and volatile drugs are inhaled and absorbed through the epithelium of the fine divisions of the lungs (alveoli)	Very fast absorption of drug into blood Pulmonary disease-drug at site of action	Poor regulation of dosage Inconvenient	Isoproterenol aerosol Nitrous oxide ("laughing gas") Ether

4. Injection				
(a) Subcutaneous (hypodermic)	Into or under the skin	Slow, even and prolonged effects Implantation pellets (months) Prevents enzymatic destruction in gastrointestinal tract	Only nonirritating drugs can be so administered Painful	Protamine insulin
(b) Intramuscular	Deep into muscle tissue	Aqueous solution: rapid absorption Oil: slow, even absorption with long duration of action Irritating substances can be used	Injection into blood vessel	Procaine penicillin
(c) Intravenous	Directly into vein	No absorption problems Immediate onset of action Exact dose enters blood Irritating solutions can be used Large volumes can be injected	Once injected, drug cannot be recalled Rapid injection: adverse circulatory effects Complete sterility essential (danger of viral hepatitis) Drug must be completely in solution	Epinephrine Thiopental (Pentothal)
(d) Intraperitoneal	Into peritoneal cavity	Rapid absorption Large volumes can be injected	Danger of puncturing the intestines (infection) Used in laboratories, rarely in humans	Peritoneal dialysis (drug poisoning)
(e) Intrathecal or intraspinal	Directly into cerebrospinal fluid (CSF)	Ensure drug enters central nervous system (brain and spinal cord)	Difficult technique	Streptomycin Spinal anesthesia (childbirth)

The diabetic is subjected to the painful inconvenience of daily injections of insulin because if taken orally, this compound is readily inactivated by the proteolytic enzymes of the gastrointestinal tract that normally digest the proteins in our food.

Surface Area

A direct relationship exists between the available *surface area* and the rate of absorption. The very extensive surface area of the small intestines provides an excellent environment for the absorption of drugs after their oral administration. In fact, most drug absorption after oral administration occurs in the small intestines. For selected drugs, inhalation is a very useful route of administration. To abort acute asthmatic attacks, patients frequently inhale epinephrine or isoproterenol. The instantaneous relief obtained can be attributed to the expansive surface area of the alveoli of the lungs and the very large number of capillaries present for drug absorption.

The rate of absorption is strongly influenced by the concentration gradient across the absorbing membrane. Drugs given in higher concentrations are more rapidly absorbed. When active transport processes are responsible for absorption, the concentration gradient has no effect on the rate of drug transport into the bloodstream.

DISTRIBUTION

Once a drug enters the bloodstream, either after absorption from its site of administration or by virtue of an injection directly into the blood, it must usually cross one or more membranes prior to reaching its ultimate site(s) of action. It should not be assumed that all the administered drug reaches this tissue site, and as a practical matter, only a very small percentage may. Large amounts of the drug may be biotransformed and inactivated, excreted without chemical change, distributed to nontarget tissue sites or concentrated in fat or bound to proteins in the plasma. All of these processes lower the concentration of free drug in the blood, thereby reducing the amount of drug available to interact at the receptor site or other loci of action. With the exception of protein-bound molecules (see below), virtually all drugs are able to filter through the relatively large pores in the capillary walls and enter the interstitial fluid that lies in the spaces between cells. Drugs must gain access to this fluid if they are to exert their effects on the cell membrane or in the cell.

It should be recalled that cell membranes have lipid characteristics. Thus, whereas lipid-soluble compounds are able to penetrate the membrane by diffusion, lipid-insoluble compounds are excluded passage via simple passive processes. Small molecules enter the cell by filtration through the pores in the membrane. Large molecules that are lipid-insoluble gain entry into the cell by active transport (see Figure 3–3).

Let us now consider how the protein binding of drugs in the plasma alters the properties of these biologically active compounds. Thereafter, we shall examine the factors that influence the distribution of drugs into the brain and across the placental barrier, and we shall briefly discuss the resulting pharmacological implications that arise from these phenomena.

Protein Binding of Drugs

The extent to which a drug is able to be distributed outside blood vessels is often modified by protein binding. Unlike most other molecules, proteins are too large to pass through the walls of the capillaries, and, as a result, when drugs are bound to proteins, they are trapped in the plasma. The chemical properties of the drug determine whether it will be bound, and to what extent. For example, after a therapeutic dose of bishydroxycoumarin (Dicumarol), an anticoagulant or drug that prevents blood clotting, we observe that 98 to 99 percent of the molecules are protein-bound; by contrast, the pain and fever-reducing agent antipyrine is virtually unbound. With few exceptions, binding is a reversible phenomenon; that is, at a given time, some finite fraction of the total number of drug molecules are bound to plasma proteins with the remainder free or unbound (Figure 3–4).

What are the pharmacological consequences of protein binding? Binding prevents the drug from leaving the plasma; thus it is biologically inactive because the bound compound is unable to gain access to and interact with its target sites at the cell. In addition, the drug is not subject to biotransformation or elimination from the body. Hence, protein binding serves as a storage depot for drugs, causing such compounds to have a long duration of action as a result of their slow release from binding sites on the protein.

Albumin is the primary protein in the plasma that binds drugs. This protein possesses only a finite number of binding sites, and, as might be anticipated, two different drugs may compete for these limited number of sites. Drugs having a stronger affinity for these sites are able to displace compounds possessing a weaker affinity. Rapid displacement of very potent drugs from albumin may abruptly elevate the amount of free biologically active drug molecules in the plasma. Displacement of the anticoagulant bishydroxycoumarin from protein binding sites has resulted in fatal internal bleeding (Figure 3–4). Moreover, this serves as an ominous warning of the possible dangers associated with the indiscriminate use of several drugs concurrently. We shall further consider drug-drug interactions in the last section of this chapter.

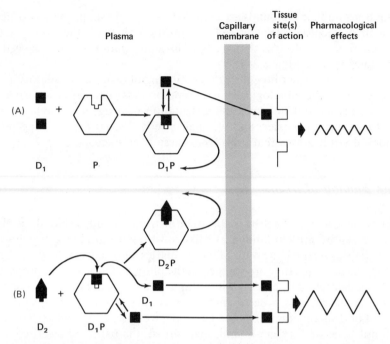

Plasma   Capillary membrane   Tissue site(s) of action   Pharmacological effects

FIGURE 3–4. Protein Binding and Displacement of Drugs. (A) Drug 1 (D_1) is administered and absorbed into the blood stream. Some fraction of the administered dose is bound (D_1P) to plasma protein (P), while the remainder is unbound or free. Unlike the protein-bound drug, the free drug molecules are able to cross the capillary membrane and exert a pharmacological effect at a tissue site. (B) Drug 2 (D_2) has a stronger affinity for the protein binding sites than does D_1. Hence, when D_2 is administered, it displaces D_1 from its protein binding sites, resulting in a high plasma concentration of free D_1 that is available to exert its pharmacological effects.

Blood-Brain and Placental Barriers

Blood-Brain Barrier

The passage of drugs to the brain and cerebrospinal fluid (CSF) differs somewhat from normal membrane transfer. The rate at which drugs enter the brain and CSF is related to their lipid solubility; lipid-soluble substances (such as general anesthetics) readily enter the brain, while lipid-insoluble compounds and charged molecules enter much more slowly (even after intravenous administration), at a rate proportional to their size. Water-soluble molecules for which active transport processes exist (glucose, amino acids) also readily enter the brain.

For a drug to enter a neuron (nerve cell) in the brain, it must first cross membranes of the capillary walls and glial cells (connective tissues of the brain), then the extracellular fluid compartment of the brain, and finally the cell membrane of the neuron. Glial cells closely surround the capillaries, thereby impeding the movement of drugs into and out of the brain; the **blood-brain barrier** is thought to be located where the cell membranes of the capillaries and glial cells meet.

Drugs can enter the brain directly or indirectly from the blood via the CSF. The CSF, formed in the cavities or *ventricles* of the brain, bathes the surfaces of the brain and spinal cord and serves to protect these structures by cushioning them against trauma. The *blood-CSF barrier* consists primarily of the epithelial cells of the choroid plexus of the ventricles.

The permeability of these barriers is modified by certain disease states. Administration of even large doses of penicillin fails to produce measurable changes in the levels of this antibiotic in the CSF of normal subjects. By contrast, penicillin readily enters the CSF of patients with meningitis (inflammation of the membranes surrounding the brain and spinal cord).

In some cases, it is desirable to modify the physical properties of certain drugs in order to convert them to charged molecules. As such, they still retain their ability to act in the periphery or outside the brain, but are markedly limited in their ability to enter the brain. On a gram-for-gram basis, heroin produces greater psychic effects than morphine. Heroin's enhanced potency has been attributed to its greater lipid solubility and the resulting facility with which it enters the brain.

Placental Barrier

Ever since the tragic thalidomide episode of the early 1960s, clinicians and scientists have shown great interest in the placental transfer of drugs and their effects upon the developing fetus. The placenta is a tissue rich in blood vessels that serves as a respiratory, digestive, and excretory organ for the fetus. Although lipid-soluble compounds preferentially cross the placenta, the placenta is permeable to most compounds having a molecular weight of less than 1000, and this includes most of the commonly used drugs. Among the many drugs capable of rapid passage from the mother to the fetus are ether, alcohol, antibiotics, barbiturates, morphine, and heroin. In one study of 382 infants born to heroin-addicted mothers, 259, or 67 percent, manifested characteristic narcotic withdrawal symptoms shortly after birth. Maternal ingestion of the antibiotic tetracycline can cause staining of fetal teeth and retardation of bone growth.

The ability of drugs to cross the placenta and enter the fetal circulation has very significant implications for the pregnant mother. Drugs that are relatively safe for the mother may have profound effects on the developing fetus. Thalidomide, a medical pariah, is a classic example. Attempted suicides by adults employing 20 to 40 times the average dose of this sedative-hypnotic have been unsuccessful, thus attesting to the very high therapeutic index (lethal dose/effective dose) of this compound. However, when taken during the first three months of pregnancy, as little as one normal dose has been shown to produce significant physical deformities of the fetus. Therefore, pregnant women should take only those drugs thought to be essential by their physicians.

BIOTRANSFORMATION (METABOLISM)

You have taken a drug which has been absorbed and subsequently distributed throughout the body; the drug has interacted with a receptor and an effect of some finite duration has resulted. Is this foreign compound doomed to sail eternally throughout your bloodstream like the legendary ship *The Flying Dutchman*? Are you obliged to harbor this drug for the remainder of your life? Biotransformation of drugs prevents our bodies from becoming a junk yard of foreign compounds.

The kidney is the most important organ responsible for the excretion of drugs from the body (Figure 3–5). If we consider that the kidney tubules have lipid cell membranes very much like those found in other tissues, it may be surmised that lipid-soluble drugs will readily diffuse across the walls of the kidney tubules, whereas water-soluble compounds will not. Thus, after a water-soluble compound is filtered through the glomerulus of the kidney, it will not be reabsorbed but rather will be excreted in the urine. By contrast, a lipid-soluble compound will be reabsorbed and returned to the plasma. In general, **biotransformation** *reactions convert lipid-soluble drugs into less lipid-soluble, more water-soluble products (metabolites),* which are more easily eliminated by the kidneys. Some drugs that are sufficiently water-soluble are eliminated without prior biotransformation.

Enzymes

Some fascinating studies have suggested that the necessity for the drug metabolism and the essential enzymes required for carrying out these chemical changes in drugs may have developed in phylogenetic succession, as a part of the evolution of land animals. Lipid-soluble compounds can readily leave the body of fish through the gills. Therefore, it could be teleologically argued that there exists no reason for a highly developed enzyme system to biotransform drugs, or any other foreign organic compounds into more water-soluble metabolites. Whereas fish are able to metabolize drugs to a limited extent, amphibia can do so more effectively. However, terrestrial animals (reptiles, birds, and mammals) were required to develop sophisticated enzyme systems or perish as the result of an accumulation of toxic materials. A further prerequisite was that these enzymes be relatively nonspecific, in order to deal with a wide variety of compounds never previously encountered by the organism or its forebears.

Some drugs can be metabolized by a small number of the more than 2000 highly specific enzymes that participate in the normal biochemical reactions of the body. These reactions of intermediary metabolism are necessary for the breakdown of foods, generation of energy, and the synthesis of tissues and other compounds required by the body for the maintenance of life. For example, alcohol (ethanol) and the skeletal muscle relaxant succinylcholine are broken down by the enzymes alcohol dehydrogenase and pseudocholinesterase, respectively.

Of far greater importance, however, are the relatively **nonspecific drug metabolizing enzymes** associated with the endoplasmic reticulum of the liver. The *liver* is the major organ of the body responsible for the biotransformation of drugs. The endoplasmic reticulum, when viewed under an electron microscope, resembles a thin tubular network. Some of the reticulum appears "rough," because of the presence of dense bodies termed ribosomes; the ribosomes are the sites of protein synthesis. Other reticulum have no ribosomes and appear "smooth." The smooth endoplasmic reticulum or *microsomes* contain the nonspecific drug metabolizing enzymes.

As a consequence of the chemical reactions occurring in the microsomal fraction of the liver (1) the drug may lose all or some of its original pharmacological activity, or (2) an inactive drug may be biotransformed into a biologically active metabolite.

Drugs are also biotransformed by enzymes in the mitochondria of the liver, as well as those found in the plasma, lung, and intestines. These enzymes assume considerably less overall significance in drug biotransformation.

Several important generalizations can be made with regard to biotransformation reactions:

1. In almost all cases, the end product is less lipid-soluble and more water-soluble, thus facilitating its urinary excretion and eventual elimination from the body.

2. In the past, these reactions were thought to be, and were even termed, "detoxification mechanisms," implying that the products were less active than the parent drug. This, clearly, is not the case in all instances! The parent compound parathion, which is used as an insecticide, is inactive; only after an appropriate biotransformation reaction involving oxidation does it become the biologically active and very toxic agent paraoxon. *Prodrug* is the term used for a biologically inactive parent compound that is metabolized to an active metabolite.

3. Drug metabolism is important because it explains, in part, why some individuals are extremely sensitive to drugs (hypersensitive), whereas others are extremely resistant. Hypersensitive individuals often biotransform drugs slowly, and consequently inactivate and eliminate them more slowly than normal, whereas persons who are more resistant to drugs rapidly biotransform and eliminate them.

4. Although most drugs are metabolized, it should not be assumed that this must always be the case. Among the types of drugs not metabolized are very water-soluble compounds, such as relatively strong organic acids and bases and charged molecules; chemically inert compounds, such as general

anesthetics (that are less than 5 percent metabolized); and insoluble compounds not absorbed from the gastrointestinal tract.

EXCRETION

The main routes of drug elimination are through the kidneys (urine), in the
bile, and via the feces. Compounds may also be eliminated through the
pulmonary epithelium (expired air), salivary and sweat glands, and mammary
glands (milk). By far, the most important of these routes of elimination is
through the **kidneys** (Figure 3-5).[3]

The glomeruli of the kidneys are capable of filtering about 4 oz (120 ml) of
plasma water per minute. It should be recalled that free unbound drugs are
filtered, whereas protein-bound compounds are not. After filtration, lipid-
soluble compounds are readily reabsorbed across the lipid membranes of the
kidney tubules and are consequently not eliminated in the urine. It should be
anticipated that in the presence of inadequate kidney function resulting from

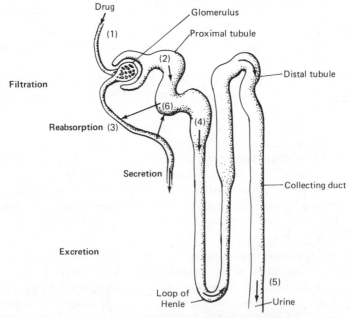

FIGURE 3-5. Urinary Excretion of Drugs by the Kidneys. Small blood vessels (1) carry
plasma-containing drugs to the glomerulus of the kidney for filtration (2). Lipid-soluble
drugs are capable of diffusing across the cell membranes of the proximal tubules (3) and
thereby escape excretion. This is termed tubular reabsorption. Water-soluble compounds do
not diffuse across the kidney tubules (4), are not reabsorbed, and are eventually excreted in
the urine (5). Some drugs and metabolites are secreted from the plasma (6) and are
thereafter eliminated from the body in the urine (5).

[3] Normal kidney physiology will be considered in detail in Chapter 21.

disease, or in very young infants, the ability of the body to excrete drugs via this route will be reduced; the possibility of drug-induced toxicity resulting from an accumulation of drugs is increased in such individuals.

The relative acidity of the urine strongly influences whether a compound will be reabsorbed or excreted. Amphetamine is excreted twenty times more rapidly in acidic urine (pH 5) than it is in more neutral urine (pH 8). "Speed freaks," high-dose users of methamphetamine or amphetamine, generally have a highly acidic urine as a consequence of drug-induced starvation. The duration of the excitatory experience they seek is markedly reduced because of the rapid excretion of the drug. When forced to eat, their urine becomes less acidic, less drug is eliminated in a fixed time, and this enables them to get a greater amphetamine-induced "high" for their money.

In the first major section of this chapter, we have considered the mechanisms responsible for the absorption of drugs into the bloodstream from their site of administration and for their distribution to target tissues, biotransformation to more water-soluble metabolites, and eventual excretion from the body. As we shall observe in the second part of this chapter, changes or abnormalities in the capacity of these mechanisms to function normally directly influence the organism's response to drugs.

FACTORS MODIFYING DRUG RESPONSES

We are tired of the lecture hall and have decided to apply some of our basic pharmacological knowledge to some practical field work. In this regard, we are particularly fortunate to have recently received a rather large sum of money from the "Zilch Pharmaceutical Company" to conduct clinical studies on their new barbiturate "Zilchital." Preliminary animal and human tests have demonstrated that this compound is relatively safe. We have complied with all the necessary legal requirements, and arrangements have been made to use a large park in the center of town for our study. This experiment is designed to determine how long subjects sleep after receiving 100 mg of "Zilchital." The first 1000 individuals who pass our location will serve as subjects, and, of course, all are extremely enthusiastic about participating in this worthy scientific endeavor. Being eager to get underway, we start our experiment at 8:00 A.M. and finish, rather wearily, at midnight that evening. Statistical evaluation of the results indicates that the average duration of sleep was 200 minutes. What magnitude of variation, that is, extreme values, might be expected? Perhaps 180–220 minutes? This is highly unlikely. A more realistic range might be 30–600 minutes.

Among the factors that might be responsible for the marked variation in drug response are age, body weight, sex, species variation, genetic factors, route of administration, time of administration, emotional factors, pre-existing disease, and patient drug history (Figure 3–6). Most of these factors have been

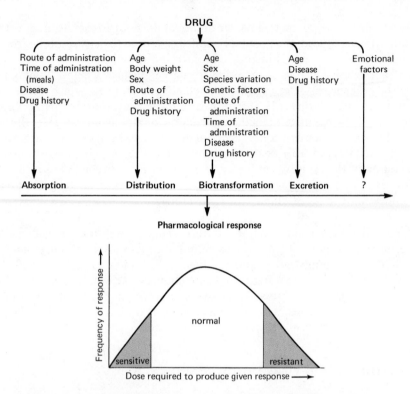

FIGURE 3-6. Pharmacodynamic Influences Modifying the Response to Drugs.

shown to influence one or more of the following pharmacodynamic parameters: drug absorption, distribution, biotransformation, and excretion. How emotional factors influence the drug response has not as yet been adequately explained in pharmacodynamic terms.

Age

If our subjects were truly chosen randomly, it might be expected that there would be extreme variation in the ages of the persons participating in this study; that is, our subjects might range from very young infants to octogenarians. It can be generally stated that infants and very senior individuals are more sensitive to drugs than normal. The "normal" or average individual is 18 to 65 years old and weighs between 60 and 90 kg (130 to 200 lb).

Over the years, many formulas ("rules") have been devised to calculate approximate infants' and children's dosages as a fraction of the average adult dose. Dosage estimates, computed on the basis of age, body weight, or body surface area, represent only *approximations* since they are predicated upon the erroneous concept that the child is a miniature adult (see below). Some of these rules continue to be widely used because, as yet, no absolute method for the determination of such dosages has been found.

Infants

Pharmacologically, infants cannot be considered small adults. This is not a mere reference to size but rather to the ability of an infant to handle drugs. *Infants (especially neonates) have very poorly developed drug metabolizing enzyme systems.* Their inability to adequately metabolize and inactivate drugs results in an intensified drug response for prolonged periods of time.

In a classical experiment,[4] white mice were given a fixed dose of a barbiturate agent (in amounts proportional to differences in their body weights), and the duration of ensuing sleep measured. As can be readily observed, the younger the animal, the longer the drug-induced sleep. These investigators were able to correlate longer sleeping times in younger mice with a reduction in the rates of metabolism and inactivation of this barbiturate.

Age (days)	Sleeping Time (minutes)
1	> 360
7	107
21	27
90 (adult)	< 5

To compound the difficulty of young infants in metabolizing drugs, their kidneys are functionally inefficient, thus impairing excretion of drugs. Prior to the recognition of these dangers, use of the antibiotic chloramphenicol (Chloromycetin) was observed to cause deaths in many very young infants. These fatalities have been attributed to inadequate metabolism (conjugation) and an inability to excrete the drug.

The practical implications of these observations are evident. In the absence of medical supervision, extreme caution should be exercised when giving drugs to the very young. What may constitute a very reasonable dose for a 3-year-old child may be totally unreasonable for a 1-month-old infant.

Elderly Individuals

It has long been recognized that elderly persons are hypersensitive to barbiturates and other central nervous system depressants. Many factors undoubtedly contribute to their increased susceptibility to drug-induced effects. In general, drugs tend to remain in the body of an elderly person for longer periods of time thus increasing the intensity of the desired clinical effects as well as the potential for toxicity.

[4] W. R. Jondorf, R. P. Maickel, and B. B. Brodie, "Inability of Newborn Mice and Guinea Pigs to Metabolize Drugs," *Biochemical Pharmacology* 1:352 (1958).

As an inevitable consequence of the aging process, the pumping efficiency of the heart is diminished as is kidney function (decreased kidney blood flow, glomerular filtration rate, and tubular secretion), and the capacity of the liver to metabolize drugs. Thus, the rate and efficiency of drug elimination processes are reduced.

Body fat as a proportion of total body weight increases with age promoting the accumulation of chronically administered, lipid-soluble drugs in fatty tissues; many such drugs are those prescribed for the treatment of behavioral disorders. Total body water, plasma volume, and the extracellular fluid all decrease relative to total body weight thus potentially affecting drug distribution. Moreover, since the concentration of plasma proteins decreases with advancing age, the amount of drug capable of binding to plasma proteins is reduced, and, conversely, the relative concentration of the unbound, biologically active drug is increased.

On the other hand, in some aged patients, absorption of drugs from the gastrointestinal tract may be reduced, which could result in a diminished therapeutic response. Poor absorption could be the consequence of reduced gastric acid secretion, decreased abdominal blood flow, and impairment of those systems responsible for the transport of drugs across the membranes of the gastrointestinal tract.

Body Weight

Placing one teaspoonful of sugar in a 4 oz versus an 8 oz cup of coffee results in a considerable difference in the concentration of sugar in the resulting beverage. Similarly, administration of 100 mg of drug to a 100 lb versus a 200 lb person will also produce marked differences in the concentration of the drug in the blood and at the site of action. In our theoretical Zilchital study, all subjects were given a fixed 100 mg dose of the drug regardless of their body weights. It might be reasonable to assume that abnormally thin persons would have greater drug-induced effects, that is, would sleep longer, than would extremely obese individuals. As a practical matter, drug dosage is generally not adjusted for small differences in body weight.

Sex

Although many animal studies, especially those in rats, have demonstrated sex-dependent differences in the response to drugs, very little good information has been documented in humans. The *general* rule states that women are more sensitive to drugs than men. However, the exceptions far outweigh this rule and, in general, both sexes respond equivalently to drugs.

Since most clinically employed drugs cross the placenta, the pregnant woman must be extremely judicious in her selection of medications (if any are taken at all) in order to protect the fetus. Harsh laxatives, such as castor oil, should be avoided because such drugs may initiate abortion. Obviously, drugs such as thalidomide that can potentially cause teratogenic effects or fetal abnormalities should not be taken during the gestational period.

Many medications ingested by the mother may be passed to her *nursing infant* through the breast milk.[5] Of the many drugs that the mother is likely to ingest, fortunately, at normal therapeutic doses, only a limited number are likely to produce adverse effects in the infant. Maternal ingestion of morphine and other narcotics, some hypnotics (sleep-producing drugs), and large amounts of alcohol are likely to produce infant sedation. The tetracycline antibiotics may cause staining of teeth and bones while cascara and danthron (laxatives) may cause infant diarrhea. Drugs taken by the mother for the treatment of thyroid disorders have been shown to have adverse effects on the infant thyroid gland.

While it would be prudent for nursing mothers to avoid ingesting any medication, health considerations may make this recommendation impossible. Mothers requiring medication should take the drug 15 minutes after nursing or three to four hours prior to the next feeding; this permits a sufficient period of time to elapse to clear the maternal serum of drug and allows drug levels in the milk to decline to low concentrations. Conversely, drugs taken 30 to 60 minutes prior to the feeding usually attain peak serum and milk concentrations during nursing.

Species Differences

Marked species variations have been observed in the response to drugs. These differences have often been correlated with different rates of metabolism; that is, the faster the rate of drug metabolism and inactivation, the shorter the duration of drug action.

The practical implications of this information are important. All preliminary evaluation of drugs is carried out in animals, and compounds deemed inactive in animal screening tests are rarely examined in humans. Only one out of every 1000 compounds tested ever reaches clinical trials. One may speculate as to how many potentially valuable therapeutic compounds have been eliminated from further study based on negative animal studies.

Species differences in drug response may also be applied to the principle of **selective toxicity** upon which chemotherapy is based (Chapter 28). Ideally, chemotherapeutic agents are toxic to the invading organism (parasite, bacterium, virus) and yet nontoxic to the host. Whereas many insecticides are poisonous to both mammals and insects, malathion is more selectively toxic to insects because of species differences in enzyme activity. Malathion is an inactive compound that is converted to an active metabolite, malaoxon, by an oxidation reaction. Both drug and metabolite are inactivated by a hydrolysis

[5] T. E. O'Brien, "Excretion of Drugs in Human Milk," *American Journal of Hospital Pharmacy* **31**: 844–54 (1974); J. A. Knowles, "Breast Milk–A Source of More than Nutrition for the Neonate," *Clinical Toxicology* **7**: 69–82 (1974).

reaction catalyzed by the enzyme carboxyesterase. Mammals have high carboxyesterase activity and are able to rapidly convert malathion into an inert
product before it can be converted to malaoxon. Insects are less fortunate
because they have low carboxyesterase activity. Thus, they are poisoned by an
accumulation of the toxic malaoxon. Insect resistance to malathion results from
increases in the activity of this hydrolytic enzyme, thus enhancing the ability of
the insect to inactivate this compound.

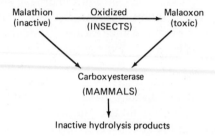

    Physiological differences between species are also an important con-
sideration. Strychnine and red squill have been used as rat poisons. Unlike
humans and household pets, the rat is unable to eliminate these compounds by
vomiting, because it lacks this protective reflex.

    A pharmacological approach to dealing with the blood-sucking vampire
bat may save Latin American cattle raisers one million head annually, valued at
$250 million. This bat feeds exclusively on vertebrate blood, and, in the process,
is capable of transmitting paralytic rabies to its prey. In the past, gassing,
poisoning, shooting, netting, trapping, and dynamiting have all been explored
in an attempt to reduce the population of these bats, unfortunately without
notable success.

    Vampire bats, however, are extremely sensitive to the effects of anti-
coagulants, drugs used therapeutically to slow the rate at which blood clots;
equivalent doses of these drugs do not adversely affect cattle. In a preliminary
experiment conducted in 1972, cattle were injected with diphenadione, an
anticoagulant. For several days after a single injection, blood levels of
diphenadione were sufficiently high that it killed bats that ingested this drug
with their normal feeding of 20 ml (2/3 oz) of blood. Two weeks after a single
treatment of 207 cattle, fresh bat bites were reduced by 93 percent.

Genetic Factors: Pharmacogenetics

    In addition to interspecies differences in the response to drugs, individual
members of the same species may also react differently. Among the newest subdivisions of pharmacology is that of **pharmacogenetics** which is the *study of the
influence of genetic factors on the drug response.* As will be seen in the following
paragraphs, speaking biologically, all people are not created equal.

There are two general types of individual variation to drugs: continuous variation and discontinuous variation. Continuous variation follows the normal or Gaussian distribution and is depicted graphically as a bell-shaped curve (Figure 3–7). Suppose we wish to determine the number of rats killed by varying doses of a new rat poison. In this example, we are asking a very straightforward question: Does the rat die at a given dose of poison or not? Let us assume that this quantal (all-or-none) response follows a normal distribution. If the mean lethal dose is 50 mg, we should anticipate that 68 percent of the animals will die from doses of 40–60 mg and that 95 percent will die from doses of 30–70 mg.

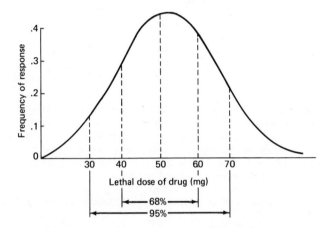

FIGURE 3–7. Continuous or Normal Variation in Drug Response. The response of animals after varying doses of a drug normally follows a normal distribution. This figure represents the dose of a poison required to kill a random group of 100 rats. If the average or mean dose required to produce death is 50 mg, then the dose required to kill 95% of the animals should lie between 30 to 70 mg. We observe from this curve that whereas some rats are quite sensitive to the lethal effects of this poison (that is, they succumb to low doses), other animals exhibit resistance (high doses of the poison are required to produce death). Fine gradations in response are noted in continuous variation.

Subtle gradations in drug response are not always seen, and, indeed, in some instances different and discrete responses are obtained (Figure 3–8). Such *discontinuous variation* has been demonstrated with isoniazid (INH), a drug widely used for the treatment of tuberculosis. Clinical studies have shown that, whereas half the white and half the black people in the United States are able to rapidly inactivate isoniazid, the other halves of these populations are slow inactivators of this compound. However, we observe that the percentage of slow inactivators is markedly different in other ethnic groups: Native Americans (21%), Japanese (13%), and Eskimos (5%). Slow inactivation has been attributed to reduced amounts of an acetyltransferase enzyme, a defect transmitted as an autosomal recessive trait. Individuals who slowly inactivate INH

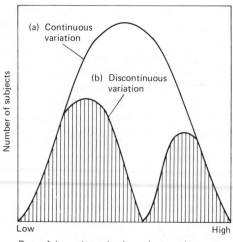

FIGURE 3–8. Continuous (Normal) and Discontinuous Variation in Drug Response.
Compare continuous variation (a), which is usually observed and which follows a normally
distributed bell-shaped curve, with discontinuous variation (b). In the latter, different and
discrete responses are obtained to the drug. As depicted in curve (b), two separate and distinct populations of subjects exist with respect to their drug response, for example, with
respect to their ability to metabolize isoniazid (see text).

are more likely to develop certain undesirable side effects affecting the nervous
system.

Very significant practical implications arise from these pharmacogenetic
studies. Traditionally, all normal 20-year-old, 150-lb male subjects are given the
same dose of a drug for the treatment of a given disease. Whereas a very
favorable therapeutic response might be obtained in one individual, another
may fail to respond, and a third suffer from drug-induced adverse side effects.
There is a growing body of evidence demonstrating that some of these differences can be attributed to variations in the manner in which the body handles
drugs, for example, differences in the extent of absorption or the speed of
metabolism. Many of these differences have been shown to have a genetic basis.
In the future, it is quite probable that simple tests will become available to
enable the physician to predict whether an individual will be highly sensitive or
resistant to drug effects.

Pharmacogenetic differences, in part, account for the development of
resistant strains of bacteria and insects. In the previous section concerning
species differences, we observed that malathion is selectively toxic to insects
because they are unable to effectively hydrolyze and inactivate this compound.
Strains of mosquitoes have emerged that are resistant to this insecticide, and
their survival has been attributed to genetically induced elevated carboxyesterase activity.

Routes of Administration

Rates of absorption, distribution, and metabolism are directly dependent upon the route of administration employed. These factors influence the onset, duration, and intensity of the drug-induced response. Whereas Zilchital might induce sleep 30 minutes after oral administration, intravenous dosage would probably produce this same response in less than one minute. The various routes of drug administration are compared in Table 3–3.

Time of Drug Administration

Meals

Drugs are more rapidly absorbed prior to a meal than after a meal. Many of us have personally observed that alcohol has more rapid and pronounced effects on an empty stomach than when imbibed in similar volume after dinner. Beer has a slower inebriating onset of action than wine, because the carbohydrates in beer delay the absorption of alcohol. Milk is frequently, but unwisely, taken with tetracycline antibiotics in order to reduce gastrointestinal upset. Whereas milk does reduce the incidence of drug-induced nausea, it also retards drug absorption, lowers plasma drug levels, and thereby reduces the desired antibacterial effect.[6]

Time of Day

Daylight has an activating influence, thereby enhancing the effects of stimulants, such as amphetamine, and reducing the effects of barbiturate depressants. Conversely, larger doses of amphetamine are required for stimulation in the evening.

Emotional Factors and Placebos

The patient's *emotional status* at the time of drug administration markedly affects the response obtained. These psychological factors are most pronounced when the patient is taking a drug capable of altering behavior, such as stimulants, depressants, tranquilizers, and hallucinogens.

The *environmental setting* can modify an individual's mood to produce markedly different effects. Consider the possible responses elicited after several glasses of wine in different settings. Contrast the jubilation at a wedding or wild party with the amorous effects at a romantic candlelit table (when accompanied

---

[6] E. A. Hartshorn, "Food and Drug Interactions," *Journal of the American Dietetic Association* **70**: 15–19 (1977).

by a seductive member of the opposite sex), or with the feelings of depression at a dark, lonely corner of a depressing bar bemoaning the loss of one's mate.

Placebos and Physician-Patient Relationship

Among the most important elements of successful therapeutic treatment is the physician-patient rapport. A French proverb tells us that, "The presence of the doctor is the beginning of the cure." By prescribing medication, physicians at least tacitly imply that they anticipate beneficial effects. In some cases, the physician may even unequivocally state that he or she *expects* favorable results. In this instance, the patient is extremely receptive to taking the medication and getting better. However, should the physician merely suggest, "Well, perhaps it may help—but then again, maybe it will not," the patient may be less than convinced about the virtues of the drug. It is well recognized that health and disease are strongly influenced by *psychic* factors and that many symptoms of disease have a psychosomatic origin. This being the case, the power of suggestion may be as potent as a pharmacologically active compound.

The term **placebo,** translated from the Latin "I will please," may be defined as any therapy (or component of therapy) that objectively lacks specific activity for the condition being treated. Its effectiveness is predicated upon the *suggestion* offered at the time of its administration.

Placebos may be of two types: pure and impure. A *pure placebo* is a substance, administered as a drug, that could have no conceivable physiological effect; the "sugar pill" and saline injection are examples of pure placebos. The *impure* or *active placebo* possesses the potential to produce physiological or pharmacological effects but has no objective beneficial effects when given for the specific medical disorder being treated—either because it inherently lacks activity or because it is being administered at a clearly subthreshold dose. Common active placebos include injections of vitamin B_{12} for the general alleviation of fatigue (in the absence of pernicious anemia) and the routine use of penicillin for the treatment of a viral infection.

Are placebos clinically effective? In a classic report by Henry Beecher in 1955,[7] data were collected on the beneficial effects of placebos, administered orally or by injection, to 1082 patients. Placebos were found to be effective for the relief of severe postoperative wound pain, cough, mood changes, headache, seasickness, anxiety and tension, and the common cold in an average of 35 percent of these patients. Other investigators have observed placebo-induced beneficial changes in blood cell count, adrenal gland secretion, gastric (stomach) secretion and motility, blood pressure, respiratory rate, remission of warts, insomnia, and schizophrenia.

The beneficial effects of a placebo are more likely to be manifested when the end point of therapy is a change in behavior (mood, level of alertness), a subjective sensation (pain, nausea), or a response that is under the control of the

---

[7] H. K. Beecher, "The Powerful Placebo," *Journal of the American Medical Assocication* **159**: 1602 (1955).

endocrine system or autonomic nervous system (constriction of the bronchioles in asthmatics, changes in blood pressure). That placebos are considerably less effective in the absence of such symptoms is vividly illustrated by their very limited effectiveness in causing joint changes in rheumatoid arthritis, regression of widespread cancers, or improvement in chronic diseases not characterized by periods of remissions.

Like all potent drugs, placebos are capable of producing adverse effects. After being warned of the side effects associated with the use of oral contraceptives, 17 percent of the women taking placebos reported experiencing nausea, vomiting, headache, dizziness, and gastrointestinal upset. As a byproduct of the powerful consumer movement of the 1970s, many patients have expressed the desire (and in some cases demanded) to know more about the drugs prescribed for them. In 1977, the Food and Drug Administration mandated that the pharmacist distribute *patient package inserts* (PPIs) when dispensing prescriptions for oral contraceptives and estrogens. The PPI is intended to describe, in language readily comprehensible to the average layperson, the potential adverse effects and dangers associated with the use of the medication. The PPI for estrogens contains the statement, "You must decide, with your doctor, whether the risks are acceptable to you in view of the benefits of treatment." It might be predicted that the reported incidence of adverse effects will substantially increase in patients after reading PPIs and that patient compliance in taking the medication, as prescribed, may decrease.

Various factors influence the "effectiveness" of the placebo, and these include the size, shape, color, and taste (slightly bitter, but not unpleasant) of the medication, and the frequency of its administration.

The high incidence of placebo-induced effects make it imperative to compare a new drug with a placebo for relative effectiveness. Moreover, to eliminate bias, it is useful to conduct *double-blind studies.* That is, neither the physician nor the patient is aware of whether the patient has received the active drug or a placebo. The physician can then objectively evaluate the patient's improvement in the absence of any preconceived bias, and only after the completion of the study does he or she learn which medication the patient has actually received.

Pre-existing Disease State

Disease modifies the patient's response to drugs, and some drugs only exert their activity in the presence of disease. Pentobarbital (Nembutal) produces more prolonged sleep in patients with liver disease. This can be readily explained on the basis of the liver's inability to biotransform and inactivate this drug. Patients with impaired kidney function may be more susceptible to drug-induced toxicity unless adjustments are made in dosage (see discussion of cumulative effects, below). Aspirin reduces elevated body temperature, but has no effect on normal temperature. Diarrhea speeds the passage of drugs through the gastrointestinal tract; less drug is absorbed, and larger than usual doses must be given orally to produce the desired therapeutic effects.

Patient Drug History

The prior use of the same or different drugs may greatly influence the quantitative response obtained after taking medication. This response may be a reduction or an intensification of the effects normally elicited. We shall now consider tolerance and tachyphylaxis, cumulative effects, and drug-drug interactions.

Tolerance and Tachyphylaxis

After repeated doses of a drug, a *diminished effect* is sometimes observed. As a consequence of this increased resistance to the usual dose, successive increases in dosage or shorter intervals of time between successive doses are required to produce the effects originally obtained. Whereas **tolerance** is said to develop after days or weeks of repeated drug administration, the term **tachyphylaxis** is used to describe a diminished response that occurs within a relatively short period of time, for example, within minutes to hours. These phenomena may result from decreased absorption of the drug, its increased metabolism or excretion, or cellular adaptation to the drug's effects.

For heroin addicts, tolerance represents a very real problem, for they are obliged to take larger and larger doses to get the same psychological response. Moreover, cross-tolerance to the effects of pharmacologically related compounds may develop, particularly those acting at the same receptor site. This is the basis for the substitution of methadone for heroin in the rehabilitation of opiate addicts. If some of our subjects were regular barbiturate users or alcoholics, their response to "Zilchital" would probably have been markedly reduced because of cross-tolerance.

Tolerance does not develop to all the effects of a given drug nor does it necessarily develop at the same rate and to the same extent to different drug-induced effects. After chronic administration of narcotic agents, considerable tolerance develops to their ability to relieve pain, cause sedation, and depress respiration, while little or no tolerance develops to drug-induced miosis (constriction of the pupils) and constipation.

Cumulative Effects

A drug may produce cumulative effects when its inactivation and/or excretion are slower than the rate at which the drug is being administered. Since more drug is entering the body than is being removed, a buildup results, causing repeated dosage of the drug to produce a more marked response than was obtained after the first dose. In congestive heart failure, a priming dose of about 2 mg of digoxin is given. Thereafter, a daily maintenance dose of 0.25 mg is given to replace the drug removed and thereby maintain optimal amounts of the drug in the body. Cumulative effects may also have dangerous consequences, as is observed in chronic lead poisoning or plumbism. Children who ingest paint chips over long periods of time accumulate lead, a metal which is eliminated very slowly from the body. Eventually nerve and brain damage results.

The *kidney* is the most important organ involved in drug elimination and, for some drugs, is the exclusive agent of drug removal. The dosage of some drugs administered to patients with impaired kidney function must often be reduced to prevent their cumulation from resulting in drug-induced toxicity. For example, kanamycin (Kantrex), an antibiotic present in the urine un-metabolized, has a low margin of safety and is capable of causing kidney toxicity and hearing losses. The *biological half-life* (time required to eliminate one-half of the drug) of this drug is 2 hours in normal individuals and about 25 hours in patients with severe kidney failure. Thus, while the normal interval between successive doses of kanamycin is 3–4 hours, in patients with severe kidney impairment this interval may be extended to every 72–96 hours.[8]

Drug-Drug Interactions

The effects of a drug may be modified by the prior or concurrent administration of another drug. These *combined effects may be greater than, equal to, or less than the effects of the individual drugs when given singly.*

Potentiation or synergism.   The response obtained is *greater* than the algebraic sum of the independent effects of each drug ("2 + 2 = 5"). Penicillin and streptomycin together are more effective for the treatment of certain bacterial infections than is the sole use of either antibiotic. Potentiation may result from two agents acting by different mechanisms or one drug facilitating the action of the other. For example, drug A may enhance the uptake of drug B into the cells or A may prevent the enzymatic inactivation of B.

Addition or summation.   The response obtained is *equal* to the algebraic sum of the independent effects ("2 + 2 = 4"). The sedation and central nervous system depression observed after a barbiturate followed by an alcohol chaser is approximately equivalent to the depression produced by each drug's individual effect. Addition is much more common than potentiation.

Antagonism.   The combined effects are *less* than the algebraic sum of their individual effects ("2 + 2 = 3"). One drug can antagonize the effects of another by four separate and distinct mechanisms—pharmacological, physiological, physical-chemical, and biochemical (Figure 3–9).

You will recall from Chapter 2 that the interaction of an agonist with its receptor results in a response, while in the presence of a receptor antagonist, the effect normally produced by that agonist is reduced or even totally antagonized; this is *pharmacological antagonism.* The adverse effects associated with allergic reactions, mediated by the release of histamine from certain tissues, are reduced or prevented by the administration of an antihistamine.

---

[8] W. M. Bennett, I. Singer, and C. J. Coggins, "A Guide to Drug Therapy in Renal Failure." *Journal of the American Medical Association* **230**: 1544–53 (1974).

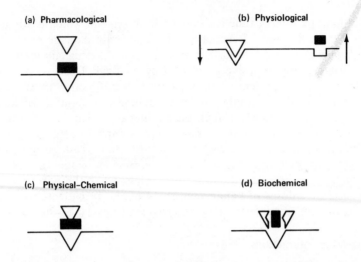

(a) Pharmacological

(b) Physiological

(c) Physical–Chemical

(d) Biochemical

FIGURE 3-9. Mechanisms Underlying Drug Antagonism. In each schematic representation, the drug that elicits an effect (agonist) is denoted by an open triangle, while the antagonizing drug is represented as a solid block. (a) *Pharmacological antagonism:* the antagonist competes with and prevents the agonist from interacting with its receptor site to elicit an effect. (b) *Physiological antagonism:* the antagonist acts at a different site and by a different mechanism to produce an effect that is opposite to and that counterbalances the effect of the agonist. (c) *Physical-chemical antagonism:* the antagonist chemically or physically interacts with and inactivates the agonist. (d) *Biochemical antagonism:* the agonist might act as an enzyme inducer, increasing the activity of liver microsomal drug-metabolizing enzymes and resulting in the more rapid metabolism and inactivation of the agonist.

Physiological antagonism is said to occur when two drugs act at different sites and by different mechanisms to produce opposite effects that counterbalance one another. Histamine and slow-reacting substance of anaphylaxis (SRS-A) cause constriction (narrowing) of the bronchioles, thus impairing normal breathing in asthmatic patients; theophylline and isoproterenol (Isuprel) produce active dilation (widening) of these respiratory airways and are highly effective and often life-saving in terminating an acute asthmatic attack.

Physical-chemical antagonism results when one drug neutralizes or inactivates another as the result of a chemical or physical interaction. Such antagonism may occur when two drugs are mixed together prior to being administered to the patient, an acidic drug neutralizing a basic drug, for example, or one drug causing the precipitation of another.[9] (The presence of a precipitate in a solution intended for intravenous administration represents a particularly hazardous situation.) The administration of chelating agents (Chapter 2) or activated charcoal in the emergency treatment of acute poisoning are common clinical applications of physical-chemical antagonism (Chapter 31).

[9] Devotees of Agatha Christie will recall that ingestion of a fine, but highly toxic precipitate of strychnine bromide was responsible for the death of Mrs. Inglethorp in *The Mysterious Affair at Styles.*

Biochemical antagonism takes place when one drug (antagonist) indirectly decreases the amount of another drug at its site of action. A drug that decreases the rate at which another drug is transported across a cell membrane, that is, that inhibits an active transport process, acts as a biochemical antagonist.

In 1954, it was observed that when mice were fed the carcinogen (cancer-producing compound) 3-methylcholanthrene, they acquired the ability to biotransform other compounds more rapidly than normal. This has been attributed to an increase in the nonspecific drug metabolizing enzymes in the microsomal fraction of the liver and has been termed *enzyme induction*. Enzyme induction has become the most extensively investigated type of biochemical antagonism.

Exposure of rodents to pesticides such as chlordane and DDT shortens the duration of action of the sleep-producing drug hexobarbital. This effect was noted after animal quarters had been sprayed with these pesticides. Over the years, hundreds of drugs (many in common use in therapeutics), insecticides, carcinogens, and other chemicals have been shown to stimulate drug metabolizing enzyme systems in man or animals. This may result in one drug activating the metabolism of another drug that is being given concurrently, thereby shortening its biological life and reducing its therapeutic effects. Repeated administration of a large number of drugs results in tolerance to their effects. Cigarette smoking enhances the metabolism of nicotine in humans, and this may account for the absence of nausea, flushing, and other unpleasant nicotine-induced effects experienced by the neophyte smoker.

In recent years, considerable attention has been directed toward the dangers associated with drug-drug interactions, especially those involving enzyme induction. Failure to appreciate this problem has had fatal consequences in many instances.

From the information presented in this section it should be luminously clear that our experimental design for the clinical evaluation of Zilchital was poor at best. By randomly selecting 1000 subjects and giving them a fixed dose of drug without regard to age, body weight, species (if we were truly random in our selection of subjects, choosing both humans and infrahuman species), routes of administration, time of drug administration, medical history, and prior drug experience, we could not hope to obtain meaningful results. Similarly, wise physicians should not give the same dose, or even the same drug, to all their patients who have the same disease.

SUMMARY

The path of a drug has been traced from the time of its introduction into the body until it is eventually eliminated. Each of the intervening steps—namely, absorption, distribution, biotransformation or metabolism, and excretion—necessitate that the drug cross one or more cell membranes.

The physical and chemical properties of the drug determine the mechanism and to what extent it will cross these membranes. Small molecules filter through the pores in the walls of the membranes; lipid-soluble compounds dissolve in the lipid membrane and pass by diffusion; large, lipid-insoluble drugs require an energy-generated active transport system. Only by the last energy-requiring process are drugs able to be accumulated against a concentration gradient. Drug absorption is dependent upon the solubility of the drug, its route of administration, and the available surface area.

Plasma protein binding limits distribution and reduces the effective amount of drug available to interact with the receptor site at any one time; it serves as a depot storage area for the slow release of drug. While bound, a drug is unable to be biotransformed or eliminated from the body; as the unbound drug is removed from the body, the bound drug is slowly freed from its protein attachment. Displacement of a drug from its binding sites may cause the sudden and massive release of the drug in a pharmacologically active form.

Lipid-soluble drugs most readily enter the brain. The placental barrier is less discriminating and most of the frequently used drugs are able to enter the fetal circulation. The pregnant woman should exercise restraint in her use of drugs, especially during the first three months of pregnancy.

Biotransformation, mainly by the relatively nonspecific drug metabolizing enzymes located in the microsomal fraction of the liver, convert lipid-soluble drugs into more water-soluble products. These metabolites may be more or less active than the parent compound. The ultimate water-soluble products are more readily removed from the body, chiefly by excretion in the urine.

When a drug is administered, a normally predictable response is anticipated based upon the experience obtained with many other subjects who have received the same compound. A large number of factors may be responsible for quantitatively modifying this "normal" response, most of which can be explained in terms of absorption, distribution, biotransformation, and excretion.

Many other factors play a role in modifying our individual response to drugs. The very young and the very old are generally highly sensitive to drugs. Often the rate of drug metabolism and inactivation differs markedly among species, thus accounting for great variation in the intensity and duration of drug action. Variation among species, based upon genetic factors, is now recognized as being an important consideration. In the future, extreme drug susceptibility and resistance will undoubtedly be explained on the basis of pharmacogenetic factors. The patient's psychological mood, the environmental setting in which the drug is taken, the patient-physician relationship, and the power of suggestion (such as accompanies the use of placebos) are all of very great significance in altering the response to drugs. The response to a drug may be markedly modified by other drugs taken either previously or concurrently with the new medication.

SUPPLEMENTARY READINGS

General References

Binns, T. B., ed., *Absorption and Distribution of Drugs.* Edinburgh: E. & S. Livingston, Ltd., 1964.

Brodie, B. B., and J. R. Gillette, eds., *Concepts in Biochemical Pharmacology. Handbook of Experimental Pharmacology.* Vol. 28, Parts 1–2. Berlin: Springer-Verlag, 1971.

Christensen, H. N., *Biological Transport.* 2nd ed. Reading, Mass.: W. A. Benjamin, Inc., 1975.

DiPalma, J. R., ed., "Modern Approaches to Pharmacology," in *Drill's Pharmacology in Medicine.* 4th ed., pp. 10–124. New York: McGraw-Hill, 1971.

Goldstein, A., L. Aronow, and S. M. Kalman, *Principles of Drug Action: The Basis of Pharmacology.* 2nd ed. New York: John Wiley, 1974.

Gorrod, J. W., and A. H. Beckett, eds., *Drug Metabolism in Man.* London: Taylor & Francis, 1978.

LaDu, B. N., H. G. Mandel, and E. L. Way, eds., *Fundamentals of Drug Metabolism and Drug Disposition.* Baltimore: Williams & Wilkins, 1971.

Tedeschi, D. H., and R. E. Tedeschi, eds., *Importance of Fundamental Principles in Drug Evaluation.* New York: Raven Press, 1968.

Testa, B., and P. Jenner, *Drug Metabolism: Chemical and Biochemical Aspects.* New York: Marcel Dekker, 1976.

Vesell, E. S., ed., "Drug Metabolism in Man," *Annals of the New York Academy of Sciences* 179: 1–773 (1971).

Specific References

Benet, L. Z., ed., *The Effects of Disease States on Drug Pharmacokinetics.* Washington, D.C.: American Pharmaceutical Association, 1976.

Boréus, L. O., ed., *Fetal Pharmacology.* New York: Raven Press, 1973.

Conney, A. H., "Pharmacological Implications of Microsomal Enzyme Induction," *Pharmacological Reviews* 19: 317–66 (1967).

Gibaldi, M., *Biopharmaceutics and Clinical Pharmacokinetics.* 2nd ed. Philadelphia: Lea & Febiger, 1977.

Hanstein, P. D., *Drug Interactions.* 4th ed. Philadelphia: Lea & Febiger, 1979.

Hartshorn, E. A., *Handbook of Drug Interactions.* 3rd ed. Hamilton, Ill.: Drug Intelligence Public., 1976.

Kalow, W., *Pharmacogenetics: Heredity and the Response to Drugs.* Philadelphia: Saunders, 1962.

Oldendorf, W. H., "Blood-Brain Barrier Permeability to Drugs," *Annual Review of Pharmacology* 14: 239–48 (1974).

Rapoport, S. I., *Blood-Brain Barrier in Physiology and Medicine.* New York: Raven Press, 1976.

Reidenberg, M. M., *Renal Function and Drug Action.* Philadelphia: Saunders, 1971.

Richey, D. R., and A. D. Bender, "Pharmacokinetic Consequences of Aging," *Annual Review of Pharmacology and Toxicology* **17**: 49–65 (1977).

Schwarz, R. H., and S. J. Yaffe, eds., *Drug and Chemical Risks to the Fetus and Newborn.* New York: Alan R. Liss, Inc., 1980.

"Symposium on Drugs and the Unborn Child," *Clinical Pharmacology and Therapeutics* **14**(4), Part 2: 619-770 (1973).

Toothaker, R. D., and P. G. Welling, "The Effect of Food on Drug Bioavailability," *Annual Review of Pharmacology and Toxicology* **20**: 173-99 (1980).

Vallner, J. J., "Binding of Drugs by Albumin and Plasma Protein," *Journal of Pharmaceutical Sciences* **66**: 447–465 (1977).

Vesell, E. S., "Relationship Between Drug Distribution and Therapeutic Effects in Man," *Annual Review of Pharmacology* **14**: 249–70 (1974).

Yaffe, S. J., ed., "Symposium on Pediatric Pharmacology," *Pediatric Clinics of North America* **19** (1): 1–259 (1972).

4

The Development
of New Drugs

No scientific discipline is currently as hotly pursued as chemistry; is one not compelled, therefore, to apply its astounding results to man? . . . Chemists concentrate the fragrance of cinnamon into a few drops; and distill from treacherous poisons and innocent plants—the most amazing medications. Yet there is more to come! If chemistry keeps its promises . . . whatever is alive, will be perfect; and, in the end, man will live for centuries, free from pain and suffering, in indestructible health, until he dissolves, serenely, in peace.

—Johannes Gaub (1734)

The **perfect drug** has absolute specificity in its action, helps all persons with the disease, has no side effects, and is completely nontoxic. At present, there are approximately 15,000 prescription products that contain one or more ingredients. Estimates of the number of nonprescription products on the market vary from 100,000 to one-half million. Are there not a sufficient number of drugs available to the consumer or for the physician to prescribe?

Even the most severe critics of the pharmaceutical industry would have to answer, "Emphatically, no." Why not? First, we should emphasize that the "perfect drug" has yet to be developed. Penicillin, in many respects, comes closest to achieving the status of the ideal drug. This antibiotic is highly effective for the treatment of a wide range of bacterial infections and is virtually nontoxic to the patient. Yet, resistant bacterial strains have progressively developed, and about 10 percent of the total population is allergic to penicillin. Millions of people are dying of cancer and heart disease each year or suffering from mental illness. Available drugs often control some of these diseases, but few patients are cured.

How many drugs are essential for the practice of medicine? In a recently completed survey,[1] a total of more than 2800 drugs were found to be listed in the hospital formularies of 52 institutions throughout the United States. Ninety percent of these formularies listed the same 230 drugs, while only 69 drug entities were considered to be essential by and were included in *all* formularies (Table 4-1). The World Health Organization maintains a list of 209 drugs that they consider to be "essential to meet the health needs of most people"; this list is one-third the size of the average American hospital formulary, which contains 712 drug entities. Hence, it would appear that only a limited number of drugs can be viewed as fundamental therapeutic agents that are essential for the prac-

TABLE 4-1. DRUG ENTITIES APPEARING IN ALL 52 AMERICAN HOSPITAL FORMULARIES

Therapeutic Category*	Specific Drug Entities
Analgesic-anti-inflammatory agents	Acetaminophen, aspirin, indomethacin
Anticonvulsants	Diphenylhydantoin (phenytoin), primidone
Antihistamines	Chlorpheniramine, diphenhydramine, promethazine
Anti-infective agents	Ampicillin,† chloromycetin, erythromycin, gentamicin, isoniazid, kanamycin, metronidazole, neomycin, nitrofurantoin, nystatin, penicillin G, procaine penicillin G, streptomycin, sulfisoxazole, tetracycline†
Autonomic agents	Atropine, epinephrine, isoproterenol, phenylephrine, pilocarpine, scopolamine
Cardiovascular agents	Clofibrate, digoxin, heparin, hydralazine, lidocaine, methyldopa, procainamide, propranolol,† quinidine, reserpine, warfarin
Gastrointestinal agents	Bisacodyl, castor oil, magnesium sulfate, sodium bicarbonate
Hormones (endocrine agents)	Chlorpropamide, dexamethasone, diethylstilbestrol, hydrocortisone, methylprednisone, testosterone
Psychotherapeutic agents	Chloral hydrate, chlorpromazine, diazepam,† imipramine, paraldehyde, prochlorperazine, thioridazine
Renal (kidney) agents	Aminophylline, ammonium chloride, ethacrynic acid,† mannitol
Vitamins and iron preparations	Ascorbic acid, cyanocobalamin, ferrous sulfate, folic acid, iron dextran injection, phytonadione, pyridoxine, thiamine

Source: Taken from report of T. D. Rucker and J. A. Visconti, *How Effective Are Drug Formularies? A Descriptive and Normative Study* (Washington, D. C.: ASHP Research and Educational Foundation, Inc., 1979).

*The therapeutic categories used in this table are not identical to those used in the original report. Some drug entities may be classified under more than one therapeutic category.

†The five most commonly prescribed single-entity drugs in 1979 (*Pharmacy Times*, April 1980), p. 34.

[1] T. D. Rucker and J. A. Visconti, *How Effective Are Drug Formularies? A Descriptive and Normative Study* (Washington, D.C.: ASHP Research and Educational Foundation, Inc., 1979).

tice of medicine. The balance constitute subtle and often not very significant modifications of these basic drug entities.

DRUGS FROM NATURE AND THE LABORATORY

> *Because the newer methods of treatment are good, it does not follow that the old ones were bad; for if our honorable and worshipful ancestors had not recovered from their ailments, you and I would not be here today.*
>
> —Confucius (551–478 B.C.)

Natural Sources of Drugs

Prior to the nineteenth century, most drugs were derived from natural sources. Plants and, less commonly, animals have provided many of the basic drugs used in modern therapeutics.[2] Moreover, some microorganisms have furnished humans with antibiotics (Table 4–2). Ethnic folklore or the empirical therapeutic use of a leaf or root has often provided the first clue that a plant contained a concealed pharmacologically active substance. The plant is ground up, digested, and treated with a variety of organic solvents (such as ether, chloroform, and alcohol), acids, and bases. Eventually, and with some good luck, a partially purified extract emerges that still retains biological activity. In the not too distant past, analytical chemical techniques were such that the scientist was obliged to be satisfied with "fraction E." However, with advances in analytical chemistry, the natural products chemist is often able to crystallize the pharmacologically active constituent.

It has been estimated that thousands of *marine species,* both plant and animal, contain pharmacologically active compounds. Of these, only a very small percentage have been actually tested for biological activity and only a mere handful of these have been chemically and pharmacologically studied intensively. Antibiotic, antitumor, fungicidal, cardiovascular, neuropharmacological, and psychopharmacological actions have been detected in natural products of marine origin. Five-hundred times more toxic than strychnine to mice, tetrodotoxin (puffer fish) and saxitoxin (shell fish) are among the most poisonous nonproteins known. In the coming decade, *marine pharmacology* will undoubtedly become one of the most active areas of investigation.

[2] The 1970s have witnessed a renaissance in interest in drugs derived from natural sources. With the resumption of diplomatic relations with the People's Republic of China, western scientists and clinicians are taking a fresh and objective look at herbal medicine, the traditional foundation of Chinese therapeutics. Hormones have historically been the primary source of drugs derived from animal sources. Laboratories around the world are now seeking to evaluate the therapeutic potential of interferon as an anticancer and antiviral agent, of prostaglandin derivatives in the treatment of bronchial asthma and gastric ulcers and to cause abortion and induce labor at term, and the role of endorphins in pain and behavioral disorders to serve as a lead in new drug development.

TABLE 4-2. CONTEMPORARY DRUGS DERIVED FROM NATURAL SOURCES

Drug	Source	Pharmacologic or Therapeutic Class
Atropine	Leaves and roots of *Atropa belladonna* (belladonna)	Parasympathetic nervous system antagonist
Bishydroxycoumarin	Sweet clover	Anticoagulant
Chorionic gonadotropin	Urine of pregnant women	Male and female sex disorders
Colchicine	Corm and seeds of *Colchicum autumnale* (meadow saffron)	Antigout
Digitalis	Leaves of *Digitalis purpurea* (foxglove)	Heart stimulant
Ephedrine	*Ephedra sinica* (ma huang)	Sympathetic nervous system stimulant
Epinephrine	Beef adrenal gland	Sympathetic nervous system stimulant
Estradiol	Mare urine	Female sex hormone
Insulin	Beef pancreas	Antidiabetic
Morphine	Juice of *Papaver somniferum* (poppy)	Narcotic analgesic
Penicillin	*Penicillium notatum* (mold)	Antibiotic
Prostaglandins	Sheep seminal vesicle	Uterine stimulation
Quinine	Bark of cinchona tree	Antimalarial
Reserpine	Roots of *Rauwolfia serpentina* (snake root)	Antihypertensive
Somatotropin	Human pituitary glands	Growth failure
Thyroid	Beef thyroid	Thyroid deficiency
Vinblastine	Leaves of *Vinca rosea* (periwinkle)	Anticancer
Vitamin C	Citrus fruits	Antiscurvy

Synthetic Organic Medicinals

The late nineteenth century saw the rise of German dye manufacturing which begot the modern pharmaceutical industry. Although drug research and development existed in the United States prior to the twentieth century, after World War II there was an enormous expansion in the breadth and depth of these operations. By far, the greatest number of new drug discoveries have resulted from research in the United States since this time.

It would be satisfying to the scientific ego to believe that the life-saving drugs currently available were the end result of brilliant conceptualization and Sherlock Holmes–like inductive and deductive reasoning. Paul Ehrlich[3] attributed his success in research to "four big *G*s" *Geduld* ("patience"), *Geschick*

[3] Paul Ehrlich (1854–1915), the "Father of Chemotherapy," was an outstanding German chemist, bacteriologist, and pathologist. He was the first to postulate that drugs interact with chemical groupings on the cell which he termed "receptors." In 1908, Ehrlich received the Nobel Prize in Medicine/Physiology, not for his work on "selective toxicity" or "magic bullets" (specific chemotherapeutic agents), but rather for studies in immunology.

("ability"), *Geld* ("money"), and *Glück* ("luck"), to which we may add a fifth G—*Geist* ("inspiration"), a quality possessed in abundance by this brilliant scientist. Most significant new drugs have been discovered fortuitously or by astute clinical observations. Before the reader becomes disillusioned, it should be added with all deliberate haste, that exceptions to this statement exist.

Generally the development of new drugs is based upon one of two basic research strategies: the modification of the structure of natural products or existing drugs, or the synthesis of a unique compound either for a specific disease or with the hope that a disease exists for which the drug will prove useful in treating.

OBJECTIVES IN THE STRUCTURAL MODIFICATION OF EXISTING COMPOUNDS

Structural modification, or less charitably, molecular manipulation of natural products or existing compounds, often patented by a rival pharmaceutical company, has a variety of objectives. These include: (1) enhancement of the primary effect, while reducing secondary effects; (2) an alteration of absorption, distribution, metabolism, or excretion of existing compounds; and (3) entrance into a financially attractive market to get a "piece of the action."

Enhancement of the Primary Effect, with Reduction in Secondary Effects

"Accentuate the positive, eliminate the negative" is probably sung today with greater gusto in the drug industry than it is on Tin Pan Alley. That is, can a compound be made that possesses more of the desired primary effects and less undesirable secondary side effects and/or toxicity? The use of corticosteroids for the treatment of rheumatoid arthritis illustrates this objective.

Rheumatoid arthritis is a chronic, painful inflammatory disease primarily affecting the joints of the hands and feet. In advanced stages, we observe progressive stiffness; the joints become distorted and deformed and eventually the patient becomes totally disabled and bed-ridden. In 1948, Philip Hench and Edward Kendall demonstrated that *cortisone*, a naturally occurring corticosteroid hormone released from the adrenal cortex, was able to produce dramatic symptomatic improvement in patients with this disease.[4] Unfortunately, cortisone is unable to cure rheumatoid arthritis, but must be used for many months or even for the remainder of the patient's life. Retention of salt and body fluids represent a major problem with this drug. As a direct result of these effects, we see occurrence of significant edema (swelling caused by accumulation of water), which impairs the ability of the heart to efficiently pump

---

[4] In recognition for this discovery, the 1950 Nobel Prize in Medicine was jointly awarded to the chemists Kendall and Tadeus Reichstein and the clinician Hench.

blood around the body. A large number of newer synthetic cortisone-like drugs are now available that are far more potent in their ability to reduce arthritic debilitation and yet retain negligible amounts of body water. These new compounds have resulted from small, but highly significant modifications of the basic cortisone molecule.

Chlorothiazide, hydrochlorothiazide, and bendroflumethiazide have a 200-fold range of potency in their ability to enhance urine output. May we assume that 5 mg of one diuretic is necessarily superior to 1000 mg of the other? Not at all. The therapeutic indexes are approximately the same, as are their side effects.

Structural modification of a basic chemical nucleus can give rise to derivatives with many diverse and often more specific effects. The *phenothiazine* nucleus has proved to be a rather versatile progenitor of pharmacologically useful compounds (Table 4-3). It is of interest to note that phenothiazine itself was used in the past as a urinary antiseptic, insecticide, and as an anthelmintic, a drug used in the treatment of worm infestations.

TABLE 4-3. PHENOTHIAZINE DERIVATIVES WITH DIVERSE PHARMACOLOGICAL EFFECTS

Name (Trade Name)	Therapeutic Class and Disease or Symptoms	R_1	R_2
Chlorpromazine (Thorazine)	Antipsychotic– Schizophrenia Antiemetic– Nausea and vomiting	$-Cl$	$-CH_2CH_2CH_2N(CH_3)_2$
Promethazine (Phenergan)	Antihistamine– Allergies	$-H$	$-CH_2\underset{\underset{CH_3}{\mid}}{CH}-N(CH_3)_2$
Trimeprazine (Temaril)	Antipruritic–Itching	$-H$	$-CH_2\underset{\underset{CH_3}{\mid}}{CH}-CH_2N(CH_3)_2$
Methotrimeprazine (Levoprome)	Analgesic–Pain	$-OCH_3$	$-CH_2\underset{\underset{CH_3}{\mid}}{CH}-CH_2N(CH_3)_2$
Ethopropazine (Parsidol)	Anti-Parkinsonism– Parkinson's disease	$-H$	$-CH_2\underset{\underset{CH_3}{\mid}}{CH}-N(C_2H_5)_2$
Propiomazine (Largon)	Sedative– Prior to surgery	$-COC_2H_5$	$-CH_2\underset{\underset{CH_3}{\mid}}{CH}-N(CH_3)_2$

Note: Subtle changes in chemical structure produce diverse changes in biological activity.

Modification of Absorption, Distribution, and Metabolism

Absorption

The "oral contraceptives" might have been called the "subcutaneous contraceptives" had it not been for chemical modifications in the structures of the natural hormones, estradiol and progesterone. These hormones are virtually inactive by mouth, perhaps as a result of their inactivation by intestinal bacteria. However, with small but highly significant changes in their molecules, the resulting products, ethinyl estradiol and norethindrone, are able to resist bacterial attack and are highly active when taken orally (Table 4-4).

TABLE 4-4. RELATIVE ACTIVITIES OF NATURAL AND SYNTHETIC ESTROGENS AND PROGESTINS AFTER THE ORAL AND SUBCUTANEOUS ROUTES OF ADMINISTRATION

Natural	Synthetic
ESTROGENS	

Estradiol / Ethinyl estradiol

Relative activity:		
Oral	1	40
Subcutaneous	500	500

PROGESTINS

Progesterone / Norethindrone

Relative activity:		
Oral	1	500
Subcutaneous	100	500

Distribution

Drugs are distributed throughout the body by crossing cell membranes. It should be recalled that in order to enter the brain, a compound must be sufficiently lipid-soluble to penetrate the blood-brain barrier. It is often desirable to prevent drugs from entering the brain in an attempt to reduce the incidence of behavioral and neurological side effects. Atropine and scopolamine are effective antispasmodic agents (relax the smooth muscles of the gastrointestinal tract) that also reduce gastic acid secretions in the stomach; these properties make these compounds useful for the treatment of ulcers. However, large doses of atropine or scopolamine cause confusion, hallucinations, and coma. When these compounds are chemically converted to their charged, lipid-insoluble, quaternary ammonium derivatives, that is, methylatropine or methscopolamine, they are unable to readily enter the brain and produce undesirable behavioral adverse effects.

Metabolism

The rate of metabolism is an important factor in determining a drug's duration of biological action. With suitable chemical changes in the drug molecule, this rate may be either increased or diminished. Penicillin is subject to inactivation in the stomach by gastric acid, and also by the enzyme penicillinase, which is produced by several strains of *Staphylococcus aureus*. When sufficient amounts of penicillinase are present, this antibiotic is rapidly broken down and inactivated, enabling these bacterial strains to become penicillin-resistant. More recent research has made available new penicillins that are resistant to acid hydrolysis and penicillinase attack, thus markedly reducing the rate of their inactivation and improving their therapeutic utility.

Financial Incentives

Perhaps the greatest incentive for molecular gymnastics on the part of the pharmaceutical manufacturer is to enter a lucrative market. All too often "me, too" products are introduced that are vigorously promoted to the medical profession on the basis of some dubious advantage over a competing product. This practice has led to an incredible multiplicity of products in the same therapeutic class, all serving the same general therapeutic objective and acting by the same basic pharmacological mechanism. Antihistamines, used for the treatment of allergic disorders, number in excess of 30. There are about at least 15 different brands of oral contraceptives; if you consider that about 10 million women take "the pill" each month in the United States, even a small piece (such as 5 percent) of the market is a rather substantial one. At present, without a prescription, we may purchase about 50 different brands of analgesics for pain or headache. All contain aspirin or an aspirin-like compound.

THE RATIONAL DEVELOPMENT OF NEW DRUGS

While a great number of drugs have resulted from modest chemical modifications and serendipity, in the interest of fair play and to restore the reader's confidence in pharmacologists and medicinal chemists, we shall now discuss the rational development of several drugs, that is, those agents that resulted from "99 percent inspiration and 1 percent perspiration." These drugs could be developed only after a fundamental understanding of the disease entity was appreciated. We shall briefly consider the background surrounding the evolution of levodopa, allopurinol, and dimercaprol.

Levodopa and Parkinson's Disease

In the 1950s, it was ascertained that patients with Parkinson's disease had very low concentrations of *dopamine*[5] in the corpus striatum and substantia nigra, which are parts of the basal ganglia in the brain. Symptoms of this disease include tremors, stiffness, and difficulties in walking. The obvious solution to the problem might be to give dopamine to replenish these deficient stores. We term this *replacement therapy*. Unfortunately, dopamine is unable to cross the blood-brain barrier; its biological precursor, **levodopa**, however, does enter the brain after oral administration. When given in rather large daily doses (4–6 g), sufficient amounts of levodopa are able to enter the brain and are converted to dopamine by the enzyme dopa decarboxylase. A large proportion of the administered dose is converted to dopamine extracerebrally (outside the brain) and is, therefore, unable to enter the brain (Figure 4–1).

Levodopa represents the most effective treatment currently available for the treatment of Parkinson's disease, notwithstanding the many undesirable secondary effects observed in virtually all patients employing this drug. Attempts have been made to reduce these side effects, as well as to lower the effective absolute dose of this very expensive drug. A partially successful approach to these problems has been accomplished by coadministering a dopa decarboxylase inhibitor such as carbidopa, which is unable to enter the brain. As a direct consequence of inhibition of this enzyme outside the brain, orally administered levodopa is not converted extracerebrally to dopamine. Because this enzyme is not inhibited in the brain, decarboxylation can and does occur. Use of levodopa with a peripheral (extracerebral) dopa decarboxylase inhibitor substantially reduces adverse side effects, while retaining the desired therapeutic properties of this drug, at a dose of about one-sixth that required when levodopa is employed alone. The dopa-carbidopa combination is mark :ted as Sinemet.

---

[5] As we shall discuss in Chapters 5 and 6, dopamine is thought to be one of the chemicals responsible for the transmission of impulses from one nerve to another. These chemicals are termed neurotransmitters.

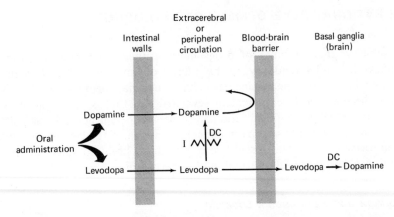

FIGURE 4-1. Rationale for the Use of Levodopa in the Treatment of Parkinson's Disease. Dopamine when given orally (by mouth) does not cross the blood-brain barrier; levodopa does enter the brain and is converted to dopamine in the basal ganglia by the enzyme dopa decarboxylase (DC). We can prevent the peripheral conversion of levodopa to dopamine with an extracerebral dopa decarboxylase inhibitor (I), which permits more levodopa to enter the brain.

Allopurinol and Gout

Allopurinol's development was based upon adequate biochemical knowledge of *gout*. This extremely painful disorder results from increased production or reduced excretion of uric acid, the end product of nucleic acid and purine metabolism. High plasma uric acid levels result in the deposition of this compound in the joints. Allopurinol (Zyloprim) was designed to inhibit uric acid synthesis by blocking the enzyme xanthine oxidase, which, in turn, reduces plasma urate levels and deposition in the joints.

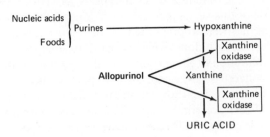

Dimercaprol and Heavy Metal Poisoning

During the early days of World War II, Stocker and Peters at Oxford began an intensive and systematic search for an antidote to the arsenic-containing war gas, lewisite. Arsenic and other heavy metals exert their toxic effects by combining with and blocking sulfhydryl (——SH) groups on essential enzymes. Dimercaprol or British antilewisite (BAL) is a chelating agent that forms a more stable complex with arsenic than arsenic forms with the ——SH groups of the cellular enzymes. Hence, the metal can be withdrawn from the cells, thereby reversing the toxic effects of this poison. An unexpected dividend derived from this work was the nonmilitary application of dimercaprol as an antidote for many metal poisons that act by combination with cellular ——SH groups. Such poisons include arsenic, mercury, gold, antimony, and bismuth.

ANIMAL AND CLINICAL EVALUATION OF NEW DRUGS

A tortuous journey lies between the time of recognition that a chemical substance possesses biological activity until the time that it is approved by the Food and Drug Administration (FDA) as a drug that can be prescribed for the treatment of a disease. Less than one out of every 1000 compounds synthesized successfully completes this journey; only one compound of every 8 that enters clinical trials will eventually reach the market. The required steps include extensive pharmacological and toxicological studies in animals followed by far more intensive, meticulous, and expensive testing in humans. It has been estimated that five to ten years elapse before a compound appears on the market, at a cost of many millions.[6] We shall now briefly trace the path a drug takes from the first time it is tested in animals until it is clinically available to the practicing physician for routine use in patients.

Animal Studies

Depending upon the structure of a newly synthesized compound and/or the objectives of the pharmaceutical company or researcher, the pharmacologist will conduct either a "blind" screen or specific tests to evaluate the compound for a particular action.

In a *general blind screen,* a range of doses of the compound are injected into test animals, usually mice or rats, and gross behavioral observations are made with an eye toward detecting *any* activity. Observations for a compound with potential central nervous system activity generally include changes in awareness, motor activity, coordination, posture, muscle tone, reflexes, and autonomic responses (pupil size, salivation, alterations in temperature or in the rate of the heart and respiration), as well as gross toxicity. The results from such a simple dose-response profile often provide clues that suggest more sophisticated tests to define the nature of the activity.

[6] Readers interested in the complex economics of drug development should consult R. W. Hansen, "The Pharmaceutical Development Process: Estimates of Development Costs and Times and the Effects of Proposed Regulatory Changes," in *Issues in Pharmaceutical Economics,* ed. R. I. Chien, (Lexington, Mass.: Lexington Books, D. C. Heath & Co., 1979), pp. 151–181.

By contrast, the screening procedure may be highly *specific,* with the investigator seeking a particular pharmacological effect. After testing 605 compounds as potential cures for syphilis, Paul Ehrlich's 606th compound, arsphenamine (Salvarsan), proved to be safe and effective. During World War II, the Japanese controlled the world's natural sources of quinine. Of the 15,000 compounds our government screened as substitute antimalarials, only two, chloroquine and primaquine, were found to be superior to quinine. In recent years, there has been very exhaustive screening of soil samples from almost all parts of the world in an attempt to discover new antibiotics or anticancer agents; more recently this search has been extended to the oceans.

The animal screening procedure employed to detect pharmacological activity should ideally bear some relationship to the disease in man that the drug is intended to treat. In some cases, this is relatively easy (for example, antibacterial activity), while for other diseases, there are no suitable animal models. What is the animal counterpart of human schizophrenia or depression? Do animals have psychotic thoughts? In such cases, only human evaluation of drugs can provide the ultimate answer as to the drug's effectiveness.

Toxicity Studies

> *Primum non nocere.* (First do not harm.)
> —Hippocrates (460?–377? B.C.)

After establishing that a chemical has desirable pharmacological properties, it is then necessary to evaluate the toxicity of this compound after repeated doses. This important facet of drug evaluation is of primary importance because all drugs exhibit undesirable effects when given in sufficiently high dosage. Acute toxicity, that is, toxicity after a single dose, has been determined as discussed above. In subacute toxicity studies, the animal is given specified doses of the drug for 14 to 21 days in order to determine the minimum lethal dose and maximum tolerated dose. Cumulative effects or tolerance are also observed. At the end of the test period, the animals are autopsied for pathological changes. Studies for chronic toxicity are of 90 days to several years in duration, and, by law, must employ several species, one of which must be a nonrodent. At regular intervals, the animals are sacrificed, and the blood and organ systems (central nervous, autonomic, cardiovascular, respiratory, gastrointestinal, renal, reproductive, and endocrine) are examined for possible drug-induced changes.

Based upon the chemical properties of the drug and/or its therapeutic indications, the compound must then be subjected to additional specific tests. Drugs to be used in women of the childbearing age are tested for possible *teratogenic* (abnormalities of fetal development) effects in several generations of rats. At parturition, litter size, fetal weight, and structural deformities are noted. Other studies look for *carcinogenicity,* that is, the ability of a drug to produce cancerous tumors, and *addiction potential.* This latter test is of particular importance when the test compound is to be used as an analgesic agent, stimulant, or sedative-hypnotic.

Human Studies (Clinical Pharmacology)

Let us assume that the pharmacological and toxicological properties of a new compound have been evaluated in several species of animals. At this point, many laboratory notebooks may be filled with qualitative and quantitative pharmacodynamic information concerning this drug's unique absorption, distribution, biotransformation, and excretion characteristics. Moreover, we may have comprehensively evaluated its effects on a variety of organs and systems, determined the mechanism(s) responsible for this drug's actions, and ascertained the toxicity associated with this drug.

While our test compound has emerged relatively unscathed from these detailed toxicity studies, it still remains to be determined whether it will prove to be a safe and effective therapeutic agent in humans. Prior to initiating studies in human subjects, the sponsor (usually a pharmaceutical manufacturer) must submit, for FDA approval, a Notice of Claimed Investigational Exemption for a New Drug. This form, commonly referred to as an IND, contains a description of the drug's composition and source, if of natural origin; information concerning its manufacture; detailed results of animal studies; the names and professional qualifications of the clinical investigators responsible for conducting the human trials; and details concerning all aspects of the experimental protocols to be conducted in volunteers, including doses, routes of administration, and clinical and laboratory observations to be performed. After being assured of the safety of the test drug and the precautions to be undertaken for the protection of the subjects participating in the study, the FDA will approve the IND, thus permitting the sponsor to conduct a three-phase evaluation of the compound.

Phase 1: Acute Human Pharmacology

Employing very small doses at the outset and gradually increasing these doses, this phase seeks to determine the absolute amount of drug required to produce pharmacological effects and adverse side effects in *disease-free humans.*

Phase 2: Exploratory Bioassay

Having established the dosage range over which the drug may be safely administered, the compound is now given to a large number of patients suffering from a disease. This phase of human studies provides the first actual indication as to whether the drug possesses actual therapeutic potential or whether it will be relegated to the category of compounds pharmacologically active only in animals.

In these first two phases, generally conducted in a limited number of patients, the clinical pharmacologist is particularly interested in detecting undesirable reactions. In some instances, we are able to predict their occurrence, whereas other reactions are unpredictable.

Predictable reactions are those that directly result from excessive doses of the drug. These adverse effects are seen in all patients, although the dosage necessary to produce such effects will vary according to the susceptibility of the individual. The therapeutic class of the drug usually provides the basis for predicting these side effects. For example, high doses of a sedative are likely to produce coma.

Unpredictable reactions are not dose-related, but are seen only in selected persons who differ from normal. In some subjects, a normal or even a small dose may produce an extreme reaction; this is termed *intolerance. Idiosyncrasies* are genetically determined quantitative or qualitative unusual drug reactions. For example, succinylcholine produces markedly extended muscle relaxation in some individuals at normal dose levels (quantitative); other patients exhibit excitement rather than depression with barbiturates (qualitative). *Hypersensitivity or allergic* reactions are observed following reexposure to a variety of drugs, among them penicillin, sulfonamides, and aspirin. The mechanism of drug allergies is similar to other allergies and is mediated by antigen-antibody reactions. We shall return to a discussion of adverse drug reactions in Chapter 31.

Phase 3: Controlled Studies

Controlled studies, the most expensive stage in drug evaluation, involve the greatest number of subjects tested over the longest period of time. The test compound is critically compared with a placebo and standard reference drugs for safety and effectiveness in patients with the disease or symptom for which the drug is intended to be used. Final approval for marketing is granted by the FDA only after the FDA is convinced that the sponsor's documentation supports claims for safety and effectiveness.

The existing three-phase system of drug evaluation is not without limitations. Some critics have argued that the FDA's demands for proof of safety and effectiveness are unduly excessive and result in inordinate delays in the availability of highly significant new drugs in the United States, drugs with a proven clinical track record in Great Britain and Western Europe.[7] By contrast, we have learned from highly painful experiences that long after completion of Phase 3 testing, previously undiscovered adverse effects may come to light. These include adverse effects manifested only after chronic drug administration over periods of many months to several years, drug-drug interactions, and relatively uncommon toxic effects that only become evident after many patient-years of drug usage.

[7] W. M Wardell, "Introduction of New Therapeutic Drugs in the United States and Great Britain: An International Comparison," *Clinical Pharmacology and Therapeutics* **14**: 773–90 (1973).

The need for and desirability of employing an additional phase in the drug evaluation process is gaining increasing favor. The proposed Phase 4, involving *postmarketing drug surveillance,* would permit the FDA to grant conditional approval for the marketing of highly important new drugs before all the traditional Phase 3 data is accumulated; at the same time the FDA would continue to gather information about adverse reactions as they are recognized and reported by practicing clinicians using the drug. Should the nature or incidence of these adverse effects outweigh the potential drug benefits, the FDA could withdraw its *conditional approval.*[8]

FDA Drug Evaluation and Drug Names

In late 1978 it was disclosed that the FDA has been silently rating new drugs approved for use. Inspection of the number-letter rating assigned reveals at a glance whether the approved drug was perceived to represent a thunderous advance in therapeutics or whether its impact on the pharmacological Richter scale was merely that equivalent to a falling parakeet feather. Drugs in the former category are currently receiving FDA approval for marketing almost one year earlier than the latter.

The *number*, from 1 to 5, assesses the drug's uniqueness; the lower the number, the more novel the drug. Totally new chemicals marketed for the first time in the United States are assigned number 1, while the number 5 is given to a "me, too" drug, an exact duplicate of a drug already marketed by another company.

Letters (A, B, C) are employed to denote the therapeutic virtues of the drug. The coveted A rating is given to a drug that is considered to be a breakthrough, a significant therapeutic gain, because it provides greater effectiveness or safety for the treatment of a disorder that is not adequately treated by available drugs. The B designation means that the drug offers modest but real advantages over existing agents because of a significant reduction in annoying side effects, greater convenience of administration, or less frequent doses. Drugs offering little or no advantage are assigned a C.

Of the 411 drugs approved for marketing by the FDA between 1973 and 1978, 60 (14.6%) received the 1-A or 1-B rating, while 194 (47.1%) were relegated to the 5-C category.[9]

After FDA approval, the manufacturer and the United States Adopted Names Council (USAN) then agree upon a descriptive *generic* (nonproprietary or official) name. The pharmaceutical manufacturer selects a *brand name (trade name),* under which the drug will be promoted and marketed. It is in the best interests of the manufacturer, who has the exclusive rights to use this name, to make it simpler, shorter, more euphonious and far easier for the physician to

[8] J. S. Welsh, "Target: Adverse Drug Reactions," *American Pharmacy* NS19: 494–97 (1979).

[9] "FDA Hastens Approval of 'Important' New Drugs," *American Pharmacy* NS19: 182–85 (1979); "How the FDA Rates Prescription Drugs," *Consumer Reports,* October 1978, pp. 578–81.

remember than the generic name. Compare the ease in saying and remembering hexocyclium methylsulfate versus Tral, or dioctyl calcium sulfosuccinate versus Surfak, or finally allylisopropylacetylcarbamide versus Sedormid.

DRUG SAFETY AND EFFECTIVENESS

What information would you request from a pharmaceutical manufacturer if it were your responsibility to approve new drugs for marketing? Would proof of safety be the only requirement or should a drug also be effective, with documented evidence available to substantiate its therapeutic claims?

The criteria for FDA approval have evolved over the years as the direct result of several notorious drug disasters. In 1937, Elixir of Sulfanilamide (an antibacterial sulfa drug in solution) was introduced. At this time, drugs could be marketed without prior review by the FDA. Within several months, 76 deaths were reported (with possibly 100 more that were unreported) before the sale of this product could be stopped. These fatalities were eventually attributed to diethylene glycol, the solvent used to dissolve sulfanilamide. To protect the consumer, the Federal Food, Drug, and Cosmetic Act was enacted the following year, which gave the FDA the authority to review the *safety* of all drugs prior to marketing.

The number and severity of adverse reactions consistent with FDA approval of a new drug depend upon the class of drugs and the disease for which the drug is intended to be used. A large number of side effects would be far more readily acceptable in a drug capable of curing lung cancer than in a new analgesic. That is, if a drug is marketed for the treatment of a relatively minor condition, such as the relief of mild pain, and many other useful products are available, there is little justification for the approval of a new drug having many undesirable and potentially hazardous side effects. Conversely, where there are no drugs available for the treatment of an otherwise fatal disease, the incidence of side effects may be of secondary importance.

The thalidomide episode (1959–1961) served as the driving force for the 1962 amendment to the Federal Food, Drug, and Cosmetic Act of 1938. This amendment empowered the FDA to review both the *safety and effectiveness* of all new drugs prior to marketing, as well as to examine the efficacy claims of those drugs introduced between 1938 and 1962. Enlisting the assistance of the prestigious National Academy of Science and National Research Council, from 1966 to 1969, the FDA sought to evaluate the effectiveness of about 3000 prescription drugs and drug combinations. The results of these studies completed in 1971 indicated that of the 3000 drugs, 15 percent were deemed "ineffective," 35 percent "possibly effective," 7 percent "probably effective," and 19 percent "effective." The remaining 24 percent were rated "effective but" with certain limitations. In reaction to a possible ban on the first two drug categories, these results have been and are presently being attacked by pharmaceutical manufacturers and by physicians who are opposed to government intervention in their prescribing practices. Undoubtedly, this controversy will continue for many years before it is satisfactorily resolved and, at which time, clinicians and patients can be assured that the prescribed drug is in fact effective for its intended therapeutic use.

OTC Drugs

In 1972, the FDA initiated a similar program intended to focus upon non-prescription or *over-the-counter* (OTC) drugs. Seventeen panels of health professional experts were assigned the arduous task of establishing standards for all the estimated 100,000 to 500,000 OTC drugs on the American market.

More specifically, the program goals included: (1) identification of safe and effective ingredients for OTC products; (2) determination of safe and effective dosage ranges of such drugs; (3) establishment of acceptable combinations of ingredients and the therapeutic rationale for their inclusion; (4) determination of acceptable indications for self-medication in accordance with the claims of the drug manufacturer; and (5) provision of readily comprehendible (but not misleading) information on the label giving the user appropriate directions for the safe use of the drug as well as warnings and cautions.

This review will probably prove considerably more arduous because of the vast number of products involved and, in many instances, the absence of definitive studies to substantiate the manufacturer's claims. Most over-the-counter drugs contain more than one ingredient, only some of which may be effective. In general, few meaningful studies have been carried out to determine whether the sum of these ingredients is more effective and/or less dangerous than each component when taken alone.

We are all cognizant of the influence of effective advertising on our purchasing habits. In most instances, misleading promotion merely results in the loss of a modest sum of money. The ego of a man wearing "Macho" aftershave lotion may be somewhat deflated when he is not attacked by hordes of beautiful women. Similar feelings of despair may exist for a woman, who, six months after using "Lady Godiva's" blond hair coloring is still waiting for a date.

Should proprietary drug manufacturers be permitted to mislead and even deceive the consumer with the "results of recent clinical tests" purporting to demonstrate the superiority of their products? As we view these advertisements, we should ask whether competent clinical investigators conducted these studies. How many patients were in the study? What controls (placebos) were employed? Did the investigators conduct a double-blind study, or did they consciously or subconsciously bias the results reported by patients? Was a clinically relevant parameter measured that bears a direct relationship to the disease symptoms for which the drug is being promoted? Are the results advertised to the public representative of the overall findings or are they taken totally out of context? Many suffering people try product after product in search of relief. Unbeknownst to the consumer, although many of these drug mixtures appear to differ markedly, in actuality their similarities are far greater than their differences. Compounding the problem of an often great expenditure of funds for the purchase of these questionably effective products is the patient's delay in seeking treatment from a qualified medical practitioner. Such extensive delays often totally alter the prognosis of the disease to the detriment of the patient.

ETHICAL CONSIDERATIONS
IN HUMAN EXPERIMENTATION

> *In the field of clinical research a fundamental distinction must be recognized between clinical research in which the aim is essentially therapeutic for a patient, and the clinical research the essential objective of which is purely scientific and without therapeutic value to the person subjected to the research.*
>
> —Declaration of Helsinki (1964)

Scientific investigators take an extensive leap when they progress from testing a new drug or medical procedure in animals to conducting studies in human subjects. There is little disagreement that the drug must be exhaustively investigated under the most ideal conditions of a hospital or clinic prior to its use in general medical practice. The fundamental problem is obtaining suitable human subjects who are cognizant of the fact that they are participating in such a clinical experiment. In some instances, we find the answer to be very straight-forward. If the patient is dying of an incurable disease and all standard therapeutic measures have failed, the patient may be most willing and eager to submit to a new drug or organ transplant or other surgical procedure. Although this previously untested procedure is an experiment and does constitute clinical research, the primary objective is to save the patient's life.

Most clinical research is not as clear-cut as indicated above. In many instances, the work has been deemed unethical, most frequently because the patients were unaware that they were participating in an experiment; that is, they did not grant their *informed consent*. Mere consent to receive a new drug is not sufficient if the patient has not been apprised of the inherent risks involved. There is a considerable difference between infecting prison *volunteers* with malarial parasites in order to evaluate antimalarial agents, and injecting live cancer cells into hospital patients, telling them only that they would be receiving "some cells," with no reference to the word cancer.

Since 1974, when the United States Congress created the National Commission for the Protection of Human Subjects of Biomedical and Behavioral Research, ethical, moral, and legal questions have been the subject of vigorous and often heated debate. These debates have resulted in the Department of

Health, Education, and Welfare issuing regulations limiting clinical trials on fetuses, pregnant women, women having a high potential for becoming pregnant, children, and prisoners.

We have indicated the importance of employing a placebo when evaluating new drugs. In some clinical research, the use of a placebo may not only be unnecessary, but more importantly, unethical. Chloramphenicol (Chloromycetin) has been shown to be effective for the treatment of typhoid fever, and a high mortality rate is observed when this antibiotic is withheld. When evaluating a new drug for the treatment of this disease, it would be unjustified to compare the new compound with a placebo. Rather this new drug should be compared with the standard product, chloramphenicol.

Beecher notes that, "An experiment is ethical or not at its inception; it does not become ethical *post hoc*—ends do not justify means. There is no ethical distinction between ends and means."

SUMMARY

At present there are about 1,600 distinct chemical compounds available for the treatment of disease. Whereas some of these compounds have been proved to have an unchallenged place in therapeutics, a far larger number are merely subtle modifications of existing compounds or lack substantial clinical merit.

Over the years, the trend has shifted away from drugs of natural origin to compounds that have been designed in medicinal organic chemistry laboratories. This statement is not intended to demean the importance of drugs derived from plants and animals, for modern therapeutics would be at a great loss without atropine, digitalis, morphine, antibiotics, and vitamins.

Most new drugs are the result of chemical modifications of pharmacologically active natural compounds or existing drugs. Such modifications in structure attempt to (1) increase the desired primary effects, while simultaneously eliminate or reduce undesirable secondary effects; (2) alter the pharmacodynamic properties of the drug in order to improve its absorption, distribution, metabolism, and excretion; and (3) design a product that will enable a company to establish a financial "foothold" in a highly profitable market. With regard to the last point, one should not lose sight of the fact that a pharmaceutical manufacturing company seeks profits and has shareholders to satisfy. Profits derived from less than revolutionary advancements in therapeutics are often reinvested in research that seeks to develop highly original and significant drugs.

It is most gratifying when a new drug is discovered based upon careful inductive and deductive reasoning. That is, a drug whose design is the logical result of in-depth knowledge of the disease state. Advancements in related medical sciences in the future will undoubtedly provide pharmacologists with the basic information they require to conceive of such compounds.

Whether the result of genius or relatively simple molecular manipulation, the compound must be thoroughly evaluated for safety and effectiveness prior to its arrival on the pharmacist's shelf. Animal studies are designed to evaluate the pharmacological and toxicological properties of the compound. Subsequent testing in humans investigates its effectiveness and potential hazards. In recent years, the Food and Drug Administration's requirements for approval of new drugs have become considerably more stringent, thus raising the costs and risks associated with the development of new medications. This has resulted in greater protection of the public and also a marked decline in the number of new single-chemical entities introduced as drugs in the United States.

SUPPLEMENTARY READINGS

Beecher, H. K., "Ethics and Clinical Research," *New England Journal of Medicine* **274**: 1354–60 (1966).

Boyd, E. M., *Predictive Toxicometrics.* Baltimore: Williams & Wilkins, 1972.

Cooper, J. D., ed., *The Efficacy of Self-Medication. Philosophy and Technology of Drug Assessment.* Vol. 4. Washington, D.C.: Interdisciplinary Communications Associates, 1973.

Gerald, M. C., "Judging OTCs: Science Narrows the Choice," *American Pharmacy* **NS19**: 242–46 (1979).

Melmon, K. L., and H. F. Morrelli, eds., *Clinical Pharmacology: Basic Principles in Therapeutics.* 2nd ed. New York: Macmillan, 1978.

Mills, D. H., "Whither Informed Consent?" *Journal of the American Medical Association* **229**: 305–10 (1974).

Nodine, J. H., and P. E. Siegler, eds., *Pharmacological Techniques in Drug Evaluation.* Vol. 1. Chicago: Year Book Medical Publishers, 1964.

Ruggieri, G. D., "Drugs from the Sea," *Science* **194**: 491–97 (1976).

Siegler, P. E., and J. H. Moyer, eds., *Pharmacological Techniques in Drug Evaluation.* Vol. 2. Chicago: Year Book Medical Publishers, 1967.

Silverman, M., and P. R. Lee, *Pills, Profits & Politics.* Berkeley: University of California Press, 1974.

Talalay, P., ed., *Drugs in Our Society.* Baltimore: Johns Hopkins Press, 1964.

Wardell, W. M., ed., *Controlling the Use of Therapeutic Drugs. An International Comparison.* Washington, D.C.: American Enterprise Institute, 1978.

Young, J. H., *Toadstool Millionaires: A Social History of Patent Medicines in America Before Federal Regulation.* Princeton, N.J.: Princeton University Press, 1961.

———, *Medical Messiahs: A Social History of Health Quackery in Twentieth-Century America.* Princeton, N.J.: Princeton University Press, 1967.

Zbinden, G., "Experimental and Clinical Aspects of Drug Toxicity," *Advances in Pharmacology* **2**: 1–112 (1963).

———, "The Significance of Pharmacologic Screening Tests in the Preclinical Safety Evaluation of New Drugs," *Journal of New Drugs* **6**: 1–7 (1966).

section two —————————

Drugs Affecting the Peripheral Nervous System

5

General Principles
of Neuropharmacology

*The power of moving in every part of the body by means of the muscles which
obey the will, or by means of others the action of which are involuntary; the
various perceptions by the five external senses; and lastly those mental powers
namely memory, imagination, attention and judgment, together with the passions of the mind; all these seem to be exercised by the ministry of the nerves;
and are impaired, disturbed, or destroyed, in proportion to any injury done to
the brain.*

—William Heberden (1710–1801)

A living organism's ability to survive in a constantly changing environment
is directly dependent upon its ability to perceive external signals and respond to
them in an appropriate manner. Plants respond to such physical stimuli as light,
touch, chemicals, and gravity; for example, we observe that a stem bends
toward a light source, a response termed positive phototropism. Amoebae are
unicellular animals that possess simple sensing mechanisms that enable these
protean creatures to move toward or away from favorable or aversive stimuli.
The amoeba is incapable of complex discrimination of these signals and yet,
notwithstanding the absence of a nervous system, is capable of simple learning.
By contrast, humans are able to discriminate and respond to extremely complex
signals, whether actual or symbolic.

Some of these perceived signals or *stimuli* are warnings that our survival is
endangered, such as a fire alarm bell, a flashing red light at a railroad crossing,
or a poison label on a medicine bottle. Others merely apprise us of a noteworthy
change in the surroundings, for example, the glimpse of an extremely attractive
member of the opposite sex. Many such stimuli require cognitive evaluation
prior to responding, while others initiate an unconscious reflex response, as illustrated by the immediate withdrawal of the bare foot after stepping on a sharp
seashell at the beach. The responses to all these stimuli are under the direct

control of the subject. Although we normally respond to pain-producing stimuli by withdrawing, acts of painful self-mutilation, as by Vincent van Gogh, have shown that this urge can be suppressed.

In addition to the readily observable external responses elicited by stimuli, *involuntary* responses occur simultaneously within the body. In response to fright, the heart rate and blood pressure increase, the respiratory rate quickens, pupils widen, and the level of circulating blood sugar increases to provide a source of energy. The sight of a Thanksgiving Day dinner at Grandmother's house evokes involuntary salivation and an increased release of gastric acid in the stomach in preparation for ingestion and digestion.

External and internal responses are all mediated by the *nervous system,* the balance and regulation of which is readily modified by a wide variety of drugs that are capable of stimulating or depressing its activity. A single drug may cause such apparently dissimilar effects as dryness of the mouth, dilation of the bronchioles, inhibition of the movement of the involuntary smooth muscles of the intestinal tract, and an increase in the heart rate. Some of these drugs have been successfully used to treat disease and prevent death in such medical emergencies as shock, while others have been employed as poisons in the form of war gases and insecticides.

Prior to considering how drugs alter the normal function of the nervous system, we shall first discuss the physiology of this system. At the outset, the student should be cautioned about the complexity of the material in this chapter. Whereas the general principles of neuropharmacology are logical and systematic, the integral component facts build rapidly. Furthermore, many new terms will be introduced as an unavoidable necessity. A glossary of terms appears at the end of this chapter (see Table 5–5). The fascinating nature of the material easily compensates for these problems.

OVERVIEW OF THE NERVOUS SYSTEM

The *nervous system* is composed of all the nerve tissues (the brain, spinal cord, nerves, and ganglia) in the body. The basic functions of these tissues are to receive stimuli, to transmit this information to nervous centers, and to initiate an appropriate response. Nerve tissues are characterized by *irritability,* the capacity to respond to stimuli, and *conductivity,* the transmission of a message along nerves from one part of the body to another. These essential properties of irritability and conductivity enable the organism to recognize external stimuli and to respond mentally and physically in a manner most advantageous for survival in a continually changing and, at times, threatening environment.

The *central nervous system* (CNS), consisting of the *brain* and *spinal cord,* collects and integrates nerve impulses arising from within and outside the body. There are about 10 billion nerve cells, or neurons, in the human nervous system. The *peripheral nervous system,* which includes all nervous tissues not in the

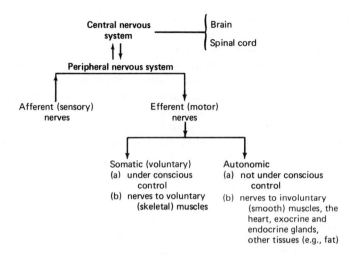

FIGURE 5-1. Divisions and Interrelationships of the Nervous System.

brain and spinal cord, serves to connect all parts of the body with the central nervous system. This peripheral system receives stimuli and initiates responses after interpretation by the central nervous system (Figure 5–1).

Neurons leaving sensory receptors, cells which detect a stimulus, are called *sensory or afferent neurons,* and those leading to effector cells (muscles, glands, or the heart) are termed *motor or efferent neurons.* Sensory and motor neurons are often separated by connecting nerve cells termed *association neurons* (Figure 5–2).

The gap or space between two neurons is termed a *synapse,* and the space between the nerve ending and an effector cell is called the *neuroeffector junction.* The existence of a space rather than physical continuity between these structures will prove to be of fundamental importance when we discuss chemical transmission of nerve impulses.

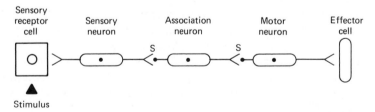

FIGURE 5-2. Typical Pathway for Conduction and Transmission of the Nerve Impulse. A stimulus (light, heat, sound, chemical) activates a sensory receptor cell, which generates the conduction of an impulse from a sensory neuron to an association neuron and finally to a motor neuron, which in turn initiates a response at an effector cell. The space between two neurons is termed a synapse (S), and the space between the end of the motor neuron and the effector cell is called the neuroeffector junction. When the effector cell is a voluntary skeletal muscle, this space is termed the neuromuscular junction.

Peripheral Nervous System

All nerves lying outside the brain and spinal cord are termed *peripheral nerves*. Throughout most of the body the nerves are mixed, containing both sensory and motor fibers. Sensory fibers convey messages from receptor cells located in the skin, muscle, or joints to the central nervous system. Motor fibers carry nerve impulses originating in the brain and spinal cord to effector cells, which in turn respond in an appropriate manner.

The efferent limb of the peripheral nervous system is subdivided into somatic and autonomic nerves (Figure 5–1). The somatic division innervates or sends nerves to skeletal muscles, while the autonomic division innervates the autonomic effector cells. The somatic nervous system controls or influences functions that are consciously influenced, for example, locomotion, posture, and respiration. Several classes of pharmacological agents are capable of modifying the function of these nerves. Local anesthetics, procaine, for one, prevent the intraneuronal conduction of nerve impulses. Neuromuscular blocking agents related to curare are used prior to surgery and act by preventing synaptic transmission of nerve impulses to voluntary (skeletal) muscles by motor neurons.

AUTONOMIC NERVOUS SYSTEM

The somatic nervous system requires conscious activation, while the autonomic nervous system (ANS) does not. This latter system controls internal tissue functions which are essential for the preservation of life. Autonomic innervation is supplied to the heart, smooth (involuntary) muscles in the chest and abdominal areas, and to exocrine glands. While we are able to decide whether or not to flex the biceps muscles of our upper arm, we have limited control over whether perspiration will occur or whether the smooth muscles of our intestinal tract will be active or inactive.

Essentially, the autonomic nervous system is a *motor system* that receives and conducts information from the brain and spinal cord to effector cells. This information is carried along two fibers which synapse at a *ganglion* or group of nerve cells. The nerve fiber that carries the message from the central nervous system to a ganglion located in the periphery is termed a *preganglionic fiber*. The nerve impulse is then transmitted from the ganglion to an effector cell via a *postganglionic fiber* (see Table 5–3, p. 108).

Sympathetic and Parasympathetic Nervous Systems

Anatomically, the autonomic nervous system is divided into two divisions, termed the *sympathetic* and *parasympathetic nervous systems*. The major physiological differences between activation of these divisions are summarized in Table 5–1.

TABLE 5-1. COMPARISON OF THE RESPONSES OF EFFECTOR SYSTEMS
TO AUTONOMIC NERVE IMPULSES

Effector System	Sympathetic (Adrenergic) Nerve Impulses (alpha [α] or beta [β])*	Parasympathetic (Cholinergic) Nerve Impulses
Cardiovascular system		
Heart		
Rate of contraction	Increase [β]	Decrease
Force of contraction	Increase [β]	Decrease
Blood pressure	Increase [α]	Decrease
Blood vessels		
Skin and mucous membranes	Constriction [α]	Dilatation
Skeletal muscle	Dilatation [β]	Dilatation
Coronary	Dilatation; constriction [α, β]	–
Smooth muscles		
Stomach and intestines (motility and tone)	Decrease [α, β]	Increase
Eye		
Radial muscle–iris	Contraction (mydriasis– widening of pupil) [α]	–
Sphincter muscle–iris	–	Contraction (miosis– pupil)
Ciliary muscle	Relaxation (focus lens for far vision) [β]	Contraction (focus lens for near vision)
Urinary bladder sphincter	Contraction [α]	Relaxation
Bronchial	Relaxation (dilatation) [β]	Contraction (constriction)
Uterus	Nonpregnant: relaxation [β]	–
Adrenal medulla	–	Secretion of epinephrine and norepinephrine
Glands		
Sweat (cholinergic)	Generalized secretion	Localized secretion
Salivary	Slight, thick secretion [α]	Profuse, watery secretion
Lacrimal	–	Increase in secretion
Gastrointestinal	–	Increase in secretion
Bronchial	–	Increase in secretion
Miscellaneous responses		
Basal metabolic rate	Increase [β]	–
Liver glycogen breakdown to blood sugar	Increase [β]	–
Male sex organs	Ejaculation [α]	Erection
Pancreas (islets)	Inhibition of insulin secretion [β]	–

*The significance of α and β is discussed on p. 107 and in greater detail in Chapter 6 on pp. 120-21.

Origin of Preganglionic Fibers

Preganglionic parasympathetic fibers arise from the cranial nerves of the brain stem and sacral (pelvic) segments of the spinal cord. Sympathetic fibers originate from the thoracic (chest) and lumbar (lower back) regions of the spinal cord (Figure 5–3).

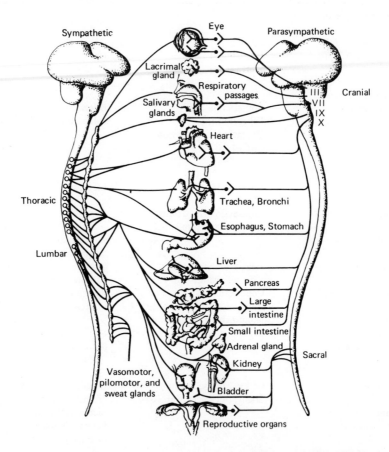

FIGURE 5–3. The Autonomic Nervous System. The sympathetic division is shown on the left and the parasympathetic division on the right. Note that (a) sympathetic preganglionic fibers arise from the thoracic and lumbar regions of the spinal cord; parasympathetic fibers originate from the cranial areas (cranial nerves denoted by roman numerals) and sacral areas; (b) sympathetic preganglionic fibers are short and postganglionic fibers are long; for the parasympathetic system the opposite relationship exists; (c) many postganglionic neurons are innervated by each sympathetic preganglionic fiber, whereas usually only one or two postganglionic parasympathetic fibers arise from each preganglionic fiber; (d) most organs are innervated by both divisions of the autonomic nervous system.

Relative Length of Autonomic Fibers

Parasympathetic ganglia are close to, or even directly on, the innervated tissue; sympathetic ganglia are in relatively close proximity to the central nervous system. Hence, it should be surmised that preganglionic parasympathetic fibers are long, while their postganglionic fibers are short; conversely preganglionic sympathetic fibers are generally short, with long postganglionic fibers arising from the ganglion to the innervated tissues.

Ratio of Preganglionic to Postganglionic Fibers

Differences exist in the ratio of preganglionic to postganglionic fibers, a factor directly accountable for the breadth of the response observed after stimulation of each division. The parasympathetic nervous system acts to conserve body resources and provide a more favorable environment for tissue repair. A preganglionic to postganglionic fiber ratio approaching 1:1 to 1:2 usually exists in the parasympathetic division. Thus, stimulation of this division produces very discrete effects limited to selected tissues.

The sympathetic division, by contrast, is a dynamic system, which when activated in response to stress, exerts a widespread influence on almost all tissues having sympathetic fibers. This difference may be better understood when we consider that one preganglionic neuron synapses with a large number of postganglionic neurons (1:10 to 1:20) thereby permitting simultaneous activation of each of the effector cells they innervate.

Physiological Functions of the Autonomic Nervous System

Most organs of the body are innervated by *both* divisions of the autonomic nervous system, with each generally, but not always, working in opposition. The sympathetic division prepares the body for vigorous muscular activity, stress, and emergencies, while the parasympathetic division is concerned with digestive processes and with the conservation and storage of bodily resources.

How might the autonomic response of an all-American quarterback competing in the last minutes of this year's Rose Bowl game differ from a long-retired desk clerk, recollecting his 1908 Model T Ford, while dozing in a rocking chair after a heavy meal? The sympathetic nervous system would be vigorously operating in our gridiron hero, causing the adrenal medulla to discharge massive amounts of epinephrine (adrenaline) into the blood. Activation of this system would increase the rate and force of contraction of the heart and cause a shunting of the blood flow into the voluntary muscles, a widening of the bronchioles, an enlargement of the pupils, and a rise in blood sugar. The sympathetic nervous system has prepared his body for fight or flight.

By contrast, our octogenarian great-grandfather has a slow heart rate. His breathing is noisy as a consequence of bronchial constriction, the pupils are small, saliva may be dropping from the corner of the mouth, and his intestinal tract would be active. Thus, we see that the parasympathetic system is active during sleep and digestion.

Both divisions evoke qualitatively the same response in some tissues (increased salivation), while other tissues receive innervation from only one division (most blood vessels, sweat glands, and the spleen). Where dual innervation of organs exists, it should not be assumed that when one system is "on," the other is "off." Rather both divisions are operating simultaneously, although one may be functioning at a lower level of activity. This is not unlike the operation of a car with both the accelerator and brake pedals depressed to a greater or lesser extent. Such a system of dual innervation permits a wider range of control of organ function.

Chemical Mediators

The chemical substances responsible for transmission of the nerve impulse across synapses and at neuroeffector junctions differ. This will be considered in detail below.

Integration of Autonomic Function by the Central Nervous System

After a peripheral sensory stimulus activates a sensory neuron, a message is transmitted to the central nervous system for integration and interpretation. This message may signal a full bladder, a drop in blood pressure after suddenly arising from a recumbent position, the need to widen the pupils of the eyes after entering a darkened theater, the requirement to adjust heat production and loss in order to maintain a constant body temperature, or an appropriate emotional response to a threatening situation.

There are no cells exclusively concerned with autonomic integration, but rather this function is carried out in many parts of the brain and spinal cord. Table 5–2 summarizes some of the different sites of autonomic integration in the central nervous system.

A large number of drugs are able to modify autonomic activity by virtue of their action on the integrative centers in the brain and spinal cord. Aspirin reduces fever by activating body temperature regulating centers in the hypothalamus responsible for heat loss. Toxic concentrations of general anesthetics, which include ether, cyclopropane, and halothane (Fluothane), stop respiration by a depressant effect on the respiratory centers in the medulla.

Thus far, we have observed that all conscious, voluntary actions and unconscious, involuntary functions of the body are controlled by the nervous system. Sensory receptor cells detect changes in the environment and transmit

TABLE 5-2. SITES OF AUTONOMIC INTEGRATION IN THE CENTRAL NERVOUS SYSTEM

Site of Integration	Autonomic Functions Influenced
Spinal cord	Sweating, blood pressure, and reflex emptying of urinary bladder and rectum
Medulla	Blood pressure and respiration
Hypothalamus	Integration of all activities for both divisions of autonomic nervous system: body temperature, water balance, carbohydrate and fat metabolism, blood pressure, emotions, feeding, sexual behavior, and sleep
Cerebral cortex	Integration of somatic and vegetative functions, both sensory and motor
Limbic system	Integration of emotional state with motor and visceral activities

this information to nervous centers by sensory (afferent) neurons. The message is integrated and interpreted in the central nervous system, which includes the brain and spinal cord, resulting in the subsequent activation of effector cells by motor (efferent) neurons. The function of internal organs is largely controlled by the autonomic (involuntary) nervous system. This motor system of neurons innervates smooth muscles, the heart, and the exocrine glands. Information is carried from the central nervous system to peripheral autonomic ganglia by preganglionic fibers, which synapse with postganglionic fibers responsible for transmitting the message to effector cells. The autonomic nervous system has two major divisions, the sympathetic and the parasympathetic.

We shall now consider the chemical mechanism by which nerve impulses cross the spaces to other neurons or to effector cells. A clear understanding of these mechanisms is essential for an appreciation of how drugs modify the activity of the autonomic nervous system.

CHEMICAL MEDIATION OF TRANSMISSION AT SYNAPSES AND JUNCTIONS

In response to a stimulus, a nerve impulse travels from sensory to motor neurons and finally to an effector cell (Figure 5-2). The space between two neurons is termed the *synapse* and that between the motor neuron and an effector cell, the *neuroeffector junction* (autonomic nervous system) or neuromuscular junction (somatic nervous system). *Conduction* is the passage of a nerve impulse in a neuron. *Transmission* is the passage of the impulse across a synapse or junction.

How is this nerve impulse transmitted across these gaps? In earlier years, one school of thought advocated an electrical hypothesis ("electrogonists"), while an opposing camp supported a chemical theory ("chemagonists"). Some have termed this the "soup versus juice" (or "spark") controversy. Today, the overwhelming body of evidence supports the concept of *chemical transmission* at mammalian synapses and junctions. Conduction of nerve impulses along the neuron is an electrical phenomenon.

Historical Development of Chemical Transmission

Isolated observations regarding the similarity between nerve stimulation and drug-induced effects were made about the turn of this century. Muscarine and stimulation of the vagus (a parasympathetic nerve) were both observed to produce a slowing of the heart rate, while injections of extracts of the adrenal gland simulated or imitated sympathetic nerve stimulation. In 1904, T. R. Elliott, while still a graduate student at Cambridge, suggested in a short paper that the effects of sympathetic nerve stimulation might be mediated by a release of *epinephrine* (also called adrenaline). This revolutionary concept was rejected by his major professor and was omitted from his doctoral thesis and the full-length paper describing these experiments that appeared the following year. In 1907, W. E. Dixon advanced the theory that transmission of impulses from parasympathetic nerves was the result of the release of a substance that might be related to choline. Dixon's theory was also dismissed by his contemporaries. There is a considerable difference between the observation that a drug mimics or imitates nerve stimulation and the notion that the effects observed after stimulation of that nerve are mediated by a naturally occurring (endogenous) chemical substance. Such proof did not come forth until Otto Loewi's classic experiments in 1920.[1]

Although Loewi had believed in the concept of chemical transmission for many years, the design of a crucial experiment to prove it conclusively was a difficult task. On the evening before Easter Sunday in 1920, Loewi awakened from his sleep and made some notes derived from a nocturnal inspiration. Arising the following morning, he found himself unable to decipher these notes. Fortunately for science, the same dream recurred the following morning at three o'clock. Before the idea could again elude him, he rushed to his laboratory. The description of this very simple, yet brilliant, experiment, illustrated in Figure 5–4, appears in his own words.[2]

> The hearts of two frogs were isolated, the first with its nerves, the second without. Both hearts were attached to Straub cannulas filled with a little Ringer solution. The vagus nerve of the first heart was stimulated for a few minutes. Then the Ringer solution that had been in the first heart during the stimulation of the vagus was

[1] Otto Loewi (1873–1961), a German physiologist-pharmacologist, was corecipient of the 1936 Nobel Prize in Physiology for his studies on chemical transmission of nerve impulses.

[2] O. Loewi, "An Autobiographic Sketch," *Perspectives in Biology and Medicine* **4**: 3–25 (1960).

transferred to the second heart. It slowed and its beats diminished just as if its vagus had been stimulated. Similarly, when the accelerator nerve was stimulated and the Ringer from this period transferred, the second heart speeded up and its beats increased. These results unequivocally proved that the nerves do not influence the heart directly but liberate from their terminals specific chemical substances which, in their turn, cause the well-known modifications of the function of the heart characteristic of the stimulation of its nerves.

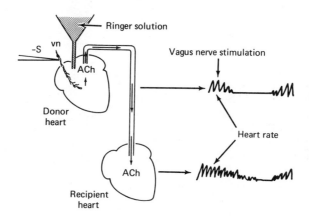

FIGURE 5–4. Loewi's Experiment Demonstrating Chemical Transmission of Nerve Impulses. The vagus nerve (vn) of the donor heart was electrically stimulated (S) causing the release of a chemical transmitter substance, which Loewi termed "vagusstoff" (acetylcholine, ACh). After the donor heart stopped, the Ringer solution (a physiological salt solution) was transferred to the recipient heart from which the vagus nerve was removed. The heart stopped just as if the nerve had been electrically stimulated. Thus, he demonstrated that neither the nerves themselves nor an electrical current were directly responsible for the effects on the heart. Rather depression of the heart could be attributed to a *chemical substance released from the nerves.*

In the 1930s, W. B. Cannon and his co-workers showed that after stimulation of sympathetic nerves, a substance resembling epinephrine was released. This compound was identified as *norepinephrine* by U.S. von Euler[3] in 1946. For many years considerable confusion existed concerning the effects produced by norepinephrine and similar compounds on receptor sites innervated by the sympathetic nervous system. This puzzle was clarified by Ahlquist's hypothesis that two distinct adrenergic (sympathetic) receptor types exist; these he designated as *alpha* (α) and *beta* (β) receptors. *Beta* receptors are now known to be of two types: β_1 and β_2.

[3] Ulf Svante von Euler (1905–), a Swedish physiologist-pharmacologist, was the 1970 recipient of the Nobel Prize in recognition of this work. He was the first to demonstrate the biological activity of the prostaglandins (Chapter 14) during the early 1930s.

TABLE 5-3. CHOLINERGIC AND ADRENERGIC NERVES

Nerve (Chemical Mediator)	Sites of Innervation	Schematic Representation
A. Cholinergic (Acetylcholine; (ACh)	1. All postganglionic parasympathetic fibers (neuroeffector junction) 2. All autonomic (sympathetic and para-sympathetic) preganglionic fibers (autonomic ganglia) 3. Preganglionic (splanchnic nerve) fibers to the adrenal medulla 4. Postganglionic sympathetic fibers to sweat glands and certain blood vessels 5. Somatic motor nerves to skeletal or voluntary muscles (neuromuscular junction) 6. Parts of the central nervous system	*Autonomic nerves* *Parasympathetic* *Sympathetic*
B. Adrenergic (Norepinephrine; NE)	1. All postganglionic sympathetic fibers (except A-4) 2. Parts of the central nervous system	*Motor nerve*

108

Adrenergic and Cholinergic Nerves

It is now established beyond a doubt that the transmission of impulses between nerve fibers or from a nerve fiber to an effector cell is accomplished by chemical substances that are released from nerve endings. These chemical mediators of transmission are called **neurotransmitters.** The nature of the released neurotransmitter is physiologically and pharmacologically of greater importance to us in our study of drug action than is the anatomical differentiation of whether a nerve is part of the sympathetic or parasympathetic division of the autonomic nervous system. Hence, we shall classify autonomic nerves functionally on the basis of the neurotransmitter substance they release.

We shall call all nerves that release the neurotransmitter *acetylcholine* **cholinergic nerves,** and those that liberate *norepinephrine* (noradrenaline) **adrenergic nerves.** *In general, all parasympathetic nerves discharge acetylcholine and nearly all postganglionic sympathetic nerves release norepinephrine.*

Since exceptions to this general rule exist, it is not entirely correct to consider parasympathetic and cholinergic nerves to be synonymous; similarly sympathetic and adrenergic nerves are not always equivalent. For example, sympathetic fibers innervate the sweat glands and certain blood vessels, but these are cholinergic in nature; that is, they release acetylcholine.

Preganglionic fibers of both the sympathetic and parasympathetic divisions of the autonomic nervous system release only acetylcholine, and, therefore, *all preganglionic nerves are considered cholinergic nerves.* Bearing in mind the exceptions noted in the preceding paragraph, we can make the following statements regarding the neurotransmitters released at postganglionic neuroeffector junctions: *those postganglionic sympathetic nerves that release norepinephrine are designated adrenergic nerves; postganglionic parasympathetic nerves all discharge acetylcholine and are termed cholinergic nerves.* The somatic motor neurons, which innervate voluntary skeletal muscle at the *neuromuscular junction,* are all *cholinergic.* Table 5-3 summarizes the location of adrenergic and cholinergic nerves.

Our knowledge of the identity of neurotransmitters in the brain, when compared to those in the periphery, has been less conclusively resolved. Among the most prominent candidates suggested as neurotransmitters in the brain are acetylcholine, norepinephrine, dopamine (a substance chemically related to norepinephrine), and serotonin. Other speculative candidates include gamma-aminobutyric acid (GABA), glycine, glutamic acid, histamine, substance P, and certain endorphins.

Criteria for Potential Neurotransmitters

Many compounds have been suggested as *neurotransmitters,* but only a few are firmly entrenched in this coveted position. While the evaluation of the credentials of compounds in the peripheral (somatic and autonomic) nervous system is relatively easy, identification and positive proof of those in the brain is a very formidable task methodologically. What criteria must a compound meet before we consider it to be a neurotransmitter?

1. The nerve must be capable of synthesizing the neurotransmitter; thus, enzymes that catalyze this manufacturing process must be available in the neuron.
2. The neurotransmitter must be demonstrated to be stored in nerve ending particles so that it will be available to be released in response to a nerve impulse.
3. Following stimulation of the nerve, the release of the neurotransmitter must be demonstrated at the synapse or junction.
4. The pharmacological effects seen after local administration of the neurotransmitter must be identical to those seen after nerve stimulation.
5. A mechanism must be present for terminating the action of the neurotransmitter after it has interacted with the receptor site.
6. An antagonist which is able to block the action of the neurotransmitter should also be capable of blocking the effects of normal nerve stimulation, thus altering normal physiological function.

Sequence of Events in Neurochemical Transmission

Based upon the criteria set forth in the previous section, the neurotransmitter initiates a physiological response by the following sequence of events (Figure 5–5).

1.   Release of the Neurotransmitter

The neurotransmitter is synthesized from naturally occurring endogenous starting (precursor) substances that are present in the neuron; these synthetic reactions are catalyzed by specific enzymes. Once formed, the neurotransmitter is stored in a *bound* inactivated form in particles or *vesicles* located in the nerve endings. A nerve impulse generates a nerve action potential which causes the release of the neurotransmitter from the vesicles through the nerve membrane into the synapse. It has been suggested that the calcium ion (Ca^{2+}) may enter the nerve ending and actively promote the release of the neurotransmitter by fostering fusion of the membranes surrounding the vesicles with the nerve cell membrane.

2.   Neurotransmitter-Receptor Interactions

The neurotransmitter, after being released from the nerve ending, crosses the junctional gap and interacts with receptors located on the membrane of the postganglionic neuron or effector cell. This interaction may produce one of two types of changes in the permeability of the postsynaptic membrane: (a) nonspecific changes causing an increased permeability to all ions (sodium, potassium, and chloride) which results in *depolarization* or an excitatory postsynaptic potential (EPSP); (b) selective permeability changes to only the smaller ions (potassium and chloride) which produces *stabilization* or *hyperpolarization* of the membrane; this is termed an inhibitory postsynaptic potential (IPSP).

3.   Initiation of Postsynaptic Effects

These different actions on membrane permeability produce opposite biological effects: (a) EPSP results in an *excitatory response* generating an action potential in a postsynaptic neuron or muscle, a contractile response in muscle, or a stimulation of glandular secretion; (b) IPSP opposes excitatory influences, thus producing an inhibitory influence of the postsynaptic structure or a marked reduction in excitation.

4.   Termination of Neurotransmitter's Action

After each impulse, it is necessary to inactivate and/or terminate the neurotransmitter's action. Acetylcholinesterase destroys acetylcholine by hydrolysis. Norepinephrine is taken back into the presynaptic neurons (re-uptake process), thus removing it from the receptor area; this neurotransmitter may also be inactivated by degradative enzymes located inside the neuron and in the synapse (extraneuronally). Furthermore, both neurotransmitters may

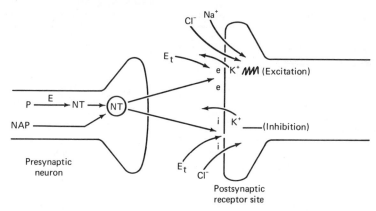

FIGURE 5–5. Sequence of Events in Neurotransmission. The endogenous precursor (P) is converted to a neurotransmitter (NT) through an enzyme (E) catalyzed reaction. The neurotransmitter is bound in a vesicle (NT) until it is released from the nerve endings by a nerve action potential (NAP). After release, it travels across the junction to interact with a postsynaptic receptor site.

An excitatory neurotransmitter (e) causes nonspecific changes in the permeability of the postsynaptic membrane, resulting in an influx of sodium (Na^+) and chloride (Cl^-) and an efflux of potassium (K^+). Depolarization of the membrane (EPSP) and an excitatory response ($\wedge\!\!\wedge\!\!\wedge$) in the tissue results from an influx of sodium.

An inhibitory neurotransmitter (i) produces specific changes in membrane permeability causing an influx of chloride (Cl^-) and an efflux of potassium (K^+). In this case the membrane is stabilized or hyperpolarized (IPSP), with inhibition of the tissue resulting (——).

The neurotransmitter's action is terminated by an enzyme (E_t), by diffusion from the receptor, or by re-uptake by the presynaptic neuron.

simply move away from the receptor site by diffusion, which also terminates their actions.

Classification and Sites of Action of Autonomic Drugs

As might be anticipated, drugs can act at different steps in the sequence of events leading to and including normal transmission of the nerve impulse. Some drugs enhance this process and produce stimulation; other compounds interfere with these events and cause inhibition of autonomic function. Table 5–4 provides examples of each.

A wide variety of compounds capable of stimulating or blocking adrenergic and cholinergic nerves has been developed, and these drugs have been utilized both therapeutically and experimentally. Drugs capable of producing effects similar to those seen when adrenergic nerves are stimulated are called *adrenergic* or *sympathomimetic* (mimic or imitate) agents. *Adrenergic blocking agents* prevent the effects normally seen after adrenergic nerve activation.

TABLE 5-4. INTERACTION OF DRUGS WITH AUTONOMIC TRANSMISSION

Site of Drug Action	Neurotransmitter (NT)	
	Acetylcholine*	Norepinephrine
Inhibits synthesis of NT	Hemicholinium†	α - Methyl tyrosine†
Inhibits intra-vesicle storage of NT	–	Reserpine
Releases NT	Carbachol	Amphetamine
		Tyramine†
		Ephedrine
Inhibits release of NT	Botulinum toxin†	Guanethidine
Activates receptors (excitatory effects)	A. Choline esters (bethanechol)	Catecholamines and related amines
	Pilocarpine	
	Muscarine†	α - stimulant: phenylephrine
	B. Nicotine†	β - stimulant: isoproterenol
	C. Nicotine†	
Blocks receptors (inhibitory effects)	A. Atropine	α - blocker: phentolamine
	B. Hexamethonium	
	C. Curare-like drugs (d-tubocurarine)	β - blocker: propranolol
Inhibits termination of NT action (enhances NT's effects)	Neostigmine	Amphetamine
	Physostigmine	Cocaine
	DFP	Imipramine

*Cholinergic sites of action: A. Parasympathetic postganglionic neuroeffector site.

B. Autonomic ganglia. C. Neuromuscular junction.

†Pharmacological tool—not employed in therapeutics.

Analogous terms are used for drugs modifying cholinergic activity, that is, *cholinergic or parasympathomimetic agents*[4] and *cholinergic blocking agents.* Since both sympathetic and parasympathetic autonomic ganglia function identically, drugs acting at these sites are termed *ganglionic stimulants* and *ganglionic blocking agents.* The next three chapters will consider examples of these drugs.

Having considered the basic principles of neurophysiology and neuropharmacology, we are now ready to specifically discuss adrenergic agents (Chapter 6) and cholinergic and cholinergic blocking agents (Chapters 7 and 8). As we shall observe, these drugs have great relevancy to society, both therapeutically and toxicologically.

SUMMARY

We are able to perceive changes in our environment, interpret the significance of these stimuli in terms of well-being and make appropriate external and internal responses in a manner most appropriate to insure our survival. The nervous system is directly responsible for these capabilities. Impairment of the function of the nervous system, whether resulting from disease, injury, or drugs, may threaten our survival.

Basic principles of neurophysiology and neuropharmacology have been considered in this chapter. (See Table 5–5 for a glossary of terms.) We have traced a stimulus from its triggering a message in a sensory receptor cell, along a sensory neuron to the central nervous system for integration and interpretation, to its initiation of a nerve impulse along a motor neuron causing a response by an effector cell.

The peripheral nervous system innervates both voluntary effector cells of the somatic nervous system and the involuntary effector cells controlled by the autonomic nervous system. In both neural systems, the transmission of the nerve impulse from neuron to neuron or from neuron to effector cell is mediated by a chemical substance termed a neurotransmitter.

The autonomic nervous system, composed primarily of motor fibers, innervates the involuntary smooth muscles of the body (those of blood vessels and others found in the chest, abdominal, and pelvic regions of the body), the heart, and the exocrine and endocrine glands. This system is divided into the sympathetic and parasympathetic divisions, each of which has a preganglionic fiber leaving the brain or spinal cord and a postganglionic fiber responsible for innervation of an effector cell.

---

[4] It has been previously noted that adrenergic and sympathetic or cholinergic and parasympathetic nerves are not exactly equivalent. However, we shall yield to the pressures of tradition and accept these designations as synonymous when we refer to drugs in these classes.

TABLE 5-5. GLOSSARY OF TERMS USED IN NEUROPHARMACOLOGY

Acetylcholine: The cholinergic neurotransmitter (see Table 5-3).

Adrenergic drug: Drug producing effects similar to those seen when adrenergic nerves are stimulated; a sympathomimetic agent.

Adrenergic nerves: Nerves that release norepinephrine; most postganglionic sympathetic nerves (see Table 5-3).

Afferent neuron: See *Sensory neuron.*

Autonomic nervous system: Involuntary division of the nervous system; nerves activate the heart, glands, and involuntary muscles that are not under conscious control.

Central nervous system: Brain and spinal cord.

Cholinergic drug: Compound producing effects similar to those seen when cholinergic nerves are stimulated; a parasympathomimetic agent.

Cholinergic nerves: Nerves that release acetylcholine; all preganglionic nerves, postganglionic parasympathetic nerves and somatic motor nerves (see Table 5-3).

Conduction: Passage of a nerve impulse down a neuron.

Effector cells or tissue: Cells capable of responding to activation by motor neurons; cells of the heart, involuntary (smooth) muscles, glands.

Efferent neuron: See *Motor neuron.*

Ganglion: A group or cluster of nerve cells lying outside the central nervous system; preganglionic fibers synapse at autonomic ganglia.

Motor neuron: A nerve cell responsible for carrying a message from the central nervous system to an effector cell.

Neuroeffector junction: The space between the end of a motor neuron and an effector cell.

Neuromuscular junction: Space between a somatic motor nerve and a voluntary (skeletal) muscle.

Neuron: A nerve cell.

Neurotransmitter: A chemical agent (norepinephrine or acetylcholine) that is responsible for transmitting impulses between nerve fibers or from a nerve fiber to an effector cell.

Norepinephrine: The adrenergic neurotransmitter (see Table 5-3).

Parasympathetic nervous system: One of two divisions of the autonomic nervous system (see Figure 5-3).

Peripheral nervous system: All nerves lying outside the brain and spinal cord.

Postganglionic fiber (neuron): A motor nerve cell of the autonomic nervous system that originates at an autonomic ganglion and terminates (but does not touch) an effector cell.

Preganglionic fiber (neuron): A motor nerve cell of the autonomic nervous system that originates in the central nervous system and terminates at an autonomic ganglion.

Sensory neuron: Nerve cell responsible for carrying messages of changes in the external environment or within the body to the central nervous system; an afferent neuron.

Sensory receptor cells: Specialized cells that are highly sensitive to changes in the environment.

114

TABLE 5-5. CONTINUED

Somatic nerves: Nerves activating voluntary muscles.

Stimulus: A change in the environment.

Sympathetic nervous system: One of two divisions of the autonomic nervous system (see Figure 5-3).

Synapse: The space between two nerve cells.

Transmission: Passage of a nerve impulse across a synapse or junction.

The sympathetic division and the adrenal medulla enable the body to successfully face stress and emergencies, while the parasympathetic division permits the body to carry out digestion and conserve energy. The activity of these divisions is under the control of the central nervous system, with the hypothalamus serving as the most important site of central integration.

Neurotransmitters are responsible for transmitting nerve impulses across synapses (space between two autonomic neurons), and at neuroeffector junctions (between a neuron and an effector tissue). Neurons that release acetylcholine are classified as cholinergic nerves, and these include: (1) all autonomic (sympathetic and parasympathetic) preganglionic fibers; (2) all postganglionic parasympathetic fibers; (3) postganglionic sympathetic fibers to certain blood vessels and to sweat glands; (4) somatic motor neurons to skeletal muscles (neuromuscular junction); and (5) parts of the central nervous system. Adrenergic fibers release norepinephrine and include all postganglionic sympathetic fibers, except those listed in (3) above. In addition, the adrenal medulla, anatomically and functionally part of the sympathetic division, secretes epinephrine (adrenaline) as well as a lesser amount of norepinephrine. Acetylcholine, norepinephrine, and dopamine are probably neurotransmitters in certain parts of the central nervous system.

The neurotransmitter is released from vesicles located in the nerve endings, interacts with a receptor to initiate a response, and is then inactivated or removed from the receptor area. In the next three chapters, we shall consider drugs that modify normal autonomic activity.

SUPPLEMENTARY READINGS

Aidley, D. J., *The Physiology of Excitable Cells.* Cambridge, England: Cambridge University Press, 1971.

Appenzeller, O., *The Autonomic Nervous System. An Introduction to Basic and Clinical Concepts.* 2nd rev. ed. Amsterdam: North-Holland Publishing Co., 1976.

Burn, J. H., *The Autonomic Nervous System for Students of Physiology and Pharmacology.* 5th ed. Oxford: Blackwell Scientific Publications, 1975.

Cooper, J. R., F. E. Bloom, and R. H. Roth, *The Biochemical Basis of Neuropharmacology.* 3rd ed. New York: Oxford University Press, 1978.

DeRobertis, E., *Synaptic Receptors. Isolation and Molecular Biology.* New York: Marcel Dekker, 1975.

Hubbard, J. I., ed., *The Peripheral Nervous System.* New York: Plenum Press, 1974.

Mayer, S. E., "Neurohumoral Transmission and the Autonomic Nervous System," in *Goodman and Gilman's The Pharmacological Basis of Therapeutics.* Edited by A. G. Gilman, L. S. Goodman, and A. Gilman, 6th ed., Chap. 4, pp. 56-90. New York: Macmillan, 1980.

McLennan, H., *Synaptic Transmission,* 2nd ed. Philadelphia: Saunders, 1970.

Rang, H. P., ed., *Drug Receptors,* Baltimore: University Park Press, 1973.

Triggle, D. J., and C. R. Triggle, *Chemical Pharmacology of the Synapse.* New York: Academic Press, 1976.

Turner, P., *Clinical Aspects of Autonomic Pharmacology.* Philadelphia: Lippincott, 1969.

6

Adrenergic (Sympathomimetic) Drugs

These changes—the more rapid pulse, the deeper breathing, the increase of sugar in the blood, the secretion from the adrenal glands—were very diverse and seemed unrelated. Then, one wakeful night, after a considerable collection of these changes had been disclosed, the idea flashed through my mind, that they could be nicely integrated if conceived as bodily preparations for supreme effect in flight or in fighting.

—Walter B. Cannon (1871–1945)

Adrenergic or **sympathomimetic drugs** elicit effects that are similar to stimulation of adrenergic nerves. After these nerves release norepinephrine from their endings, this neurotransmitter travels across the neuroeffector junction and interacts with the adrenergic receptor site to initiate an effect. Adrenergic agents may act indirectly by stimulating the release of norepinephrine from nerve endings or may directly stimulate the adrenergic receptor.

Therapeutically, members of this class are used to combat life-threatening disorders, which include acute attacks of bronchial asthma, shock, and cardiac arrest. These drugs are also employed for more common everyday purposes such as nasal decongestion and appetite suppression, and for allergic disorders.

ADRENERGIC TRANSMISSION

Norepinephrine is the naturally occurring adrenergic neurotransmitter. *Dopamine* is a biosynthetic precursor of norepinephrine and is generally believed to be a neurotransmitter in the central nervous system of mammals. *Epinephrine* is formed from norepinephrine in the adrenal medulla and acts as the primary hormone in that endocrine gland. Dopamine and epinephrine share some of the actions of norepinephrine. Because of their chemical structures, all three are frequently referred to as **catecholamines.** The chemical interrelationships among these compounds and the pathways for their synthesis within the body are depicted in Figure 6-1.

Norepinephrine, the most widely studied adrenergic neurotransmitter, is bound in nerve ending granules in association with an adenosine triphosphate (ATP)-protein complex. After its release from the nerve ending in response to a nerve impulse or drug, it interacts at an adrenergic receptor site. Its action is terminated primarily by its recapture by nerve endings, a process termed reuptake. Of lesser importance is its enzymatic inactivation by catechol-O-methyltransferase (COMT) extraneuronally and by oxidative deamination by monoamine oxidase (MAO) with the neuron (Figure 6-2).

Mechanism of Action of Adrenergic Agents

Adrenergic or sympathomimetic agents elicit effects that are identical to those observed after stimulation of adrenergic (postganglionic sympathetic) nerves. Experimental evidence has shown that these drugs may have a direct, indirect, or mixed mechanism of action.

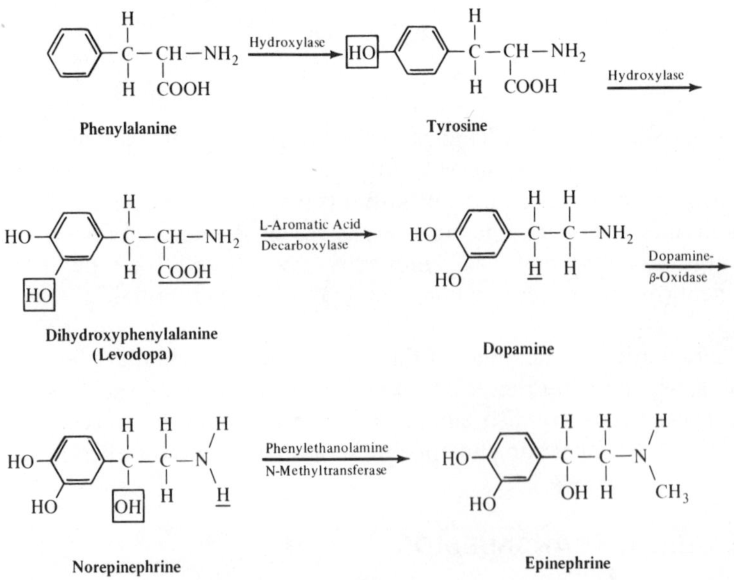

FIGURE 6-1. Biosynthesis of Biogenic Catecholamines. Phenylalanine is an essential amino acid that is ingested as a normal constituent of the diet. It is converted in the body to tyrosine, an amino acid capable of entering the neuron. From tyrosine, via the intermediate compound levodopa, the neurotransmitters dopamine and norepinephrine and the adrenal hormone epinephrine are synthesized in the appropriate cells.

Direct.   Drugs such as epinephrine, norepinephrine, isoproterenol (Isuprel), and phenylephrine (Neo-Synephrine) activate the adrenergic receptor directly. That is, their action is not dependent upon the release of norepinephrine.

Indirect.   Amphetamine and the experimental agent tyramine act indirectly by causing the release of norepinephrine from postganglionic sympathetic nerve endings. It is the released norepinephrine that is responsible for the pharmacological effects.

Mixed.   Ephedrine acts directly on the adrenergic receptor and indirectly by a release of norepinephrine.

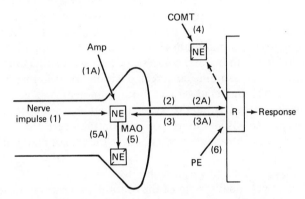

FIGURE 6–2. Action and Inactivation of Norepinephrine with Modes of Action of Direct (Phenylephrine) and Indirect (Amphetamine) Acting Adrenergic Agents. Norepinephrine is bound in a physiologically inactive state in a nerve ending granule $\boxed{NE}$. A nerve impulse may cause its release (1) from the nerve ending, resulting in its interaction with an adrenergic receptor site (R), (2) and with the initiation of a biological response. Norepinephrine's action is terminated by re-uptake (3) or it is chemically inactivated $\boxed{NE}$ by the enzymes catechol-O-methyltransferase (COMT) (4) and monoamine oxidase (MAO) (5).

   Adrenergic agents may cause stimulation directly or indirectly. Amphetamine (Amp) acts indirectly by increasing the release of norepinephrine from nerve ending granules (1A, 2A), preventing its re-uptake (3A), and inhibiting its breakdown by MAO (5A). Phenylephrine (PE) has a direct action at the adrenergic receptor site (6).

These mechanisms of action are significant both pharmacologically and therapeutically. Frequent repeated administration of indirect adrenergic agents causes a successively diminished response. This phenomenon, termed *tachyphylaxis,* results from a depletion of norepinephrine from the nerve endings more rapidly than it can be replenished.

If we refer again to Figure 6–2, we observe that amphetamine (best known as an appetite suppressant and drug of abuse) may produce stimulation of the brain by several mechanisms, while phenylephrine (a drug widely employed for the relief of nasal congestion) has only one primary mode of action. Amphetamine may act by (1) increasing the release of norepinephrine by the nerve endings; (2) prevention of the re-uptake of norepinephrine by the nerve endings, thereby prolonging its action at the adrenergic receptor site; and (3) inhibiting the norepinephrine-inactivating enzyme MAO. Phenylephrine has a direct action at the adrenergic postsynaptic receptor site.

PHYSIOLOGICAL AND PHARMACOLOGICAL EFFECTS OF CATECHOLAMINES

In the periphery, the naturally occurring catecholamines norepinephrine and epinephrine act to maintain the body's normal physiological balance and to prepare the animal for "flight or fight." *Norepinephrine* is normally released from adrenergic nerves to maintain the function of the sympathetically innervated tissues, as well as to make the necessary circulatory adjustments required in exercise and when assuming an erect position. In response to emotional stress, pain, trauma, and emergencies both imminent and actually present, *epinephrine* is discharged from the adrenal medulla to mobilize the body's defenses. Epinephrine has stimulatory effects on the heart; that is, it increases the rate and force of contraction, and enhances the rate of metabolism as well.

Dopamine is thought to be an inhibitory neurotransmitter in the basal ganglia and extrapyramidal system of the brain. Low levels of dopamine in the basal ganglia have been causally related to Parkinson's disease. This neurological condition, commonly referred to as "the shaking palsy," is characterized by rigidity, stiffness of voluntary muscles, tremors of the fingers and hands, and flexion of the head, body, arms, and knees.

Adrenergic Receptors: Alpha and Beta

For many years, it was observed that no single adrenergic blocking agent was capable of antagonizing all the actions of norepinephrine and epinephrine. Ahlquist, in 1948, suggested that there were two types of adrenergic receptors, and these have been designated *alpha* (α) and *beta* (β). Some adrenergic drugs preferentially act at only one of these sites, while other agents are capable of activating both. Moreover, adrenergic blocking agents primarily block either α- or β-adrenergic receptors. Norepinephrine primarily acts on α-receptors and isoproterenol (a synthetic catecholamine) is a selective β-receptor stimulant. Both receptors are activated by epinephrine, but because of the greater sensitivity of β-receptors to this catecholamine, the effects resulting from the activation of β-receptors predominate. The existence of two subtypes of β-

receptors (β_1-, β_2) has been established, and it now appears that there are also subtypes of α-receptors.[1]

Stimulation of α-receptors is associated with constriction of small blood vessels (vasoconstriction), widening or dilation of the pupils (mydriasis), and relaxation of the involuntary smooth muscles of the gastrointestinal tract. Activation of β_1-receptors results in an increase in the rate and force of contraction of the heart and increase in free fatty acids (lipolysis). Beta$_2$-activation causes relaxation of the smooth muscles of the bronchioles (bronchodilation), gastrointestinal tract, and uterus, vasodilation of the blood vessels in skeletal muscles, and an increase in skeletal muscle contractility causing muscle tremors. Beta-receptor activation also results in a rise in blood glucose levels resulting from a breakdown of liver glycogen (glycogenolysis) (Table 6-1).

TABLE 6-1. COMPARISON OF THE PHARMACOLOGICAL EFFECTS OF NOREPINEPHRINE, EPINEPHRINE, AND ISOPROTERENOL

Effect On	Norepinephrine (α)	Epinephrine ($\alpha + \beta$)	Isoproterenol (β)
Heart			
Rate	Slowed (due to a reflex rise in blood pressure)	Increased (direct action)	Increased (direct action)
Force of contraction	Little effect	Increased	Increased
Cardiac output	Little effect	Increased	Increased
Mean blood pressure	Increased	No change	Decreased
Blood flow to:			
Muscle	Decreased	Increased	Increased
Skin	No change or decreased	Decreased	Increased
Brain	No change or or increased	Increased	Increased
Total peripheral resistance	Increased	Decreased	Decreased
Metabolic effects			
Oxygen consumption	Little effect	Increased	Increased
Blood glucose	Little effect	Increased	Increased
Bronchial smooth muscle	Little effect	Relaxed (dilated)	Relaxed (dilated)

Note: Effects listed are those produced by moderate doses of these drugs administered by a slow intravenous infusion.

[1] The postulation or even demonstration of additional subclassifications is generally not greeted with enthusiasm by neophyte readers in any disciplines. In pharmacology, however, such subclassifications have led to the development of more specific therapeutic agents with fewer adverse side effects. For example, during the 1970s a series of relatively specific β_2-agonists have been developed that are quite useful for the treatment of bronchial asthma (Chapter 27). These drugs have minimal effects on β_1-receptors and, therefore, cause few undesirable effects on the cardiovascular system.

Biological Effects of Catecholamines

To permit us an appreciation of the therapeutic applications of the cat-echolamines, let us first look briefly at some of the more significant effects that might result after the intravenous injection of a moderate dose of each of these compounds to healthy human subjects (Table 6–1).

Epinephrine (Adrenaline)

Cardiovascular system. The β-stimulatory effects cause an increase in the rate and force of contraction of the heart, resulting in an increase in the amount of blood leaving the heart (cardiac output). Blood flow is diverted from relatively nonactive parts of the body, which include the spleen and kidneys, to areas that actively participate in the body's reaction to stress, for example, skeletal muscles, brain, and liver. No overall significant changes in blood pressure are observed.

Bronchial muscle. The bronchi of the lungs are widely dilated, thus facilitating respiration.

Metabolic effects. Epinephrine causes a breakdown in liver glycogen (glycogenolysis), the body's storage form of glucose, thus markedly elevating blood sugar (hyperglycemia). In addition, free fatty acids are released from adipose or fat tissue and oxygen consumption is elevated. As a result, the body has raw materials at its disposal for an increased expenditure of energy.

Norepinephrine (Noradrenaline, Levarterenol)

Since this compound is physiologically concerned with circulatory adjust-ments, and not with responses to emergency situations, norepinephrine's effects are different from those seen with epinephrine. Moreover, this compound almost exclusively possesses α-adrenergic activity.

Cardiovascular system. Although norepinephrine directly increases the heart rate (β_1), the net overall effect is a slowing of this rate because of a reflex mechanism resulting from drug-induced general vasoconstriction, and an increase in the resistance of the flow of blood through these vessels which causes an increase in total peripheral resistance. These latter effects cause a significant elevation in blood pressure in the arteries, but no significant changes occur in cardiac output (Chapter 19).

Isoproterenol (Isuprel)

Whereas norepinephrine has almost exclusive α-activating activity and epinephrine has both α-and β-activity, isoproterenol, a synthetic catecholamine, has virtually selective β-stimulatory properties. This compound causes bronchodilation as well as marked stimulatory effects on the rate and force of contraction of the heart. In this regard, it should be observed that isoproterenol's actions more closely resemble epinephrine than norepinephrine.

Table 6-1 compares these three catecholamines and illustrates the differences resulting from α (norepinephrine), β (isoproterenol), and $\alpha + \beta$ (epinephrine) activation.

Therapeutic Uses of Catecholamines

Epinephrine, norepinephrine, and isoproterenol are inactivated in the gastrointestinal tract and cannot be given orally. They must be given by injection or, in the case of epinephrine and isoproterenol, can also be administered by inhalation.

Bronchial Asthma

This respiratory disease, afflicting 5 million Americans, results from a spasmodic contraction of the smooth muscles of the bronchi (bronchoconstriction), causing an impairment in the ability to inhale air into the lungs. There is, also, an increase in the quantity and thickness of bronchial secretions of mucus. In an acute asthmatic attack, manifested by great difficulties in breathing, epinephrine or isoproterenol is administered by injection or inhalation. These drugs widen the bronchioles (bronchodilation) by relaxing the smooth muscles of these tissues, a β-effect. In addition, by an α-stimulating action, epinephrine constricts the blood vessels in the bronchial mucosa decreasing congestion and edema, inhibits mucus secretions, and reduces the thick liquidy mechanical obstruction. The drug treatment of bronchial asthma will be discussed in Chapter 27.

Allergic Disorders

Epinephrine usually produces prompt relief in life-threatening allergic reactions such as serum sickness and angioneurotic edema. These conditions will be considered in Chapter 27.

Cardiac Arrest

Viewers of television's medical heroes are familiar with epinephrine's ability to stimulate the heart after it has failed. The injection of this drug directly into the heart often dramatically restores its beat after stoppage due to drowning, suffocation, shock, electrocution, and anesthesia (Table 6-2).

TABLE 6-2. COMMONLY EMPLOYED SYMPATHOMIMETICS

Type and Use	Generic Name	Selected Trade Names
Epinephrine-like cardiac stimulants (β_1- adrenergic effects)	Epinephrine	Adrenaline
	Isoproterenol	Isuprel
	Dobutamine	Dobutrex
Norepinephrine-like agents used for vasopressor effects to increase blood pressure (α-adrenergic effects)	Levarterenol (norepinephrine)	Levophed
	Dopamine	Intropin
	Ephedrine	
	Metaraminol	Aramine
	Methoxamine	Vasoxyl
	Phenylephrine	Neo-Synephrine

Shock

In this poorly defined syndrome, which results from a myriad of causes, the circulatory system does not function adequately enough to supply the tissues with their requirements of oxygen and nutrients. Norepinephrine has been used to restore and maintain sufficient blood pressure and ensure adequate blood flow to the vital organs. These effects are produced by an increase in total peripheral resistance, without the necessity of stimulating a heart that may be weakened by disease (Table 6–2).

Use with Local Anesthetics

Local anesthetics reduce or eliminate pain in a specific or localized area of the body. Those who have faced a dentist drill-to-tooth are well aware of these effects. Epinephrine is frequently used in conjunction with these agents to constrict the blood vessels at the area of the injection preventing the drug diffusion from the site of action. This vasoconstriction prolongs the duration of action of local anesthetics and also reduces the possibility of toxicity when they travel to other parts of the body.

NONCATECHOLAMINES: EPHEDRINE AND AMPHETAMINE

General readings may have acquainted you with the catecholamines epinephrine and norepinephrine, but personal experience may have introduced you to the noncatecholamines ephedrine and amphetamine. Ephedrine and biologically related drugs are extensively used as nasal decongestants for symptomatic relief of the common cold and as bronchodilators for the treatment of bronchial asthma (Chapter 27). In addition to their surreptitious use by amateur athletes in search of gold medals and professional athletes attempting to land seven-figure contracts (Chapter 10), amphetamine and related drugs are used as appetite suppressants and for the treatment of hyperkinetic disorders in children and narcolepsy. Moreover, at the end of the semester, amphetamine use (or misuse) markedly increases on campuses around the country by countless students attempting to avoid sleep in an effort to complete term papers and cram for final examinations. The uses, misuses, and abuses of amphetamine and other central nervous stimulants will be considered in Chapter 15.

Noncatecholamines, a major group of adrenergic agents, differ in several major respects from the catecholamines. Because noncatecholamines are less potent than the catecholamines, greater absolute amounts of the former drugs are required to produce their effects. Their greater stability in the body permits the noncatecholamines to have a longer duration of action. In addition, the noncatecholamines are effective when given by mouth and are capable of producing central nervous system stimulation.

The catecholamines (norepinephrine, epinephrine, and isoproterenol) all have a direct action at the adrenergic receptor site. By contrast, the noncatecholamines may have direct (phenylephrine), indirect (amphetamine), or mixed (ephedrine) actions. Noncatecholamines may be α- or β-adrenergic stimulants. We shall now briefly consider the pharmacology of ephedrine and amphetamine, two prototype noncatecholamine adrenergic stimulating agents.

Ephedrine

Ma huang has been used by Chinese physicians for over 5,000 years for the improvement of circulation, to stop coughs, and for the reduction of fever. Ephedrine, the active constituent of this plant, was introduced into Western medicine in 1924 and has since been employed for its peripheral adrenergic stimulatory effects. This compound has mixed actions, and, like epinephrine, is both an α-and β-adrenergic stimulant.

Therapeutic Uses

Ephedrine is currently employed for the treatment of mild-to-moderate cases of bronchial asthma, as well as to relieve nasal congestion. Although ephedrine is 100 times less potent than epinephrine, its prolonged bronchodilatory effects after oral administration make it a valuable drug for the prevention of asthmatic attacks. However, its relatively slow onset of action precludes ephedrine's usefulness in arresting acute attacks of this disease.

Oral or local administration in the form of spray or drops for nasal decongestion is predicated upon the ability of this drug to constrict the small blood vessels of the mucous membranes, as well as its inhibitory effect on secretions from the upper respiratory tract. Unfortunately, the relief produced by the shrinkage of swollen nasal membranes is merely temporary and is followed by rebound congestion. Nasal decongestants will be considered in greater detail in Chapter 27.

Side effects after oral administration of ephedrine can be predicted on the basis of this drug's adrenergic activating effects. Undesirable effects include a rise in blood pressure and an increase in heart rate. Moreover, the central stimulatory effects may cause insomnia, irritability, nervousness, and anxiety.

Dextroamphetamine (Dexedrine)

Although dextroamphetamine and related compounds have peripheral sympathetic activating activity, their therapeutic importance and abuse potential is based upon the ability of these agents to profoundly stimulate the central nervous system to produce a feeling of well-being. In this regard, it should be observed that these drugs are the most potent clinically employed stimulants of the highest centers of the brain, located in the cerebral cortex, and are capable of causing increased physical and mental activity.

Dextroamphetamine and other central nervous stimulants will be considered in detail in Chapter 15. For the present then, let us merely summarize what effects might be observed if we were to take a normal therapeutic dose of about 10 mg. We would be more alert, have a decreased feeling of fatigue, an elevated mood, enhanced initiative, confidence, and the ability to concentrate. Appetite is suppressed and physical and verbal activities are increased.

Amphetamine is clinically employed as an appetite suppressant, as a stimulant to prevent attacks of uncontrollable sleep in narcolepsy, and for its paradoxical calming effects in hyperkinetic disorders in children.

SUMMARY ─────────────────────────────

Adrenergic or sympathomimetic drugs produce the effects one would observe after stimulation of the postganglionic sympathetic (adrenergic) nerves. Catecholamine and noncatecholamine adrenergic stimulants are widely used in therapeutics. These drugs may act by a direct action on the adrenergic receptor (α, β_1, β_2) indirectly via the release of norepinephrine, or by both mechanisms.

Alpha-adrenergic activation, with norepinephrine, primarily causes a rise in blood pressure. Epinephrine and isoproterenol administration results in a stimulation in the rate and force of contraction of the heart, a redistribution of blood flow to the action organs (skeletal muscles and brain), and a relaxation of bronchial smooth muscle. In addition, epinephrine produces metabolic changes that prepare the body for mobilization when confronted with emergencies. These drugs have been used for the management of acute bronchial asthmatic attacks, allergic disorders, cardiac arrest, and shock. Ephedrine is used to prevent the respiratory difficulties associated with bronchial asthma and as a nasal decongestant.

Dextroamphetamine, a potent central nervous stimulant and antifatigue agent, has been shown to be effective for the treatment of behavioral disorders (hyperkinesia) in children, for its alerting effects in narcolepsy, and as an appetite suppressant.

SUPPLEMENTARY READINGS

Aviado, D. M., *Sympathomimetic Drugs.* Springfield, Ill: Charles C Thomas, 1970.

Blashko, H., and E. Muscholl, eds., *Catecholamines. Handbook of Experimental Pharmacology.* Vol. 33. Berlin: Springer-Verlag, 1972.

Burnstock, G., and M. Costa, *Adrenergic Neurons: Their Organization, Function, and Development in the Peripheral Nervous System.* New York: John Wiley, 1975.

Iverson, L. L., S. D. Iverson, and S. H. Snyder, eds., *Biochemistry of Biogenic Amines. Handbook of Psychopharmacology.* Vol. 3. New York: Plenum Press, 1975.

Langer, S. Z., "Presynaptic Receptors and Their Role in the Regulation of Neurotransmitter Release," *British Journal of Pharmacology* **60**: 481–97 (1977).

Lefkowitz, R. J., "β-Adrenergic Receptors: Recognition and Regulation," *New England Journal of Medicine* **295**: 323–28 (1976).

Szabadi, E., C. M. Bradshaw, and P. Bevan, eds., *Recent Advances in the Pharmacology of Adrenoceptors. Proceedings of a Satellite Symposium of the 7th International Congress of Pharmacology held at Owens Park, Manchester, on 24th–26th July 1978.* Amsterdam: Elsevier North-Holland Biomedical Press, 1978.

Weiner, N., "Norepinephrine, Epinephrine, and the Sympathomimetic Amines," in *Goodman and Gilman's The Pharmacological Basis of Therapeutics.* Edited by A.G. Gilman, L.S. Goodman, and A. Gilman, 6th ed., Chap. 8, pp. 138–75. New York: Macmillan, 1980.

7

Cholinergic Agents, Chemical Warfare Agents, and Insecticides

Acetyl-cholin[e] . . . is a substance of extraordinary physiological activity. In fact, I think it safe to state that, as regards its effect upon the circulation, it is the most powerful substance known.

—R. Hunt and M. Taveau (1906)

Cholinergic or parasympathomimetic agents are compounds capable of imitating acetylcholine or intensifying the effects of endogenous acetylcholine at its receptor sites. In either case, the end results are actions that are qualitatively similar to those observed after activation of cholinergic nerves. *Cholinergic blocking agents* are antagonists of acetylcholine at its receptor sites. These drugs will be discussed in Chapter 8.

Cholinergic agents are employed for the treatment of glaucoma—a major cause of blindness—and myasthenia gravis, a neurological disease affecting voluntary muscles. Moreover, drugs in this class are of great contemporary interest because of their use as insecticides and for their potential employment in chemical warfare.

CHOLINERGIC TRANSMISSION

In Chapter 5, we briefly touched upon the importance of **acetylcholine** as a neurotransmitter. We observed that acetylcholine is the chemical mediator of nerve impulses at all (sympathetic and parasympathetic) autonomic ganglia, at the postganglionic parasympathetic neuroeffector junction, at the neuromuscular junction, and in some parts of the central nervous system.

Acetylcholine's synthesis is controlled by the enzyme choline acetyl-transferase, which mediates the transfer of an acetyl group from acetyl coenzyme A to choline, a normal constituent of the diet. This synthetic reaction (1) is depicted as going from left to right.

$$CH_3\overset{\displaystyle O}{\overset{\|}{C}} - \; + \; HO-CH_2CH_2\overset{+}{N}(CH_3)_3 \quad \underset{\xleftarrow{\hspace{2cm}}}{\xrightarrow{\hspace{2cm}}} \quad CH_3\overset{\displaystyle O}{\overset{\|}{C}}-OCH_2CH_2\overset{+}{N}(CH_3)_3$$

(1) Choline acetyl-transferase

(2) Acetylcholin-esterase

Acetyl group   Choline   Acetylcholine

Following its release from vesicles at the nerve endings, acetylcholine interacts with the cholinergic receptor to initiate a response. Acetylcholine is then very rapidly hydrolyzed and inactivated by the enzyme acetylcholinesterase. This inactivation reaction (2) is depicted as going from right to left. Choline, one of the products of this reaction, is taken up by the nerve endings responsible for its release, and is reused for the synthesis of new molecules of acetylcholine.

Prior to our discussion concerning the modes by which drugs modify cholinergic transmission, we should point out that a body of evidence exists suggesting that the cholinergic system may play a role in the acquisition of learning.

CHOLINERGIC AGENTS: SITES AND MODES OF ACTION

Classification of Cholinergic Agents

Let us now turn our attention to the pharmacology of cholinergic agents. We may conveniently divide cholinergic agents into two major categories on the basis of whether they act by a direct or indirect mechanism;[1] by indirect we mean by inhibition of the enzyme cholinesterase.

Direct-acting agents activate receptor sites innervated by cholinergic nerves. In this regard they mimic the effects of acetylcholine. *Cholinesterase inhibitors* do not directly interact at the cholinergic receptor, but rather act indirectly by preventing acetylcholinesterase from inactivating acetylcholine. This inhibition permits the buildup of acetylcholine at the receptor site causing more intensive and prolonged cholinergic activation. The resulting pharmacological effects are qualitatively similar to those observed after stimulation of cholinergic nerves, although quantitatively of far greater magnitude. Whereas in certain cases this action may be highly desirable, as in the treatment

[1] We use the term *indirect* to refer to the mechanism of action of both adrenergic (Chapter 6) and cholinergic agents. Indirect-acting adrenergic compounds cause the release of norepinephrine, while cholinergic drugs, having an indirect action, prevent the enzymatic breakdown of acetylcholine. Thus, although these mechanisms of action are very different, in both cases we see enhanced neurotransmitter-induced effects.

of glaucoma, when cholinesterase is inhibited for long periods of time, toxic effects resulting from overstimulation ensue. We shall see that this action is the basis for the use of cholinesterase inhibitors as nerve gases or insecticides.

Cholinergic Receptor Sites: Muscarinic and Nicotinic

So far, we have tacitly assumed that all cholinergic receptor sites are biologically equivalent. If this were the case, it would not be unreasonable to assume that an effective cholinergic blocking agent such as atropine would be able to effectively antagonize acetylcholine at all these sites. This has not been shown to be the case.

Whereas atropine is a potent acetylcholine antagonist at the neuroeffector junction, it is a relatively ineffective antagonist at the autonomic ganglia and at the neuromuscular junction. We find *d-tubocurarine,* a curare-like skeletal muscle relaxant, antagonizes acetylcholine most effectively at the neuromuscular junction, while the antihypertensive agent hexamethonium, used to reduce high blood pressure, is active only at autonomic ganglia.

Muscarine is a naturally occurring alkaloid[2] obtained from mushrooms. Its cholinergic stimulatory properties are limited to the neuroeffector junction. *Nicotine,* a constituent of tobacco, acts at both the neuromuscular junction and autonomic ganglia, producing initial stimulation followed by depression; it is not active at the neuroeffector junction (Chapter 32).

Although we observe that all three sites are responsive to acetylcholine-induced activation, they differ with respect to their anatomical locations, physiological functions, responsiveness to antagonists, and, most fundamentally, in the three-dimensional structure of the receptor site. Thus, we find it useful to subdivide cholinergic receptors into two categories: *muscarinic* (neuroeffector junction) and *nicotinic* (autonomic ganglia and neuromuscular junction) (Table 7-1).

TABLE 7-1. PHARMACOLOGICAL CHARACTERISTICS OF CHOLINERGIC RECEPTORS

Cholinergic Receptor	Junction	Stimulated by	Blocked by
Muscarinic	Neuroeffector	Acetylcholine Muscarine	Atropine
Nicotinic	Autonomic ganglion	Acetylcholine Nicotine	Hexamethonium
	Neuromuscular	Acetylcholine Nicotine	*d*-Tubocurarine

[2] An alkaloid is a nitrogen-containing organic basic compound naturally occurring in plants. Many very common drugs are alkaloids, some of which include morphine, quinine, caffeine, cocaine, physostigmine, and nicotine. See T. Robinson, "Alkaloids," *Scientific American* **201**(1):113-21 (1959).

Effects of Cholinergic Stimulation

Although acetylcholine has a paramount role in neurophysiology, it is not used therapeutically for several reasons. These include rapid inactivation by acetylcholinesterase and lack of specificity of action. Synthetic cholinergic agents currently employed for therapeutic purposes have generally surmounted these shortcomings.

Let us now briefly outline some of the major effects that might be observed after an injection of acetylcholine or after exposure to nerve gases or cholinesterase inhibitor insecticides. It should be noted that many systems are profoundly affected.

Cardiovascular System

The major effect on the cardiovascular system is vasodilation or a widening of the blood vessels. This results in a drop in blood pressure, flushing of the face, and a rise in skin temperature. Furthermore, the heart rate may be slowed or transiently stopped.

Smooth Muscles

A wide variety of highly unpleasant effects result from an activation of smooth muscles. Constriction of the bronchioles, coupled with an increased secretion of mucus by the glands of the respiratory tract, causes mechanical obstruction to breathing, eliciting asthmatic-like attacks. Intestinal cramps and diarrhea result from an increase in peristaltic activity of the gastrointestinal tract. Contraction of the muscles of the bladder causes urination.

Exocrine Glandular Secretions

Acetylcholine markedly stimulates secretions from cholinergically innervated glands, as evidenced by salivation, sweating, and tearing (lacrimation). Glands responsible for the digestion of food are also activated, and these include secretions from the stomach (gastric acid), intestines, and pancreas.

Eye

Cholinergic stimulation causes constriction of the pupils and a reduction in the intraocular pressure. We shall find these effects to be of great significance when we consider the use of pilocarpine in the treatment of glaucoma.

The aforementioned effects occur within minutes after a moderate dose of acetylcholine is injected subcutaneously (under the skin) and end within five minutes. By contrast, exposure to toxic amounts of a cholinesterase inhibitor insecticide produces similar effects that persist for many hours. Administration of atropine prior to the injection of acetylcholine would prevent or at least markedly reduce most, but not all, of these effects.

COMMONLY USED CHOLINERGIC AGENTS

Direct-Acting Agents

Muscarine

The prototype of this class, muscarine, is an alkaloid that is present in certain poisonous mushrooms, in particular the fly mushroom, *Amanita muscaria.* Muscarine has enjoyed a long history of successful use by professional poisoners. Among the more notable victims were the wife and children of the Greek poet Euripides (480?-406? B.C.). The Viking Berserkers "psyched up" for war by eating modest amounts of poisonous mushrooms which may have included *A. muscaria.* The Berserkers were "filled with a great rage under which they howled as wild animals, bit the edge of their shields, and cut down everything they met, without discriminating between friends or foe."[3] Some authors have speculated that the mushroom in *Alice in Wonderland* ("One side will make you grow taller, and the other side will make you grow shorter") may have been the fly mushroom, which was popularized almost one century later in Walt Disney's classic film *Fantasia.* Accidental ingestion of these mushrooms continues to be a medical problem with a high incidence of mortality in the absence of suitable treatment such as atropine. Muscarine is only employed as an experimental agent and has no therapeutic uses.

Bethanechol (Urecholine)

Following abdominal surgery, the intestines may lose their muscle tone (normal tension), resulting in distention of the intestinal walls and an impairment in normal peristaltic activity. In such situations, we observe that food and other contents are not propelled down the gastrointestinal tract. Another unpleasant consequence of abdominal surgery may be a loss of tone in the smooth muscle of the bladder, causing swelling and an inability to urinate. Bethanechol and related cholinergic activating agents are used to restore parasympathetic tone to the smooth muscles of the intestinal tract and bladder. Unlike acetylcholine, bethanechol is not subject to hydrolysis and inactivation by cholinesterase.

Pilocarpine and Glaucoma

Diaphoretic agents, drugs that promote sweating, were formerly used to rid the body of excessive water.[4] With the introduction of highly effective diuretics (drugs that increase urine output; Chapter 21), pilocarpine and other diaphoretics ceased to be clinically employed for this purpose. The use of locally applied pilocarpine to stimulate sweating for the diagnosis of pancreatic cystic fibrosis has rescued the diaphoretics from a category of historical obscurity.

---

[3] Quotation cited without providing original source by H. B. Murphree in *Drill's Pharmacology in Medicine.* 4th ed., ed. J. R. DiPalma, New York: McGraw-Hill, 1971, p. 430.

[4] A reliable source states that a single injection of pilocarpine could stimulate the excretion of several liters of sweat.

Pilocarpine is more widely employed to constrict the pupils and reduce intraocular pressure in *glaucoma*. This common disease of the eyes is a major cause of blindness in persons over 40 years of age. Let us now consider glaucoma and the mechanism underlying pilocarpine's beneficial effects.

The eye is filled with fluids that maintain sufficient pressure in the eyeball to permit it to keep its shape. Aqueous humor is a fluid formed in the posterior chamber of the eye, which passes through the pupil and into the anterior chamber. Normally, the fluid is then drained from the anterior chamber through the canal of Schlemm; the rate of fluid inflow into the canal is equal to the outflow, with a constant pressure of 15 mm of mercury (Hg) created. In certain types of glaucoma there is a constriction of this canal causing inadequate drainage and reduced fluid outflow. Intraocular pressure is increased to more than 100 mm Hg, leading to compression of the optic nerve and eventual blindness. When applied as drops to the eye, pilocarpine and cholinesterase inhibitors constrict the pupil, cause contraction of the ciliary muscle, and as a result widen the canal. Drainage of the aqueous humor is increased and intraocular pressure reduced (Figure 7–1).

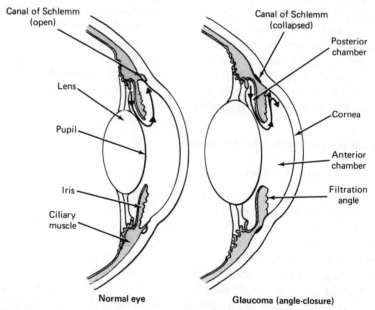

Canal of Schlemm (open)

Canal of Schlemm (collapsed)

Posterior chamber

Lens

Pupil

Cornea

Anterior chamber

Iris

Filtration angle

Ciliary muscle

Normal eye   Glaucoma (angle-closure)

FIGURE 7–1. Abnormal Changes in the Eye in Glaucoma. Aqueous humor is formed in the posterior chamber of the eye, passes through the pupil into the anterior chamber, and is drained through the canal of Schlemm (as depicted by arrows). In glaucoma (angle-closure) the pupil is dilated, increasing the base of the iris and narrowing the filtration angle. This restricts drainage of the aqueous humor and results in an increase in intraocular pressure because of the accumulation of this fluid.

Pilocarpine and similar cholinergic agents constrict the pupil and contract the ciliary muscle, thus withdrawing the iris. This permits drainage of the aqueous humor through the canal of Schlemm and reduces the markedly elevated intraocular pressure associated with glaucoma.

Cholinesterase Inhibitors (Anticholinesterases)

While you are reading this chapter, acetylcholine is being released from the cholinergic nerve endings in your body; it interacts with a receptor and is very quickly inactivated. For the normal, healthy individual this breakdown of acetylcholine is highly desirable. In certain diseases such as myasthenia gravis the cholinergic receptor located on skeletal muscle is inadequately stimulated by acetylcholine. In such cases, it is advantageous to prevent the rapid breakdown of acetylcholine so as to permit the buildup of the neurotransmitter and increase cholinergic activation. However, we should emphasize that excessive accumulation of acetylcholine has deleterious toxicological consequences.

Cholinesterase inhibitors act by combining with and tying up the enzyme so effectively that it is unable to inactivate acetylcholine. Anticholinesterase agents are classified as being reversible or irreversible inhibitors of acetyl-cholinesterase.

When cholinesterase is able to hydrolyze slowly the anticholinesterase agent, the enzyme inhibitory effects are gradually reduced. Such *reversible inhibitors,* physostigmine (eserine) and neostigmine (Prostigmin), for example, act for several hours after a single dose. On the other hand, organophosphorous inhibitors, such as the nerve gas Sarin, are active for several weeks. Normal cholinesterase activity is restored only after the synthesis of new enzyme molecules, or when a cholinesterase reactivator, notably pralidoxime (2-PAM), is used as an antidote. The tenacious attachment of the organophosphorous inhibitors to cholinesterase, with the resulting long duration of action, has caused these agents to be termed *irreversible* inhibitors.

Reversible Cholinesterase Inhibitors

Physostigmine (Eserine)

Physostigmine is an alkaloid derived from the Calabar bean or ordeal bean of West Africa, a plant used by some tribes for the trial of witches by ordeal. It was hypothesized that an innocent person, with nothing to fear, would rapidly ingest the beans. A large, single dose induces vomiting, rapidly removing this compound from the system without causing poisoning. By contrast, the guilty person, afraid of being poisoned, would nibble slowly at the bean. Because a massive single dose was not administered, vomiting would not occur. This would permit the poison to be retained in the body and absorbed, with death the inevitable outcome.

Physostigmine was used in the past for the treatment of myasthenia gravis, but has since been replaced by neostigmine and other safer drugs. It is currently used in the treatment of glaucoma, acting by constricting the pupils and reducing intraocular tension, as well as for its ability to reverse atropine-induced mydriasis or widening of the pupils.

Neostigmine and Myasthenia Gravis

Neostigmine is a synthetic compound which differs from physostigmine in two major respects. Whereas physostigmine acts exclusively as a cholinesterase inhibitor, neostigmine induces both anticholinesterase activity as well as direct action on the cholinergic receptor site. A more important difference is the relative ability of these two compounds to enter the brain. Neostigmine is a lipid-insoluble quaternary ammonium compound which poorly crosses the blood-brain barrier. Thus, in contrast to physostigmine which readily enters the brain, neostigmine produces little or no adverse side effects in the central nervous system. This latter difference served as the rationale for its therapeutic introduction in 1931.

The most important medical use of neostigmine is for the diagnosis and treatment of *myasthenia gravis*. This disease primarily, although not exclusively, affects women, most frequently between the ages of 20 and 50. Skeletal muscles become weak and readily fatigued. In the early stages of the disease, weakness is restricted to the muscles of the eye, producing a characteristic drooping of the eyelids. As the disease progresses, weakness spreads to the facial muscles (causing difficulties in chewing, swallowing, and talking), to the upper limbs and abdomen, and to the muscles of respiration. In the absence of adequate treatment, death may result from respiratory failure.

Determination of the exact cause of myasthenia gravis has been the subject of considerable speculation and study. Normally, the numbers of acetylcholine-cholinergic receptor interactions are far more than adequate to trigger a postsynaptic action potential at the neuromuscular junction resulting in skeletal muscle contraction (Chapter 5); this excess has been referred to as the "safety margin" in neuromuscular transmission.

The results of recent studies reveal that while the presynaptic motor terminals of myasthenic patients contain the normal numbers of acetylcholine vesicles, the clinical symptoms associated with the disease appear to result from a reduction in the number of acetylcholine receptors. As a consequence, there is a decrease in the "safety margin" in neuromuscular transmission, with frequent transmission failures and manifested by voluntary muscle weakness. This decrease in receptor number appears to be the result of an *autoimmune* attack by antibodies directed specifically against the acetylcholine receptors. These antibodies (which have been found in the serum of 90 percent of patients with myasthenia gravis) are thought to act by blocking the active site of the receptor molecule as well as by increasing the degradation of the receptors. Neostigmine (Prostigmin) has been used to diagnose and treat this disorder. Within 10 to 30 minutes after a subcutaneous injection, there is a dramatic temporary reversal of the symptoms. Moreover, this drug is employed orally for the treatment of the disease, with favorable results. Other cholinesterase inhibitors used for the chronic treatment of myasthenia gravis include ambenonium (Mytelase) and pyridostigmine (Mestinon).

Irreversible Cholinesterase Inhibitors: Organophosphates

Organophosphates are characterized by a firmer attachment to cholinesterase, inhibiting this enzyme for extensive periods of time. Their name derives from their chemical classification as organic alkylphosphate esters. Medically, organophosphate compounds are used for the treatment of glaucoma. Reversible inhibitors, such as physostigmine, must be instilled into the eyes as drops two to four times daily. The long duration of action of the irreversible inhibitors, such as echothiophate, requires administration only once or twice weekly. In addition, organophosphates have gained the public's interest as insecticides and potential nerve gases.

Echothiophate (Phospholine)	**Sarin (GB)**	**Parathion**
(Treatment of glaucoma)	(Nerve gas)	(Insecticide)

Pharmacology and Toxicology

Organophosphates have never actually been employed in chemical warfare. In 1968, 6,000 sheep were accidentally killed in Utah, allegedly as the result of exposure to the war gas VX that was being tested by the Army about 17 miles away. This serves as an excellent testimonial to the extreme toxicity of VX and other similar nerve gases.

A very real problem is the incidence of toxicity to farm workers who employ organophosphate insecticides. In California, there are about 200 cases of organophosphate poisoning annually. Exposure may result from inhalation, absorption through the unbroken skin, and by ingestion. Aircraft sprayers and other handlers are most frequently exposed; contamination also results from residues on work clothing or after the conveyance of these compounds in the air, as noted by the extensive sheep kill. Other causes of organophosphate poisoning include accidents while transporting these chemicals or after ingestion by children.

After a single acute exposure, death may occur in as little as one or two minutes or as long as 24 hours, depending upon the dose, the route by which the compound enters the body, and the specific properties of the poison. Nerve gas poisons such as Sarin (GB) or Soman (GD) are odorless and colorless and, therefore, provide no advance warning of their presence. What kinds of toxic effects might we expect to see after exposure to these compounds? Sublethal concentrations produce constriction of the pupils, a watery discharge from the nose, and great difficulty in breathing as a result of bronchoconstriction. With higher concentrations, we note profuse salivation, nausea, vomiting, diarrhea, mental confusion, muscle twitching and weakness, paralysis, convulsions, and eventual death from respiratory failure. It should be observed that these symptoms all arise from excessive cholinergic activation resulting from the high concentrations of acetylcholine at its receptor sites.

The only effective preventive measures are immediate use of a gas mask, if a nerve gas is being used, and protective clothing. After exposure, the victim should be removed from the toxic environment, or the contaminated areas of the skin should be washed with water, and artificial respiration initiated.

Atropine is highly effective in antagonizing the muscarinic actions (salivation and gastrointestinal and respiratory problems) and other symptoms adversely affecting the central nervous system. As we have previously indicated, atropine is ineffective in blocking the nicotinic actions of acetylcholine at the autonomic ganglia and neuromuscular junction, resulting in muscle paralysis. Atropine prevents acetylcholine from gaining access to the muscarinic receptor sites located at the neuroeffector junction.

Another approach in an effort to antagonize the effects of the irreversible organophosphate cholinesterase inhibitors has been the *reactivation* of the enzyme cholinesterase. A reactivating agent such as pralidoxime acts by combining with the organophosphate and "pulling" it away from the enzyme at both muscarinic and nicotinic sites in all parts of the body. Because these organophosphorous compounds persist in the body for days or even weeks and are still capable of inhibiting cholinesterase for this period of time, atropine and/or pralidoxime therapy may have to be continued for several weeks. Figure 7–2 summarizes the mode of action of organophosphorous inhibitors and the mechanism of atropine and pralidoxime as antidotes.

Organophosphates do not come to the mind of the public when they think of common therapeutic agents. It is most probable that the existence of organophosphates is known to you because of their important place in two controversial classes of compounds: chemical warfare agents and insecticides. In this regard, we shall digress now and survey the major members of each of these classes rather than restrict our discussion exclusively to the organophosphates.

AGENTS EMPLOYED IN CHEMICAL WARFARE

Chemical warfare is the direct use of chemicals as weapons. These chemicals, employed as solids, liquids, or gases, are capable of producing lethal, injurious, irritating, or incapacitation effects to personnel. The ignoble history of chemical warfare can be traced to ancient times and primitive civilizations where poisonous arrows were employed. The Spartans used the irritating gases

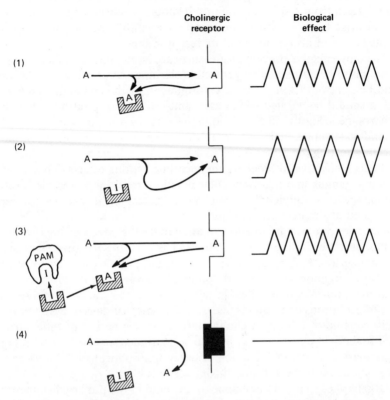

FIGURE 7–2. Mechanism of Action of Organophosphate Cholinesterase Inhibitors and Antidotes. (1) Acetylcholine (A) is released from the nerve endings and interacts at the cholinergic receptor site to produce a biological effect. It is then inactivated by the enzyme cholinesterase ( ), as is some fraction of acetylcholine liberated from the nerve endings.

(2) In the presence of an organophosphate cholinesterase inhibitor (I), the enzyme is inhibited ( ), and inactivation of acetylcholine does not occur. This makes more acetylcholine available at the receptor, resulting in a marked intensification of the biological effects.

(3) Pralidoxime (PAM) is capable of reactivating cholinesterase by pulling away the inhibitor. The enzyme is again functional and is able to inactivate acetylcholine.

(4) Atropine ( ), a cholinergic blocking agent, antagonizes acetylcholine by occupying the cholinergic muscarinic receptor, thereby preventing an acetylcholine-receptor interaction. It should be noted that even in the presence of atropine, cholinesterase still remains inhibited by the organophosphate agent.

TABLE 7-2. AGENTS USED IN CHEMICAL WARFARE

Class	Examples
Organophosphorous nerve gases	Sarin (GB)* Soman (GD) Tabun (GA) VX*
Vesicants or blistering agents	Lewisite Sulfur mustard (mustard gas)
Irritating agents (Tear gases)	Chloroacetophenone (Mace, CN)* Chlorobenzylidene malononitrite (CS)* Diphenylaminochloroarsine (DM)*
Mental incapacitants (Psychochemicals)	LSD-type (?)

*Agents of contemporary importance.

of sulfur in their siege of Athenian cities in 400 B.C. Many armies over the ages have resorted to poisoning the food and water of their enemies. The modern age of chemical warfare began in World War I when the Germans used chlorine gas against the French and Canadian troops in Ypres, Belgium. Taken by surprise, the troops suffered 20,000 casualties. Although gases were used to a limited extent in the 1936 Italian invasion of Ethiopia, chemicals have not been widely employed since World War I. Notwithstanding this, major powers all over the world have been developing and stockpiling poisonous compounds as deterrents.

Chemical weapons can be divided into four major categories: nerve gases, vesicants, irritants, and mental incapacitants (Table 7-2). We shall emphasize that these categories of agents are both chemically and pharmacologically dissimilar.

Organophosphate Nerve Gases

By far the most effective chemical weapons are the organophosphorous derivatives first prepared by the Germans during World War II.[5] These *irreversible cholinesterase inhibitor nerve gases* are odorless, colorless, and provide no advance warning. They are effective in very low concentrations and are capable of causing death within minutes after exposure. We have already considered the pharmacological and toxicological aspects of these drugs.

[5] Soviet troops reportedly employed a nerve gas (said to be Soman) in their invasion of Afghanistan, which began in late 1979.

Vesicant or Blistering Agents

Sulfur mustard or mustard gas and similar agents were used during World War I and were reported to account for 25 percent of all the casualties suffered by the Allied Expeditionary Force. Several hours after exposure, irritation and burning of the eyes and skin are experienced. Higher concentrations cause nausea, vomiting, abnormal heart beats (cardiac arrhythmias), and shock. Long-term effects on survivors include ulceration of the gastrointestinal tract and a reduction in white blood cells. This latter effect was recognized several years after the "Great War," and resulted in the use of nitrogen mustard in the treatment of cancer (Chapter 30).

Lewisite is an arsenic-containing vesicant capable of producing immediate pain, inflammation, and permanent damage to the eyes. We have already discussed the rational development of dimercaprol (BAL or British antilewisite) as a specific antidote to this liquid vesicant (Chapter 4).

Irritating Agents

Irritating agents, commonly referred to as tear gas, are used mainly for riot control but have also been employed in combat, most recently in Vietnam. Generally delivered as an aerosol, these agents produce almost immediate irritation to the eyes, profuse tearing, coughing, nausea, vomiting, and cause difficulties in breathing. Although some members of this class (diphenylaminochloroarsine [DM]) may incapacitate an individual for up to two hours, Mace (chloroacetophenone) produces irritation for only a few minutes.

Mace does not usually produce permanent eye damage, although lesions on the cornea have occurred when sprays have been fired at very close range. There is no specific treatment, but eyes should be washed as rapidly as possible. Victims should avoid rubbing their eyes; topical or local anesthetics should not be applied because these agents slow the healing process.

Mental Incapacitants or Psychochemicals

Mental incapacitants cause confusion and produce changes in behavior, impairing an individual's ability to respond normally to stimuli or command. In addition, they can produce fear and destroy the will to fight. Such drugs investigated by the military and the Central Intelligence Agency (CIA) have included or are related to LSD-25.

INSECTICIDES

There are approximately 80,000 species of insects in the United States, of which 10,000 produce some injury to humans, crops, forests, and livestock. Of these, approximately 300 constitute a real problem. Amidst the furor regarding the dangers of *insecticides and pesticides* to humans, wildlife, and the balance of nature, we should consider that these chemicals have also proved to be of great benefit.

Insecticides affect the insect after ingestion (systemic or stomach poisons), absorption (contact poisons), or inhalation (fumigants).

1. *Systemic poisons.* These insecticides, also termed stomach poisons, are ingested by the insect and absorbed into the bloodstream from the stomach. The insecticide is then transported in the blood to its site of action in the insect's nervous system.

2. *Contact poisons.* Compounds of this type exert their lethal action after passing through the insect cuticle or exoskeleton and entering the bloodstream. Others cause suffocation of the insect.

3. *Fumigants.* Applied in a gaseous form, they readily enter the breathing pores of the insect.

Control of agricultural pests has enabled the farmers of this country to produce high quality, low cost foods in surplus quantities. Pesticides are used to destroy disease-bearing, destructive, and annoying bacteria, insects, and rodents that prey on crops, plants, livestock, pets, and people. Moreover, pesticides control over twenty diseases, two of which are malaria and typhus. Although these diseases are virtually unknown in the United States, many parts of the developing world are still scourged by their presence.

The major concerns regarding the use of some of these agents is focused upon residues in the soil and water causing lethal effects to fish and other marine life, as well an interference with the normal hatching of birds. Moreover, residues have been detected in the dairy products, meat, fish, poultry, fruits, and vegetables that eventually find their way to our dinner table. We shall now consider the use and dangers associated with three major classes of insecticides: organophosphorous compounds (malathion), chlorinated hydrocarbons (DDT), and natural products (pyrethrins). (See Table 7–3.)

Organophosphorous Compounds

Organophosphorous compounds act as both contact and systemic poisons. The precise mechanisms by which these agents produce their lethal effects in insects is poorly understood, especially when compared with the large volume of information available on their toxicity to mammals. It is generally thought that

TABLE 7-3. INSECTICIDES

Class	Examples
Organophosphates (cholinesterase inhibitors)	Parathion (Thiophos; E605) Malathion TEPP (tetraethylpyrophosphate) EPN (O-ethyl-[4-nitrophenyl]-phenyl-phosphonothioate) OMPA (octamethylpyrophosphor-amide) Systox
Chlorinated hydrocarbons	DDT (chlorophenothane) Lindane (gamma-benzene hydrochloride) Chlordane Dieldrin Aldrin Endrin
Natural products	Pyrethrins Rotenone Nicotine

agents such as parathion, malathion, and the other members of this class act by an inhibition of cholinesterase, causing the buildup of acetylcholine. Symptoms of toxicity in the insect include excitability, tremors, paralysis, and eventual death. The immediate cause of death remains obscure.

Parathion

Parathion is a widely used insecticide that is itself relatively nontoxic. It must be converted to an active metabolite, paraoxon, before it exerts its insecticidal action. Occupational exposure by farm workers and accidental ingestion by children have resulted in a large number of poisonings and deaths.

Malathion

Malathion has greater selective toxicity to insects than to man, other mammals, and birds. For example, the LD50 of malathion after oral administration is about 1,500 mg/kg in rats and mice, 1,100 mg/kg in ducks, and 275 mg/kg in chickens. By contrast, its topical LD50 to the housefly, American cockroach, and pea aphid are 30, 8.4, and 0.75 mg/kg, respectively.

With the exception of parathion and systox, members of this class are not stable in water and are, therefore, not persistent. Parathion and systox may be present for several weeks after application to crops and have been found as residues on harvest food. The incidence and quantities of organophosphorous residues detected on foods is generally low and is not thought to constitute a hazard. Furthermore, animal studies have failed to detect any major teratogenic potential associated with these compounds.

Chlorinated Hydrocarbons

In previous years, DDT (chlorophenothane) has produced a major revolution in agriculture; more recently, we have seen this revolution spread to ecology. DDT is the best-known, cheapest, and most effective insecticide.[6] Its popularity stems from its very low cost, stability, potency, persistency after application to plants, and relatively low toxicity. Whereas the persistency of DDT residues for long periods of time after a single application is extremely advantageous for the farmer, these same residues in animal tissues and foods have generated considerable apprehension in the minds of the public. The ecological hazards associated with this agent and the development of insect resistance have reduced the popularity that DDT once enjoyed.

Toxicity

Chlorinated hydrocarbons are very lipid-soluble and, as a result, are highly effective in penetrating the insect cuticle. Fortunately, absorption through the skin of mammals is relatively poor, and, therefore, the toxicity of DDT from external application is quite low. For both mammals and insects, the site of toxicity is the nervous system. Following an initial period of tremors and an increase in activity, the insect's nervous system becomes disorganized; a loss of motion, paralysis, and death ensue. Poisoning in humans is characterized by feelings of apprehension, confusion, numbness, tremors, convulsions, muscle weakness, with death resulting from respiratory failure.

Human deaths have been reported after the accidental or suicidal ingestion of 10–20 g of DDT dissolved in oil. The lethal dose of this compound is sufficiently high that it is not deemed a significant danger, and there are very few well-documented cases of fatal DDT poisoning. Virtually all deaths have resulted from the ingestion of DDT in an oily solution and often death has been attributed to the solvent vehicle. When ingested as a powder, this compound is very poorly absorbed. In one study, 51 human volunteers ate 35 mg (0.5 mg/kg) of DDT per day for eighteen months without any adverse effects. This dose is 200 times the amount generally present in the diet. Pesticide handlers have been studied over the last 30 years, and although their fat contains 50 times the normal levels of DDT, no adverse effects to their health have been demonstrated. In addition, there is no evidence available at present that in-

---

[6] Although DDT was first synthesized in 1874, its insecticidal properties were not observed until 1939. In recognition for his pioneering work on DDT, Paul Müller, a Swiss chemist, was awarded the Nobel Prize in 1955.

dicates any undesirable effects in human fetuses resulting from maternal exposure to these insecticides during pregnancy.

Ecological Hazards

While mammals must be exposed to rather large doses to produce toxic effects, fish are very susceptible to chlorinated hydrocarbons. From 1960 to 1963, several million fish of many species were killed as a result of the runoff of endrin and similar insecticides from the northern farmlands into the Mississippi River. The hatching ability of some birds—including eagles, falcons, pelicans, and pheasants—is adversely altered by DDT. In an attempt to eradicate gnats from Clear Lake, California, the lake was sprayed with DDT on three occasions from 1949 to 1957. Of the thousand nesting pairs of grebes residing there, not even one grebe was hatched from 1950 to 1961. Following exposure to DDT, egg shells became thinner, more fragile, and susceptible to breakage during the period of maternal nesting. It has also been suggested that insecticides produce abnormal maternal behavior, resulting in intentional egg-breakage and egg-eating. Earthworms are a major source of DDT poisoning for robins. These considerations led to the banning of DDT in the United States in 1972 for all but a limited number of agricultural uses for which effective substitutes are not available.

DDT in Perspective

Is DDT completely devoid of saving graces? Consider, if you will, that *malaria* is the most common disease affecting human beings, claiming several hundred million victims throughout the world and constituting the greatest public health problem facing the human race. In certain tropical regions virtually all inhabitants are infected with malaria from the time they are a few days old until they die. DDT has been effectively used to control the carrier *Anopheles* mosquito and has been responsible for the eradication of malaria in several parts of the world.

Typhus caused more deaths during World War I than any other single cause, including battle injuries. During World War II, the application of DDT to the clothing of over one million persons averted a major typhus epidemic in Naples. This insecticide kills the lice that carry typhus.

There is little argument that the indiscriminate use of DDT should be immediately discontinued. At this time, however, a worldwide ban on DDT and related agents appears unrealistic. Continued use should be predicated upon the benefits to public health and agriculture obtained. In regions where DDT has been shown to endanger wildlife and disrupt the ecological balance, its use should be terminated, or, where clearly benefiting the public health, very carefully controlled.

Scientists are continuing their search for safer, more effective insecticides. In recent years, biological alternatives to the chemical control of insect pests are being actively investigated. These include the use of sex attractants and the fostering of natural enemies to destroy the insects.

Natural Insecticides

A group of commonly used household and garden products may be conveniently grouped together under a miscellaneous category of natural insecticides. Unlike the organophosphates and chlorinated hydrocarbons, which are synthetic products, the members of this category of insecticides are all derived from plants.

Pyrethrins

Pyrethrins, common components of household spray products, are derived from pyrethrum (chrysanthemum) flowers. Pyrethrins cause paralysis of insects or a "knock-down effect." They possess only brief residual effects and are nontoxic to humans and animals. Skin contact should be avoided because these compounds cause skin irritation (contact dermatitis) in allergic individuals.

Rotenone

Over 100 years ago, it was suggested that a Malayan fish poison might be an effective insecticide. The poison, containing the active chemical rotenone, was extracted from the roots of the leguminous plant *Derris*. Rotenone's paralyzing effects to insects are slower than the pyrethrins but are more reliable and result in fewer recoveries. In addition to being sprayed on plants and crops, it is also employed to combat animal parasites such as lice, ticks, and fleas.

Nicotine

An alcoholic solution of tobacco leaves was used as an insecticide in colonial America to combat a beetle which showed a preference for plums. The active constituent in these leaves is nicotine. This alkaloid is a highly effective contact poison used to control plant lice. Nicotine-induced tremors and convulsions are followed by paralysis, effects probably resulting from actions at the insect ganglia. This agent is not selective and is also toxic to man and animals. In vertebrates, nicotine acts at the autonomic ganglia and in the central nervous system to produce convulsions and respiratory failure. We shall discuss nicotine in Chapter 32.

SUMMARY

In this chapter, we have explored the pharmacology and toxicology of cholinergic agents. These drugs produce their effects by directly activating the cholinergic receptor site (pilocarpine) and/or by inhibiting cholinesterase (physostigmine). Inhibition of this enzyme permits the buildup of acetylcholine, which in turn enhances activation of the cholinergic receptor site.

Although Gertrude Stein once observed that "a rose is a rose is a rose," we cannot say that a cholinergic receptor is a cholinergic receptor is a cholinergic receptor. Rather we see that acetylcholine activates several different types of cholinergic receptor sites. These include the muscarinic receptor (neuroeffector junction) and the nicotinic receptor (autonomic ganglia and neuromuscular junction).

The varied effects of cholinergic stimulation can be best illustrated by examining the toxicological consequences associated with poisoning by a cholinesterase inhibitor. These effects include a marked stimulation of secretions from exocrine glands (tearing, salivation, sweating), constriction of the smooth muscles of the bronchioles, a drop in blood pressure, depression of the heart rate, and paralysis of the respiratory muscles. Whereas therapeutic doses increase the muscle strength of a person with myasthenia gravis, toxic doses produce convulsions and paralysis. Antidotes for poisoning by organophosphorous cholinesterase inhibitors are atropine, which blocks the cholinergic receptor, and/or pralidoxime (2-PAM), which reactivates cholinesterase.

Cholinergic agents are used therapeutically for the treatment of glaucoma and myasthenia gravis. They have also been found useful as activators of peristalsis and urination postoperatively.

Organophosphates are prominent members of a class of agents used in chemical warfare and as insecticides. Compounds used in chemical warfare include the organophosphates (Sarin or GB); the vesicants or blistering agents of World War I infamy (mustard gas); irritating agents such as tear gas and Mace, which are used in riot control; and mental incapacitants or psychochemicals which impair a combatant's normal behavior.

Insecticides gain access to the insect's nervous system either by absorption through the exoskeleton (contact poisons), by ingestion of plants and other foodstuffs (systemic poisons), or by inhalation (fumigants). Common classes of insecticides include the organophosphates (parathion), chlorinated hydrocarbons (DDT), and a group of natural insecticides commonly used in the home and garden. The chlorinated hydrocarbons have been subjected to the greatest public attack because of their well-documented effects on the disruption of the ecological balance.

Whether by accidental ingestion by children or through the gross negligence of adults, pesticides represent an important human poison. Of the 156,330 individual poison reports submitted in 1977 to the National Clearinghouse for Poison Control Centers, 9,099 or about 6 percent were caused by pesticides. Of these, 5,316 or 58 percent were accidental ingestion accidents by children under 5 years of age. Although most of us generally recognize the hazards associated with the more potent agricultural pesticides, we are often cavalier in our handling and storage of products commonly used in the home.

SUPPLEMENTARY READINGS

Brimblecombe, R. W., *Drug Actions on Cholinergic Systems*. Baltimore: University Park Press, 1974.

Cohen, J. B., and J. P. Changeux, "The Cholinergic Receptor Protein and Its Membrane Environment," *Annual Review of Pharmacology* 15: 83–103 (1975).

der Marderosian, A. H., "Pesticides," in *Remington's Pharmaceutical Sciences*. 15th ed., Chap. 65, pp. 1182–207. Easton, Penn.: Mack Publishing Co., 1975.

Drachman, D. B., "Myasthenia Gravis," *New England Journal of Medicine* 298: 136–42, 186–93 (1978).

Durham, W. F., and C. H. Williams, "Mutagenic, Teratogenic and Carcinogenic Properties of Pesticides," *Annual Review of Entomology* 17: 123–48 (1972).

Grob, D., ed., "Myasthenia Gravis," *Annals of the New York Academy of Sciences* 214: 1–682 (1976).

Havener, W. H., *Ocular Pharmacology*. 4th ed. St. Louis: C. V. Mosby, 1978.

Matsumara, F., *Toxicology of Insecticides*. New York: Plenum Press, 1975.

Pharmacology Society Symposium, "Riot Control Agents," *Federation Proceedings* 30: 84–99 (1971).

Sidel, V. W., and R. M. Goldwyn, "Chemical and Biological Weapons—A Primer," *New England Journal of Medicine* 274: 21–27 (1966).

Waser, P. G., ed., *Cholinergic Mechanisms*. New York: Raven Press, 1975.

Watson P. G., ed., "Glaucoma," *British Journal of Ophthalmology* 56 145–318 (1972).

Wright, R. H., "Why Mosquito Repellents Repel," *Scientific American* 233 (1): 104–11 (July 1975).

Zaimis, E., ed., *Neuromuscular Junction. Handbook of Experimental Pharmacology*. Vol. 42. Berlin: Springer-Verlag, 1976.

8

Cholinergic Blocking Agents and Neurotoxins

Certain edibles, such as mandragora (mandrake) and hyoscyamus (henbane),[1] induce madness; but these affections are never called mania; for springing from a temporary cause, they quickly subside, but madness has something confirmed in it.

—Aretaeous of Cappadocia (81-138?)

In Chapter 7 we considered drugs capable of activating tissues innervated by cholinergic nerves. *Cholinergic blocking agents or anticholinergic agents* are drugs that prevent acetylcholine from stimulating the cholinergic receptor site. The designation "cholinergic blocking agent" is a relatively imprecise term that does not tell us where the antagonism is taking place. That is, are we blocking acetylcholine at the postganglionic parasympathetic neuroeffector junction (muscarinic receptor) or at the autonomic ganglia or at the neuromuscular junction? Hence, to preclude ambiguity, these drugs should be more definitively designated as *antimuscarinic agents, ganglionic blocking agents, and neuro- muscular blocking agents,* respectively.

Our discussion in this chapter will be restricted mainly to atropine, a widely used antimuscarinic agent. In addition, we shall briefly survey some fascinating natural products that act as therapeutic agents, experimental tools, and nervous system poisons by virtue of their interference with normal cholinergic transmission. Let us first consider the potato family, the natural source of atropine and related antimuscarinic agents.

THE POTATO FAMILY

The potato or *Solanaceae* family is a very versatile group of plants. Some members are ornamentals (petunia, matrimony vine), while others are foods

[1] Plants containing atropine-like substances.

(potato, tomato, eggplant, peppers), and some are even drugs (past or present), such as atropine, scopolamine, hyoscyamine, stramonium, and mandrake. You may recall that the potato, or more correctly, the absence of the potato, was largely responsible for the Irish immigration to the United States in the middle of the nineteenth century.

The leaves and roots of the belladonna plant are sources of atropine, scopolamine (hyoscine), and hyoscyamine, alkaloids having far greater pharmacologic similarities than differences. **Belladonna** is the most important member of the *Solanaceae* family, unless, of course, you come to this book as a biased potato farmer. "Belladonna," or beautiful lady, was the laudable objective of sixteenth-century Italian women who squeezed the berries of these plants into their eyes in order to widen and brighten their pupils. The belladonna alkaloids were well known to, and respected by, the ancient Hindus and Greeks, who employed them for medicinal purposes, as well as to medieval poisoners who used these compounds to ply their profession. Linnaeus (1707–1778), the famous Swedish naturalist, scientifically classified this plant (commonly called the deadly nightshade), *Atropa belladonna,* in honor of Atropos, the oldest of the three Fates, who cut the threads of life. Prior to considering atropine, the reference antimuscarinic agent, let us remain in the pharmacological archives for several minutes more.

Atropa belladonna played an integral role in the celebration of the *Sabbat* or Black Mass. At this ritual gathering, witches of the Middle Ages worshipped Satan, performed lewd and macabre acts, and desecrated Christianity. Traditionally, witches flew to the Sabbat on brooms, cats, and other animals. They "acquired" this power of flight by liberally covering themselves with a soot-containing ointment having as its active ingredient *belladonna.* The effects of this drug on behavior and on the heart conveyed to these susceptible individuals the sensation of flying. This sensation was so realistic that, at their trials, many accused witches testified about the vivid nature of this experience with absolute sincerity.

Hyoscyamus niger or henbane has a long history as a narcotic agent used to produce sleep and relieve pain. The sorcerer of the Middle Ages found this plant to be of inestimable value in interactions with demons and to facilitate soothsaying. Although visual hallucinations may result from its use, it has not become a "street drug." This is not at all unfortunate because henbane is quite toxic to humans and is reported to cause permanent insanity. Claudius was supposed to have used henbane to kill his brother, Hamlet's father. Whereas considerable literary scholarship has been generated by this play, medical science has turned a deaf ear to the suggestion that the intra-aural route might prove useful for the systemic administration of drugs to sleeping patients. Henbane should not be confused with wolfsbane *(Aconitum napellus).* Students of literature know wolfsbane to be a useful vampire-repellent;[2] however, we should point out that double-blind studies demonstrating the effectiveness of this plant have not as yet been conducted.

[2] B. Stoker, *Dracula,* 1897.

In recent years, many young nonasthmatics have taken to smoking Asthmador cigarettes, a product intended to relieve the symptoms of asthma. This product contains an atropine-like compound, *stramonium,* which is derived from the Jimson or Jamestown weed (*Datura stramonium*). The mind-alerting effects of this plant were long known to Indian tribes who inhabited Mexico and the United States and who used this plant in rites dealing with puberty in young men. South American witch doctors employ *Datura* to communicate with spirits who assist them in properly diagnosing disease and to uncover thieves and foretell the future of the tribe. The ancient Chibcha gave *Datura* to the wives and slaves of dead chieftains. Experience demonstrated to these inhabitants of the Bogota area of Colombia that after drug-induced lethargy, the survivors were far more "receptive" to the prospects of being buried alive with their deceased master. The New World had no monopoly on *Datura.* The dried leaves and seeds were brought into Europe from Asia during the Middle Ages by the gypsies, "who employed their smoke to intoxicate and delude their dupes." In the eighteenth century, one Baron Storck of Vienna advocated stramonium for the treatment of mania, melancholia, and epilepsy.

ATROPINE AND RELATED ANTIMUSCARINIC AGENTS

Therapeutically, antimuscarinic drugs, such as atropine, are used for gastrointestinal disorders, Parkinson's disease, eye examinations, motion sickness, and, until recently, as a component of nonprescription sleep-inducing preparations. Let us first consider the mechanism of action and pharmacological effects of atropine that account for these diverse therapeutic uses.

Mechanism of Action

Atropine blocks the actions of acetylcholine at the postganglionic parasympathetic junction (muscarinic receptor). This antagonist interacts with the same receptor groups on effector cells normally activated by the agonist acetylcholine. While atropine is able to combine with this receptor, it is incapable of activating the receptor site (Figure 8–1). Moreover, as a result of atropine's occupancy of this site, endogenous acetylcholine is unable to interact with and produce normal cholinergic stimulation. We observe, in effect, a chemically induced paralysis of tissues with muscarinic receptor sites (Chapter 7). It should be emphasized that atropine does not prevent the release of acetylcholine nor does it interact chemically with acetylcholine to inactivate this neurotransmitter. At present, it is not well understood why normal therapeutic doses of atropine only antagonize acetylcholine at the muscarinic receptor while not at the nicotinic receptors.

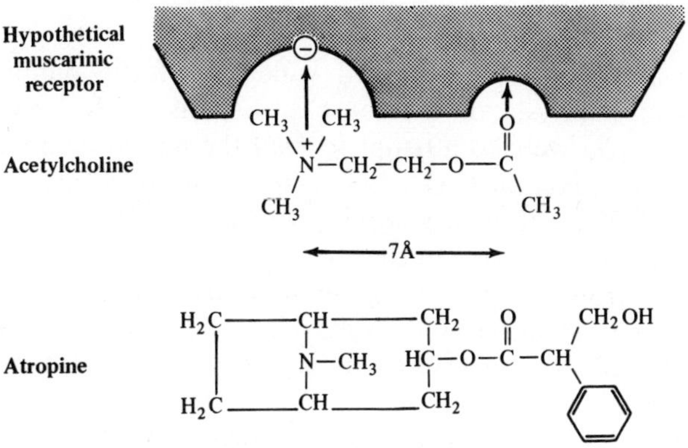

FIGURE 8-1. Atropine, Acetylcholine, and the Hypothetical Muscarinic Receptor Site. Atropine bears some distinct chemical similarities to acetylcholine; for example, the distance between the nitrogen (N) and the carbonyl oxygen (C=O) is 7Å. The figure depicts the interaction between the agonist (acetylcholine) or antagonist (atropine) and the hypothetical muscarinic receptor site.

Pharmacological Effects

We may summarize the pharmacological properties of atropine by stating that this drug antagonizes all the muscarinic effects of acetylcholine. Specifically, we might observe the effects described below after giving 0.5 mg of atropine to a normal healthy subject.

Exocrine Glands

Secretions from exocrine glands are inhibited by atropine. Salivation is prevented; indeed, dryness of the mouth is one of the most common side effects associated with the use of antimuscarinic agents. The sweat glands are also inhibited. The inability to sweat accounts in part for the marked rise in body temperature (hyperthermia) frequently observed after toxic doses of atropine in young children and infants; body temperature may reach or exceed 109°F. Secretions of gastric acid in the stomach are reduced somewhat, while there is a marked decrease in other gastrointestinal secretions and in the secretion of mucus from the bronchioles.

Smooth Muscles

The normal tension (tone) and spontaneous movements (motility) of the smooth muscles of the gastrointestinal tract and bronchioles are reduced. This is an *antispasmodic* effect. Atropine has no effect on the production of urine, but does interfere with its elimination by depressing the tone and motility of the urinary bladder.

Eye

Antimuscarinics produce marked widening of the pupils of the eye (mydriasis) and paralysis of the muscles responsible for accommodation (cycloplegia). If you were to attempt to read the names of the States of the Union that are found on the back of a five-dollar bill, your small muscles of accommodation (ciliary muscles) would contract. This muscle contraction produces changes in the shape of the lens and permits you to visualize objects only a few inches from your eye. Atropine-induced cycloplegia prevents the eyes from focusing on near objects and results in blurred vision. However, changing the shape of the lens is not necessary for the perception of distant objects, and such vision remains clear even after the administration of atropine.

Atropine does not alter the intraocular pressure of the normal eye. Where resistance to the outflow of aqueous humor exists, such as caused by a preexisting constriction of the canal of Schlemm, these drugs increase intraocular pressure. Therefore, atropine-like drugs should be avoided by persons with glaucoma (Chapter 7).

Central Nervous System

Acetylcholine is considered by most investigators to be a neurotransmitter in the central nervous system. Hence, it should not be surprising that cholinergic blocking agents are able to affect behavioral changes, presumably by modifying cholinergic transmission in the brain. Whereas normal therapeutic doses of atropine have minimal effects on the central nervous system, toxic doses produce *excitation*. This is manifested by euphoria, restlessness, irritability, hallucinations, and delirium. At these higher doses, the respiratory centers become depressed, and death may result from respiratory failure.

Scopolamine or hyoscine, a compound closely resembling atropine, produces *drowsiness,* amnesia, and dreamless sleep in normal doses. Nonprescription sleep-facilitating products formerly contained this antimuscarinic agent. In the past, scopolamine was used with morphine for obstetrical anesthesia, a state referred to as "twilight sleep." This drug combination produced marked drowsiness, but consciousness was maintained, and the patient was capable of following instructions. When the woman awakened, she had no unpleasant recollection of the traumas of childbirth. The major shortcoming of "twilight sleep" is the variation in the response obtained; for example, in some instances, the patients become delirious or maniacal. Large doses of scopolamine produce the same peripheral and behavioral effects that are seen after toxic amounts of atropine.

Both muscarinic and nicotinic receptor sites are present in the brain. Cholinergic blocking agents are able to antagonize acetylcholine at these sites. Whether the behavioral aberrations produced by these drugs are a direct consequence of this blockade has not been resolved to date. Moreover, because of our uncertainty as to the nature of the antagonism, that is, whether we have muscarinic or nicotinic blockade, for the present time it is prudent to refer to such drugs by the general designation of cholinergic blocking agents.

Therapeutic Uses of Antimuscarinic Agents

Many of atropine's diverse pharmacological effects have proved medically useful, causing this drug to enjoy very widespread popularity over the years as a therapeutic agent. A great many synthetic antimuscarinic agents have been introduced into clinical medicine (Table 8–1). In most cases, when compared with atropine, they have been shown to possess few significant advantages and cost considerably more. Many of these synthetic products are quaternary ammonium compounds, which are lipid-insoluble, and, therefore, do not easily enter the brain. The absence of behavioral and neurological side effects is, however, often compensated for by undesirable effects resulting from the quaternary structure, such as some ganglionic and neuromuscular blocking effects.

Preoperative Medication

Atropine inhibits secretions from exocrine glands. This drug is frequently used prior to surgery to prevent salivary and bronchial (mucus) secretions stimulated by general anesthetics. The dangers associated with the possible

TABLE 8-1. SELECTED ATROPINE-LIKE DRUGS COMMONLY EMPLOYED IN THERAPEUTICS

Generic Name	Selected Trade Names
Antisecretory-antispasmodic (Ulcer therapy)	
Belladonna alkaloids (mixture)	Donnatal
Glycopyrrolate	Robinul
Methscopolamine	Pamine
Oxyphencyclimine	Daricon
Propantheline	Pro-Banthine
Mydriasis and cycloplegia (Eye disorders)	
Cyclopentolate	Cyclogyl
Eucatropine	Euphthalmine
Homatropine	—
Parkinson's disease	
Benztropine mesylate	Cogentin
Biperiden	Akineton
Procyclidine	Kemadrin
Trihexyphenidyl	Artane

blockage of respiratory airways and the resulting impairment of breathing caused by excessive fluid accumulation are thereby precluded.

Gastrointestinal Disorders

Reduction in the motility of the smooth muscles of the stomach and the inhibition of gastric acid secretions *(antisecretory effect)* serve as the basis for the wide utilization of antimuscarinic agents in the management of *gastric ulcers.* Their use for the treatment of diarrhea is predicated upon the ability of these drugs to reduce spasms and excessive motility in the gastrointestinal tract *(antispasmodic effects).* The use of antimuscarinic agents for the treatment of ulcers and diarrhea will be discussed in Chapters 25 and 26, respectively.

Uses in Ophthalmology

Atropine and related drugs are administered as drops to produce mydriasis and cycloplegia prior to diagnostic examination of the eye. Mydriasis, or a widening of the pupils, is desirable when the retina is being studied for signs of disease. The eye specialist often uses a cycloplegic prior to diagnostic examinations of the eye for the purpose of fitting proper corrective lenses to remedy nearsightedness (myopia) or farsightedness (hyperopia).

Parkinson's Disease

Prior to the introduction of levodopa in the late 1960s, cholinergic blocking agents were the most widely used drugs for the reduction of the tremors and stiffness associated with Parkinson's disease. Success with these agents is modest, since less than half of the cases are substantially improved, and the use of these drugs is limited by a large number of side effects common to this class, including dry mouth, blurred vision, an inability to urinate, confusion, dizziness, and the danger of provoking a glaucoma attack in patients with elevated intraocular pressure.

Motion Sickness

For violent trips of short duration, characterized by vigorous activity, scopolamine has been shown to be effective in averting the nausea and vomiting associated with motion sickness. Several antihistamines are also of value for the prevention of motion sickness. Antihistamines such as dimenhydrinate (Dramamine) are preferred for less vigorous trips of longer duration (Chapter 27). At present, the mechanism underlying the actions of these two classes of drugs is obscure.

Nonprescription Sleeping Preparations

Proprietary sleep aids formerly contained scopolamine in combination with an antihistamine. Many of the effects—including excitement, confusion, and hallucinations—observed in suicide attempts with high doses of these agents were the result of scopolamine toxicity. In the late 1970s, the Food and Drug Administration, after careful review of the documented evidence, concluded that scopolamine, at the doses used, was neither safe nor effective for use in nonprescription sleep-facilitating products and withdrew its approval for the inclusion of this drug in such products.

NEUROTOXINS AND CHOLINERGIC TRANSMISSION

Nature has provided us with a rather large number of poisonous compounds whose beneficial and toxic properties may be attributed to effects on cholinergic transmission. In particular, these *neurotoxic agents* act on motor neurons, at the neuromuscular junction, and also at the neuroeffector junction. Some of these agents are used in purified form as experimental tools to better understand nerve conduction and transmission. Sources of such poisons include (but are no means limited to) bacteria, fish, snakes, and plants.

Botulinum Toxin

All too often we are frantically warned by the news media to return a can of soup or vegetables to the market because of reports of botulism resulting from the ingestion of its contents. *Botulism* is a disease that almost always results from eating improperly preserved foods; frequently these foods are bottled in the home. The disease is caused by *botulinum toxin,* an extremely poisonous protein substance released by the bacterium *Clostridium botulinum.* Type A toxin is the most toxic substance known to man; 1mg (1/30,000 oz) is capable of killing 20 million mice! Botulism has a mortality rate of about 65 percent in humans. It is characterized by visual disturbances, muscular weakness, respiratory paralysis, and eventual death. The toxin acts by preventing the release of acetylcholine from all cholinergic nerve endings, thus preventing transmission of the nerve impulse to muscles and, in particular, those required for breathing.

Tetrodotoxin and Saxitoxin

The dangers associated with ingestion of selected parts of the puffer fish were appreciated by the ancient Egyptians (2700 B.C.) and Chinese (200 B.C.). Among the more illustrious near-victims were Ian Fleming's secret agent, James Bond (007), and Captain James Cook. Cook described his epicurean disaster in a journal recounting his second voyage around the world. He and Mr. Forster, the ship's naturalist, ate the liver and roe (fish eggs) of the unfamiliar fish in New Caledonia in 1774.

About three to four o'clock in the morning, we were seized with most extraordinary weakness in all our limbs attended with numbness of sensation like to that caused by exposing one's hands and feet to a fire after having been pinched much by frost. I had almost lost the sense of feeling nor could I distinguish between light and heavy objects, a quart potfull of water and a feather was the same in my hand. We each took a vomit and after that a sweat which gave great relief. In the morning, one of the pigs which had eaten the entrails was found dead.[3]

Tetrodotoxin, the puffer fish poison, is the same as tarichatoxin, a poison obtained from egg clusters of a California salamander. The action of tetrodotoxin is similar to that of local anesthetics such as procaine and cocaine but nearly 100,000 times more active. Tetrodotoxin acts on the outside surface of cell membranes of sensory and motor nerve fibers blocking sodium pores. This interferes with the movement of sodium into the nerve and thereby prevents the generation of an action potential. As a consequence, conduction along nerve fibers is blocked, resulting in a loss of sensation and paralysis of voluntary muscles.

Saxitoxin, a neurotoxin isolated from the Alaskan butter clam, is the causative agent of paralytic shellfish poisoning, which in turn is associated with the red tides of the west coast of North America. The *red tide* is the outward manifestation of a massive bloom of a dinoflagellate (algae), *Gonyaulax catenella,* which synthesizes the toxin. The appearance of a red tide occurs when the algae count exceeds 20,000 cells/ml, while the infested shellfish becomes too toxic for human consumption at counts of only 100–200 cells/ml. The potency, mechanism of action, and symptoms of saxitoxin and tetrodotoxin toxicity are similar, namely, progressive muscle paralysis with death resulting from respiratory failure.

In 1568 the French naturalist Jacques Grevin ascribed a divine rationale for the existence of poisonous fish in *De Venenins:* "He who oversees everything also created very many poisonous fish, and in this way he punishes those who seek them."

Venoms

While the terms *venomous* and *poisonous* are generally used interchangeably, a distinction should be made between these terms. A *venomous animal* has a secretory gland or group of highly specialized secretory cells, sometimes (but not always) a venom duct, and a structure for delivering the venom, such as a sting, spine, jaw, tooth, or fang. *Poisonous animals* are those whose tissues, in part or in their entirety, are toxic. Thus, all venomous animals are poisonous but not all poisonous animals are venomous.

Poisonous or venomous animals are found in almost every phylum. Representative venomous animals are listed in Table 8–2. Although the venom of some animals may produce adverse effects that are primarily exhibited on one

[3] J. Cook, *Journal of Captain James Cook on His Voyages of Discovery,* 2nd ed., ed. J. C. Beaghehole (London: Cambridge University Press, 1961), pp. 534–35.

TABLE 8-2. REPRESENTATIVE VENOMOUS ANIMALS

Classification	Animals	Primary Clinical Symptons
Marine organisms		
Coelenterates (Cnidaria)	Fire or stinging coral	Inflammation, extreme pain, respiratory distress, collapse, death from cardiac arrest
	Portuguese man-of-war	
	Jellyfish	
Molluscs	Cones	Muscle weakness, respiratory paralysis*
Fish	Stingrays	Cardiovascular toxicity, cardiac arrest*
	Scorpion fish	
	Weeverfish	
Arthropods		
Insects	Bees	Pain, inflammation, cardiac arrest in sensitized individuals*
	Wasps	
	Yellow jackets	
	Hornets	
	Fire ants	Extreme pain
Spiders	Scorpions	Skeletal muscle weakness, respiratory arrest*
	Black widow spiders	Muscle spasms*
	Tarantulas	Red blood cell destruction (hemolysis), internal bleeding
	Ticks	Muscle weakness and paralysis (tick paralysis)*
Snakes		
Elapids	Kraits	Primarily neurotoxic effects including blockade of nerve conduction, neuromuscular transmission, and direct effects on skeletal muscle; respiratory failure*
	Cobras	
	Eastern coral snakes	
Crotalids	Rattlesnakes	Severe internal bleeding, cardiovascular collapse, shock*
	Copperheads	
Viperids	Russell's viper	Similar to crotalids*
	Puff adder	
	Jumping viper	
Amphibians		
	Newts	Destruction of red blood cells
	Tree frogs	

*Neurotoxic effects of venom responsible to some degree for observed effects in victims.

system—such as on the nervous system and skeletal muscle (neurotoxins), blood cells (hemotoxins), or the cardiovascular system (cardiotoxins)—it should be noted that venoms are complex mixtures of compounds having several or many biological activities.

Among the numerous compounds identified in the venom of the Southeast Asian krait *Bungarus multicinctus* are two proteins, α-bungarotoxin and β-bungarotoxin. The former irreversibly binds to and blocks the postsynaptic cholinergic (nicotinic) receptor at the neuromuscular junction; this compound produces neuromuscular blockade and skeletal muscle paralysis by a curare-like action (see below). Beta-bungarotoxin prevents the release of acetylcholine from motor nerve endings. These two compounds, isolated as pure chemicals from the elapid venom, are employed as experimental tools in studies designed to investigate the normal physiology of neuromuscular transmission, the mechanisms by which drugs modify neuromuscular function, and disease states (such as myasthenia gravis) which interfere with normal skeletal muscle function.

Coniine

Students of history and philosophy are well acquainted with Socrates' death, after imbibing an extract of *hemlock*. The major toxic compound in this plant is *coniine*, an alkaloid that acts like nicotine. This compound produces paralysis of sensory and motor nerve endings and the central nervous system. Death results from respiratory failure.

A partial description of the toxic effects of hemlock, as experienced by Socrates, is described by his student Plato:[4]

> You [Socrates] have only to drink this, he [Crito] replied, and to walk about until your legs feel heavy, and then lie down, and it will act of itself. . . . And the man who gave the poison began to examine his feet and legs, from time to time: then he pressed his foot hard, and asked if there was any feeling in it, and Socrates said no; and then his legs, and so higher and higher, and showed us that he was cold and stiff. And Socrates felt himself, and said that when it came to his heart, he should be gone . . . the man uncovered him, and his eyes were fixed. Then Crito closed his mouth and his eyes.

Curare

> *The essence of a fruitful experimental approach is the design of relatively simple questions which the research worker can ask of his material in such a way as to yield an answer which is clear, unambiguous, and suggests fresh questions of a similar kind. In the application of this method Claude Bernard was a master.*[5]
>
> —L. Shuster (1962)

[4] Plato, "Phaedo," in *The Trial and Death of Socrates*, ed. E.J. Church, (London: Macmillan, 1896), pp. 211–13.

[5] *Readings in Pharmacology* (Boston: Little, Brown, 1962), p.73.

Curare is among the most widely known and fascinating neurotoxic drugs. Curare-like drugs are widely used to produce skeletal muscle relaxation and paralysis during surgical anesthesia, as well as to prevent the convulsions associated with tetanus. Prior to the introduction of more exotic toxic substances during World War II, curare was among the most commonly employed chemical murder weapons in mystery stories, causing death by respiratory failure.

Curare is a term that refers to crude extracts of the root bark of *Chondodendron* and *Strychnos,* vines ("bushropes") indigenous to the Upper Amazon and Orinoco rivers and regions of nations formerly called the Guianas. The special techniques involved in the preparation of curare was a well-guarded secret entrusted only to the tribal witch doctors. It appears likely that the active principles were extracted in water and that resins and gums were added to permit the product to adhere to the weapon tips.

The first samples of curare were brought back from Guiana to England by Sir Walter Raleigh in 1595. For many centuries prior to his arrival, South American Indians used the dark brown plant extract as an arrow poison in battle and to kill wild animals for food. Two centuries later, during the course of his expedition to South America, the German explorer-scientist Humboldt studied the preparation and field use of this poison. In his published chronicles, he noted that the flesh of animals poisoned by curare could be safely eaten and that wounds made by poisoned arrows could be sucked out without hazard.[6]

In a classic series of studies conducted during the 1840s and 1850s, the brilliant French physiologist Claude Bernard (1813–1878) sought to determine the mechanism by which curare caused skeletal muscle relaxation. In these experiments, he studied the effects of curare on contractions of the gastrocnemius (calf) muscle removed from large frogs. In the absence of curare, direct electrical stimulation of the muscle or of the attached sciatic (motor) nerve caused contractions of the muscle. After exposure to curare, the muscle continued to contract when directly stimulated but failed to respond to nerve stimulation. Bernard then performed experiments establishing that curare did not interfere with the ability of nerve to conduct impulses. On the basis of these studies, he correctly concluded that the failure of the muscle to respond to nerve stimulation was caused by the effects of curare at the site of the nerve-muscle junction.[7] We now know that **d-tubocurarine,** the active constituent in curare, prevents acetylcholine from interacting with and activating cholinergic

---

[6] While curare effectively enters the blood after injection (from the tip of an arrow or dart, for example), it is not absorbed to any appreciable extent after oral administration.

[7] The implications arising from these studies were of far greater significance than the mere discovery of the site of action of curare. They led to an intensive investigation of the nature and function of the junction between nerves and muscles and the manner by which nerve stimulation results in muscle contraction. The search for and discovery of "vagusstoff" by Loewi (Chapter 5) was one of many byproducts arising from Bernard's work.

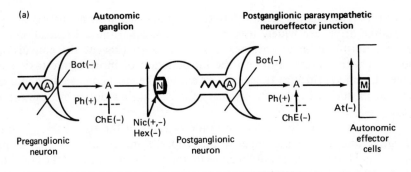

(a) Autonomic ganglion Postganglionic parasympathetic neuroeffector junction

Preganglionic neuron Postganglionic neuron Autonomic effector cells

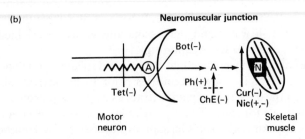

(b) Neuromuscular junction

Motor neuron Skeletal muscle

FIGURE 8–2. Sites of Action of Drugs Altering Cholinergic Transmission. Drugs may act on (a) autonomic or (b) motor cholinergic nerves or at acetylcholine's site of action on effector cells. Acetylcholine (A) activates muscarinic (M) receptor sites, located on autonomic effector cells, and nicotinic (N) receptor sites, located at the autonomic ganglion and neuromuscular junction. Drugs may produce stimulatory (+) or inhibitory (−) effects. Tetrodotoxin (Tet) interrupts the conduction of the nerve impulse (/\/\/\ ) down motor neurons innervating skeletal muscle. Botulinum toxin (Bot) prevents the release of acetylcholine from nerve endings. At all sites, physostigmine (Ph) inhibits the inactivation of acetylcholine by cholinesterase (ChE). Nicotine (Nic) has both stimulatory and inhibitory effects on the autonomic ganglion and neuromuscular junction. Hexamethonium (Hex), atropine (At), and curare (Cur) specifically antagonize acetylcholine at cholinergic receptors located at the autonomic ganglion, postganglionic parasympathetic neuroeffector junction, and neuromuscular junction, respectively.

(nicotinic) receptor sites on the surface of skeletal muscle; neuromuscular paralysis and respiratory failure result.

SUMMARY

Drug interference with the process of cholinergic transmission may be highly desirable for the successful treatment of disease. In other instances we find that the chemical slave of humans becomes their master. There are three anatomically and physiologically different cholinergic receptor sites and different antagonists of acetylcholine at each of these sites.

Atropine, the reference standard for all other antimuscarinic drugs, blocks the cholinergic receptor site at the postganglionic parasympathetic junction. A normal therapeutic dose of this alkaloid inhibits secretions from exocrine glands (dryness of the mouth and inhibition of sweating), reduces the tone and motility of the smooth muscles of the stomach and intestines, and induces mydriasis and cycloplegia of the eye. Higher doses cause marked changes in behavior. Curare blocks acetylcholine at the neuromuscular junction producing skeletal muscle relaxation. Ganglionic blocking agents such as mecamylamine (Inversine) and hexamethonium (Methium) prevent cholinergic transmission at the autonomic ganglia (Chapter 21). Atropine specifically prevents innervation of postganglionic effector organs innervated by cholinergic neurons, while ganglionic blocking agents prevent activation of organs by preganglionic neurons arising from both the sympathetic and parasympathetic divisions. Although these latter drugs have been employed for the treatment of high blood pressure, their therapeutic utility has been limited by the many adverse side effects which result from the relative lack of specificity in their action.

Microorganisms, animals, and plants are all potential sources of neurotoxic agents. Bacterial products (botulinum toxin) and compounds derived from fish (tetrodotoxin from the puffer fish), snakes, insects (venoms), and plants (curare and physostigmine from the ordeal bean) all act by modifying normal cholinergic neurotransmission. Figure 8–2 depicts the site of action for many of these drugs.

SUPPLEMENTARY READINGS

Argov, Z., and F. L. Mastaglia, "Disorders of Neuromuscular Transmission Caused by Drugs," *New England Journal of Medicine* **301**: 409–13 (1979).

Baslow, M. W., *Marine Pharmacology.* Baltimore: Williams & Wilkins, 1969.

Bettini, S., ed., *Arthropod Venoms. Handbook of Experimental Pharmacology.* Vol. 48. New York: Springer-Verlag, 1978.

Brimblecombe, R. W., *Drug Actions on Cholinergic Systems.* Baltimore: University Park Press, 1974.

Bücherl, W., E. E. Buckley, and V. Deulofeu, eds., *Venomous Animals and Their Venoms.* Vols. 1 and 2. New York: Academic Press, 1968 and 1971.

Cheymol, J., ed., *Neuromuscular Blocking and Stimulating Agents. International Encyclopedia of Pharmacology and Therapeutics.* Sec. 14. Oxford: Pergamon Press, 1972.

Covino, B. G., and H. G. Vassallo, *Local Anesthetics: Mechanisms of Action and Clinical Use.* New York: Grune & Stratton, 1976.

Greenblatt, D. J., and R. I. Shader, "Anticholinergics," *New England Journal of Medicine* **288**: 1215–19 (1973).

Habermann, E., "Bee and Wasp Venoms," *Science* **177**: 314–21 (1972).

Lee, C.-Y., ed., *Snake Venoms. Handbook of Experimental Pharmacology.* Vol. 52. New York: Springer-Verlag, 1978.

Rašková, H., ed., *Pharmacology and Toxicology of Naturally-Occurring Toxins. International Encyclopedia of Pharmacology and Therapeutics.* Vols. 1-2, Sec. 71. Oxford: Pergamon Press, 1971.

Simpson, L. L., ed., *Neuropoisons—Their Pathophysiological Actions. Poisons of Animal Origin.* Vol. 1. New York: Plenum Press, 1971.

Zaimis, E., ed., *Neuromuscular Junction. Handbook of Experimental Pharmacology.* Vol. 42. Berlin: Springer-Verlag, 1976.

section three

Drugs Affecting the Central Nervous System

9

Introduction to the Central Nervous System

From the brain, and from the brain only, arise our pleasures, joys, laughter and jests, as well as our sorrows, pains, griefs and tears. . . . It is the same thing that makes us mad or delirious, inspires us with dread or fear, whether by night or by day, brings sleeplessness, inopportune mistakes, aimless anxieties, absent-mindedness, and acts that are contrary to habit.

—Hippocrates (460?–377? B.C.)

The central nervous system consists of the brain and the spinal cord and serves to coordinate and direct the functions of all tissues of the body. Such control enables the organism to adapt by maintaining a relatively constant internal environment (*homeostasis*) in a constantly changing external environment. How is this accomplished?

The peripheral nervous system receives thousands of *sensory inputs* (sight, smell, taste, touch, and sound) and transmits these stimuli to the spinal cord and brain. These latter nervous structures, in particular the brain, are able to process this incoming information. As the result of a highly efficient filtering process, 99 percent of the sensory information received is discarded as being unimportant or irrelevant. After information has been evaluated and deemed pertinent, selected areas of the central nervous system initiate a nerve impulse in motor fibers, which activate an effector organ or tissue to make an appropriate response to promote the best interest of the organism.

The activity and function of the central nervous system is subject to a wide range of chemical influences which are capable of producing a myriad of effects. To illustrate the diversity of these chemicals and effects, let us consider a few examples that will serve as prelude to the third major section of this book. All drugs of abuse and many commonly misused drugs have their primary sites of action in the central nervous system, for example, heroin and other opiates, barbiturates, cocaine, marijuana, alcohol, amphetamine, hallucinogens (LSD, peyote, mescaline), tobacco, and caffeine. Morphine relieves pain and aspirin reduces fever by their actions in the central nervous system. Chronic exposure to mercury and lead adversely affects the brain, and these metals produce behavioral and neurological dysfunctions. Deficiencies of pyridoxine (vitamin B_6) and niacin cause convulsions in infants and pellagra, respectively. In the not too distant past, niacin deficiency was a major cause of severe behavioral aberrations and hospitalization in mental institutions in the southern United States.

When we consider the actions of drugs on the central nervous system it should be strongly emphasized at the outset that in almost all cases drugs act at more than one anatomical and functional site. It should not be necessarily inferred that the drug is differentially concentrated in a particular area of the brain, but rather that some sites are more susceptible than others to the drug. Whereas low doses of a drug may preferentially act at one locus, additional parts of the central nervous system are affected as the dose is progressively increased. Furthermore, because our understanding of the functions of the different regions of the brain is limited and our knowledge of neurotransmitters in the brain is relatively rudimentary, our explanations of the mechanisms of drug action in the central nervous system may be necessarily vague.

To provide some background for the subsequent chapters in this section, let us briefly review the physiological functions of the major areas of the central nervous system. These are shown in Figure 9-1. Although we shall discuss each site separately, we should bear in mind that there are extensive neural connections permitting communication, feedback, and interactions among these sites.

FOREBRAIN

Cerebrum (Cerebral Cortex)

Hawks have keener vision, cheetahs have fleeter feet, and elephants are far more massive and powerful, but humans are the preeminent creatures on earth. A one-pound mass of protoplasm called the **cerebrum,** containing 9 billion neurons, separates us from all other living organisms. The cerebrum is the site of consciousness, the highest neural center for the coordination and interpretation of external events and internal stimuli. Removal of the entire frog cerebrum produces no behavioral changes and this amphibian can see as well as before. By contrast, humans become totally blind, extensively paralyzed and, while they can carry out primitive vegetative functions such as breathing, they soon die.

The cerebral cortex contains sensory, motor, and association areas that receive information; after processing these stimuli, signals are transmitted to appropriate parts of the body along effector neurons. The *sensory* areas of the cortex are concerned with sight, smell, taste, and sound. *Motor* areas are

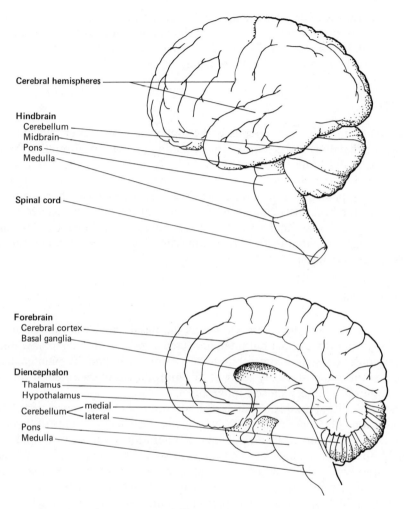

Cerebral hemispheres

Hindbrain
Cerebellum
Midbrain
Pons
Medulla

Spinal cord

Forebrain
Cerebral cortex
Basal ganglia

Diencephalon
Thalamus
Hypothalamus
Cerebellum — medial
          — lateral
Pons
Medulla

FIGURE 9–1. The Human Brain. Top: lateral view; bottom: sagittal section through midline of the brain.

responsible for the direction of all voluntary muscle movements and speech. The most sophisticated portions of the cerebral cortex are the *association areas.* These areas, distributed throughout the cortex, establish relationships from among the many sensory inputs; the cortex collects, interprets, and integrates information transmitted to it from all other parts of the central nervous system. The association areas direct the highest mental activities—namely, memory, learning, reasoning, judgment, imagination, and prudence—that differentiate humans from all other forms of life. Thus, inspired by the most noble intentions or base malice, brilliance or abysmal ignorance, love or hate, we are able to perform voluntary and purposeful acts, as well as refrain from carrying out such deeds.

A wide variety of drugs is capable of directly or indirectly altering cerebral function. These include the stimulants amphetamine and caffeine; the depressants alcohol, barbiturates, and ether; and drugs such as phenytoin (Dilantin), which are used to prevent epileptic seizures.

Thalamus

In lower animals the thalamus is the highest sensory center, whereas in humans the thalamus and cerebral cortex function as a unit. Information from the periphery and brain is relayed to the sensory areas of the cerebral cortex after traversing the thalamus. Crude sensations such as undiscriminating consciousness, pain, pressure, and temperature are interpreted by the thalamus. This part of the brain participates in the emotional responses associated with feelings of pleasantness and unpleasantness. Finally, the thalamus plays an important part in maintaining and regulating the extent of one's consciousness, alertness, and attention.

Basal Ganglia

The region of the forebrain known as the basal ganglia is composed of several anatomically distinct but interconnected structures that direct involuntary (not under conscious control) muscle function, including the maintenance of muscle tone and posture. By contrast, the motor areas of the cerebral cortex take charge of voluntary muscle movements.

Patients with Parkinson's disease have been shown to have very low concentrations of dopamine in the basal ganglia. Deficient amounts of this inhibitory neurotransmitter are associated with alterations in muscle tone and abnormal movements. This neurological disease is characterized by at-rest tremors, rigidity, and difficulties in initiating movement. We have previously discussed the therapeutic use of levodopa to replenish the deficient stores of dopamine in the basal ganglia (Chapter 4). A parkinsonian syndrome is commonly associated with the administration of antipsychotic agents.

Limbic System

Emotions involve both mental and physical elements. That is, we become aware of the sensation, have a desire to act, and finally express our feelings both internally and externally. We have already considered the influence of the autonomic nervous system upon our internally manifested emotional responses. The *hypothalamus* and other parts of the *limbic system* are intimately involved with the expression of emotions. The limbic system consists of about one dozen structures that are connected by neurons to each other and also to the cerebrum. Some of the more prominent and better studied components of this system are the septal areas, amygdala, and hippocampus. After a brief mention of these structures we shall discuss the functions of the hypothalamus in some detail.

The *septal areas* of the limbic system exert an inhibitory influence on the hypothalamus and reticular activating system (see below), as well as modify behavioral arousal and emotions. The *amygdala* receives neural signals from all parts of the limbic system and transmits impulses to the cortex, hippocampus, and hypothalamus. Hypothalamic activity is enhanced by the amygdala. Memory and emotional behavior are influenced by the *hippocampus.*

Hypothalamus

Although the hypothalamus occupies a relatively small area of the total brain, its influence on normal body physiology and behavior is colossal. In Chapter 5 we discussed the hypothalamus as the major site responsible for the central control of both the sympathetic and parasympathetic divisions of the autonomic nervous system. The hypothalamus also influences many vegetative functions, that is, those activities of the body essential for the maintenance of life. These functions include regulation of the cardiovascular system (blood pressure and heart rate), maintenance of body temperature and body water content (influencing both water consumption and excretion), and control of feeding behavior, as well as the central control of carbohydrate and fat metabolism. The hypothalamus also modulates the activity of the pituitary gland which in turn controls the activity of endocrine glands.

Among the most fascinating functions of the hypothalamus and limbic system are those involved with the *subjective appreciation of sensations,* that is, whether we consider external stimuli to be pleasant or unpleasant. Among the first to report in this area were James Olds and Neal Miller who made their earliest reports in the 1950s. It was observed that rats with permanently implanted electrodes could be trained to press a lever that would activate an electrical shock to be delivered to specific areas of their brains. When the electrodes were placed in the ventromedial nuclei of the hypothalamus, Olds noted that the rats would respond up to 5000 times an hour for 24 consecutive hours in an attempt to receive a rewarding or pleasurable electrical stimulus. This has been termed approach behavior. Hungry animals continued to self-stimulate themselves rather than take time out to eat. What effects might we observe if the electrodes are inadvertently or purposefully placed in the periventricular structures of the hypothalamus and thalamus? In this instance, the rat would only press the lever once and never again. Stimulation of this aversive region of the brain produces pain or punishment.

The *reward system* is located in the medial forebrain bundle, which consists of a group of nerve fibers connecting the forebrain, midbrain, and hypothalamus. There is considerable experimental evidence to suggest that these structures are innervated by adrenergic neurons; that is, norepinephrine is the neurotransmitter responsible for nerve transmission between neurons (Chapter 6). Drugs capable of causing the release of norepinephrine, or preventing its enzymatic destruction or re-uptake into neurons, or those able to directly activate the adrenergic receptor site are able to increase the rate of self-stimulation when electrodes are placed in the reward center. Drugs that deplete the brain of norepinephrine or block norepinephrine at its receptor sites depress the rate of self-stimulation. Thus, amphetamine and cocaine enhance the rate of bar pressing leading to electrical self-stimulation, while reserpine (a norepinephrine depleter) and chlorpromazine (a blocker) depress this rate.

The *punishment center* is under the influence of cholinergic neurons (Chapter 7). Hence, cholinomimetic agents such as carbachol or physostigmine enhance behavioral responses that promote the avoidance of punished behavior. As we might expect, cholinergic blocking agents, atropine for one, disrupt behavior that would normally prevent punishment. This same atropine-like response has been observed after administration of the antianxiety drugs, for example, antianxiety agents such as meprobamate and the benzodiazepine derivatives (chlordiazepoxide).

It would be tempting to extrapolate from these animal studies to humans and hypothesize that our motivated behavior is influenced by similar reward and punishment centers. When the human reward center is in fact stimulated electrically, the subjects report feeling more relaxed. Conversely, activation of the punishment regions evokes sensations ranging from fear to terror. These two centers may function reciprocally, so that stimulation of the reward system may simultaneously inhibit the punishment system.

Psychosomatic Disorders

> *A bodily disease, which we look upon as whole and entire within itself, may, after all, be but a symptom of some ailment in the spiritual part.*[1]
>
> —Nathaniel Hawthorne (1850)

Periodically, we all observe the strong influence of our emotions upon physiological function. How did you feel the last time you were subjected to some stressful situation, for example, an important job interview, or getting ready to give an oral presentation to your class and hostile professor on a topic for which you were inadequately prepared? When we are faced with such unpleasant predicaments, our hearts may beat somewhat faster than normal, our stomachs feel as if they were being used as trampolines, our palms and underarms get wet, and our mouths become dry.

It has been estimated that of all the patients who call upon a general medical practitioner, one-third have no actual organic pathologic change that explains their illness. In another equal number of patients the symptoms complained of are totally out of proportion or cannot be explained by the organic

---

[1] *The Scarlet Letter.*

disease discovered. Thus, although such patients (constituting about two-thirds of all patients) may come to their physician with very real physical symptoms of disease, psychic factors frequently play a causative or contributory role in these conditions. Some such typical diseases include peptic ulcers, ulcerative colitis, bronchial asthma, various skin reactions, hay fever, high blood pressure, menstrual disorders, headache, muscle cramps, and so forth.

Some of these diseases can be better understood by looking at the influence of the hypothalamus on peripheral tissues. The hypothalamus provides the central control of autonomic nervous system function, skeletal muscle activity, and also release of hormonal secretions from the adrenal cortex and thyroid gland, among other endocrine glands. Some of the consequences of unpleasant emotional sensations as mediated by the hypothalamus are outlined in Figure 9–2.

An understanding of the influence of psychic factors on the actually observable physical symptoms of disease helps us to appreciate the importance of the placebo (Chapter 3) and the psychoactive agents. This latter category of drugs, to be discussed in the subsequent chapters of this section, include narcotic and nonnarcotic drugs for the relief of pain, sedatives, tranquilizers, and antidepressants.

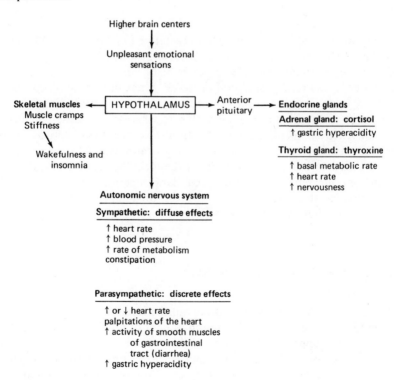

FIGURE 9–2. Psychosomatic Disorders: Influence of Emotional Factors on the Origin of Physical Symptoms.

HINDBRAIN

The cerebellum, medulla, pons, and midbrain are the four structures comprising the hindbrain or brain stem. We shall only concern ourselves with the first two.

Cerebellum

The cerebellum is responsible for coordinating the fine movements of our voluntary muscles throughout the body, permitting us to perform smooth and accurate body movements. The cerebellum modulates neural impulses arising from the motor areas of the cerebral cortex, basal ganglia, and spinal cortex that are involved with voluntary movements. In conjunction with the cerebrum and vestibular system of the inner ear, posture and body equilibrium are maintained. Drugs that interfere with the function of the cerebellum cause a loss of balance, dizziness, and uncoordinated jerky movements.

Medulla

Many of the body's most essential vegetative functions are controlled by the medulla. The *respiratory* center and those concerned with *heart rate* and *blood pressure* are frequently referred to as being *vital,* because destruction of these sites generally results in a fatal outcome. Many depressant drugs, having their primary site of action at the cerebrum and other forebrain sites, have secondary toxic effects on the medulla. Hence, whereas low doses of alcohol, general anesthetics, morphine, and barbiturates act therapeutically by modifying the activity of forebrain areas, high doses cause death by depressing the respiratory and cardiovascular centers in the medulla. In addition, the *cough and vomiting centers* are found in the medulla. Coughing and vomiting are two related activities that are controlled by the medulla and that involve the participation of the respiratory muscles.

RETICULAR ACTIVATING SYSTEM

We have already discussed the ability of the cerebral cortex to receive sensory stimuli, to evaluate this information in light of previous experiences, and then to initiate an appropriate response. When we are asleep such sensory information is not consciously perceived, and is, therefore, useless to us. The *ascending reticular activating system* serves to arouse the cortex and maintain a state of consciousness. Direct stimulation of the cortex will not awaken us. The RAS is a diffused network of nerve fibers located in the central portion of the brain stem that travel from the lower medulla to the midbrain. Neurons also maintain two-way communication between the RAS and the cerebral cortex (Figure 9–3).

Depression of the RAS results in sedation and loss of consciousness, while irreversible coma is a consequence of severe injury or destruction of the RAS. It might be inferred that the activity of the RAS is very susceptible to drug-induced influences, and, in fact, such is the case. General anesthetic agents, ether and halothane, for example, sufficiently inhibit the RAS, resulting in the loss of consciousness. Barbiturates depress many areas of the central nervous system; however, we find that the RAS is most susceptible to these drugs. These sedative-hypnotic agents reduce the sensitivity of the RAS to sensory stimuli. By contrast, we observe that amphetamine and the endogenous catecholamines are able to lower the threshold of the RAS to sensory stimulation. Such an action would account for amphetamine's ability to increase alertness, attentiveness, and awareness of the environment. LSD also enhances the susceptibility of the RAS to receiving sensory input; this mechanism apparently differs from that produced by amphetamine.

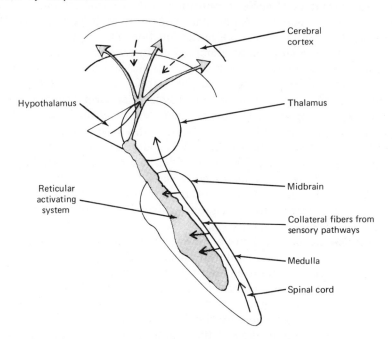

FIGURE 9–3. Arousal of Cerebral Cortex by the Reticular Activating System (RAS).
Neural pathways from the RAS are responsible for activating the cortex. In turn the cortex sends messages back to the RAS.

SPINAL CORD

The spinal cord serves as a conduit for the transfer of information between the peripheral nerves and the brain. That is, ascending nerves transmit sensory impulses up the spinal cord, whereas descending tracts send instructions to effector cells via motor fibers. Simple reflex functions such as the familiar knee jerk are controlled solely by the spinal cord, as well as those reflexes concerned with locomotion and the male sexual act of ejaculation. Muscular activity is also modulated by the spinal cord.

CHEMICAL TRANSMISSION IN THE CENTRAL NERVOUS SYSTEM

How do drugs modify normal or abnormal behavior? Perhaps a more fundamental question to pose is what are the factors responsible for abnormal behavior? For about one-quarter of a century, biologically oriented scientific investigators have actively sought to find these answers by examining the chemical mediators of nerve transmission in the central nervous system.[2]

It has been suggested that mental disease may be the consequence of some irregularity in normal neurotransmitter function. That is, too much X, or too little Y, or the formation of an abnormal neurotransmitter Z may be the cause of schizophrenia, anxiety, mania, or depression. Consider a logical corollary. If neurotransmitters are required for normal behavior and aberrations in these endogenous chemicals are responsible for abnormal behavior, might we not attempt to explain drug-induced changes in behavior in terms of a drug-neurotransmitter interaction? The pursuit of this avenue of research has been greatly retarded by an inadequate understanding of chemical transmission in the central nervous system. The pieces of this puzzle are slowly fitting into place, giving us a glimpse of the final picture here and only an outline there.

Positive identification of neurotransmitters in the central nervous system has proved far more abstruse than were similar efforts in the peripheral nervous system (Chapter 5). What criteria must a compound meet before being seriously considered a chemical mediator of nerve transmission? (1) The suspected neurotransmitter should be nonuniformly distributed throughout the brain nerve endings. (2) The enzymes required for the synthesis and inactivation of the neurotransmitter must also be differentially located to parallel high and low concentrations of the chemical mediator: (3) If the neurotransmitter is responsible for regulating behavior, we should observe alterations in behavior with changes in the concentration of the neurotransmitter. (4) Strong supportive

---

[2] The author is aware of strong arguments suggesting that abnormal behavior may result from the learning of inappropriate responses and that the successful treatment of mental illness should revolve about a relearning process. Nevertheless, most of our attention will be focused upon biological factors.

TABLE 9-1. SCOREBOARD OF EVIDENCE SUPPORTING SELECTED SUSPECTED NEUROTRANSMITTERS IN THE CENTRAL NERVOUS SYSTEM

Criteria	Acetylcholine	Norepinephrine	Dopamine	Serotonin (5-Hydroxy-tryptamine)	Gamma-amino-butyric acid (GABA)	Glycine
Uneven distribution	+	+	+	+	+	+ (spinal cord)
Enzymes-synthesis	+	+	+	+	+	+
Enzymes-inactivation	+	+	+	+	+	Uptake
Presence in nerve endings	+	+	+	+	+	+ (?)
Release demonstrated	+	+	+	+	+	+ (?)
Changes in neuronal activity after local administration	+	+	+	+	+	+
Proposed physiological/pathological function	NT-Renshaw cell of spinal cord Levels of activation of the cortex Extrapyramidal system—activation Water intake Learning and memory	Manic-depression Emotions RAS activity Food intake Body temperature	Motor activity (Parkinson's disease) Psychoses Secretion of hormones from anterior pituitary gland (prolactin)	Biological rhythms (pineal gland—melatonin) Sleep Body temperature Emotions	Inhibitory NT	Inhibitory NT in spinal cord
Drugs whose effects are attributed to neurotransmitter interaction	Oxotremorine DFP Physostigmine	Chlorpromazine Reserpine Amphetamine Cocaine Antidepressants (desipramine, tranylcypromine)	Levodopa Chlorpromazine Apomorphine Bromocriptine Amphetamine	LSD p-Chlorophenylala-nine (synthesis of serotonin) Reserpine (?) MAO inhibitors Imipramine	Diazepam Vitamine B_6 (pyridoxine) Thiosemicarbazide (convulsant) Anticonvulsants	Strychnine
Drug antagonists	Atropine Scopolamine Ditran	Chlorpromazine Dibenamine Yohimbine	Chlorpromazine Haloperidol	Methysergide	Bicuculline Picrotoxin	Strychnine

Note: Great restraint should be exercised in reading this table, because many of the entries (especially the proposed physiological and pathological functions) are not accepted by all (or, in some instances, even by most) investigators.

evidence is also provided by detecting the release of the suspected neuro-transmitter after nerve stimulation and (5) by demonstrating neurotransmitter-induced changes in the activity of single nerve cells after local administration of this chemical.

Table 9-1 summarizes some evidence suggesting that acetylcholine, nor-epinephrine, dopamine, serotonin, gamma-aminobutyric acid (GABA), and glycine are neurotransmitters in the central nervous system. The opioid peptides (endorphins and enkephalins) are discussed in Chapter 13. We shall return to a consideration of some of these chemical mediators in subsequent chapters in this section. The interested reader should consult the references at the end of the chapter for a comprehensive consideration of this subject.

SUMMARY

The central nervous system receives sensory messages signaling changes in the external or internal environment, interprets this information in terms of previous experiences, and initiates an appropriate response. Drugs are capable of favorably or unfavorably modifying these processes.

Just as drugs cause behavioral aberrations, the imbalance of endogenous compounds may also be a cause of behavioral and neurological disease. Con-duction and transmission of nervous impulses require the movement of ions, neurotransmitters, and sufficient raw material to supply energy and rebuild cells. Excessive or deficient quantities of such biologically essential compounds, even one such compound, can prove disastrous.

The disease phenylketonuria, resulting from an inborn or genetically deter-mined error of the metabolism of the amino acid phenylalanine, illustrates this principle. With apologies to George Herbert:

> For want of a normal gene the enzyme was lost,
> For want of an enzyme the metabolism was lost,
> For want of the metabolism the brain function was lost,
> For want of the brain function the intellect was lost,
> For want of the intellect the child was lost.

From the discussion in this chapter, it should not necessarily be concluded that the defective neurotransmitter or chemical is present throughout the entire brain. Just as we have observed that a drug may preferentially affect one brain part or, more precisely, a selected group of neurons in one part of the brain, so might a defective endogenous compound. The very extensive degree of direct and indirect interconnections and interrelationships among the neurons of the brain often cause drug effects at one site to reverberate throughout the rest of the brain and body.

In the following chapters of this section, we shall consider drugs capable of enhancing or depressing the functions of the central nervous system, as well as initiating or supressing abnormal behavior.

SUPPLEMENTARY READINGS

"The Brain," *Scientific American* **241** (3): 44–232 (1979).

Carpenter, M. B., *Human Neuroanatomy*. 7th ed. Baltimore: Williams & Wilkins, 1976.

Cooper, J. R., F. E. Bloom, and R. H. Roth, *The Biochemical Basis of Neuropharmacology*. 3rd ed. New York: Oxford University Press, 1978.

Eccles, J. C., *The Understanding of the Brain*. New York: McGraw-Hill, 1973.

Krnjević, K., "Chemical Nature of Synaptic Transmission in Vertebrates," *Physiological Reviews* **54**: 418–540 (1974).

Kuhar, M. J., and S. F. Atweh, "Distribution of Some Suspected Neurotransmitters in the Central Nervous System," *Reviews of Neuroscience* **3**: 35–76 (1978).

Lipton, M. A., A. DiMascio, and K. E. Killam, eds., *Psychopharmacology—A Generation of Progress*. New York: Raven Press, 1978.

Montcastle, V. B., ed., *Medical Physiology*. 15th ed., Vol. 1. St. Louis: C. V. Mosby, 1974.

Siegel, G. J., R. W. Albers, R. Katzman, and B. W. Agranoff, eds., *Basic Neurochemistry*. 2nd ed. Boston: Little, Brown, 1976.

Snyder, S. H., "Brain Peptides as Neurotransmitters," *Science* **209**: 976-83 (1980).

10

Drug Abuse
in Today's Society

As scientists involved in drug phenomena, we are in somewhat the same dilemma that faced the nuclear physicists who split the atom. We have their example before us, and we should profit by it. No amount of breast-beating and cries of "mea culpa" will put the stopper back on the pill bottle any more than it put the old-fashioned atom together again.

—Stanley F. Yolles (1970)

In common parlance the term addiction ... carries moral implications, without regard to the relative capacity of the drug to induce dependence, or to its relative effects on the individual and society. For example, some crusaders against tobacco apply the term addiction with equal force and stigma to cigarette smokers as to heroin-dependent persons. ... It is a common designation by those in the communications media and public forum who wish to stir the emotions or exploit the spectacular by painting a grim picture of all drug abuse.

—Maurice H. Seevers (1972)

[T]he complete elimination of drug abuse is not a realistic objective. . . . In our modern society, it is unlikely that the drug problem is going to go away no matter how effective our approaches may be. The public is eager to be told that we will solve the problem—that it will go away. . . . the drug abuse problem can be limited; we can achieve realistic and important objectives, but elimination . . . is not . . . one of these.

—Robert L. DuPont (1978)[1]

As we consider the pharmacological effects of drugs that have their primary action in the central nervous system, when applicable we shall discuss

[1] Director, National Institute on Drug Abuse.

the unique characteristics of the use, misuse, and abuse of these drugs. This chapter will present some general concepts concerning the nonmedical use of drugs. After considering an overview of the problem, we shall explore some theories concerning psychological dependence, tolerance, and physical dependence. The chapter concludes with a discussion of the use of drugs in sports and a retrospective and prospective view of drug abuse.

DRUG ABUSE: AN OVERVIEW

Hardly a day passes when the mass media does not include news about drugs and some aspect of their abuse. We read that a heroin ring is smashed in New York City; our government warns that nations who fail to stop the exportation of illicit drugs into this country will face the loss of military and economic aid; an athlete has been disqualified because of use of drugs during athletic competition. Many readers of this book may have been initially interested in learning more about drugs of abuse and subsequently realized that drugs have a profound impact on society in many other ways that are totally unrelated to abuse. It is unfortunate that some individuals think of abuse as being synonymous with drugs and overlook the highly beneficial effects many of these compounds have had on our health and well-being.

> The effects of drug abuse on our countries and our communities are partly determined by the biological action of the chemicals we call "drugs." This biological effect does not depend upon one's age, sex, race, culture, or national origin. This means that no person and no country is immune from drug abuse. Drug abuse is not a unique characteristic of any particular segment of society, any particular geographic region, or any particular nation. It is a global human problem. Certainly demographic, geographic, political, and social factors do influence the levels of drug abuse throughout the world. However, it is important to recognize that none of these factors eliminates drug abuse problems and that epidemic spread of drug abuse is no longer infrequent, even in areas once thought to be safe from drug abuse.[2]

Drug Use, Misuse, and Abuse

What is **drug abuse?** A simple and universally acceptable definition of this term is difficult to obtain. Depending upon our unique orientation, and often colored by our conscious and subconscious biases, we may view drug abuse from medical, sociological, psychological, legal, moral, or philosophical vantage points. One authority defines drug abuse as "the use, usually by self-administration, of *any drug* in a manner that deviates from the approved

[2] R. L. DuPont, "International Challenge of Drug Abuse: A Perspective from the United States," in *The International Challenge of Drug Abuse.* NIDA Research Monograph 19 (Washington, D.C.: U.S. Government Printing Office, 1978), p. 7

medical or social patterns within a given culture." Others view drug abuse as the use of any drug to such an extent that it interferes with the health, economic, or social function of the individual. To many persons, this definition mainly denotes the illicit use of heroin, cocaine, LSD, and marijuana by members of the drug culture.

Drug misuse falls within the boundaries of our broad definition of drug abuse. Drug misuse may be said to occur when drugs are used in the absence of therapeutic or rational considerations, on a routine basis for the management of trivial disorders, or at dosage levels or for periods of time that exceed those generally recommended. We should recognize, however, that the use, misuse, and abuse of drugs lie on a continuum, with grey areas lying at their interphases. Depending upon the patterns of drug usage, a single compound can be placed in any of these three categories. The question of whether a drug is legal or illegal should not, in this author's opinion, confuse the issue. For example, if a physician has prescribed one capsule of a barbiturate for sleep and the patient takes two, is this use or misuse? When an individual smokes one marijuana "joint" at home, is he or she a drug abuser?

The misuse of drugs is far more subtle than flagrant drug abuse, and it is also far more prevalent. Within the purview of drug misuse we may appropriately include: the indiscriminate use of tranquilizers at the first sign of stress; the use of laxatives when one has not had a bowel movement for 24 hours; sharing antibiotics with members of one's family when the common cold appears; and the use of weight-reducing products for months or years in the absence of a positive and continuous loss of weight. The heavy and compulsive cigarette smoker is rarely branded a drug misuser by society, and yet such an individual falls within the limits of our definition. Drug use in sports has aroused the interested concern of many individuals, even those who are totally apathetic to athletic competition. As we shall observe, drug use by athletes may be viewed as use or misuse depending upon the particular situation and perhaps upon our biased loyalty toward the individual competitor or team.

ADDICTION, HABITUATION, AND DEPENDENCE

For many years the terms *addiction* and *habituation* have been loosely and often interchangeably used by the lay person as well as by the scientist. These terms differ with respect to the relative magnitude of the psychological dependence, tolerance, and physical dependence drugs produce after chronic administration, as well as the effects of the chronic usage of these compounds on the individual and society. Table 10–1 summarizes these differences. Some drugs clearly fall into one category or another. Whereas the chronic and continuous use of heroin leads to addiction, the heavy and repeated use of coffee (caffeine) often results in habituation. But what is the appropriate category for cocaine, a drug which produces strong psychological dependence with no tolerance or physical dependence? Amphetamine use results in psychological dependence and tolerance but only questionable physical dependence (Table 10–2).

TABLE 10-1. CHARACTERISTICS DISTINGUISHING ADDICTION AND HABITUATION

Characteristics	Addiction	Habituation
Psychic dependence – need to continue to take the drug	Overwhelming desire or compulsion to obtain the drug by any means	Desire to continue to take the drug
Tolerance – tendency to increase the dose	Generally present	Slight or absent
Physical dependence and abstinence syndrome	Generally present	Absent
Detrimental effects to individual and society	Present	If any, on the individual
Examples	Heroin, alcohol	Marijuana, coffee

In 1964, the World Health Organization's Expert Committee on Addiction-Producing Drugs recognized that their earlier criteria inadequately distinguished addiction and habituation. Moreover, new drugs with unique pharmacological properties appeared on the drug scene which did not appropriately fall into either category. They recommended the abandonment of these older terms and substituted *dependence* as an all-inclusive term. **Drug dependence** may be defined as a *state of psychic or physical dependence, or both, on a drug, resulting from the use of that drug on a periodic or continuous basis.* Furthermore, since the specific characteristics differ for each class of drugs, specific types of drug dependence are described, for example, dependence of the opiate type, the alcohol-barbiturate type, the amphetamine type, the hallucinogen (LSD) type, the *Cannabis* type. This flexible system permits a new drug category to be readily established as new drugs of abuse become recognized.

The general term "dependence" directs our attention to the characteristics common to all drugs of abuse (Table 10–1) and yet clearly differentiates, by an exact description, those specific characteristics that are unique for each drug-dependent state. We should also note that the attempt to fit all drugs of abuse into the rigid compartments of addiction or habituation has had a prejudicial effect on the emotions and attitudes of society regarding the use of certain drugs, as well as the treatment of dependent persons. To some, "addiction" to LSD or marijuana is as dangerous as addiction to heroin. Such misconceptions in part account for equivalent legal penalties for the sale of narcotics, psychomimetics, and marijuana in certain states.

Let us now examine the fundamental characteristics used to describe all types of drug dependence, be it dependence upon a cigarette or upon heroin. These characteristics are psychological dependence, tolerance, and physical

TABLE 10-2. CHARACTERISTICS ASSOCIATED WITH COMMONLY USED AND MISUSED DRUGS

Name	Street Names	Route of Administration	Effects Sought	Psychological Dependence	Tolerance	Physical Dependence
Narcotic analgesics Heroin	H, Horse, Junk, Smack, Harry, Stuff, Scag	Injected or sniffed	Euphoria; relief of mental anguish; prevention of withdrawal symptoms	Marked	Marked	Marked
Morphine	M, White Stuff	Injected or oral				
Barbiturates	Goofballs, Barbs	Oral or injected	Reduction of anxiety and tension; euphoria	Marked	Marked	Marked
Pentobarbital (Nembutal) Amobarbital (Amytal) Secobarbital (Seconal) Secobarbital + Amobarbital (Tuinal)	Yellows, Yellow Jackets Blues, Blue Devils, Blue Heavens Reds, Red Devils, Redbirds Rainbows					
Nonbarbiturate sedative-hypnotics	See Table 11-1	Oral	Reduction of anxiety and tension; euphoria	Marked	Marked	Marked

Alcohol	Booze, Juice	Oral	Reduction of anxiety and tension; euphoria	Marked	Marked	Marked
Amphetamines	See Table 17-1	Oral or injected	Euphoria; alertness	Marked	Marked	Questionable
Cocaine	C, Coke, Flake, Gold Dust, Stardust, Charlie, Candy	Injected or sniffed	Euphoria; intense stimulation	Marked	No	No
Cocaine and heroin	Speed Ball					
Psychotomimetics	See Table 17-1		See Table 17-1	Yes	Yes	No
Marijuana	See Table 17-1		See Table 17-1	Yes	Yes; reverse tolerance	No
Tobacco	Coffin Nail, Fag	Smoked or chewed	Reduction of anxiety and tension	Yes	Yes	Yes
Caffeine		Oral	Mental and physical stimulation	Yes	Yes	Very mild
Glue (toluene)		Inhaled	Euphoria	Yes	No	No

dependence. While psychological dependence is greatly influenced by subjective factors, tolerance and physical dependence are pharmacological phenomena amenable to *objective* analysis and are largely independent of emotional influences. That is, when sufficient amounts of certain drugs are administered repeatedly, drug tolerance and physical dependence will be observed in all persons, regardless of their behavioral state.

Psychological Dependence

Persons who feel that they must continue using a drug to maintain a normal state of well-being are said to be *psychologically (psychically, emotionally) dependent* upon that drug. Some people feel they need a morning cup of coffee or a cigarette. If these drugs are unavailable, the user may become annoyed and somewhat irritable or nervous. In the absence of a sleeping pill, the regular user may have great difficulty in falling asleep. By contrast, the heroin-dependent person or the chronic alcoholic does not simply "need" these drugs but rather has an overwhelming and compulsive desire to obtain them. Daily activities for the heroin user revolve about the drug. This pattern of activity, termed *compulsive drug-seeking behavior,* involves obtaining money, most often by the commission of crimes, evading the police, finding a drug pusher, using the drug, and then returning to the streets several hours later in an attempt to get more money. Hence, we observe that there is a broad spectrum of psychological dependence ranging from "I sure hope Joe has an extra cigarette" to "Don't get in my way, I will stop at nothing to get that drug."

Drug-seeking behavior can be demonstrated in infrahuman species. Monkeys and rats have been trained to perform complex behavioral tasks in order to receive a drug injection as a reward. Schuster and Thompson explain the basis and rationale for conducting such studies:

> The literature regarding the behavioral aspects of drug dependence can most profitably be interpreted within the framework of operant conditioning principles. The fundamental principle underlying operant conditioning is that certain aspects of behavior are controlled by their consequences. Past occurrence of certain behavioral consequences controls the future frequency of recurrence or pattern of behavior or both which produced those consequences. Behavior controlled by its consequences is deemed operant behavior and controlling consequences are reinforcers. A drug serving as a controlling consequence for the operant behavior leading to its administration is, therefore, defined as a reinforcer. The principal goal of the experimental analysis of the behavioral aspects of drug dependence is to determine the biological and environmental variables which modify a drug's reinforcing efficacy, that is, the extent to which a drug is self-administered.[3]

Among the drugs shown to be reinforcers of operant behavior in animals are the opiates, barbiturates, alcohol, stimulants, and nicotine.

[3] C. R. Schuster and T. Thompson, "Self Administration of and Behavioral Dependence on Drugs," *Annual Review of Pharmacology* **9**:483 (1969).

Theories of learning involving operant behavior have been postulated to explain the development of psychological dependence in humans. Let us assume that an individual who is faced with a stressful and anxiety-producing situation discovers his or her anxieties are reduced or eliminated most effectively by a drink or a tranquilizer. When the stress reoccurs, the individual again uses this drug, which has become a reinforcer. In time, drug use continues even in the absence of stress.

Drugs may be repeatedly used because their effects are perceived as good or pleasurable. For example, amphetamines uplift the spirits; this is termed *positive reinforcement* or a *positive pleasure.* Other drugs, such as heroin, erase feelings of frustration or dissatisfaction, and thereby provide a *negative pleasure.*

Three factors contribute to the initial use of drugs for nonmedical purposes and may subsequently contribute to the development of psychological dependence. These strongly interrelated factors are the drug, the individual, and the setting or environment in which the drug is taken.

Drug

The repeated use of some drugs, such as the narcotics, produces physical dependence and a very distressful abstinence syndrome after abrupt cessation of drug administration. To preclude the onset of the abstinence syndrome, the user continues to take these drugs. The cocaine or amphetamine user is not confronted with withdrawal symptoms, but continues using these drugs for the "flash" or euphoric feeling. Others desire the behavioral and perceptual changes produced by marijuana or mescaline. This author once employed an individual who steadfastly contended that he was incapable of doing a good day's work without his morning vitamin capsule.

The magnitude of psychological dependence is directly influenced by the pharmacological properties of the specific drug, the dose employed, the intervals between drug administration, and the duration of drug usage.

Individual

Many individuals begin to use illicit drugs in search of pleasure, out of curiosity, or with the hope that the drug will provide them with a greater insight. Other reasons for the nonmedical use of drugs include enhancement of self-confidence, greater courage, facilitation of self-appraisal, search for religious or mystical experiences, relief of boredom, alleviation of depression, reduction of nervousness, improvement of interactions with the opposite sex, and enhancement of mental and physical performance.

Setting

For some, drugs are perceived as solvents that are capable of dissolving mental pains associated with society's misery, injustice, loneliness, frustration, and interpersonal conflicts. Drugs transform their thoughts from insoluble worldly problems to an ethereal setting.

> Widespread criticism of . . . modern social structure is pervasively encountered among drug users. Although such criticism has been encountered in every generation, young people of our time speak with a greater sense of urgency, convinced that human survival is at stake. Much of the criticism is coupled with a search for a new society free of middle-class values which are seen as competitive, aggressive, materialistic, and acquisitive. They speak with undisguised anxiety about rapidly advancing technological change, with genuine foreboding about pollution, racism, nuclear power, over-population and the general aggressive-competitive, middle-class lockstep life directed toward security and affluence at the expense of humanistic concerns.[4]

Initial drug usage is also strongly influenced by group identification and peer group pressures. Individuals who are uncertain about their identity often attempt to conform to the mores of their friends. Nonconformity with the group, they fear, may result in alienation and rejection.

Tolerance

Many of you may recall the profound effects of your first smoke or alcoholic beverage. With repeated use of these compounds, the intensity of the initially experienced effects diminished. A similar reduction in pharmacological response is observed after the repeated use of many drugs, a phenomenon called *tolerance*. In order to maintain the drug's original quantitative effects, it is necessary for the user to continuously elevate the dose employed.

Tolerance is not an all-or-none phenomenon; that is, it may develop to some of the drug's effects, while not to others. Moreover, when it develops, tolerance may only partially reduce the magnitude of a drug's effect, but not eliminate it. For example, tolerance develops to morphine's sedative and respiratory-depressing effects, thus markedly elevating the normal lethal dose, yet morphine-induced pinpoint pupils and constipation continue. Chronic administration of the barbiturates and alcohol results in tolerance to the sedation produced by moderate amounts of these drugs, but it does not substantially elevate the lethal dose.

As tolerance is developing to the individual drug being repeatedly used, simultaneously, *cross-tolerance* is being established to other compounds in the

---

[4] E. Lipinski, "Motivation in Drug Misuse," *Journal of the American Medical Association* **219**:173 (1972).

same class and even to other compounds in closely related drug classes. Cross-tolerance between two drugs or between two drug classes is generally considered to be highly suggestive of a common mechanism of action. For example, cross-tolerance is observed among narcotic agents, among barbiturate and nonbarbiturate sedative-hypnotics and alcohol, and among certain psychotomimetic agents (LSD, mescaline). We do not, however, see cross-tolerance among these different drug classes.

Mechanisms of Tolerance

Many theories have been proposed which attempt to explain the underlying mechanisms responsible for tolerance. These theories fit into two general categories: dispositional tolerance, involving changes in the manner in which the body handles drugs; and functional tolerance, producing physiological or behavioral adaptations to the presence of the drug. Let us briefly consider each of these theories.

Dispositional tolerance.   The magnitude of drug-induced effects are directly related to the concentration of the drug at the receptor site of drug action. Thus it follows that if this concentration of drug is reduced, the magnitude of the drug effect will also be reduced. Theories predicated upon dispositional tolerance suggest that repeated drug administration may cause changes in the normal absorption, distribution, metabolism, or elimination of drugs so that less drug reaches the site of action. The end result of dispositional tolerance should be the uniform development of tolerance to all the effects of the drug. When, on the other hand, tolerance is acquired to only some of the drug's effects, it is highly unlikely that altered biological disposition is the only mechanism responsible for tolerance.

What general changes in biological disposition might produce tolerance? Less drug may be *absorbed* into the blood from the intestines. Chronic administration of a drug, such as a barbiturate, may cause an increase in the rate of *metabolism* and inactivation of that compound by the drug-metabolizing enzymes in the liver. Alterations may occur in the *distribution* of the drug to its ultimate site of action, for example, an increase in the relative proportion of drug molecules bound to plasma proteins. Finally, the drug may be *excreted* or otherwise eliminated from the body more rapidly.

Functional tolerance.   Theories of dispositional tolerance are based upon changes in the way the body *handles* the drug, either prior to or after reaching the site of drug action. Mechanisms concerning functional tolerance are predicated upon a reduction in the sensitivity of cells, tissues, organs, or systems to the drug after its chronic administration. When viewed at a cellular level, it has been suggested that the *receptor sites* may become less responsive to the action of the drug. Based upon our discussion of drug-receptor interactions (Chapter 2), repeated use of a drug may reduce the number of available unoccupied receptor sites, or reduce the rate at which the drug interacts with the receptor site. Some drugs do not directly interact with a receptor site but rather cause the release of a chemical mediator substance which activates the receptor. Depletion of this chemical mediator after chronic drug administration would also produce tolerance.

Tolerance may also be the consequence of *physiological adaptations* of the individual that serve to counterbalance the effects of the drug. That is, if the initial effect of the drug was an increase in blood pressure, certain cardiovascular responses might be activated that tend to restore blood pressure to its normal level. Individuals might also learn to change their *behavior* or acquire new skills to compensate for deficits produced by the drug, thus enabling them to restore their predrug performance.

Physical Dependence

When we stop taking antihistamines, vitamins, antibiotics, oral contraceptives, aspirins, or most other drugs after weeks or months of continuous daily administration, no adverse effects result that can be attributed to drug withdrawal. However, chronic administration of some drugs, virtually all of which are central nervous system depressants, causes adaptive physiological changes in the individual such that normal tissue function is maintained only in the presence of the drug. The presence of the drug becomes normal, and its absence, abnormal. Viewed simply, we may consider that the body has reset its "normal" control value to a new level, just as you might set the thermostat in your home to 65° instead of 74°.

Abrupt withdrawal of the drug disrupts this readjusted level, resulting in adverse changes in physiological function. These changes are termed the *abstinence syndrome,* and when they can be demonstrated, the individual is said to be physically dependent upon the drug. Administration of that drug, or a compound that shows cross-dependence with the original drug, restores the normal balance and rapidly terminates the abstinence syndrome.

Unequivocal physical dependence has been demonstrated to develop after chronic administration of such central nervous system depressants as the narcotic analgesics, the barbiturate and nonbarbiturate sedative-hypnotics, and alcohol. There is no evidence to suggest that the psychotomimetics, marijuana, cocaine, or glue cause physical dependence. This issue has not been resolved for amphetamine.

Many theories have been proposed which attempt to link drug tolerance and physical dependence. In general, we observe that these drugs initially cause depression of the activity of an organ or physiological function. After chronic administration of the drug, function returns to normal; this we have termed tolerance. Abrupt withdrawal of the drug results in exaggerated or supernormal tissue function, which manifests itself as part of the abstinence syndrome.

DRUG USE IN ATHLETIC COMPETITION

Considerable attention has been focused upon the use of drugs as an artificial means of enhancing athletic performance by humans (amateur and professional) and animals (the horse). Gilbert notes that:

> The notion that some place there is a compound . . . that will automatically convert bronze metals into gold is a general one confined to no one nation, sport or class of competitors. This conviction that there is the athletic equivalent of the philosopher's stone sought by ancient alchemists, and the terrible fear that somebody else may have already found it, is the rationale—or irrationale—behind many of the current athletic drug practices. It is used as a justification by physicians and trainers for prescribing drugs that cannot be justified on conventional medical grounds. . . . It is the reason athletes carry their own little black drug bags, endanger their health, risk their reputations, and break oaths and laws to get and use bizarre pharmaceuticals. It explains the ever-multiplying rumors about records being set and games being won by doped competitors.[5]

Therapeutic and Ergogenic Drugs

Depending upon their intended use, drugs employed by athletes may be classified as therapeutic or ergogenic agents. *Therapeutic* or *restorative drugs* are employed for the treatment of a pathological condition in order to restore health, while *ergogenic* or *additive drugs* are employed to increase physical or mental capacity to enhance athletic performance.

Therapeutic agents are used for the treatment of athletic injuries (abrasions, strains, sprains, dislocations, and fractures), to relieve excessive anxiety or nervousness, and for the management of other medical problems. Drugs used for the relief of pain and discomfort associated with athletic injuries include analgesics (aspirin, codeine), anti-inflammatory agents (aspirin, phenylbutazone [Butazolidin], steroids), local anesthetics (ethyl chloride, procaine [Novocaine], lidocaine [Xylocaine]), muscle relaxants (diazepam [Valium], meprobamate [Equanil]), and proteolytic enzymes. Other medical disorders for which the athlete may receive drug therapy include sunburn, athlete's foot, and swimmer's ear (problems arising directly from practice and competition), respiratory infections, diarrhea and other disturbances of the gastrointestinal tract, and pre-existing conditions such as asthma, diabetes, and epilepsy.

A wide variety of mechanical approaches and nutritional and pharmacological substances have been and continue to be used by athletes seeking to enchance their performance in athletic competition; this use of *ergogenic aids* is

[5] B. Gilbert, "Drugs in Sports. Problems in a Turned-On World," *Sports Illustrated*, p. 72. June 23, 1969.

commonly referred to as *doping*. While some ergogenic aids are effective and their use is subject to universal condemnation in amateur athletics, other aids are undoubtedly of little or no value and improve performance by a placebo mechanism.

Amphetamine is the most widely publicized ergogenic agent; its pharmacological effects have found many useful applications in athletic competition, for example, to increase the aggressiveness and physical performance of football and hockey players, to reduce the fatigue and increase the stamina of runners and cyclists, and to suppress the appetite and facilitate weight loss in boxers and jockeys. Other commonly used ergogenic drugs are the anabolic steroids, testosterone-like compounds intended to increase body weight, muscle mass, and strength. Considerable controversy exists regarding the effectiveness of these drugs.

Use of the following categories of drugs prior to or during competition has been banned by the International Olympic Committee (IOC): psychomotor stimulants (amphetamine-like compounds and cocaine, but not caffeine), sympathomimetic amines (ephedrine and related drugs), miscellaneous central nervous system stimulants (amiphenazole, leptazole [pentylenetetrazol or Metrazol], strychnine), narcotic analgesics (morphine-like compounds), and the anabolic steroids.

Whereas there is general denunciation of the use of ergogenic drugs to artificially elevate amateur athletic performance (and lip service is paid to their proscription in professional athletics such as football), a far more controversial issue involves the use of an ergogenic agent for therapeutic purposes. At the 1972 Olympic Games in Munich, the gold medal winner in the 400-meter freestyle swimming competition was disqualified after his urine was found to contain ephedrine, a drug he was employing to alleviate the respiratory difficulties associated with asthma.

Theoretical Benefits of Drugs in Sports

There are many physical and psychological factors that contribute to success in athletic competition. In order to assess the potential benefits a drug might confer on an athlete, one must first identify those factors influencing performance in that sport. For example, the demands placed upon the individual competitor in golf, in the 100-meter run, and in football are substantially different. While an amphetamine-related stimulant might improve the performance of an athlete on the gridiron, an antianxiety agent might be more beneficial to a golfer. Reversing this choice of drugs, by contrast, might cause a significant deterioration in performance. While it is far beyond the scope of this text to critically evaluate the use and established benefits (if any) obtained from the use of specific drugs in different athletic activities, drugs might theoretically enhance performance on a number of sports-related dimensions.

Hand-foot-eye coordination.   Sports such as golf, archery, tennis, racket-ball, and place kicking in football all require the coordination of muscular activity to visual cues. The use of antianxiety agents prior to or during the event might reduce tension and thus enhance coordination.

Expenditure of energy stores.   In sports involving massive expenditures of energy and maximum oxygen consumption such as cycling and long distance running, heart stimulants, vasodilators, and oxygen carriers have been used. Stimulants have been employed to reduce feelings of fatigue and increase alertness.

Aggressive behavior.   Sports involving extensive and intensive physical contact, pain, aggressive behavior, and the need for feelings of supreme self-confidence include football, hockey, and soccer; amphetamine and cocaine purportedly improve performance in these sports.

Reaction time.   Activities placing a great premium upon rapid responses to ever-changing environmental differences include auto and motorcycle racing, alpine skiing, and boxing. Amphetamine, caffeine, and other stimulants have been reported to enhance the rate of reaction response.

Muscle mass.   In competitions such as weight lifting and throwing where there is a strong relationship between muscle mass and strength, the use of anabolic steroids is not uncommon. These drugs are sometimes employed by female athletes.

Menstrual cycle.   The use of appropriate hormones (such as estrogen-progestin-containing oral contraceptives) can be employed by female athletes to regulate the onset of their menstrual period. Moreover, analgesic agents and diuretics are often employed to control pain and fluid accumulation during the menstrual cycle.

DRUG ABUSE: IN RETROSPECT AND IN PROSPECT

Regardless of our markedly divergent formal training and philosophical outlook and with the exception of a few controversial areas, it is relatively simple for us to agree upon the contents of an outline defining the specific characteristics associated with different drug-dependent states. However, it would probably be far more difficult for us to agree upon the underlying causes of drug abuse, the most appropriate treatment for an individual, and what measures can be taken to prevent more persons from abusing drugs. Our answers to these problems significantly differ depending upon whether we choose to view the nontherapeutic use of drugs medically, psychosocially, or morally.

Let us consider heroin dependence from each of these three positions. An advocate of the *medical* view would state that the heroin addict is a patient suffering from a chronic disease having an undetermined, preexisting cause. Treatment involves drug withdrawal, with the possible use of methadone. If we adopt a *psychosocial* position, we consider the addict to be an individual suffering from a preexisting personality disorder and one who may be the innocent victim of social injustice. Treatment objectives include the psychological, social, and vocational rehabilitation of the addict, as well as an overall attempt to correct the underlying detrimental social factors. Finally, the *moralist* views the addict as a wrongdoer or criminal who must personally assume the responsibility for his or her drug-dependent state. Incarceration and abrupt drug abstinence or "cold turkey" withdrawal without the benefit of methadone are generally considered to be the most appropriate "treatments."

Thus, we can appreciate the quandary among individuals who view heroin dependence as a disease, as a byproduct of society with its inherent shortcomings, or as a crime. This author finds it difficult to accept the premise that the nonmedical use of drugs is a criminal act, regardless of whether the drug is a legal or illicit compound. History has repeatedly shown us that jailing the alcoholic or heroin addict has not altered the course of these problems for the individual or society.

Vigorous debate has been generated as to whether an individual should be permitted to freely use drugs, as long as no one else is injured as a consequence. Does your fundamental right to use your body supersede society's obligation to protect you from harming yourself or society's right to protect itself from the necessity of supporting an unproductive individual? Moreover, should the masses be denied the use of a drug in an attempt to protect a few who will abuse this compound if it becomes readily available? Some individuals are apparently eager to self-administer *any* drug, on an empirical basis, in search of a unique behavioral effect. A better fundamental understanding of the interacting psychological and social factors leading to a heavy drug involvement is essential to the development of a rational approach to modifying or preventing such drug-using behavior and effectively treating such individuals. It seems unlikely, however, that the nonmedical use of drugs will cease to exist even if our imperfect society is transformed into a utopia.

SUMMARY

All types of drug-taking behavior may be viewed as a spectrum ranging from medical use, to misuse, to abuse. Whereas some drug-taking situations are easy to categorize objectively, others are influenced by our background and biases. The use of drugs in athletic competition serves as a contemporary example of this conflict.

Since 1964, the term *dependence* has been preferred to the older designation of *addiction* and *habituation*. Drug-dependent states are described in terms of the relative tendency to produce psychological dependence, tolerance, and physical dependence. A summary of the distinguishing characteristics of common drugs of abuse and misuse was presented in Table 10–2.

Individuals are said to be psychologically dependent on a drug when they feel that they need that compound to maintain a state of well-being. This state is influenced by the interrelated factors of the drug, the drug user, and the environment or setting.

Tolerance is a term used to describe a reduction in pharmacological effect after repeated drug administration. This phenomenon may be the consequence of an alteration in the manner in which the body handles the drug (dispositional tolerance), resulting in a reduction in the concentration of drug reaching its site of action; or the result of functional tolerance, where the body makes appropriate physiological or behavioral adaptations to compensate for the drug's effects.

Physical dependence is said to have developed when the body requires the drug to maintain normal physiological function. Withdrawal of the drug precipitates an abstinence syndrome which can be promptly terminated by administering the same drug or a related compound. Theories have been proposed that attempt to explain concurrent development of drug tolerance and physical dependence; however, these two phenomena do not always both occur with a given drug (for example, amphetamine).

Drug abuse may be viewed as a medical, psychosocial, or moral problem. This author believes that the solution to the problem requires multidisciplinary cooperation and more effective educational efforts to permit individuals to evaluate both the benefits derived from drugs and their potential dangers.

SUPPLEMENTARY READINGS

Brecher, E. M., and the Editors of Consumers Reports, *Licit and Illicit Drugs.* Mt. Vernon, N.Y.: Consumers Union, 1972.

Dupont, R. L., A. Goldstein, and J. O'Donnell, eds., *Handbook on Drug Abuse.* Washington, D.C.: U.S. Government Printing Office, 1979.

Jaffe, J. H., "Drug Addiction and Drug Abuse," in *Goodman and Gilman's The Pharmacological Basis of Therapeutics.* Edited by A. G. Gilman, L. S. Goodman, and A. Gilman. 6th ed., Chap. 23, pp. 535-84. New York: Macmillan, 1980.

Kalant, H., A. E. LeBlanc, and R. J. Gibbins, "Tolerance to and Dependence on Some Non-Opiate Psychotropic Drugs," *Pharmacological Reviews* **23**: 135–91 (1971).

Krasnegor, N. A., ed., *Behavioral Analysis and Treatment of Substance Abuse.* NIDA Research Monograph 25. Washington, D.C.: U.S. Government Printing Office, 1979.

Lettieri, D. J., M. Sayers, H. W. Pearson, eds., *Theories on Drug Abuse. Selected Contemporary Perspectives.* NIDA Research Monograph 30. Washington, D.C.: U.S. Government Printing Office, 1980.

Mulé, S. J., and H. Brill, eds., *Chemical and Biological Aspects of Drug Dependence.* Cleveland, Ohio: Chemical Rubber Co. Press, 1972.

Pradhan, S. N., and S. N. Dutta, eds., *Drug Abuse: Clinical and Basic Aspects.* St. Louis: C.V. Mosby, 1977.

Richter, R. W., *Medical Aspects of Drug Abuse.* New York: Harper & Row, 1975.

Vesell, E. S., and M. C. Braude, eds., "Interactions of Drugs of Abuse," *Annals of the New York Academy of Sciences* **281**:1–489 (1976).

Williams, M. H., *Drugs and Athletic Performance.* Springfield, Ill.: Charles C Thomas, 1974.

11

Sedative-Hypnotic and Antiepileptic Agents

It appears that every man's insomnia is as different from his neighbor's as are their daytime hopes and aspirations.

—F. Scott Fitzgerald (1896–1940)

Not poppy, nor mandragora,
Nor all the drowsy syrups of the world,
Shall ever medicine thee to that sweet sleep
Which thou ow'dst yesterday.[1]

—William Shakespeare (1604)

Central nervous system depressants are among the most widely used class of therapeutic agents and include a great number of drugs subject to misuse and abuse. Within the general classification of central nervous system depressants are the sedative-hypnotics (barbiturates), antiepileptic agents, tranquilizers (antianxiety and antipsychotic agents), narcotic analgesics (morphine), and the general anesthetics (ether); this subdivision of depressants is predicated upon their therapeutic applications. We shall observe that, depending upon the dosage employed, any single drug in this class may produce varying degrees of depression ranging from slight drowsiness to profound coma and even death (Figure 11–1). This dose-response phenomenon has best been studied with respect to the general anesthetic agents used in surgery.

In this chapter we shall focus our attention upon the general anesthetics, barbiturate and nonbarbiturate sedative-hypnotics (drugs used to relieve anxiety or induce sleep), and the antiepileptics. Subsequent chapters of this section will discuss other central nervous system depressants.

[1] Othello, act 3, scene 3.

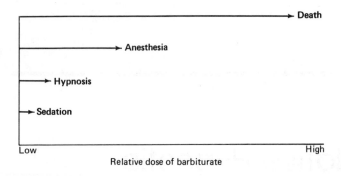

FIGURE 11-1. Relative Degree of Depression Produced by Increasing Doses of a Typical Barbiturate.

GENERAL ANESTHETICS

The discovery of general anesthetics represents one of the most significant contributions of pharmacology to the practice of medicine. Prior to 1846 and the first public demonstration of ether's anesthetic[2] properties, opium and alcohol were the only drugs available for the relief of pain during surgery. General anesthetic agents produce muscle relaxation, loss of consciousness and pain (analgesia), with minimal depression of respiration and cardiovascular functions (blood pressure and heart rate). Moreover, anesthesia prevents emotional distress by abolishing the patient's perception of aversive external stimuli associated with surgical procedures.

The magnitude of central nervous system depression is directly proportional to the dose of anesthetic used. At the lowest concentrations, the reticular activating system[3] is depressed, producing analgesia and loss of consciousness. As the higher cortical centers become depressed, a second stage of anesthesia ensues, characterized by delirium, excitement, and increased motor activity. The *third stage,* that of **surgical anesthesia,** is manifested by loss of muscle tone and complete muscle relaxation, and is the consequence of depression of the midbrain and spinal cord. Further increases in the concentration of the anesthetic agent progressively paralyze the cardiovascular and respiratory centers of the medulla, resulting in a drop in blood pressure, a rapid and abnormal heart beat, and respiratory depression and death. As might be surmised, the level of anesthesia produced in the early phase of the third stage is most useful during most types of surgery.

On the basis of their physical properties, general anesthetic agents fall into two major categories: inhalation and nonvolatile. **Inhalation** types include *volatile liquids* such as ether, chloroform, and halothane (Fluothane), and *gases*

---

[2] Anesthesia denotes without sensation or feeling.

[3] The physiological functions of the different parts of the central nervous system are discussed in Chapter 9.

such as cyclopropane and nitrous oxide ("laughing gas"). **Nonvolatile** anesthetics include the intravenously administered barbiturate thiopental (Pentothal). The general anesthetics listed and other members of this class have their own distinctive advantages and disadvantages, but almost all have adverse effects on the respiratory and cardiovascular systems in high doses.

Abuse of Inhalants

A large number of heterogeneous *volatile solvents* and chemicals employed as propellants in aerosol cans are inhaled by some individuals to produce an inebriated condition. These compounds are chemically and pharmacologically similar to alcohol, ether, and chloroform. Benzene, toluene, naphtha, carbon tetrachloride, acetone, methyl ethyl ketone, and the Freons are examples of only a fraction of the chemicals inhaled from airplane glues,[4] lighter fluids, gasoline, paint and lacquer thinners, varnish removers, cleaning fluids, refrigerants, and aerosols.

The population of individuals abusing inhalants is generally more homogeneous than that using other classes of abused substances. The typical user is a male in his early teens from a socioeconomically disadvantaged background. Reports of the faddish but transitory use of inhalants in group settings among middle-class youths in communities throughout the United States are not uncommon. Heavy inhalant users generally abandon this habit in their middle or late teens; solvent sniffing by adults is somewhat unusual.

Inhalation of fumes to produce an altered state of consciousness has its origins in antiquity. The Oracle of Delphi, an ancient Greek priestess, proclaimed her prophetic messages while in a trance-like state elicited by inhalation of carbon dioxide. Many a nineteenth-century college student, in search of mirth, participated in ether frolics, chloroform jags, and laughing gas demonstrations. After attending a public demonstration of the effects of nitrous oxide[5] for which he paid 25 cents, the Hartford, Connecticut dentist Horace Wells was inspired to employ this gas to achieve the painless extraction of teeth.

The inhalant user generally puts the cleaning fluid (carbon tetrachloride) or airplane glue (toluene) in a bag, holds the bag over his nose, and deeply inhales the fumes. Initial effects include an alcohol-like euphoria, ringing in the ears, double vision, and, occasionally, hallucinations; speech is slurred and

---

[4] Among the varied approaches taken to deal with the abuse of airplane glue (toluene) is to incorporate synthetic oil of mustard (allyl isothiocyanate) in commercial products in amounts that will not interfere with model toy construction but that will produce nausea if inhaled in high concentrations.

[5] Wells attended the demonstration undoubtedly lured by an advertisement in the December 10, 1844, issue of the *Hartford Courant* which read in part: "THE EFFECT of the GAS is to make those who inhale it either Laugh, Sing, Dance, Speak or Fight, &c., &c., according to the leading trait of their character. They seem to retain consciousness enough not to say or do that which they would have occasion to regret." Quoted in H. R. Raper, *Man Against Pain* (Englewood Cliffs, N.J.: Prentice-Hall, Inc., 1945), p. 70.

coordination becomes impaired, producing a drunk-like stagger. Within 30 to 45 minutes, such an individual falls into a state of stupor or unconsciousness. Overinhalation can produce coma and death as a consequence of depression of the medullary centers controlling breathing and circulation. In addition, carbon tetrachloride is directly toxic to the heart muscle, liver, and kidney. Use of these inhalants on a chronic basis may cause abnormal heart beats, and liver and kidney damage, with possible failure of these organs.

SEDATIVE-HYPNOTICS

Hypnotics *are drugs used to induce a state resembling natural sleep.* In smaller doses, these same drugs have been employed as **sedatives,** *compounds capable of calming the individual, and thereby relieving existing anxiety and tensions.* However, the practice of using these drugs to produce sedation and thereby relieve anxiety is becoming obsolete. As will be noted in Chapter 16, antianxiety agents such as diazepam (Valium) are now available that are more specific and effective than the sedatives in their ability to relieve anxiety and tension; moreover, they cause considerably less generalized depression that impairs the daytime performance of mental and physical activities. Hence, we shall emphasize the *hypnotic* use of the sedative-hypnotic agents.

Based upon the chemical properties of these drugs, they are classified as barbiturates or nonbarbiturates. You will observe that many pharmacological properties are common to both classes of drugs. Several barbiturates are effective antiepileptic agents, and it is therefore appropriate that we also discuss this class of drugs in the present chapter.

Sleep

When the electrical brain waves of normal adults are monitored as they are falling asleep, we can note that sleep consists of two phases: a sleep phase characterized by rapid eye movements (*REM sleep*) and a non-rapid eye movement (NREM) phase. The stages of NREM range progressively from drowsiness to deep sleep (stages 1 to 4).

REM sleep has been demonstrated in all species of mammals and in birds. Humans aroused at a time when their brain waves exhibit the unique characteristics of REM sleep report that they were dreaming. Although its physiological function is not well understood, dreaming appears to be essential. If humans are repeatedly awakened every time they lapse into REM sleep, they become anxious and irritable and, within several days, may exhibit severe behavioral aberrations.

Regular use of therapeutic doses of most hypnotic agents causes suppression of REM sleep. After the chronic use of such drugs is discontinued, the body attempts to catch up for lost REM sleep by increasing the amount of this sleep phase. The "REM rebound" is generally associated with restlessness, vivid nightmares, and more intense insomnia. To counteract these sleep disturbances, the patient commonly turns again to the hypnotic agent leading in time to the development of a drug dependent state. One of the major advantages of the benzodiazepine hypnotics is that these drugs do not appear to significantly suppress REM sleep even when administered on a daily basis for several weeks.

NONBARBITURATES

Nonbarbiturates were employed as sedative-hypnotics several decades prior to the introduction of the barbiturates in the early years of this century. Then, for many years, these older agents were totally eclipsed by the barbiturates. More recently, newer nonbarbiturates have appeared on the clinical scene, ostensibly devoid of undesirable barbiturate properties such as abuse potential and a low margin of safety when taken in excessive doses. Unfortunately, in most cases these tumultuously proclaimed and promoted advantages have proven to be illusionary after extensive clinical drug usage.

Let us now consider some representative nonbarbiturates. These include the bromides and chloral hydrate (which predate the barbiturates), glutethimide, methaqualone, flurazepam, and some nonprescription products. Depending upon the particular compound, the justification for inclusion in this chapter may be therapeutic effectiveness, widespread use, or purely historical interest.

Classical Nonbarbiturates

The classical nonbarbiturates include the bromides and chloral hydrate.

Bromides

As is usual in the history of medicine, the virtues of bromide of potassium were discovered accidentally. The price of iodide of potassium, which is so largely used in the treatment of constitutional syphilis, caused a trial to be made of the bromide in the hope that it might serve as a substitute for the more costly salt. The result showed that the scientific anticipation was totally unfounded, but at the same time, revealed the sedative-anaesthetic and hypnotic virtues of the medicine, and led to its more suitable use in therapeutics, at first in allaying priapism [6] and other forms of sexual excitement, then in hysteria and in hystero-epilepsy, and finally in epilepsy itself.

---

[6] This condition, characterized by a persistent erection of the penis, usually in the absence of sexual arousal, was undoubtedly more embarrassing during the Victorian period of this quotation than in our present, more liberated, era.

Bromide of potassium . . . even when freely used by healthy persons, blunts, or suspends, both sexual desire and power. . . . [It is also effective in preventing] nocturnal seminal emissions, especially as they occur in young men of chaste life and sedentary habits, and in those who have been more or less addicted to self-abuse. . . . It has also been used with excellent results in those cases of hysteroidal excitement which verge on nymphomania.[7]

—A. Stille and J.M. Maisch (1879)

The popularity once enjoyed by the bromides as sedative-hypnotic agents is long past; however, their virtual departure from modern therapeutics should evoke little nostalgic remorse. The irritating properties of bromides in the gastrointestinal tract, with consequent vomiting, is a built-in safeguard against acute poisoning by these drugs. Chronic bromide intoxication, or *bromism*, was not uncommon in earlier years when these drugs were widely used. Among the symptoms of bromism are a skin rash that is indistinguishable from acne, gastrointestinal disturbances, and behavioral and neurological aberrations. These latter effects include motor incoordination, an impairment of memory and thought, hallucinations, delirium, and mania—which have, on occasion, been incorrectly diagnosed as mental disease.

Chloral Hydrate

Chloral hydrate was synthesized in 1832 by the famous chemist Liebig and introduced as a hypnotic agent in 1869. At this time, the competition in the hypnotic market place was very limited, with chloral hydrate's only rivals being alcohol, opium, and *Cannabis* (marijuana, hashish).

$$\begin{array}{c}
\quad\; Cl \;\; H \\
\quad\; | \quad\; | \\
Cl-C-C-OH \\
\quad\; | \quad\; | \\
\quad\; Cl \;\; OH
\end{array}$$

Chloral Hydrate

In the body, chloral hydrate is converted to trichloroethanol, a hypnotic agent. The infamous "Mickey Finn" or "knockout drops" alluded to in movies and mystery novels is prepared by adding chloral hydrate to alcoholic beverages. After an oral dose of 1 or 2 g of chloral hydrate, sleep occurs within 30 minutes and lasts for about four or five hours. Normal therapeutic doses do not produce a hangover, nor do they depress respiration and blood pressure. The major objection to the use of this product is the relatively high incidence of gastric disturbances. Chloral hydrate–induced psychological and physical dependence is relatively rare. The abstinence syndrome resembles that seen after chronic alcohol usage (Chapter 12).

[7] *The National Dispensatory* (Philadelphia: Henry C. Lea, 1879), pp. 1112–14.

Newer Nonbarbiturates

The well-publicized reports of the abuse potential of the barbiturates in the early 1950's served as a powerful impetus for the development of new classes of sedative-hypnotics. Virtually all of these nonbarbiturate compounds have been initially promoted as being nonhabit-forming, as well as having lower toxicity, fewer side effects (hangover), and the capacity to induce a more "natural" sleep than the barbiturates. The early enthusiastic clinical reports have been generally superseded by less emotional, more objective studies showing fewer significant differences between the new wonder sedative-hypnotics and the older barbiturates.

In Table 11-1, we observe that with the exception of the antihistamines and to some extent flurazepam, most of the other nonbarbiturate sedative-hypnotic agents produce a barbiturate-like abstinence syndrome after the abrupt cessation of chronic drug administration. These nonbarbiturates also produce *intoxication,* a general term referring to drowsiness, impairment of normal thought and speech, and motor incoordination, all resulting from high doses of these drugs on an acute or chronic basis. Behavioral signs of intoxication include disorientation, deficiencies in memory, confusion, impaired vision, and wide fluctuations in mood. The abstinence syndrome is characterized by convulsions and psychotic behavior. Let us now consider glutethimide, methaqualone, and flurazepam, three interesting nonbarbiturates employed as hypnotic agents.

Glutethimide

At the time if its introduction in 1954, glutethimide (Doriden) was thought to be devoid of the characteristic barbiturate shortcomings, most notably, abuse potential. Unfortunately, clinical experience over the years has failed to show that this compound has any clearly demonstrable advantages when compared with the barbiturates. Moreover, treatment of acute glutethimide toxicity poses a particularly thorny problem. In an analysis of 68 cases of acute glutethimide poisoning, the mortality rate was 21 percent, four times higher than is generally observed with barbiturates. About 5 g of glutethimide, ten times the usual hypnotic dose, produces severe intoxication; 10 g has a mortality rate of 45 percent. Severe acute drug intoxication is often characterized by recovery with a return to consciousness followed by unanticipated coma and death. Mechanical removal of glutethimide from the body is generally accomplished by means of the artificial kidney (hemodialysis).

In passing, we should point out that there is a close chemical similarity among glutethimide, phenobarbital, and thalidomide. Notwithstanding the structurally similar elements shared by glutethimide and thalidomide, drug-induced fetal abnormalities have not been associated with glutethimide. Different metabolic pathways are responsible for the biotransformation of each

TABLE 11-1. NONBARBITURATES EMPLOYED AS SEDATIVE-HYPNOTIC AGENTS

Primary Classification	Generic Name	Selected Trade Names	Comments*
Sedative-hypnotics	Bromide salts		L-A; rarely used; chronic toxicity
	Chloral hydrate	Noctec	S-A; gastric upset; low abuse potential
	Ethchlorvynol	Placidyl	S-A; P-D
	Ethinamate	Valmid	S-A; P-D
	Flurazepam	Dalmane	Hyp; no REM sleep decrease
	Glutethimide	Doriden, Rolathimide	I-A; P-D; acute poisoning difficult to treat
	Methaqualone	Mequin, Parest, Quaalude, Sopor	S-A; P-D
	Methyprylon	Noludar	S-A; P-D
	Paraldehyde		S-A; offensive odor; low abuse potential
"Minor tranquilizers" (Antianxiety agents)	Meprobamate	Miltown, Equanil	I-A; P-D (best studied)
	Chlordiazepoxide	Librium	Sed; P-D
	Diazepam	Valium	Sed; P-D
	Oxazepam	Serax	Sed
Antihistamine (Sleep aid)	Pyrilamine	Cope, Compoz, Nervine, Nytol, Quiet World, Sleep-Eze, Sominex	Nonprescription ingredient; questionably effective at recommended doses

*Key to abbreviations: S-A, short-acting; I-A, intermediate-acting; L-A, long-acting; Sed, sedative primarily; Hyp, hypnotic primarily; P-D, physical dependence with barbiturate-like withdrawal syndrome well documented.

of these compounds, and it has been suggested that a metabolite of thalidomide is the teratogenic-inducing culprit (Chapter 3).

Phenobarbital   **Glutethimide**   **Thalidomide**

Methaqualone

Lacking the prophetic powers of Delphi (or, more precisely, Cassandra) as late as 1970, one of the authors (M. C. G.) during the course of his basic phar-macology lectures, brushed aside methaqualone as "just another nonbarbiturate not worthy of any special discussion." Since this time, "Sopors" have been among the most widely discussed drugs in this geographic area. Although the local Chamber of Commerce proudly proclaim Columbus [Ohio] to be the "All-American City," among the drug culture it is said to be the "Sopors Capital of the World."[8]

—M. C. Gerald and P. M. Schwirian (1974)

The methaqualone story began in India where it was synthesized as a potential antimalarial agent. Animal studies reported in 1955 revealed that it possessed hypnotic activity. One decade later it was being widely promoted in Great Britain and Western Europe as a safe and effective nonbarbiturate devoid of abuse liability and capable of producing natural sleep. This illusion persisted in the United States until 1973 in spite of an ever-increasing volume of reliable reports from Great Britain and Australia (Mandrax,[9] Melsedin), Germany and other European nations and Japan (Hyminal) documenting methaqualone's strong abuse potential and dangers when taken in acute overdosage.

Methaqualone first appeared on the American scene in 1965 under the trade name of Quaalude. Over the years sales of this product increased steadily and by as much as 360 percent in 1972 making it the sixth most popular sedative-hypnotic in the United States. Eagerness for a piece of a highly lucrative market and the absence of patent protection constraints led to the proliferation of generic equivalents of methaqualone including Sopor, Parest, Optimil, and Somnafac.

Some of the methaqualone that made its way to the street was manufactured by an informal cottage industry employing modest facilities and

---

[8] "Personalities and Attitudes of Nonmedical Users of Methaqualone," *Archives of General Psychiatry* **30**: 530 (1974).

[9] Mandrax, the most famous (notorious) methaqualone-containing compound marketed outside the United States, contains the antihistamine-depressant diphenhydramine (Benadryl).

expending little for quality control. Most, however, was legally manufactured by pharmaceutical companies and then diverted from legal channels of distribution or obtained from pharmacies by legitimate or forged prescriptions. Street acceptance of "ludes" (from Quaalude), "sopors," "sopes," "A/S" (all from Arnar-Stone's Sopor), and the "love drug" were based upon the desire to experience euphoria or an alcohol-like high, achieve relaxation, and/or facilitate sexual interactions via its purported aphrodisiac properties, all in the absence of serious toxicity. Unbeknownst to most nonmedical users was the fact that the world's literature contained reports of 2,825 cases of methaqualone poisoning and 106 suicides from 1960 to March 1973. The avalanche of reports in the scholarly and lay American literature in 1973 describing the dangers associated with the acute toxicity or chronic use of methaqualone and the adverse publicity heaped upon this drug by the mass media lead to the dubious honor of methaqualone being the first drug to be reclassified from an uncontrolled prescription drug to a Schedule II agent;[10] this reclassification has resulted in a substantial reduction (but not elimination) of its use for nonmedical purposes.

Flurazepam

Flurazepam (Dalmane) is a **benzodiazepine** derivative that is chemically related to the very widely used antianxiety agents diazepam (Valium) and chlordiazepoxide (Librium). In 1976 approximately one-half of all prescriptions for hypnotic agents filled in American retail pharmacies were for flurazepam; this drug is not used to produce daytime sedation. While not demonstrated to be clearly superior to other sedative-hypnotics in its ability to induce or maintain sleep, flurazepam does possess a number of significant advantages when compared with barbiturates or other nonbarbiturate sedative-hypnotics.

Repeated administration of this drug on a regular basis does not cause suppression of REM sleep nor is its discontinuation after prolonged usage associated with a significant increase in this sleep pattern; that is, there is no "REM rebound." This drug does, however, reduce the time spent in deep sleep (stage 4); the physiological significance of this observation has not been ascertained.

Unlike other hypnotics, flurazepam has a very high therapeutic index (toxic dose/hypnotic dose). Individuals have survived after the ingestion of massive amounts of this drug, when taken in the absence of other depressants. Tolerance develops much more slowly to the hypnotic effects of flurazepam than to the barbiturates and, unlike the latter drugs, after chronic administration, does not increase the rate of metabolism of coadministered drugs; that is, this benzodiazepine is not an enzyme inducer (Chapter 3). Additional research

---

[10]Drugs classified in Schedule II of the Controlled Substance Act of 1970 are the most rigorously controlled substances with accepted therapeutic usage and include morphine and many related narcotics, cocaine, amphetamine, and many barbiturates.

studies are required to more fully assess the abuse potential of chronically administered flurazepam.

Nonprescription Sleep Aids

In recent years, increasing concern has been expressed about the safety and effectiveness of nonprescription products containing "special calming and tension-relieving ingredients" or others designed to "lull you to sleep naturally." Compoz, promoted in 1973 to be the "largest-selling nonprescription sedative for temporary relief of simple nervous tension," was found to be no more effective than a placebo in a double-blind trial, yet not totally devoid of pharmacological activity—it caused adverse side effects in 38 percent of the patients!

Almost all these proprietary products formerly contained scopolamine and methapyrilene. The anticholinergic *scopolamine* was discontinued when experts deemed it neither safe nor effective at the recommended doses. Moreover, accidental or intentional acute overdosage of Sominex or similar products caused scopolamine-induced fever, hallucinations, and coma.

The antihistamine *methapyrilene* has been used for 25 years in cough, cold, and allergy products and as the most common ingredient in over-the-counter daytime sedatives and sleep aids (Compoz, Cope, Nervine, Nytol, Sleep-Eze, Sominex). At the doses used, this drug was questionably effective in its ability to induce sleep, but capable of producing only drowsiness at best. In June 1979, methapyrilene was voluntarily withdrawn from use when a study by the National Cancer Institute's Clearinghouse on Environmental Carcinogens showed it to be a potent liver cancer-causing agent in rats "with potential human risk." Within weeks of this finding, these proprietary products were reformulated to contain *pyrilamine maleate* or doxylamine succinate, other antihistamines with modest methapyrilene-like depressant activity but devoid of the latter's cancer-causing activity (or so it would seem, at this time).

BARBITURATES

The first useful sedative-hypnotic barbiturate appeared in the clinic in 1903, but their history and rather confusing etymology began in Munich on December 4, 1862 (other sources indicate that the year was 1864). On that day, St. Barbara's Day, the young chemist Adolph von Baeyer entered a tavern to celebrate his successful synthesis of malonylurea. Legend has it that this tavern was a favorite of artillery officers and that St. Barbara was their patron saint. We can readily appreciate the blending of Barbara and urea to give us barbituric acid, or *barbiturates,* as derivatives of this acid are called. We should point out that some authors have suggested that the Barbara alluded to was not Saint Barbara, but rather a barmaid in whom von Baeyer had some romantic or scientific interest. Let us now go to 1903, the year in which the great chemist Emil Fischer[11] and physician Josef von Mering introduced barbital into medicine. Unlike its parent compound, barbituric acid, barbital possessed hypnotic activity. Again, we are faced with an etymological controversy surrounding the derivation of barbital's trade name Veronal. Perhaps the source of this name was the Latin word *verus,* meaning truth, an obvious allusion to barbital as being a true hypnotic; or, perhaps, it refers to the Italian city of Verona, a resting place for von Mering.

Chemistry and Biological Activity

Barbital was widely used for about a decade until the introduction of phenobarbital (Luminal) in 1912. Over 2000 derivatives of barbituric acid have been synthesized over the years, and about one dozen of these are currently used as sedatives, hypnotics, anesthetics, and anticonvulsives. The chemical structures of several representative barbiturates are depicted below. Note that the only differences among these drugs are the dissimilar chemical groupings on carbon 5. Administration of a fixed dose of each barbiturate can produce marked differences in the onset and duration of action among these drugs. Table 11–2 summarizes some of the more frequently employed barbiturates with respect to their time-response patterns. Table 11–2 should be considered in relative terms rather than as an absolute guide. Many physical-chemical variables contribute to the observed differences among these barbiturates, some of which include plasma protein binding, relative distribution to the brain, accumulation in fat depots, and rates of biotransformation, inactivation, and elimination from the body (Chapter 3).

Barbituric Acid   **Phenobarbital**   **Pentobarbital**
                             (Luminal)   **(Nembutal)**

Amobarbital   **Secobarbital**
(Amytal)   **(Seconal)**

[11] Adolph von Baeyer and Emil Fischer independently received the Nobel Prize in Chemistry, although in neither case was it in recognition for their work on barbiturates.

TABLE 11-2. CLASSIFICATION OF BARBITURATES ACCORDING TO ONSET AND DURATION OF ACTION AND THERAPEUTIC USES

Classification Based on Duration of Action	Onset	Duration (Half-life)*	Uses	Representative Examples
Ultrashort	Seconds	Minutes (3-8 hr)	Intravenous anesthesia	Methohexital (Brevital) Thiopental (Pentothal)
Short	20-30 min	3-4 hours (14-42 hr)	Insomnia Preoperative sedation	Pentobarbital (Nembutal) Secobarbital (Seconal)
Intermediate	40-60 min	4-6 hours (14-42 hr)	Insomnia	Amobarbital (Amytal) Butabarbital (Butisol)
Long	1-2 hours	6-12 hours (24-96 hr)	Continuous sedation Anxiety and tension Hypertension Epilepsy	Mephobarbital (Mebaral) Phenobarbital (Luminal)

*The time required for plasma concentrations to be reduced by one-half.

Actions

The barbiturates generally depress most cells of the body, although when employed at therapeutic doses, depression of the central nervous system is the predominant effect observed. This results from the extreme sensitivity of the neurons of the brain to the actions of these drugs. As we have previously indicated, these effects may range from barely perceivable sedation through profound coma and death.

Many diverse mechanisms have been postulated in an attempt to account for the actions of barbiturates. These theories and explanations deal with barbiturate-induced changes in ion movements across the cell membrane; interactions with cholinergic and noncholinergic receptor sites in the brain; impairment of the biochemical reactions in the brain required to provide adequate energy for normal function; and a depression of selected areas of the brain. Among the most susceptible parts of the brain are the multisynaptic pathways of the ascending reticular activating system. Depression of the RAS prevents activation of the cerebral cortex, thereby making the cortex less responsive to the external stimuli of the environment and leading to sedation and sleep.

Therapeutic Uses

Although steadily losing ground to safer benzodiazepines with antianxiety and hypnotic properties, barbiturates continue to be used in conditions when it is desirable to produce depression of the central nervous system (Table 11–2). These drugs are used as *sedatives* in low doses to calm the anxious patient suffering from neurotic disorders or for the hypertensive patient whose mild high blood pressure is partly attributed to nervousness. In somewhat higher doses, the barbiturates are used as *hypnotics* to induce sleep. These drugs are valuable *preoperative sedatives,* providing a restful night's sleep prior to surgery. Ultrashort-acting barbiturates such as thiopental are utilized as surgical anesthetics because of the ease and rapidity with which they induce sleep.

Barbiturates are of value in *psychiatry* in narcoanalysis and narcotherapy. Deep sedation is induced by the intravenous injection of amobarbital (Amytal) or pentobarbital (Nembutal). Inhibitions are suppressed, and the patient becomes relaxed and more receptive to effectively communicating with the physician, thus permitting psychotherapy or the diagnosis of psychiatric conditions to be carried out more expediently.

Selected members of this class have been used as *anticonvulsant* agents to prevent or control seizures associated with tetanus and for strychnine and nicotine poisoning. In addition, as we shall discuss in the last major section of this chapter, selected barbiturates, phenobarbital most notably, are valuable agents for the prevention of grand mal epileptic seizures.

Side Effects and Toxicity

The most common side effects associated with the barbiturates are collectively referred to as "hangover symptoms" the morning after their use. The "hangover" is characterized by motor incoordination, listlessness, prolonged depression, nausea, and emotional disturbances. Certain individuals, especially older patients, may manifest idiosyncratic reactions to barbiturates, and these are characterized by hyperexcitability, bad dreams, delirium, and hallucinations. Skin rashes, spread widely over the trunk and limbs, also may occur.

Whether it be the result of accidental or intentional overdosage, acute barbiturate poisoning represents one of the leading causes of drug-induced toxicity.[12] Consider the statistics from New York City for the period of 1957 to 1963: There were 8,469 cases of barbiturate poisoning, of which 1,165 had a fatal outcome. Of the total cases, about half were suicide attempts and less than one in ten accidental ingestions. Accidental poisonings may result from *automatism,* where the patient after ingesting one or two doses of the barbiturate, still awake, becomes confused and inadvertently takes an overdose. Severe acute toxicity results after ingestion of five to ten times a hypnotic dose; a lethal dose is generally ten to fifteen times the concentration required for a hypnotic effect.

[12] Barbiturate-related suicides and accidental deaths have been decreasing since 1971 at a rate that is comparable to the decline in the number of prescriptions written for these drugs as hypnotic agents. During the first quarter of 1976, barbiturates were implicated in 14.5 percent of all drug-related deaths.

Symptoms of acute barbiturate toxicity include confusion and excitement prior to deep sleep and coma; at this time, respiration becomes very slow and shallow. Death results from depression of the respiratory and cardiovascular centers in the medulla. Treatment includes removal of the unabsorbed drug from the stomach and the maintenance of respiration and circulation. The use of the artificial kidney has been reported to remove the drug 10 to 45 times faster than by normal biological processes. In previous times, central nervous system stimulants (analeptic agents) were extensively used to stimulate respiration (Chapter 15). Many experts now believe that their potential dangers, such as convulsions, outweigh any benefits that they might confer. Investigators in Copenhagen have obtained highly successful results by treating barbiturate poisoning without analeptics but rather by utilizing mechanical support of respiratory functions.

Misuse and Abuse of Barbiturates

The misuse of barbiturate or nonbarbiturate sedative-hypnotics is thought to be extensive. In this context, we consider individuals who have been habitually using these drugs for years to relieve anxiety or combat insomnia. It would be far more rational to determine the underlying basis for these complaints rather than escape from them with drugs.

Abuse

The barbiturate abuser may be arbitrarily considered an individual who takes about five or ten times the usual dose over the course of a day. Let us now consider the consequences associated with such drug usage. Without any further delay, it should be strongly emphasized that barbiturates are unquestionably dangerous drugs when abused. The "barbital habit" was reported in 1905 only two years after the clinical introduction of barbiturates. Whereas society has roundly denounced the opiate and hallucinogen abuser, barbiturate abuse has not received its "fair share" of notoriety. This lack of "bad press" is unfortunate, because their abuse constitutes a far greater danger to the life of the dependent person than most other classes of drugs. The incidence of the abuse of "downs," which include barbiturates and nonbarbiturate sedative-hypnotics and antianxiety agents (meprobamate), exceeds that of the opiates. It has been estimated that between 2.75 and 4.5 million young American adults (18 to 25 years old, the population at greatest risk) nonmedically use sedative-hypnotics, while between 2 and 3.5 million use antianxiety agents for nonmedical purposes.

"Downs" or "goofballs" are taken for a variety of reasons, at different intervals, either alone or simultaneously with other drugs. The opiate-dependent individual may take a barbiturate to enhance the effects of substandard heroin. Such a practice may result in physical dependence to both drug classes. Alcohol and sedative-hypnotic agents exhibit cross-tolerance; some alcoholics employ these drugs to prevent the symptoms of alcohol withdrawal. Patterns of barbiturate abuse may range from weekend bouts of gross intoxication to chronic daily use of large doses. Short-acting barbiturates such as pentobarbital ("yellow jackets") and secobarbital ("red devils") are preferred to such long-acting agents as phenobarbital because of the rapid onset of action of the former.

The consequences of high doses of barbiturates and related sedative-hypnotics closely resemble the effects observed after alcohol intoxication. Users experience a euphoric feeling, reported as being "high," "calm," or "away." They are generally sluggish, both mentally and physically; thoughts, speech, and comprehension come slowly. Memory, judgment, attention span, emotional stability, and motor coordination are all impaired. Gross signs of drug intoxication are characterized by a staggering gait, falling, injury without recognition of its occurrence, paranoid ideas, difficulty in working or in operating a motor vehicle, and impulsive or belligerent behavior. By contrast, heroin induces drowsiness but not marked motor incoordination. In this respect, then, the consequences of high doses of sedative-hypnotics are potentially more hazardous to the individual and society than is opiate abuse.

Physical dependence generally develops after four to six times the average hypnotic dose (400—600 mg) of the barbiturate has been taken daily for several months. This state will probably not evolve when normal therapeutic doses (100 mg) are taken for years, although psychological dependence may be present; that is, the individual feels he or she "needs" the drug to go to sleep.

Significant *tolerance* develops to the intoxicating effects of these drugs permitting the daily ingestion of 1,000 to 2,500 mg. It should be strongly emphasized, however, that *as with alcohol and the nonbarbiturate sedative-hypnotics, the lethal dose of barbiturate agents is not much greater for the chronic user than for the nonuser.* This is in sharp contrast to the narcotics (heroin) where the lethal dose is considerably higher in the addict than in the nonuser. It should be noted that cross-tolerance and cross–physical dependence develops to barbiturate and nonbarbiturate sedative-hypnotics, antianxiety agents, and alcohol.

Minor and major symptoms are associated with the sedative-hypnotic *abstinence syndrome.* About twelve hours after the abrupt withdrawal of drug administration, the dependent person becomes progressively less sedated and appears to be returning to a normal, nonintoxicated state. However, over the next twelve hours, nervousness, weakness, insomnia, nausea, and tremors of the extremities are experienced. Within two or three days the withdrawal symptoms become markedly intensified and are characterized by nausea, vomiting, a drop in blood pressure, extreme weakness, delirium, hyperexcitability, fever, and convulsions. From the fourth through the seventh days, these last four named effects can lead to exhaustion, cardiovascular collapse, and death. Barbiturate withdrawal with convulsions is more dangerous than narcotic withdrawal (Chapter 13). Fatalities have been reported after abrupt withdrawal of barbiturates, meprobamate, and methyprylon. After about the eighth day, the withdrawal symptoms begin to subside, even in the absence of treatment.

Barbiturate withdrawal is extemely dangerous and should be carried out in a hospital where the patient's medical progress can be carefully monitored. In the hospital, sufficient pentobarbital is administered until the patient is mildly intoxicated. Once the patient has been stabilized, the dosage is reduced by 100 mg a day. The time required for complete withdrawal varies depending upon the original stabilizing dose but may generally be consummated in less than two weeks.

EPILEPSY AND ANTIEPILEPTIC AGENTS

Many present-day physicians object to the term "epilepsy" because they do not like to pronounce sentence on a patient by using a word with such unpleasant connotations. The concise Anglo-Saxon "fits" is likewise out of favor. . . . The word "convulsive" centers attention on the worst aspect of the seizure. . . . "Epilepsy" is a deep-rooted word. Its unpleasant implications will not be eradicated by official pronouncement, but only by slow alteration of the connotations of the word.[13]

—William B. and Margaret A. Lennox (1960)

Epilepsy is a neurological disorder requiring the chronic administration of barbiturates or other anticonvulsant drugs for years or even for the remainder of the patient's life.

Epilepsy is not a single disease but rather a symptom. It is a general term referring to brief and periodic episodes characterized by one or more of the following symptoms: a change in the normal state of consciousness; convulsions; a loss of muscle tone; and, sensory or behavioral alterations. These episodes are associated with a sudden and excessive firing of the neurons in the brain. By attaching electrodes to the skull of an epileptic at the time of a seizure, we can detect abnormal electrical brain waves on an electroencephalographic (EEG) recording. The specific pattern of the EEG recording serves to fingerprint the specific type of epilepsy, and such tracings can be used for diagnostic purposes. This is of crucial practical importance, because there are no "broad-spectrum" anticonvulsants useful for suppressing all types of epilep-

[13] *Epilepsy and Related Disorders* (Boston: Little, Brown, 1960), p. 41.

tic seizures. The particular drug selected depends upon the specific type of convulsive disorder. The wrong drug may provoke rather than prevent seizures.

The *antiepileptics* or *anticonvulsants* are drugs that selectively depress the central nervous system, and, in particular, prevent epileptic seizures at dosage levels that do not impair consciousness.

The ignorance, fear, superstition, and inaccurate information surrounding epilepsy is nearly as evident today as it was almost 2500 years ago among Hippocrates' fellow Greeks. Epilepsy is not a rare disorder; indeed it has been estimated that at least one million persons in the United States are currently or have been previously subjected to seizures. It ranks after apoplexy (stroke) as the second most common neurological disorder. Wheras anticonvulsants do not cure this condition, appropriate medication completely suppresses or markedly reduces the incidence of seizures for about 80 percent of the patients.

Historical Background

Among the ancient Greeks, it was generally accepted that the epileptic was possessed by spirits and gods. Hippocrates argued against this concept and attempted to offer a physical explanation, which in modern terms would ascribe a convulsion as resulting from a deficiency in the oxygen supply to the brain. For the next 2000 years, the etiology of epilepsy was variously attributed to supernatural forces, humors, and toxins.

Few of us now accept the notion that supernatural forces are responsible for causing epilepsy, and yet many persons still harbor many misconceptions and fears concerning this disorder. Epilepsy does not shorten life, nor does it cause insanity, nor do epileptics necessarily have subnormal intelligence. One writer goes further and postulates that epilepsy and leadership may be related.[14] He suggests that the "cerebral irritation" leading to seizures may also be a driving force compelling such individuals to work up to or even beyond their normal capacity. Whereas this author cannot accept a direct causal relationship between epilepsy and greatness, it is of interest to point out that some of the most famous and most provocative individuals who have figured in the pages of human history on earth were supposed to have been epileptics. These include the religious leaders Moses, St. Paul, Luther, and Mohammed; the military geniuses Alexander the Great, Julius Caesar, Napoleon, and the Duke of Wellington; the writers and poets Socrates, Dante, Lord Byron, Flaubert, Guy de Maupassant, and Dostoyevsky; and the musicians and painters Beethoven, Berlioz, Paganini, and van Gogh.

---

[14] O. Temkin, *The Falling Sickness: A History of Epilepsy from the Greeks to the Beginnings of Modern Neurology,* 2nd rev. ed. (Baltimore: Johns Hopkins Press, 1971).

Past Treatment of Epilepsy

Medical management of epilepsy for over two millenniums centered upon combating supernatural forces (by prayer or by trephining, the boring of holes in the skull), by avoiding contact with or antagonizing bad humors, or by inactivating toxins. The hot blood of a dying gladiator, the liver obtained from a wolf or vulture, and plants, herbs, and many other rational and irrational treatments were used for the treatment of epilepsy. Until the middle of the nineteenth century, it was generally agreed that the successful management of epileptic seizures lay beyond human reach.

Then, in 1857, Sir Charles Locock, the attending physician for the birth of all Queen Victoria's nine children, suggested potassium bromide for the treatment of epilepsy. Why potassium bromide? We have previously alluded to the therapeutic value of bromides for the management of intemperate sexual preoccupations, both contemplated and attempted. One of the postulated causes of epilepsy at this time was sexual excesses or stresses, such as menstruation. The drug class was obvious—employ an anaphrodisiac such as potassium bromide. Notwithstanding the erroneous reasoning, bromides were widely accepted and remained the principal anticonvulsive agent until 1912. The bromides were effective, but produced excessive drowsiness, gastrointestinal upset, skin rashes, and other symptoms associated with the chronic ingestion of these compounds. For the last 70 years, phenobarbital has been used very successfully for the treatment of grand mal epilepsy. Although phenobarbital also produces some drowsiness, its relatively low incidence of serious side effects marked the end of the extensive use of bromides. The introduction of diphenylhydantoin (Dilantin) in 1938 culminated a long and systematic search for an effective anticonvulsant agent. However, the importance of this drug extends far beyond the mere discovery of a new and effective antiepileptic agent. Diphenylhydantoin was the first drug found to be effective in preventing seizures that did not cause drowsiness. Unlike the bromides and phenobarbital that were found to be effective fortuitously after a clinical trial, diphenylhydantoin was predicted to have anticonvulsant activity prior to its first trial in human subjects, on the basis of laboratory studies conducted in animals.

Classification of Seizures

Seizures may be of unknown origin or "idiopathic," while in other instances we can point to a specific precipitating injury or disease. Some of the known causes include brain tumors, injuries (some at birth), or infections (meningitis, encephalitis, malaria, syphilis, rabies, tetanus), metabolic disturbances, high fever, drugs (Metrazol, strychnine), drug withdrawal after the development of physical dependence (alcohol, barbiturates, nonbarbiturate sedative-hypnotics), and the inadequate supply of oxygen or sugar to the brain.

Epilepsy, we have previously indicated, is not a disease but rather a symptom. Periodically there is an alteration in the state of consciousness, in the absence or presence of convulsions. Seizures may be classified on the basis of gross observations, as well as by unique changes in the patterns of brain waves.

An international classification[15] places the epilepsies into two major categories: partial and generalized seizures. *Partial seizures*, including focal motor and psychomotor (or temporal lobe) seizures originate locally, that is, in one part of the body. *Generalized seizures* are bilaterally symmetric in origin and include tonic-clonic seizures (grand mal), absences (petit mal), and a variety of other seizure types. Patients may experience more than one type of seizure or have mixed seizures on a given occasion.

Tonic-Clonic (Grand Mal) Seizures

Tonic-clonic seizures are the most common type of seizure. Prior to the loss of consciousness, about half of all seizure patients experience an unusual sensory sensation or *aura*. While the patient is unconscious, contraction of the muscles of the back and limbs and then jerking movements of the arms and legs occur, often with loss of bladder and bowel control. The patient regains consciousness several minutes after the onset of an attack, exhausted and with no recollection of the events that have transpired. In a life-threatening condition termed *status epilepticus,* there are a series of consecutive grand mal convulsions, without the intervening restoration of consciousness. This may occur during alcohol and barbiturate withdrawal.

Absences (Petit Mal Seizures)

Petit mal seizures occur most frequently in children and generally disappear after adolescence. These seizures, of 1–30 seconds in duration, do not result in falling but only in a brief lapse in consciousness during which the patient is motionless, exhibits no facial expression, and does not respond to commands.

Focal Seizures

The focal seizure orginates in one part of the body and may or may not spread to the entire body. As long as the seizure is restricted to a specific area of the body, there is no loss of consciousness.

---

[15] H. Gastaut, "Clinical and Electroencephalographical Classification of Epileptic Seizures," *Epilepsia* **11**: 102–13 (1970).

Focal motor or *Jacksonian seizures*[16] may begin with the twitching of the muscles of the fingers and wrist, which then progresses to the elbow, the shoulder, and leg on the same side. *Focal sensory seizures* cause numbness, tingling ("pins-and-needles" feeling), and heaviness of one part of the body, which progressively spreads. In addition to tactile sensations, visual (colors, stars, moving lights), auditory, and olfactory hallucinations are also experienced.

Psychomotor Seizures

. Psychomotor or temporal lobe seizures, extremely variable in nature, are characterized by periods in which consciousness is temporarily clouded, and the patient carries out inappropriate automatic acts or movements. During this period, which lasts about one or two minutes, patients are out of contact with their surroundings and are incapable of effectively communicating or responding to instructions.

General Characteristics of Anticonvulsant Agents

Let us now examine the properties of drugs used for the treatment of epilepsy. The perfect antiepileptic agent would be effective against all types of seizures and act directly at the source of the seizures. Such a drug would be totally effective in suppressing seizures without clouding consciousness or causing any other signs of central nervous system toxicity. Because the drug must be used for many years, it should be devoid of chronic toxicity, tolerance, and physical dependence.

From our previous discussion of seizures, it may be validly inferred that there are marked differences underlying the initiation of each type of seizure. Hence, it is understandable that no single drug is effective for the prevention of all types of seizures, not does any agent meet all of the above-listed criteria.

Anticonvulsive drugs are thought to act by three general mechanisms. These include: (1) an action on nonneuronal cells, such as blood vessels or extracellular electrolytes, thereby indirectly influencing the epileptic focus; (2) a direct effect on the epileptic focus to suppress excessive discharges; and (3) effects on normal neurons that surround the epileptic focus, thus preventing the spread of hyperexcitable discharge to other parts of the motor cortex. Most of the available antiepileptic agents act by this last mechanism.

Table 11-3 lists the commonly used antiepileptic agents. Observe the structural similarity that is common to these different classes of drugs. Let us now briefly examine the general pharmacological properties associated with a prototype drug from each anticonvulsant class.

---

[16] Focal and psychomotor (temporal lobe) seizures are now formally classified as partial seizures with elementary symptomatology and partial seizures with complex symptomatology, respectively.

TABLE 11-3. SELECTED ANTIEPILEPTIC AGENTS

O=C——NH
H₅C₂—C   C=O
(benzene ring)
O=C——NH

Phenobarbital
(Barbiturate)

H
N
C   C=O
(two benzene rings)
O=C——NH

Phenytoin
(Hydantoin)

O
H₃C—C   C=O
H₃C
O=C——N—CH₃

Trimethadione
(Oxazolidine)

Class and Drugs	Selected Trade Names	Seizures*
Barbiturates		
Mephobarbital	Mebaral	TCF
Phenobarbital†	Luminal	TCF
Primidone	Mysoline	TCF, PM
Hydantoins		
Phenytoin†	Dilantin	TCF, PM
Oxazolidine		
Paramethadione	Paradione	A
Trimethadione†	Tridione	A
Succinimides		
Ethosuximide†	Zarontin	A
Methsuximide	Celontin	A
Phensuximide	Milontin	A
Miscellaneous drugs		
Acetazolamide†	Diamox	A
Carbamazepine	Tegretol	TCF, PM
Clonazepam	Clonopin	A
Diazepam †	Valium	SE
Valproic acid	Depakane	PM

*Key to abbreviations: TCF = tonic-clonic (grand mal) and focal seizures; PM = psychomotor seizures; A = absences (petit mal seizures); and SE = status epilepticus.
†Most significant drugs.

Barbiturates

Phenobarbital is the oldest, safest, and most effective drug available for the treatment of tonic-clonic (grand mal) and focal seizures. All barbiturates are capable of suppressing convulsions when administered in sufficiently high doses, yet only a few members of this class have been shown to be satisfactory antiepileptic agents in nonsedative doses. The precise mechanism responsible for phenobarbital's anticonvulsant action is not known, but this drug causes greater depression of the motor areas of the cortex than the sensory areas.

This drug is not useful for absences (petit mal) or psychomotor seizures and may even worsen these conditions. The usual antiepileptic doses (100–200 mg) rarely cause addiction or barbiturate intoxication. Some tolerance and physical dependence have been shown to develop; abrupt drug withdrawal precipitates seizures and even status epilepticus.

Hydantoins

The hydantoin derivatives, such as phenytoin[17] (Dilantin), bear a close chemical similarity to the barbiturates and yet cause only mild sedation when administered at the highest therapeutic doses. Phenytoin is among the most widely used drugs for the treatment of tonic-clonic seizures and is often employed in combination with phenobarbital; it is also useful against psychomotor seizures.

Phenytoin alters the movement of ions across the nerve membrane in a manner that stabilizes the membrane, thereby reducing the tendency of the nerve cell to become excited. In this manner it prevents the spread of hyperexcitability from the epileptic focus to normal motor areas of the cerebral cortex.

There are many adverse side effects associated with the clinical use of phenytoin, although in most instances the benefits derived from the use of this drug clearly outweigh the disadvantages. These undesirable effects are on the central nervous system in the form of nystagmus or rapid involuntary oscillation of the eyeballs, dizziness and double vision; gastrointestinal upset, skin and blood disorders, and hepatitis may also occur. About 20 to 30 percent of all patients experience gingival hyperplasia, an overgrowth of the gums after the chronic administration of phenytoin. This condition, most commonly occurring in young patients, is cosmetically unsightly but does not require the discontinuation of drug therapy. The mechanism responsible for the growth of connective tissue of the gums is not known, but it can be prevented by scrupulous attention to oral hygiene.

Oxazolidines and Succinimides

Trimethadione (Tridione) was originally synthesized as an aspirin substitute; however, its lack of dependable analgesia caused it to be rapidly discarded for this purpose. In 1946, it was the first agent found useful for the suppression of absences (petit mal seizures); it is not effective for the treatment of tonic-clonic seizures. The mechanism of action of this drug is not well understood. Trimethadione causes many serious side effects as well as a high incidence of drowsiness and hemeralopia, a blurring of vision in bright light. The

[17] Phenytoin, formerly designated diphenylhydantoin, is also clinically employed for the treatment of cardiac arrhythmias (Chapter 20).

latter effect is seen in 50 percent of the patients, who report that objects viewed outdoors look as though they are covered with snow.

Ethosuximide (Zarontin) is a succinimide that is considered by many experts to be the drug of choice for the treatment of absences. It is an effective drug that does not cause serious adverse effects.

SUMMARY ――――――――――――――――――――

In this chapter we have considered three types of central nervous system depressants: general anesthetics, sedative-hypnotics, and antiepileptics. At normal therapeutic concentrations, the general anesthetics depress both sensory and motor function, producing analgesia, loss of consciousness, and muscle relaxation. The inhalant hydrocarbons (carbon tetrachloride and toluene) are extremely dangerous drugs of abuse which are pharmacologically related to the volatile anesthetics. The sedative-hypnotic agents depress sensory functions at low doses, motor functions at moderate doses, and vital functions (respiration and cardiovascular activity) at the highest doses. Every year thousands of Americans intentionally or unintentionally demonstrate that severe depression of vital functions is an irreversible pharmacological effect. Antiepileptic agents, unlike the sedative-hypnotics, are not general depressants. These drugs prevent epileptic seizures by primarily depressing the motor areas of the cortex with minimal impairment of consciousness.

We have subdivided sedative-hypnotic agents into two classes, namely, the barbiturates and nonbarbiturates. This distinction is of far greater importance chemically than it is pharmacologically. Thus, we may make some general statements that are equally applicable to both these classes of sedative-hypnotics. We observe that with progressively increasing doses, sedation and antianxiety effects are followed by sleep and the relief of insomnia, which are succeeded by a state of depression not unlike surgical anesthesia from which the patient cannot be awakened. Doubling or tripling this anesthetic dose generally causes death.

While the benzodiazepine derivative flurazepam (Dalmane) is not any more effective than the barbiturate or nonbarbiturate hypnotics in inducing or maintaining sleep, it does enjoy the following advantages: It does not suppress REM sleep nor cause REM rebound after drug withdrawal; it has a very high margin of safety when taken in massive overdosage; tolerance does not readily develop to its hypnotic effects; it is not an enzyme inducer.

Contrary to the original aspirations, most of the nonbarbiturates have been shown to possess side effects and an abuse potential that is very similar to the barbiturates. Misuse of these drugs by anxious individuals, with or without insomnia, is very widespread. Chronic flagrant abuse by individuals taking five to ten times the daily hypnotic dose is not uncommon. Tolerance develops to the intoxicating effects of these drugs, and yet there is no substantial elevation of the lethal dose. Cross-tolerance exists among the barbiturates, nonbarbiturate sedative-hypnotics and alcohol. Physical dependence develops after chronic use of these drugs for several months at daily dosage levels about four to six times the normal hypnotic dose. The withdrawal symptoms associated with these drugs are characterized by delirium and convulsions, and, therefore, withdrawal should always be undertaken under direct medical supervision.

Epilepsy is a collective term referring to the symptoms of many neurological diseases, all characterized by an alteration in normal conscious-ness and a sudden change in brain function. Antiepileptic agents serve as a prominent example of the significant benefits derived from the use of drugs for the treatment of disease; about 80 percent of all epileptics employing these drugs are either seizure-free or have a very marked reduction in the incidence of seizures. In some instances, drugs can be withdrawn after a patient has been seizure-free for several years, while other patients require these agents for the remainder of their lives. Among the safest and most effective drugs are phenobarbital and phenytoin (Dilantin) for tonic-clonic (grand mal) and focal seizures, ethosuximide (Zarontin) for absences (petit mal seizures), primidone (Mysoline) and phenytoin for psychomotor seizures, and diazepam (Valium) for status epilepticus.

SUPPLEMENTARY READINGS

Sleep

Holman, R. B., G. R. Elliott, and J. D. Barchas, "Neuroregulators and Sleep Mechanisms," *Annual Review of Medicine* **26**: 499–520 (1975).

Kales, A., and J. Kales, "Sleep Disorders: Recent Findings in the Diagnosis and Treat-ment of Disturbed Sleep." *Journal of the American Medical Association* **290**: 487–99 (1974).

Williams, R. L., and I. Karacan, eds., *Pharmacology of Sleep.* New York: John Wiley, 1976.

General Anesthetics

Adriani, J., *The Pharmacology of Anesthetic Drugs: A Syllabus for Students and Clini-cians.* 5th ed. Springfield, Ill.: Charles C Thomas, 1970.

DiPalma, J. R., ed. *Drill's Pharmacology in Medicine.* 4th ed., pp. 127–89, 211–24. New York: McGraw-Hill, 1971.

Dripps, R. D., J. E. Echenhoff, and L. D. Vandam, *Introduction to Anesthesia. The Princi-ples of Safe Practice.* 5th ed. Philadelphia: Saunders, 1977.

Eger, E. I., II., *Anesthetic Uptake and Action.* Baltimore: Williams & Wilkins, 1974.

Goodman, L. S., and A. Gilman, eds., *The Pharmacological Basis of Therapeutics.* 5th ed., pp. 53–101. New York: Macmillan, 1975.

Sharp, C. W., and M. L. Brehm, eds., *Review of Inhalants: Euphoria to Dysphoria.* Washington, D.C.: U.S. Department of Health, Education and Welfare, 1977.

Sedative-Hypnotics

Cooper, J. R., ed., *Sedative-Hypnotic Drugs: Risks and Benefits.* Washington, D.C.: U.S. Department of Health, Education and Welfare, 1977.

Gerald, M. C., and P. M. Schwirian, "Nonmedical Use of Methaqualone," *Archives of General Psychiatry* **28:**627–31 (1973).

Hartmann, E., *The Sleeping Pill.* New Haven, Conn.: Yale University Press, 1978.

Harvey, S. C., "Hypnotics and Sedatives," in *Goodman and Gilman's The Pharmacological Basis of Therapeutics.* Edited by A. G. Gilman, L. S. Goodman, and A. Gilman, 6th ed., Chap. 17, pp. 339–75. New York: Macmillan, 1980.

Insight Team of *The Sunday Times* of London, *Suffer the Children: The Story of Thalidomide.* New York: Viking Press, 1979.

Institute of Medicine, *Sleeping Pills, Insomnia, and Medical Practice.* Washington, D.C.: National Academy of Sciences, 1979.

Kagan, F., T. Harwood, and others, eds., *Hypnotics: Methods of Development and Evaluation.* New York: Spectrum Publications, 1975.

Antiepileptic Agents

Aird, R. B., and D. M. Woodbury, *Management of Epilepsy.* Springfield, Ill.: Charles C Thomas, 1974.

Ferriss, G. S., ed., *Treatment of Epilepsy Today.* Oradell, N.J.: Medical Economics, 1978.

Lennox, W. G., and M. A. Lennox, *Epilepsy and Related Disorders.* 2 vols. Boston: Little, Brown, 1960.

Woodbury, D. M., J. K. Penry, and R. P. Schmidt, eds., *Antiepileptic Drugs.* New York: Raven Press, 1972.

12

Alcohol
and Alcoholism

The tranquilizer of greatest value since the early history of man, and which may never become outdated, is alcohol, when administered in moderation. It possesses the distinct advantage of being especially pleasant to the taste buds.

—Nathan Masor (1904–)

We may not be able to quantify the violated quality of life incurred by alcohol abuse and alcoholism, but we know that many tens of millions of individuals and families are directly and indirectly affected by the 9 million persons with alcohol-related problems.

—Merlin K. Duval (1971)

In the past decade considerable attention has been focused upon the general problem of drug abuse and, more particularly, upon the drug abuser and the illegal supplier of abusable compounds. We have become noticeably alarmed by reports of the illicit use of heroin, barbiturates, amphetamine, hallucinogens, and marijuana in our own community. With the possible exception of marijuana, these fears may be well justified.

There is another drug whose use, misuse, and abuse dates back to prehistoric times. Public interest in this compound has been, like the orbits of space satellites, now in apogee, now in perigee. The compound is **alcohol.** In the 1970s, the Federal Government launched an extensive educational effort in an attempt to apprise the citizens of the magnitude of the problem of *alcohol abuse and alcoholism.* This campaign goes far beyond the traditional holiday warnings about the dangers associated with driving while under the influence of alcohol. With the realization that 9 to 10 million Americans are chronic alcohol abusers or alcoholics (7 percent of all individuals 18 years of age and older), we reach the inescapable conclusion that alcohol is the most significant drug of abuse in this country.

Let us now consider an overview of alcoholic beverages and the pharmacology of alcohol. Many of the fundamental pharmacodynamic principles
to be presented (absorption, distribution, metabolism, and elimination) are
worthy of our consideration, because when equipped with this information, we
can better comprehend the effects, both desirable and undesirable, produced by
alcohol. This information will also provide a basis for appreciating how drugs
are used for the treatment of alcoholism.

ALCOHOL AND ALCOHOLIC BEVERAGES: AN OVERVIEW

The general term **alcohol** is used in chemistry to designate a class of compounds that are hydroxy (—OH) derivatives of aliphatic hydrocarbons. There
are many common alcohols—methyl alcohol (methanol or wood alcohol),
isopropyl alcohol, the antifreeze diethylene glycol, and glycerin. In this chapter,
however, when we use the term alcohol without additional qualification, we are
referring specifically to **ethyl alcohol,** a liquid also known as *ethanol,* grain
alcohol, or proof spirit.

The alcoholic content of distilled beverages (whisky, rum, vodka) is
expressed by the designation *proof.* This term originated from the old English
custom of testing the alcoholic content of whisky by pouring it over gunpowder
and igniting it. Only whisky containing in excess of 50 percent alcohol would ig-
nite. Proof is equivalent to twice the alcoholic content by volume; for example,
100 proof whisky contains 50 percent alcohol.

Eight to ten thousand years ago, some of our Stone Age forebears chewed on
some berries. We might imagine that their stomachs became heavy and their
heads light. What happened? All alcoholic beverages arise from the process of
fermentation. In the presence of water, yeasts are able to convert the sugar
(glucose) of plants into alcohol, as depicted by the following chemical reaction.

$$C_6H_{12}O_6 \xrightarrow{\text{+ yeast}} 2C_2H_5OH + 2CO_2$$

Glucose   Alcohol   Carbon
                                          Dioxide

After the accidental discovery of alcohol, the intentional manufacture of
alcoholic beverages was "but a small step for man and a giant leap forward for
mankind." A wide variety of plants have proved to be useful substrates or substances for the action of yeast, and this is reflected by the different types of
beverages used throughout the world. By 3000 B.C. the art of the manufacture
of beer and wine was perfected in Egypt and other parts of the Middle East. The
rise and fall of the art of winemaking in the Mediterranean countries temporally
paralleled the rise and fall of the Roman Empire. Wine temporarily lost favor
and was replaced by mead, which is obtained from honey, and also by simple

beers and wines obtained from the fermentation of wild fruits. The Middle Ages brought a cultural and grape-cultivating renaissance to Europe. After the twelfth century, giant strides were made in perfecting the manufacture of wine, most notably in monasteries.

Nature alone cannot produce spirits or hard liquor by the simple process of fermentation. Yeast will continue to ferment a plant until the alcoholic content reaches about 15 percent. Thereafter, the high concentration of alcohol kills the yeast and fermentation stops. The process of *distillation,* developed in Arabia 300 years earlier, was a great tool for the twelfth-century European alchemist. Distillation was rapidly adapted to produce beverages with higher concentrations of alcohol; while nondistilled beverages do not generally have alcohol concentrations much in excess of 15 percent, distilled products range from 40 to 55 percent. The popularity of hard liquor today bears testimony to the relevancy of this old Arabian discovery. In 1975 in the United States, persons 15 years of age or older imbibed an average of 2.6 gallons of distilled spirits.

PHARMACOLOGY OF ALCOHOL

We shall now consider the pharmacology of alcohol, a compound that has been described by some observers as being "most healthful," while to others "the devil in solution."

Absorption, Distribution, Metabolism, and Excretion

Absorption

After its ingestion, alcohol is rapidly absorbed into the blood stream from the stomach and small intestines. The rate of alcohol absorption can be delayed by the presence of food or milk in the stomach. It is a common observation that when several drinks are taken on an empty stomach, a far more rapid and profound effect is observed than when an equivalent amount of alcohol is imbibed after dinner. On an empty stomach, most of the ingested alcohol is absorbed into the blood within 30 to 60 minutes.

Distribution

Alcohol gains access to all the tissues and fluids of the body. We should point out that the concentrations of alcohol in the brain rapidly approach those levels in the blood because of the very rich blood supply to this organ. This is of obvious significance, because it is the alcohol-induced effects on the brain which are of primary importance when considering the pharmacology of this compound. Alcohol very readily crosses the placental barrier potentially causing the fetal alcohol syndrome (see below).

The uniform distribution of alcohol throughout the body is of very practical legal importance to us. Tests for drunkenness generally involve an analysis of the expired air or the urine for their alcohol content. After appropriate mathematical gymnastics, these values can be converted into blood-alcohol equivalents, which, if sufficiently high, can serve as prima facie evidence that the driver is legally intoxicated.

Metabolism

Between 90 and 98 percent of the total alcohol ingested is ultimately oxidized to carbon dioxide and water, with the release of 7 kilocalories of energy per gram of alcohol (or 200 kcal per oz). These breakdown reactions, carried out primarily in the liver, can be shown to consist of three separate steps.

I.   In the presence of the hydrogen acceptor nicotinamide adenine dinucleotide (NAD),[1] alcohol is reduced to acetaldehyde by the enzyme alcohol dehydrogenase. This reaction is relatively slow and proceeds at a fixed rate,[2] regardless of the amount of alcohol present. The rate at which this reaction occurs determines the speed at which alcohol is removed from the body, and hence this reaction is termed "the rate-limiting step."

$$\text{(I)} \quad \underset{\text{Alcohol}}{CH_3-\underset{\overset{|}{H}}{\overset{\overset{\displaystyle H}{|}}{C}}-OH} + NAD \xrightarrow[\text{dehydrogenase}]{\text{Alcohol}} \underset{\text{Acetaldehyde}}{CH_3\overset{\displaystyle H}{C}=O} \quad NADH^+ + H^+$$

There are many legal, medical, and behavioral reasons why an individual would find it advantageous to hasten the rate of alcohol disappearance from the body. About 60 compounds have been studied in this regard, as have a variety of physical and physiological factors. With the exception of administration of the sugar fructose, most other chemical, physical, and biological attempts to increase the rate of alcohol metabolism have not been successful. Fructose does enhance this rate, but the high doses required, about 100 g (almost ¼ lb), cause nausea and gastric pain. Many intoxicated individuals resort to a breath of fresh air to "clear their head." Notwithstanding strong testimonial evidence attesting to the highly beneficial effects obtained, the improvement reported is purely subjective. Blood alcohol concentrations or alcohol-induced impairment

---

[1] NAD was formerly referred to as diphosphopyridine nucleotide (DPN) or coenzyme I. NADH is reduced NAD.

[2] The following simple, but not recommended, experiment illustrates this point. Let us assume that you have precisely determined the specific rate at which you metabolize alcohol. Most individuals weighing about 150 pounds break down 10 ml or ⅓ oz of alcohol (or about ⅔ oz of whisky) per hour. If you were to consume this amount of alcohol every hour, 24 hours a day for the remainder of your life, you would not become intoxicated. Suppose, as the result of a minor error, you were to take 2 oz of whisky per hour. Within four hours, your blood-alcohol level would be approximately 150 mg%. This means there are 150 mg of alcohol in every 100 ml of blood, a value also expressed as a percent, namely, 0.15%. Levels in excess of 150 mg% constitute legal drunkenness in every state, with most states now setting an upper limit of 100 mg%.

of physical and mental activities are not altered by black coffee, cold air, cold showers, or exercise.

   II.   In the second step in the sequence, acetaldehyde is rapidly converted to acetate, a reaction catalyzed by the enzyme aldehyde dehydrogenase.

$$(II) \qquad \underset{\text{Acetaldehyde}}{CH_3\overset{\displaystyle H}{C}=O} \quad \xrightarrow[\text{dehydrogenase}]{\text{Aldehyde}} \quad \underset{\text{Acetate}}{CH_3COO^-}$$

   Normally, this reaction occurs so rapidly that no acetaldehyde tends to accumulate. Inhibition of this enzyme results in the buildup of acetaldehyde, which is capable of producing extremely distressing adverse effects. We shall return to the consequences of aldehyde dehydrogenase inhibition when we discuss the use of disulfiram (Antabuse) as an alcohol deterrent.

   III.   The acetate formed from acetaldehyde mixes with the acetate derived from other biochemical reactions and undergoes the same ultimate fate; namely, it enters the Krebs cycle and is, many steps later, converted to carbon dioxide and water. Carbon dioxide is removed from the body in the exhaled air.

Excretion

   After the moderate consumption of alcohol, only 2 percent of the total is eliminated from the body without undergoing any chemical change. This value can reach 10 percent when large amounts of alcohol are imbibed. Most unoxidized alcohol is removed from the body in the exhaled air or urine, although smaller amounts are also present in the sweat, tears, and saliva.

Effects of Alcohol on the Central Nervous System

> *What wonders does not wine! It discloses secrets; ratifies and confirms our hopes; thrusts the coward forth to battle; eases the anxious mind of its burden; instructs in arts. Whom has not a cheerful glass made eloquent! Whom not quite free and easy from pinching poverty!*
>
> —Horace (65–8 B.C.)

   Although alcohol is transported to all parts of the body after its ingestion, the effects of this compound on the brain are most evident. The brain is extremely sensitive to the effects of alcohol, even in relatively low concentrations. Contrary to popular belief, the increased activity, laughter, and voluble speech witnessed after modest imbibing of alcoholic beverages is not a consequence of central nervous stimulation. *Alcohol is always a central nervous system depressant.*

   What accounts for the apparent stimulation observed with low concentrations of alcohol and for the depression after higher doses? Some areas of the brain have a lower threshold to alcohol-induced depression than others. That is, those areas of the brain that have been most recently molded as the result of rigorous and extensive education and training are the first to become depressed. Among the most sophisticated of these areas are those concerned with the restraint of natural impulses. Training is so complete that we are often cognitively unaware that these impulses are being suppressed. To a large measure, success in life may depend upon our ability to don a mask that is socially acceptable. By depressing or inhibiting these inhibitory centers of the brain with alcohol, the mask falls and so does self-restraint, producing apparent stimulation.

In small quantities, alcohol produces a feeling of euphoria and good fellowship, with increased, albeit unjustified self-confidence. Larger amounts produce excitement characterized by laughter, loquacity, and lively gesticulation. The face is observed to be hot and flushed, the eyes brighter, and the pulse rate quickened. Coupled with the shattering of the shackles of restraint, alcohol also depresses the reticular activating system, thus interfering with the normal processing of information integration by the cerebral cortex. Thinking ceases to be systematic and tends to become confused and disorganized. Subtle grades of memory, concentration, judgment, and perspective become blunted and then dissipated.

The use of sensitive testing devices has demonstrated slight impairment of motor coordination even at low blood-alcohol levels. With progressively larger amounts of alcohol, movements become uncertain, the walk degenerates into a staggering gait, followed by a total inability to locomote. Table 12–1 summarizes the correlation between blood-alcohol concentrations and behavioral deficits.

The acute toxicity resulting from alcohol ingestion should not be ignored. About one out of every three deaths from alcohol are the result of acute alcoholism. Alcohol is the second leading cause of death from poisons in the United States, closely following carbon monoxide. Fatalities from these two poisons are greater in number than the total of all other poisons. The potential dangers associated with the use of alcohol in combination with other drugs is discussed below.

From our discussion thus far, we may generally conclude that even relatively small amounts of alcohol reduce both mental and physical efficiency. This is contrary to the usual subjective self-evaluation of superior capabilities. We should point out that in selected instances modest alcohol consumption can overcome inhibitions that serve as barriers to the successful performance of certain tasks. For many individuals, alcohol is an effective defroster or catalyst for promoting sexual activities.

A word of caution should be offered to the overly enthusiastic student. Whereas one or two drinks may make lovers more receptive and amorous, five or six drinks will not transform you or your date into Don Juan or Casanova or Aphrodite, Venus, or Lolita. Quite the contrary! Large amounts of alcohol cause a deterioration of sexual performance, a fact well appreciated by Shakespeare:

**TABLE 12-1. CORRELATION OF BLOOD-ALCOHOL CONCENTRATIONS
WITH BEHAVIORAL EFFECTS**

Approximate Intake (ml spirits*)	Blood-Alcohol Levels† mg%	%	Behavioral Effects
	up to 10	up to 0.01	Effects doubtful
Up to 60	10-50	0.01-0.05	Effects slight
60	50	0.05	False sense of well-being; some impairment of vision
60-120	60-100	0.06-0.10	Effects definite, but not pronounced
120	100	0.10	Some impairment of reaction time; motor incoordination; legally considered to "be driving under the influence" in many states
180	150	0.15	Clearly intoxicated; very marked impairment of reaction time; behavioral changes; legally intoxicated in all states
Over 240	Over 200	Over 0.20	Very marked impairment to fatal outcome
240	200	0.20	Emotional instability; physical and mental depression
240-420	200-350	0.20-0.35	Confusion; slurred speech; staggering gait; blackout
360-480	300-400	0.30-0.40	Stupor
420-540	350-450	0.35-0.45	Coma
540-	450-	0.45-	Fatal outcome

Note: Underlined entries are major subdivisions of Table. They describe what effects occur at blood-alcohol levels within that range. Effects not underlined refer to effects observed at specific blood-alcohol levels.

*These approximate volumes of imbibed spirits required to produce the indicated blood levels refer to a 150 lb man. About 30 ml = 1 oz. A "shot" of spirits containing 45 ml or 1.5 oz (40-50% alcohol), a 5 oz glass of wine (12% alcohol), and 16 oz of beer (5% alcohol) all provide 0.75 oz of alcohol.

†mg % = milligrams of alcohol per 100 ml blood; % = grams of alcohol per 100 ml blood. Conversion: % x 1,000 = mg %.

"Lechery, sir, it provokes and unprovokes; it provokes the desire, but it takes away the performance."[3]

Effects of Alcohol on Other Organs and Systems

Although alcohol exerts its most pronounced effects by far on the central nervous system, we should not overlook its influence on other parts of the body. We shall briefly consider some selected actions of alcohol on the cardiovascular

[3] *Macbeth*, act 2, scene 3.

system and kidney at this time and return later to other actions when we consider the health hazards associated with chronic alcoholism.

Cardiovascular System

We have all seen westerns where the familiar frozen cowboy or gold prospector enters the town saloon and orders a shot of whisky, presumably to "defrost" his blood. Does drinking actually warm up our protagonist, or does this scene merely serve as a prelude to the next one where he meets and falls in love with a dance hall beauty?

Alcohol is a peripheral vasodilator which, by widening the blood vessels of the skin, causes flushing and a feeling of warmth. Now, let us play that reel in reverse. What would happen if our movie hero took several drinks prophylactically to fortify himself against the raging elements? A happy Hollywood ending would be far less likely. The body's normal response to cold is vasoconstriction of the surface blood vessels thereby reducing the loss of body heat. Alcohol has the opposite effect, namely, by dilating the blood vessels, body heat is lost. As might be surmised, it is far easier to "freeze to death" when grossly intoxicated than when sober.

Kidney

Some of us have undoubtedly made the personal observation that after drinking two or three bottles of beer the output of urine approaches or even surpasses the intake. Alcohol exerts a very definite diuretic effect. The antidiuretic hormone, vasopressin, secreted by the posterior pituitary gland, is responsible for the conservation of body fluids. Alcohol is able to inhibit the release of this hormone, thus resulting in the enhanced flow of urine. This effect is not sufficiently pronounced to permit the use of alcohol as a diuretic agent for the treatment of edema. The dry mouth experienced the "morning after" may be the result of alcohol-induced cellular dehydration, that is, a loss of intracellular water, rather than a deficit of total body water.

ALCOHOL-DRUG INTERACTIONS

> *The physical and behavioral effects of drugs and alcohol in combination are important considerations . . . whether the patients . . . are occasional or moderate drinkers or chronic alcoholics. Of the 100 most frequently prescribed drugs, more than half contain at least one ingredient known to interact adversely with alcohol. Most adverse effects due to alcohol-drug interactions are accidental, but the medical toll is high, including an estimated 2,500 deaths a year and 47,000 emergency room admissions a year.*[4]
>
> —FDA Drug Bulletin (1979).

[4] "Alcohol-Drug Interactions," *FDA Drug Bulletin* 9(2): 10 (1979).

A variety of potential dangers are associated with the all too frequent use of alcohol in combination with other drugs. While it is beyond the scope of this text to present a detailed catalog of such drugs, or the mechanisms underlying alcohol-drug interactions, it should be noted that problems most commonly occur when alcohol is taken with other drugs possessing central nervous system depressant properties. These drugs include barbiturate and nonbarbiturate sedative-hypnotics, antianxiety agents, some antidepressants, narcotic analgesics, and antihistamines; additive depression results from such combinations (Table 12–2). As a consequence, the ingestion of relatively reasonable volumes of an alcoholic beverage taken with the normal dose of a depressant drug may

TABLE 12-2. POTENTIAL ALCOHOL-DRUG INTERACTIONS

Interacting Drug/Class	Examples	Potential Consequences
Analgesics, nonnarcotic	Aspirin	Gastrointestinal bleeding; reduced blood clotting may lead to hemorrhage.
Antianginal/ antihypertensive agents	Nitroglycerin Methyldopa (Aldomet) Hydralazine (Apresoline) Guanethidine (Ismelin)	Hypotensive effect leading to orthostatic hypotension, faintness, loss of consciousness.
Anticoagulants	Warfarin (Coumadin)	Anticoagulation may lead to hemorrhage.
Anticonvulsants	Phenytoin (Dilantin)	Alcohol speeds metabolism of phenytoin with increased risk of seizures.
Antidepressants, monoamine oxidase inhibitors	Tranylcypromine (Parnate)	Tyramine-containing wines (Chianti) may lead to hypertensive crisis.
Antidiabetic/ hypoglycemic agents	Tolbutamide (Orinase) Chlorpropamide (Diabinese)	Reduction in blood sugar.
Antimicrobial/ anti-infective agents	Chloramphenicol (Chloromycetin) Metronidazole (Flagyl)	Disulfiram (Antabuse)-like reaction.
Central nervous system depressants	Analgesics, narcotics Anesthetics Antianxiety agents Antidepressants, tricyclics Antihistamines Antipsychotic agents Sedative-hypnotics, barbiturates, nonbarbiturates	Increases CNS depression, leading to mental and/or motor impairment, loss of consciousness, impaired respiration, coma, death.

produce profound and often unexpected impairment of mental and physical performance.

Many successful suicides, both accidental and intentional, have been attributed to the combined use of alcohol and a barbiturate. Unlike almost all other classes of central nervous system depressants, *antihistamines* are readily available without direct medical supervision and are extensively used in nonprescription cough, cold, antiallergy, and sleep-facilitating products. If you are in doubt about the relative safety or wisdom associated with taking a given drug with alcohol, consult your physician or pharmacist for advice.

ALCOHOL ABUSE AND ALCOHOLISM

Chronic abuse of alcohol has far-reaching ramifications: It produces a progressive deterioration of physical and mental health, as well as psychological and physical dependence upon alcohol. It may destroy the family unit, resulting in a broken home. It may directly or indirectly lead to one-half of all auto fatalities and homicide victims in a given year. An accountant has reported that alcohol abuse drained the economy of this country of $43 billion in 1975. Prior to examining some of these problems, let us discuss what we mean by alcohol abuse, the patterns of abuse, and the theories attempting to explain the cause(s) of alcoholism.

Patterns of Alcohol Use and Abuse

Approximately one-third of all Americans 18 years of age and over drink alcoholic beverages at least once a week, another third primarily restrict their drinking to special occasions, while the remaining third have always been or are currently abstainers. In 1975 there were an estimated 9.3–10 million problem drinkers[5] or approximately 7 percent of the adult population; an estimated 10 percent of the adult male population and 3 percent of the adult female population are problem drinkers.

There are thought to be an estimated 3.3 million problem drinkers in the 14- to 17-year-old range, one-fifth of the 17 million individuals in this age category. Unlike alcohol abuse in adults, alcohol problems among youths are more likely to be acute rather than chronic and primarily involve driving while intoxicated and belligerence rather than alcohol-induced medical and behavioral illnesses. Nevertheless, there is considerable concern about youthful drinking, since early drinking behavior serves as a predictor of drinking habits in later life.

[5] A *problem drinker* is an individual who drinks alcohol to such an extent or in a manner that results in an alcohol-induced disability; this designation includes but is not limited to alcoholics. U.S. Department of Health, Education and Welfare, *Third Special Report to the U.S. Congress on Alcohol and Health* (Washington, D.C.: 1978).

Special population groups appear to have a higher incidence of problem drinkers than the general population at large. Conservative estimates suggest that 1.5 to 2.25 million adult *women* have alcohol problems. Under 35 years of age, those women who are divorced or separated have the highest incidence of heavy and problem drinking; a higher incidence is also seen in married women under 65 who are working. Problems also occur in the *elderly*; 10 percent of males and 2 percent of females over 60 years are heavy or problem drinkers.

Among all special populations in the United States, *Native Americans* have the highest incidence of alcohol-related problems.

> "Why Indians drink" has been widely addressed by the research literature. The "firewater" myth, that Indians are predisposed genetically to pathological responses to alcohol, has become thoroughly entrenched in folk wisdom despite the lack of any scientific basis for the assertion. Currently, social and cultural explanations for high rates of problems with alcohol are predominant. . . . [Cultural] explanations range from a claim that moderate intoxication is a substitute for lost traditions to the assertion that drunkenness relieves the anxieties and frustrations caused by competition between historical tradition and pressures for integration into the dominant culture.[6]

Among *black* males, the rates of both drinking and heavy drinking are somewhat less than for white males. While a smaller proportion of black females drink than white females (39% versus 51%), of those who drink a higher incidence of heavy drinking is observed in black females (11% versus 4%). The *Spanish-speaking* population is the second largest ethnic minority in the United States. While a lack of homogeneity exists among these people, there is a greater incidence of problem drinking than is observed in the general population, and this has been attributed, at least in part, to acculturation stress.

For many of us, it would be comforting to believe that most alcoholics are skid row derelicts. Such people are often considered to be nameless and faceless rejects of society, with whom we are unable to identify; that bearded, raggedly clothed derelict is nobody we know, or moreover, anyone we care to know. How alarming it is to discover that these skid row residents comprise only 3- to 5 percent of the total alcoholic population in this country. Five percent of the nation's workers are alcoholics, with an equal number of serious alcohol abusers. In short, these people are members of our families, our friends and neighbors, our business associates—individuals with real names and faces, whom we know, and like, and even love.

There is no universal definition of what "alcoholism" is or who is "an alcoholic." Some definitions are based upon the volume consumed or whether intake exceeds that amount considered socially acceptable by members of the community. The American Medical Association defines alcoholism as

> . . . an illness characterized by preoccupation with alcohol and loss of control over its consumption such as to lead usually to intoxication if drinking is begun; by

[6] *Third Special Report to the U.S. Congress on Alcohol and Health*, p. 22.

chronicity; by progression; and by tendency toward relapse. It is typically associated with physical disability and impaired emotional, occupational, and/or social adjustments as a direct consequence of persistent and excessive use of alcohol.[7]

Causes of Alcoholism

Just as we have difficulty in adequately defining alcoholism and are not certain as to whether alcoholism is a specific disease or the symptom of some underlying behavioral disorder (psychopathology), similarly, we do not know the basic cause of this condition. Contemporary theories have been predicated upon biological (physiological-biochemical), psychological, and sociological abnormalities, with no single theory supplying a totally satisfactory answer. Assessment of the relative importance of genetic and family (environmental) factors has proved to be difficult. The available evidence suggests that *genetic* influences are involved but it is not clear how such a predisposition to alcoholism is transmitted. Male children of alcoholic parents are more likely to have a drinking problem.

Dangers of Alcohol Abuse to the Individual and Society

The acute and long-term effects of alcohol consumption serve as one of the most vivid examples of the impact of drugs on the individual and society. Areas of interest in alcohol research transcend the traditional boundaries of the effect of a drug on enzymes, organs, and systems, and even the whole individual. Moreover, investigators with expertise in the social and behavioral sciences are concerned with the interactions of alcoholics with their family units their associates, the community, and the entire nation.

Characteristics of Alcohol Dependence

In this section, we shall consider the characteristics of alcohol dependence and the effects of intemperate chronic alcohol ingestion on the individual's health. Unfortunately, alcoholism is not a personal problem; it directly or indirectly influences all other members of society.

In Chapter 11, we pointed out that there are great similarities between dependence produced by the sedative-hypnotics and by alcohol. Alcohol produces psychological and physical dependence and tolerance. Patterns of alcohol consumption may range from its occasional use to relieve emotional stress; to periodic "spree" drinking, at which time large amounts of alcohol are consumed; to extreme cases where the alcoholic has little or no control over the

---

[7] American Medical Association, *Manual on Alcoholism,* 1968, p. 6.

amounts consumed, or has lost the ability to abstain from alcoholic beverages for even a single day. In this case, abstinence results in withdrawal symptoms.

Not every drinker develops a serious drinking problem. Some drinkers never progress beyond the first stage, namely, occasional drinking to escape or relieve tensions. Ten percent of all adult drinkers are problem drinkers and an additional 26 percent have potential problems.

Psychological Dependence

Whereas many of us think a glass of cold beer might be refreshing on a hot afternoon in July, the alcoholic's desires are far more intensified. Such an individual has an intense craving for alcohol, with a greater concern about how daily activities will interfere with drinking than how drinking will adversely alter the performance of these activities. Alcohol becomes the motivating force and perhaps the only interest in life. Family, friends, and business are relegated to subordinate roles.

Tolerance

It has been appreciated for hundreds of years that the chronic drinker can readily consume amounts of alcohol that would severely intoxicate the occasional drinker. We may account for this observation by one of two very general mechanisms. First "dispositional tolerance" may develop, which results in changes in the rates at which alcohol is absorbed, distributed, metabolized, or eliminated from the body. The net effect of these changes is a reduction in the intensity and duration of alcohol's effects on the tissues, most notably the brain. Other investigators have stressed a mechanism of "functional" or "tissue" tolerance rather than dispositional tolerance. This concept describes tolerance in terms of changes in the functions or properties of tissues so as to render them less susceptible to drug-induced effects. The ultimate explanation may be a combination of some essential elements from both disposition and functional tolerance theories.

Regardless of the final explanation underlying the development of tolerance, several interesting generalizations can be made. The chronic alcoholic can consume relatively large amounts of alcohol and yet not manifest obvious signs of intoxication. However, relatively small increases in the amount of alcohol above these levels is capable of causing impairment. As an extension of this observation, the amount of alcohol that proves lethal for the alcoholic is not substantially higher than that capable of killing the occasional drinker.

Physical Dependence

Chronic ingestion of large volumes of alcohol produces unequivocal physical dependence, with the intensity of the withdrawal symptoms proportional to the degree of intoxication and its duration. The morning-after "hangover" is the usual consequence of intensive drinking for several hours. By contrast, the chronic alcohol abuser experiences seizures ("rum fits") and delirium trements (dt's) after heavy daily drinking for several weeks. Intermediate levels of drinking produce withdrawal symptoms characterized by tremors ("the shakes"), gastrointestinal upset, nervousness or "the jitters," and insomnia.

Delirium tremens, the most extreme form of alcohol withdrawal, is potentially more dangerous to the abuser than opiate abstinence symptoms. Several hours after the last drink, tremors, restlessness, headache, nausea, weakness, anxiety, and perspiration begin. These effects generally serve as an impetus for the initiation of alcohol-seeking behavior. Tremors become so severe that the drinker has difficulty successfully navigating the glass to the mouth. In the early stages, patients become extremely restless and hyperactive, and very often suffer from visual and auditory hallucinations. They may complain about bugs crawling upon them, they may see pink elephants, and they may believe that they are being attacked by menacing objects, animals, or people. Moreover, they are totally disoriented, losing track of their location and the time of day or month.

As the syndrome progresses, patients become weaker, more confused, disoriented, and agitated. By the third day after the last drink, they may be confronted with very realistic persecutory hallucinations. These symptoms and those of fever, exhaustion, cardiovascular collapse, and occasional grand mal seizures are termed "tremulous delirium." If the alcoholic does not fatally succumb, the symptoms subside within five to seven days, even in the absence of medical treatment. Treatment of delirium tremens includes the use of sedative-hypnotic agents or antianxiety agents ("minor tranquilizers") to reduce the agitation and intravenous administration of fluids, electrolytes, and vitamins (thiamine, nicotinic acid, and ascorbic acid).

Medical and Psychological Problems Associated with Alcoholism

The excessive consumption of alcohol on a chronic basis has been shown to directly or indirectly adversely modify the physical and mental health of the drinker and the pregnant female's fetus. Some of these problems will now be considered.

Nervous System

Alcoholic polyneuropathy is a disease characterized by weakness, numbness, and pain in which the patient suffers from sensory and motor impairment of the limbs. Even the mildest cases may require years for recovery; permanent changes are frequent.

The most serious consequences of chronic alcoholism are Wernicke's syndrome and Korsakoff's psychosis. *Wernicke's syndrome* is characterized by dizziness, paralysis of the nerves of the eyes, and mental confusion. The mental changes include confusion with apathy, drowsiness, inattention, lack of spontaneity, and marked disorientation. When the patient begins to recover from the confusional state, memory impairment becomes more obvious, and the symptoms of Korsakoff's psychosis then predominate.

Korsakoff's psychosis is manifested by a severe impairment of memory and learning. To compensate for an inability to remember, the patient often resorts to substituting imagined events. Although a small number of alcoholics recover from this mental disorder, for the majority the ultimate prognosis is poor.

Alcohol-induced *blackouts* are one of the danger signs associated with the excessive use of alcohol. During an alcohol blackout, the individual acts and appears normal but, at a later time when sober, is incapable of recalling the activities that have transpired.

Digestive System and Liver

A glass of wine or cocktail before dinner improves digestion. This beneficial effect has been attributed to alcohol's sedative properties as well as its ability to stimulate the secretion of gastric acid in the stomach. By contrast, the ingestion of large amounts of alcohol have a direct irritating effect on the cells lining the stomach. Stomach ulcers and gastritis (inflammation of the stomach) are frequent consequences of alcohol abuse. Among the most commonly observed diagnostic symptoms of the alcoholic are nausea and vomiting in the morning. Unfortunately, the alcoholic finds that these problems can be relieved by a few drinks.

About 75 percent of all alcoholics develop some loss of liver function. One in ten get *cirrhosis,* a disease characterized by widespread scarring of the liver. Damage to the liver prevents the production of proteins that are essential for the coagulation of blood. In advanced cases, death often results from uncontrolled bleeding, liver failure, or infections. The exact cause of cirrhosis is not known, but it is thought to result from excessive consumption of alcohol, complicated by dietary deficiencies. Treatment requires total abstinence from alcohol, and a nutritious, high-calorie, high-protein diet.

Heart

Alcohol and its metabolic product acetaldehyde exert adverse effects on the heart. Alcoholic *cardiomyopathy* is characterized by chronic shortness of breath and the signs of congestive heart failure (Chapter 20). Irregularities in the heartbeat, in particular ventricular fibrillation and palpitations caused by alcohol intoxication, are common. Atrial fibrillation is frequently seen in otherwise healthy individuals coming to emergency rooms between Sunday and Tuesday after a weekend of heavy drinking; this condition has been dubbed the "holiday heart syndrome." Whereas some reports indicate that heavy chronic drinking predisposes the drinker to coronary artery disease, the risk of heart attacks and other coronary artery diseases may be less in *light* drinkers (2.5 oz of absolute alcohol per day) than in abstainers.

Cancer

Alcohol is indisputably involved in the causation of cancer, and its consumption is one of the few types of exposure known to increase the risk of cancer at various sites in the human body. [8]

—U.S. Department of Health, Education and Welfare (1978)

Heavy drinking increases the risk of developing cancer of the mouth, tongue, pharnyx, esophagus, larnyx, and liver. Moreover, users of both alcohol and tobacco are at far greater risk to develop head, neck, and esophageal cancers. All alcoholic beverages contain chemicals in addition to alcohol, and some of these compounds are carcinogenic.

Psychological Problems

Whether you consider alcoholism to be a disease or a symptom of an underlying psychiatric disorder, it is now generally accepted that the chronic alcoholic can be only effectively treated by emotional rehabilitation and not by incarceration in the city "drunk tank." Alcoholics often have inadequate ego function (poor self-image), poor control of their impulses, unsatisfactory relationships with others (such as family, friends, and business associates), wide mood swings, sexual immaturity, emotional dependence, and a low tolerance for anxiety and frustration. Whether these problems are the cause or effect of alcoholism has not been fully determined. Alcoholics use alcohol as an escape mechanism to shield themselves from the pressures and problems frustrating them when they are sober.

Fetal Alcohol Syndrome

Behold, thou shalt conceive, and bear a son; and now drink no wine or strong drink. . . .

—Judges 13:7

While the relationship between excessive maternal alcohol consumption and aberrations in fetal development have only recently come into prominence in the United States, the concept is by no means of contemporary origin. Classical Greek and Roman mythology suggested that maternal alcoholism at the time of conception could lead to disorders in the normal development of the fetus. These thoughts undoubtedly served as the basis for the Carthaginian [9] edict forbidding the drinking of wine by newlyweds on the wedding night to prevent the conception of deformed children. In testimony presented to a commit-

---

[8] *Third Special Report to the U.S. Congress on Alcohol and Health,* p. 32.

[9] Students of ancient history will recall that Carthage, an ancient city-state of North Africa, was engaged in a series of three contests with Rome for domination of the Mediterranean. The second and most famous of these so-called Punic Wars (218-201 B.C.) involved Hannibal's unsuccessful invasion of Italy after crossing the Alps with elephants.

tee of the British House of Commons investigating "drunkenness" prior to the enactment of the Alcohol Licensure Act of 1834, infants born to alcoholic mothers were described as sometimes having a "starved, shriveled and imperfect look."

In recent years it has become well accepted that excessive consumption of alcohol by women during pregnancy can result in a group of characteristic congenital abnormalities that are collectively referred to as the **fetal alcohol syndrome** (FAS). First brought to the attention of the American health community in 1972, FAS is characterized by prenatal and postnatal growth deficiencies, delay in motor development, and anomolies of the head and face (microcephaly, short fissures of the eyelids, midfacial defects), hands, heart, and external genitalia. The IQs of affected children average 35 to 40 points below the normal scores.

The risk and extent of these abnormalities appears to be related to the amount of alcohol intake. The average daily maternal consumption of alcohol does not appear to be as significant in the etiology of FAS as high blood alcohol levels during critical stages of embryonic development; thus, pregnant women should avoid binge drinking. High blood alcohol levels may produce physical malformations during the first trimester of pregnancy, while causing growth retardation during the third trimester. Some authorities estimate the risk of FAS in chronically alcoholic mothers to range from 35 to 50 percent.

At this time no absolutely safe level of maternal alcohol consumption has been established. It would appear that there is a definite risk to the fetus with the maternal ingestion of 3 oz of absolute alcohol or about six drinks per day. Since peak blood alcohol levels are probably the most critical teratogenic factor, pregnant women should be strongly advised not to consume more than two drinks on any single day.

The Alcoholic and Society

Alcohol abuse and alcoholism cost the American society $43 billion in 1975. Of this total $19.6 billion resulted from lost production, $12.7 billion were expended for alcohol-related health and medical services, $5.1 billion in motor vehicle accidents, $2.9 billion in violent crimes, $0.4 billion in alcohol-related fire losses, and $1.9 billion in "social responses." Such responses include programs established to detect, prevent, and treat alcoholism, to rehabilitate alcoholics, to conduct research and education programs dealing with alcoholism, and to provide welfare services to the alcoholic and family. How does one place a dollar figure on deteriorated family relationships, broken homes, wasted lives, and human suffering and misery? (See Figure 12-1.) Alcoholism has reached epidemic proportions among the Native Americans, where the rate is twice that seen in the general population. On some reservations, the rate of alcoholism is as high as 25 to 50 percent.

Highway Accidents

The best-documented evidence of the detrimental effects of alcohol on society comes from the very strong relationship between traffic accidents and drinking. It has been estimated that alcohol contributes to, or is associated with, about 60 percent of all auto fatalities each year, a figure approaching 23,000. Alcohol impairs motor skills, but more significantly, it impairs judgment in relation to actual ability. Intoxicated individuals are more aggressive and impulsive in their driving and tend to exercise less caution and drive faster. This deterioration of a safe driving attitude, coupled with a slower reaction time, and impaired vision and motor coordination, produces a dangerous combination of forces with which the sober driver must contend.

Crimes, Violence, and Suicide

By depressing normal inhibitions, alcohol releases suppressed feelings of aggression and hostility, often resulting in violent behavior. Drinking offenders perpetrate a high percentage of crimes which often involve a drinking victim: robbery (72%), rape (50%), assaults (72%), and homicide (86%).

In 1975, approximately 27,000 deaths in the United States were reported to be suicides. It is estimated that as many as 10,000 of these deaths were alcohol-related.

Treatment of Alcoholism

The etiology of alcoholism is unknown. The social scientist contends that this state arises from some preexisting personality disorder. At the opposite end of the spectrum, many biological scientists maintain that a genetically determined or subsequently acquired aberration exists in the body, increasing the body's need for alcohol. These latter scientists search for metabolic disorders, enzyme deficiencies, or an imbalance in minerals or neurotransmitters. Hence, in the absence of a specifically defined cause of alcoholism upon which attention can be directed, present-day treatment must be restricted to empirical methods seeking to provide symptomatic relief, with little immediate hope of a dramatic, immediate cure rate.

One of the most basic premises underlying the successful treatment of alcoholism is the realization by patients that their drinking is beyond their control and that they must initiate effective measures to help themselves. All too often, alcoholics are unwilling to face the issue squarely and to freely admit that they are more than heavy drinkers. The importance of making this admission is embodied in the self-introduction by members of Alcoholics Anonymous: "I am an alcoholic." The road to recovery for the alcoholic is a long one, with frequent relapses. We shall now discuss two general types of treatment: emotional rehabilitation and deterrent drugs. Of these, the former has been far more successful. When drugs are used, if at all, they are generally employed in conjunction with some form of psychiatric treatment.

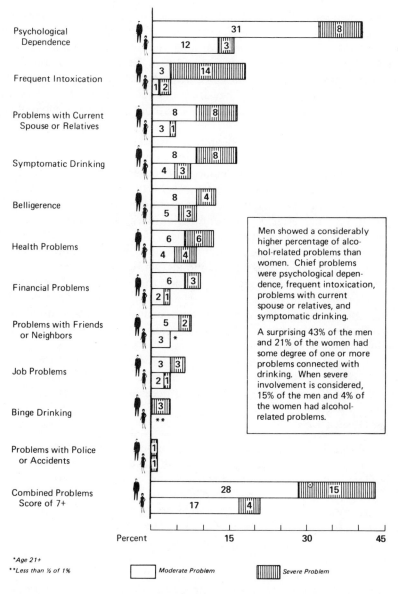

Men showed a considerably higher percentage of alcohol-related problems than women. Chief problems were psychological dependence, frequent intoxication, problems with current spouse or relatives, and symptomatic drinking.

A surprising 43% of the men and 21% of the women had some degree of one or more problems connected with drinking. When severe involvement is considered, 15% of the men and 4% of the women had alcohol-related problems.

*Age 21+
**Less than ½ of 1%

☐ Moderate Problem   ▥ Severe Problem

FIGURE 12–1. Prevalence of Alcohol-Related Problems among Adults in the United States during Three Years prior to 1967. (Adapted from U.S. Department of Health, Education and Welfare, *Alcohol and Health*, Washington, D.C.: U.S. Government Printing Office, 1971, p. 31.)

Emotional Rehabilitation

Emotional rehabilitation may be conducted in many settings, for example, individual or group psychotherapy, counseling of various types, family therapy, and psychodrama, to name a few. All have the same basic objective: to help alcoholics find and adjust to a new way of life in the absence of alcohol. These treatments attempt to reorient patients, helping them to deal with, and adjust to, the normal pressures of life. They are brought to realize that their existence can be far more rewarding and satisfying without resorting to alcohol as an escape.

Group psychotherapy with alcoholics has been found to be more effective than individual therapy. The problems common to alcoholics are often more freely brought to the surface in the company of other alcoholics, where each can empathize with the obstacles facing the others. In such a setting, rationalizations, denials, and weak excuses for relapses are vigorously attacked by the group and, yet, such attacks are counterbalanced by sympathetic understanding and strong support to continue fighting.

The most successful organization has been Alcoholics Anonymous (AA), an informal fellowship of sober alcoholics whose goal is the sobriety and rehabilitation of other alcoholics. Based upon the principle that alcoholics are powerless over alcohol, they attempt to set a goal of abstinence for only the next 24 hours. Some view their program as a resocialization process attempting to develop individual maturity. This is accomplished by the members first assuming greater responsibility for themselves and later assisting others. Although accurate statistics are lacking, it has been estimated that half the members who enter the program have no relapses and that a large number of others eventually recover, notwithstanding occasional backsliding.

Deterrent Drugs

Disulfiram is a compound once used in the rubber industry as a vulcanizing agent. This compound produced no undesirable effects except when the workers in the factory drank; then they reported being very sensitive to the effects of alcohol. This observation went unrecognized until 1948. In that year, disulfiram was being tested by some Danish investigators as an anthelmintic agent, a drug used for the treatment of worm infestations. They took some of this compound themselves to study its safety in human subjects. Then, by chance, these scientists became very ill after a few cocktails. They astutely surmised that their illness was not the result of the drug or of the alcohol but rather of the combination. Disulfiram (Antabuse) was soon introduced for the treatment of chronic alcoholism.

Disulfiram is no cure of alcoholism but is merely a crutch for the sporadic or spree drinker who is likely to relapse from abstinence impulsively, when suddenly confronted with pressure. Patients are forewarned of the consequences of drinking while under treatment with disulfiram (see below) and are, therefore, generally able to overcome their normally uncontrollable urge to have "just one drink." What are these effects and what is the mechanism responsible for their occurrence?

It should be recalled that alcohol is converted to acetaldehyde and that acetaldehyde is very rapidly converted to acetate, as mediated by the enzyme aldehyde dehydrogenase. Disulfiram inhibits this enzyme, and, as a consequence, acetaldehyde concentrations in the blood build up to levels up to ten times greater than normal. What effects are experienced when alcohol is imbibed after this drug? Within 5 to 10 minutes after a drink, the face becomes hot and then flushed; this flushing quickly spreads over the rest of the body. Thereafter, the drinker experiences dizziness, pounding of the heart, a drop in blood pressure, headache, difficulty in breathing, nausea, and vomiting. These effects, initiated by less than 2 teaspoonsful of alcohol, may last from 30 minutes up to several hours. At the end of this time, the patient is exhausted and generally goes to sleep.

In the past, the alcoholic was generally hospitalized and after several days of abstinence, warned about the consequences of drinking while taking disulfiram. To reinforce this admonition, an alcoholic beverage was given several days after the institution of drug administration. After experiencing the dramatic effects described above, the patient became understandably more reluctant to imbibe. To preclude any potentially dangerous effects, the practical demonstration has been omitted in recent years. The previous discussion should make it obvious that the use of disulfiram is not employed in the absence of a clear medical warning and should be restricted for use only for those patients truly resolute in their desire to abstain. As with the use of methadone for the treatment of opiate dependence, success with disulfiram requires supportive emotional rehabilitation. Several drugs have been shown to cause disulfiram-like reactions when taken with alcohol (Table 12–2).

SUMMARY

Alcohol has been used by the people of the world for thousands of years. In the United States, two of every three adults, 21 years of age or over, drink at least occasionally. Some report their reasons for imbibing as being merely "social," others state that "it makes me feel good," and some simply say, "I like it."

After its absorption across the walls of the stomach and small intestines, alcohol is distributed to all the tissues and fluids of the body. However, it is primarily the effects of alcohol on the brain that are of interest to us. Notwithstanding the apparent "stimulatory" effects of alcohol, this compound is unequivocally a central nervous system depressant. The commonly observed excitatory effects are the result of suppression of the inhibitory or restraining centers of the brain. The unfounded mental and physical superiority experienced, coupled with the actual mental and physical impairment, create problems for drinkers and anyone who crosses their path. Large amounts of alcohol produce clearly manifested depression and coma; death results from respiratory failure. Recent estimates suggest that 2500 deaths result annually from adverse alcohol-drug interactions. Extreme caution should be exercised when alcoholic beverages are taken concomitantly with other central nervous system depressants.

There are 9.3–10 million problem drinkers in the United States. In terms of the sheer number of individuals involved, and the amount of public and private dollars directly or indirectly expended as the result of intemperate alcohol use, alcohol is undoubtedly the most significant drug of abuse in the United States as well as in many other countries throughout the world. The alcoholic is psychologically and physically dependent upon alcohol. Chronic heavy alcohol consumption has been established to cause diseases involving the nervous system, digestive system, liver, and heart, and to increase the risk of cancer, especially in the cigarette smoker. The alcoholic's lifespan may be shortened by as much as ten to twelve years. Excessive alcohol ingestion by pregnant females may result in physical and mental abnormalities in her fetus; this is termed the fetal alcohol syndrome. There is a strong relationship between the use of alcohol and highway accidents and the commission of crimes and suicide.

Current objectives in the fight against alcoholism include its prevention or early detection, and treatment and rehabilitation of the alcoholic. There is increasing concern about the rising rate of problem drinking in teenagers. To date, the use of deterrent drugs such as disulfiram (Antabuse) in the treatment of alcoholism has not proved to be notably successful.

SUPPLEMENTARY READINGS

Forney, R. B., and F. W. Hughes, *Combined Effects of Alcohol and Other Drugs.* Springfield, Ill.: Charles C Thomas, 1968.

Israel, Y., and J. Mardones, eds., *Biological Basis of Alcoholism.* New York: John Wiley, 1971.

Kissin, B., and H. Begleiter, eds., *The Biology of Alcoholism.* Vols. 1–4. New York: Plenum Press, 1971–1974.

Mello, N. R., and J. H. Mendelson, eds., *Recent Advances in Studies of Alcoholism.* Washington, D. C.: U.S. Government Printing Office, 1971.

Noble, E., ed., *Biochemical Pharmacology of Alcohol.* New York: Plenum Press, 1977.

Seixas, F. A., ed., "Nature and Nurture in Alcoholism," *Annals of the New York Academy of Sciences* 197:1–229 (1972).

Seixas, F. A., and S. Eggleston, eds., "Alcoholism and the Central Nervous System," *Annals of the New York Academy of Sciences* 215:1–389 (1973).

Sellers, E. M., and H. Kalant, "Alcohol Intoxication and Withdrawal," *New England Journal of Medicine* 294:757–62 (1976).

Streissguth, A. P., S. Landesman–Dwyer, J. C. Martin, and D. W. Smith, "Teratogenic Effects of Alcohol in Human and Laboratory Animals," *Science* **209**:353–61 (1980).

Trémolières, J., ed., *Alcohols and Derivatives, International Encyclopedia of Pharmacology and Therapeutics.* 2 vols. Oxford: Pergamon Press, 1970.

U.S. Department of Health, Education and Welfare, *Alcohol and Health.* Washington, D.C.: U.S. Government Printing Office, 1971.

U.S. Department of Health, Education and Welfare, *Third Special Report to the U.S. Congress on Alcohol and Health.* Washington, D. C.: U.S. Government Printing Office, 1978.

Wallgren, H., and H. Barry, III, *Actions of Alcohol.* 2 vols. New York: American Elsevier Pub., 1970.

13

Narcotic
Analgesics

Without opium the healing art would cease to exist.
—Thomas Sydenham (1624–1689)

Thou hast the keys of Paradise, oh, just subtle, and mighty opium.[1]
—Thomas De Quincey (1822)

*Throw out opium, which the Creator himself seems to prescribe . . . and I firm-
ly believe that if the whole materia medica, as now used, could be sunk to the
bottom of the sea, it would be all the better for mankind,—and all the worse for
the fishes.*
—Oliver Wendell Holmes (1809–1894)

Drugs used for the relief of pain are generally categorized as being *narcotic
or nonnarcotic analgesics.* The narcotic agents, morphine for one, are derived
from the opium poppy or are synthetic derivatives possessing morphine-like
properties. The nonnarcotic agents, such as aspirin, are not chemically related
to the opium alkaloids. We are more concerned with the pharmacological distinctions between these two classes of analgesics than we are with their chemical
differences.

The **narcotic agents** (also referred to as **opiates**) are potent analgesics effective for the relief of severe pain. Moreover, drugs of this class possess potential
for abuse and are consequently subject to federal laws controlling their distribution from the manufacturer to the patient. By contrast, the **nonnarcotics** are only effective for the mitigation of mild-to-moderate pain and these drugs do not
have any abuse potential. Some authors prefer to classify narcotic and nonnarcotic analgesics as *strong* and *mild analgesics,* respectively. This chapter will

[1] *Confessions of an English Opium-Eater,* p. 179. Originally published in 1822. Republished in
1907 by E.P. Dutton & Co., New York.

focus upon the narcotic analgesic agents, while the next will consider nonnarcotic agents. Let us first consider the nature of pain and endogenous opiates.

PAIN AND ENDOGENOUS OPIATES

> *The mind is seldom quickened to very vigorous operations but by pain or the dread of pain.*
>
> —Samuel Johnson (1758)

Analgesia denotes the insensitivity to pain and **analgesic agents** are used for pain relief or mitigation. But what is pain? How do you accurately describe this sensation to a friend? Adam Smith[2] (1723–1790), in his *Theory of Moral Sentiments,* noted that, "A man may sympathize with a woman in childbed, though it is impossible that he should conceive himself as suffering her pains in his own proper person and character."

Physiological and Emotional Aspects of Pain

The dictionary tells us that pain is "a distressing feeling due to disease, bodily injury, or organic disorders; a distressing uneasiness of mind; grief." Unfortunately, this vague definition does not really help us to better appreciate its meaning. Moreover, there are many classifications of this sensation: pricking, burning, and aching pain, and throbbing or sharp pain, and so forth.

Pain is a protective mechanism alerting us that our tissues are being damaged. It provides us with a signal to separate ourselves from the pain stimulus. Prolonged, intensive pain, especially when associated with a chronic disease such as terminal cancer, serves no useful purpose and has, in fact, a damaging effect on the body.

Pain receptors are present in the skin and other tissues. Their activation generates a nerve impulse that travels along sensory pain nerve fibers to the spinal cord, up the lateral spinothalamic tract, along the reticular activating system, and into the thalamus and cerebral cortex. The thalamus furnishes us with a crude awareness of pain, whereas activation of the cortex provides a sharper perception of the nature of this sensation. The "pain experience" consists of the sensation of pain as well as emotional components.

The *emotional aspects of pain* are strongly colored by many factors. Under normal circumstances when we accidentally cut ourselves with a knife or suffer a burn, we perceive the pain as being excruciating. However, it has been observed that soldiers in battle frequently do not complain about their injuries, notwithstanding their incurrence of a severe wound. Perhaps this failure to perceive pain is the result of the combatant's feeling of relief at surviving combat. These subjective psychological factors are significant to us because they

[2] The same Scottish economist who authored *An Inquiry into the Nature and Causes of the Wealth of Nations* (1776) and who postulated the theories of the divisions of labor and laissez faire.

complicate an objective evaluation of the intensity of pain and the degree of relief obtained with an analgesic agent.

Opiate Receptors and Endogenous Opiates

The opiates (narcotic analgesics) are the most effective class of drugs available for the relief of severe pain. In this section we shall consider recent evidence that opiate-induced effects result from the interactions of these drugs with specific receptors which primarily serve as receptors for naturally occurring (endogenous) morphine-like substances. Since their discovery in the early 1970s, the physiological and possible pathological role of such compounds has remained the subject of the most enthusiastic investigation and speculation.

Opiate Receptors

While proof for the existence of opiate receptors was only recently established, their presence in the central nervous system and peripheral tissues had been postulated several decades ago. These earlier suggestions were predicated upon the potency and stereospecific actions of narcotic agonists (morphine-like drugs) and the blockade of their effects by highly specific antagonists (naloxone).

All opiates exhibit great similarities in their basic chemical structures (Figure 31-2, p. 251); relatively modest alterations in selected parts of their molecular structure often causes marked changes in their potency and even total loss of morphine-like activity. Synthetic derivatives have been prepared that are considerably more potent than the naturally occurring opiate morphine.[3]

Opiates exhibit *stereospecific actions,*[4] with the levorotatory (but not the dextrorotatory) isomer capable of effectively relieving pain and producing euphoria (a feeling of well-being). The stereospecificity of drug isomers has long

[3] Etorphine (M-99), for example, is at least 1000 times more potent than morphine and is capable of relieving pain in humans at doses of 0.1 mg (0.0001 g). The high potency of etorphine permits it to be administered in relatively small volumes and makes it useful in veterinary medical practice for the immobilization of large wild animals.

[4] Stereoisomers refer to compounds that have identical chemical and physical properties but that rotate polarized light in opposite directions; such compounds are referred to as *optical isomers.* Compounds that rotate polarized light to the left are designated levorotatory isomers, while those rotating such light to the right are called dextrorotatory. This ability to rotate light in opposite directions, which is used to distinguish between optical isomers, results from differences in their three-dimensional structures, that is, the way their atoms are arranged in space. The chemist would say that optical isomers are mirror images of one another. Our left and right hands are mirror images of one another; however, one hand cannot be superimposed over the other when both are placed with the palms facing down. When two isomers are mirror images, their three-dimensional structures are such that one isomer cannot be superimposed over the other with a perfect correspondence of all parts of the molecule.

been considered to be evidence for drug actions that are mediated via interactions with specific receptor sites located at a cellular level.

Very slight modifications in the chemistry of opiate agonists can transform such compounds into highly specific opiate antagonists, drugs devoid of analgesic properties but extremely effective and highly specific in their ability to block the effects of morphine and other agonists. Antagonists, such as naloxone (Narcan), are clinically employed as specific antidotes for the reversal of respiratory depression resulting from opiate poisoning. The extreme specificity of their actions, the low dose required, and rapid onset of action (within one minute), all suggest that they are competing with the narcotic agonists for common receptor sites.

In 1973, several laboratories[5] independently demonstrated the existence of opiate receptors in the nervous system and gastrointestinal tract. In these studies, opiate agonists and antagonists were demonstrated to stereospecifically bind to homogenates of the mammalian brain and compete for common binding sites. Moreover, a generally good correlation was demonstrated between the ability of various opiates to bind to the brain and their clinical potency as analgesic agents. As you might predict, the nonnarcotic analgesic agent aspirin did not bind to brain homogenates.

Opiate receptors are not uniformly distributed throughout the mammalian central nervous system. In general, those areas that are associated with *pain perception* are rich in opiate receptors; for example, the dorsal horn of the spinal cord (the first site in the central nervous system that conducts sensory information relating to pain up to the brain), the periaqueductal gray area (gray matter core in the brainstem that is highly responsive to experimentally induced pain stimuli and the acute and chronic effects of opiates), and the thalamus (the primary area of the brain concerned with the integration of pain stimuli). Some of the richest concentrations of opiate receptors are found in the amygdala and other selected parts of the limbic system, regions of the brain concerned with the *emotional control of behavior.* This is highly significant because, as will be discussed below, a major component of opiate-induced analgesia is an alteration in the patient's emotional reaction to pain; moreover, even in the absence of pain, the opiates cause marked alterations in mood and behavior. Opiate receptors are also found in those areas of the brainstem involved with the central regulation of respiration and nausea and vomiting.[6]

Opiate receptors have been identified in the brains of all vertebrates tested to date. No evolutionary trends have been recognized, with the same degree of

[5] Among the neuroscientists involved in the discovery of the opiate receptor were Solomon Snyder and Candace Pert at Johns Hopkins University School of Medicine, Eric Simon at New York University School of Medicine, Avram Goldstein at Stanford University and the Addiction Research Center, and Lars Terenius at Uppsala University in Sweden.

[6] The opiates produce dose-related depression of respiration and commonly cause nausea and vomiting.

opiate-receptor binding observed in primitive vertebrates (such as the hagfish and dogfish shark) as in monkeys and humans. By contrast, opiate receptors are conspicuously absent from the invertebrate brain.

Endogenous Opiates

> *It seemed unlikely, a priori, that such highly stereospecific receptors should have been developed by nature to interact with alkaloids from the opium poppy. On the contrary, the history of pharmacology, from the time of Claude Bernard's and Langley's "curare receptors," taught that most drug receptors were really receptors for endogenous ligands.*[7]

—Avram Goldstein (1976)

The presence of specific opiate receptors in vertebrates, as established by pharmacological and binding studies, suggests that endogenous opiate-like chemicals that normally interact with such receptors must exist in the body. If this were not the case, why then would such opiate-binding receptors have survived evolution? In 1974–1975, John Hughes and Hans Kosterlitz of the University of Aberdeen, Scotland, reported that they had isolated a substance from animal brain which possessed opiate-like activity, effects that were readily reversed by the specific narcotic antagonist naloxone. Further work revealed that this endogenous substance consisted of two closely related pentapeptides (simple proteins consisting of five amino acids) which differed from one another only in their terminal amino acid. These compounds, named methionine-enkephalin and leucine-enkephalin,[8] exhibit a distribution pattern in the body that generally parallels that of the opiate-receptor binding sites.

Methionine-enkephalin

H-Tyrosine-Glycine-Glycine-Phenylalanine-Methionine-OH

Leucine-enkephalin

H-Tyrosine-Glycine-Glycine-Phenylalanine-Leucine-OH

The discovery of these enkephalins sparked renewed interest in the pituitary hormone β-lipotropin whose isolation and amino acid sequence had been determined a decade before but whose biological function had not been clearly established. Among the 91 amino acids in β-lipotropin are methionine-enkephalin (amino acids 61–65), β-endorphin (61–91), α-endorphin (61–76), and γ-endorphin (61–77).[9] β-Endorphin and the enkephalins would appear to belong to two anatomically and functionally different systems.

---

[7] "Opioid Peptides (Endorphins) in Pituitary and Brain," *Science* **193**, 1081–86 (1976).

[8] Endogenous substances with morphine-like activity are generally referred to as *endorphins* or *opioid peptides,* while the term *enkephalin* is used to designate these two pentapeptides.

[9] These endorphins elicit a variety of diverse effects when administered to laboratory animals: β-endorphin produces deep analgesia of the entire body and prolonged muscle rigidity and immobility; α-endorphin causes calming (tranquilization) and analgesia of the head and neck; γ-endorphin lacks analgesic properties and causes agitation.

As will be discussed below, one of the major challenges in contemporary drug development is the discovery of highly potent and effective analgesics. useful for the relief of severe pain, and devoid of abuse potential. While it was hoped that the natural opiates would be found to lack abuse liability, the results of early studies suggest that this is not the case.

Endorphins: Possible Physiological Roles

The discovery of the opiate peptides has had a tremendous impact upon virtually every facet of neurobiology. A better understanding of these compounds may serve as a neuroscience Rosetta stone that will provide clues for the solution of mysteries that have long shrouded many aspects of nerve function. Considerable attention has been directed toward determining the role of endorphins in pain, behavior and mental disease.

Pain.   The enkephalins and β-endorphin have been shown to bind to the opiate receptor. While readily inactivated after their administration, β-endorphin and, to a lesser extent, the enkephalins have been shown to possess analgesic activity in both humans and animals.

If, as these results suggest, these peptides are endogenous analgesics (perhaps our private supply of morphine ready to be released when we are subjected to severe pain), then naloxone administration should increase our sensitivity to painful stimuli. While a number of studies have failed to demonstrate that naloxone is capable of modifying experimentally induced pain, this antagonist has been shown to increase the sensitivity of patients experiencing "natural" pain arising from tooth extractions. Thus, endorphins may only be released when the individual is subjected to highly painful and emotional situations.

Approximately one of three of us would obtain significant relief of pain if given (surreptitiously, of course) a placebo (Chapter 3); that is, we are placebo responders. The results of recent studies[10] suggest that endorphin release may be responsible for mediating *placebo relief of pain*. Patients administered naloxone reported significantly greater postoperative dental extraction pain than those individuals given a placebo. Moreover, while the naloxone failed to alter pain sensitivity in placebo nonresponders, this drug increased the pain levels of placebo responders.

Among the most fascinating health-related byproducts of the resumption of cultural exchanges with the People's Republic of China has been our exposure to *acupuncture*. Although Western physicians initially attributed acupuncture analgesia to placebo effects, the power of suggestion, or hypnosis, it is now generally accepted that the relief of pain obtained by this ancient method is real and can be profound. The ability of naloxone to significantly reduce the

[10] J. D. Levine, N. C. Gordon, and H. L. Fields, "The Mechanism of Placebo Analgesia," *Lancet* **2**: 654–57 (1978).

analgesic effects of acupuncture suggests that this procedure relieves pain by stimulating the release of endogenous opiates.

At this time it is not clear whether enkephalins are true neurotransmitters or whether they function as *neuromodulators,* that is, substances that regulate the release of neurotransmitters. Opiate receptors have been found to be localized on the endings of sensory nerves in the spinal cord. Experimental evidence suggests that enkephalin may act by inhibiting the release of an excitatory sensory neurotransmitter (such as substance P), thus interfering with the transmission of pain impulses (Figure 13-1). Such an action could account for the analgesic effects of these peptides at the level of the spinal cord.

Behavioral Roles. In addition to their ability to relieve pain, morphine and related drugs produce profound changes in the behavior and mood of humans (see below). The endorphins have been found to produce similar effects and may play a physiological role in the control of emotional behavior and possibly also appetitive drives (hunger, water intake, sex).

It has been postulated that aberrations in endorphin system function might be responsible for the etiology of or symptoms associated with certain mental illnesses, in particular schizophrenia. Supporting this hypothesis are reports that naloxone reduces hallucinations in some schizophrenic patients and the presence of abnormally increased concentrations of opiate peptides in their cerebrospinal fluid. Other investigators claim to have successfully treated schizophrenia by means of the artificial kidney (hemodialysis), implying that blood-carried substances are involved in schizophrenia; analysis of substances removed from the blood and present in the dialysate reportedly contain high concentrations of opioid peptides. Since many laboratories have failed to obtain analogous results supporting a role for the endorphins in mental illness, this exciting hypothesis remains highly controversial.

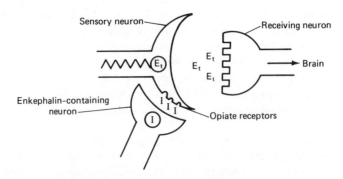

FIGURE 13-1. Enkephalin-Containing Neurons and Pain. A painful stimulus activates the release of an excitatory neurotransmitter (E_t), possibly substance P, from sensory nerve endings. This neurotransmitter stimulates a receiving neuron which conveys information about pain to specific areas of the brain. Enkephalin (I) is postulated to interact with the opiate receptor causing an inhibition of the release of the excitatory neurotransmitter thus preventing the transmission of information about pain and its perception by the individual.

CLASSIFICATION OF NARCOTIC AGENTS

Narcotic agents[11] may be classified into four categories (Figure 13-2; Table 13-1): (1) the natural alkaloids of opium (opiates), which include morphine and codeine; (2) the semisynthetic derivatives of morphine, compounds that are chemical modifications of the morphine structure; (3) synthetic narcotic agents or *opioids,* which bear only highly subtle similarities to the structure of morphine; and (4) narcotic antagonists, drugs used primarily as antidotes to antagonize the respiratory depression caused by an overdose of the narcotic analgesics.

NATURAL AND SEMISYNTHETIC NARCOTIC ANALGESICS

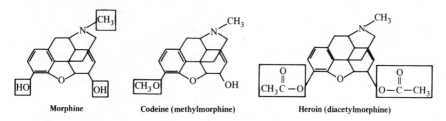

Morphine   Codeine (methylmorphine)   Heroin (diacetylmorphine)

SYNTHETIC NARCOTIC ANALGESICS

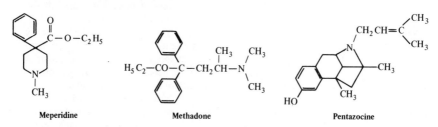

Meperidine   Methadone   Pentazocine

NARCOTIC ANTAGONISTS

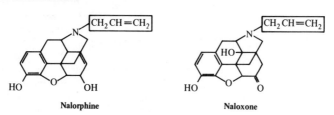

Nalorphine   Naloxone

FIGURE 13-2. Structures of Representative Narcotic Agents.

[11] The term *narcotic* has been loosely used to variously denote: illicit drugs employed for nonmedical purposes (heroin, cocaine, marijuana); central nervous system depressants; and drugs possessing both sedative and analgesic effects (morphine-like drugs). In this text, the term *narcotic* will only be employed to refer to drugs with morphine-like properties.

TABLE 13-1. REPRESENTATIVE NARCOTIC ANALGESICS OF INTEREST

Generic Name	Selected Trade Names	Remarks
Natural opium alkaloids		
Morphine		The standard against which all other narcotic agents are compared. Highly effective for relief of severe pain and suppression of cough (antitussive).
Codeine (methylmorphine)		About 1/12 analgesic potency of morphine. Useful for relief of mild pain and as antitussive agent. Much less addiction liability than morphine.
Semisynthetic derivatives of morphine		
Heroin (diacetylmorphine)		Most popular drug of abuse among narcotic addicts. Effective analgesic, but produces marked euphoria. Illegal in the U.S.
Hydromorphone (dihydromorphinone)	Dilaudid	Ten times as active as morphine, but produces proportionally greater respiratory depression. Faster onset but shorter duration of action than morphine.
Hydrocodone	Hycodan	Similar to codeine but more potent analgesic and antitussive actions.
Synthetic agents (opioids)		
Meperidine (pethidine)	Demerol	Among the most commonly used narcotic analgesics; has an analgesic potency 1/10 of morphine, with a shorter duration of action. No antitussive activity.
Methadone	Dolophine	Orally active analgesic agent with potency equivalent to morphine, but longer duration of action. Used for the treatment of narcotic dependence. It, too, is addicting.
Pentazocine	Talwin	Less active than morphine and less addictive. Weak antagonist activity.
Butorphanol	Stadol	Potent new pentazocine-like analgesic, with low abuse liability. Available only in parenteral preparations.
Propoxyphene	Darvon Darvon-N	Very widely used drug possessing modest analgesic properties. Acute toxicity of concern; not infrequently used for suicidal purposes.
Narcotic antagonists		
Nalorphine	Nalline	Antagonizes respiratory depression and other effects resulting from poisoning by narcotics. Precipitates withdrawal symptoms in dependent individuals. Produces behavioral disturbances. No longer marketed in the United States.
Naloxone	Narcan	No morphine-like effects; a pure antagonist. No analgesia, respiratory depression, or behavioral disturbances. Effective narcotic antagonist. Blocks euphoric effect of heroin when given before this agent.
Naltrexone		Has analgesic and narcotic antagonistic effects; produces physical dependence. Blocks euphoric effects of heroin; used for treatment of narcotic dependence.

The first three categories are all employed as analgesic agents for the relief of severe pain. Although there are differences in the potency of these agents— that is, different absolute amounts of these drugs must be employed to produce equivalent analgesia—and differences exist in the duration of action, the general pharmacological properties of these drugs are similar. Thus, we shall concentrate most of our attention upon morphine, the prototype narcotic analgesic, and comment on the other members of this class when the individual drugs possess properties of particular interest to us.

OPIUM

Opium has held an esteemed place in therapeutics since the first days of recorded history. Even up to the early 1800s, opium was one of the few truly effective and reliable drugs available for the treatment of pain, insomnia, cough, and diarrhea. Today, morphine, the active constituent of opium, still remains the standard against which all other analgesic agents are compared.

We shall discuss the pharmacological effects and therapeutic uses of the opiates, as well as the characteristics associated with narcotic dependence and abuse. Although the major emphasis will be on morphine, other narcotics of contemporary interest will be discussed; these include heroin, codeine, meperidine, and methadone. In addition, the narcotic antagonists warrant our attention because of their specific therapeutic applications for the management of narcotic poisoning and use for the treatment of opiate dependence. The narcotics are among the most effective and widely used drugs available for suppression of cough and the treatment of diarrhea; we shall consider cough remedies and antidiarrheal agents in Chapters 27 and 26, respectively.

We shall first consider only selected aspects of the history of opium use and abuse, since this single topic could readily constitute the subject matter of a volume of considerable size if dealt with in its entirety.

History of Opium

Opium was among the earliest drugs recorded in human history. Its behavioral effects are described in Sumerian records dating back to 4000 B.C. The medical writings of the ancient Assyrians, Greeks, and Romans all refer to opium's wondrous properties for the relief of pain and the induction of sleep. Homer's *Odyssey* may be the first reference to an opium party, where Helen, the daughter of Zeus, attempted to relieve the feelings of depression of her guests with a drug many think to be opium.

In the Middle East, followers of Mohammed learned of opium and hashish and employed these natural drugs for their psychically satisfying effects, perhaps as substitutes for alcohol, which was forbidden by the Koran. Islamic traders introduced opium to China in the ninth century where it was employed for the next 800 years for medicinal purposes to relieve the diarrhea resulting from dysentery.

China was the first country to experience a serious widespread opium abuse problem. The roots of this problem can be traced to the seventeenth century, when Portuguese and Dutch merchants began exporting tobacco to China. Over the years, it was recognized that the pleasures derived from smoking could be markedly enhanced by the addition of opium to the tobacco. English traders realized the great mercantile potential of this commodity and, in the middle of the eighteenth century, began shipping large amounts of opium into China from India. In an attempt to curb the extensive opium smoking habit among its nationals, in 1839 the Manchu government seized the opium cargo of a British ship. Objecting to the measures taken and possibly fearing the loss of a highly profitable business, the British engaged the numerically superior Chinese troops and defeated them in 1842 in the first short-lived "Opium War." Among the provisions of the Treaty of Nanking was cession of the island of Hong Kong to Great Britain. In the face of the powerful British and French forces and notwithstanding the protestations of the Manchus, the Chinese were obliged to permit the legalization of opium importation in 1858.

Over a century later, the issues of opium exportation as well as importation again became the focus of attention. Of the opium employed for the manufacture of heroin that is ultimately used in the United States, the Bureau of Narcotics and Dangerous Drugs in 1970 estimated that 80 percent was grown in Turkey, 15 percent in Mexico and 5 percent in the Far East. In response to the subtle diplomatic pressures exerted and financial incentives offered by our government, the president of Turkey decreed that the cultivation of the opium poppy and production of opium be forbidden after 1972. Thus, when considering the relevancy of pharmacology to society, we might also appropriately include drugs and international relations.

In 1806, Friedrich Sertürner, a 23-year-old German pharmacist's apprentice, isolated the active ingredient from opium. After observing the profound hypnotic effect of this alkaloid upon himself and some volunteer friends, he termed it **morphine,** after Morpheus, the Greek god of sleep. In addition to the monumental significance of this discovery for the practice of medicine, Sertürner's extraction of morphine marked the origin of the chemistry of the alkaloids. The application of morphine as an analgesic agent was greatly advanced by Wood's perfection of the hypodermic syringe in 1853.

The significant rise of morphine abuse in the second half of the nineteenth century has been attributed to such diverse confederates as literary and military factors and the promotion of patent medicines.

Several years prior to Sertürner's experiments, Thomas De Quincey purchased laudanum, an opium-containing mixture in a wine vehicle, for the relief of a toothache. The effects, described in his famous and widely read book

Confessions of an English Opium-Eater, were far more profound than he had anticipated.

> I took it: and in an hour, O heavens! What a revulsion! what a resurrection from its lowest depths, of the inner spirit! what an apocalypse of the world within me! That my pains had vanished was a trifle in my eyes; the negative effect was swallowed up in the immensity of those positive effects which had opened up before me, in the abyss of divine enjoyment thus suddenly revealed. Here was a panacea . . . for all human woes; here was the secret of happiness, about which philosophers had disputed for so many ages, at once discovered; happiness might now be bought for a penny, and carried in the waistcoat-pocket. . . .[12]

Not appreciating the potential dangers associated with the chronic use of morphine, this drug was carelessly administered to wounded soldiers in the American Civil War (1861–1865), the Prussian-Austrian War (1866), and the Franco-Prussian War (1870). The prevalence of postwar morphine addiction among these veterans was so high that this condition was termed the "army disease" and the "soldier's disease."

This was also the age of patent medicines. Prior to 1906 no legal constraints were placed upon proprietary manufacturers either with respect to the nature of the ingredients in their products or in the claims set forth for their products. Secret formulas were commonplace and often large amounts of the opiates and alcohol were the major active constituents. Extravagant claims for the cure of all diseases imaginable were made, with only one ultimate objective—to sell the product. These abuses were corrected by the Pure Food and Drug Act of 1906, and the 1914 Harrison Narcotic Act.

We shall return to contemporary aspects of opiate abuse in a subsequent section of this chapter. Let us now leave the historial aspects of opiates and consider the pharmacological properties of the opium alkaloids.

Source and Composition of Opium

Opium is obtained from the poppy, *Papaver somniferum,* a plant found in Pakistan, India, Turkey, Iran, China, the Soviet Union, Southeast Asia, and Mexico. This plant consists of a main stalk, three to four feet in height, with five to eight egg-shaped capsules on top. The poppy generally blooms in June; ten days thereafter, incisions are made in the capsule permitting a milky fluid to ooze out. The following day, the gummy mass, which has now turned brown, is carefully scraped off the capsule, pressed into cakes of raw opium, and allowed to dry. The cultivation of the poppy and collection of opium is a very tedious task, and it has been estimated that between 175 and 250 hours of labor are required to obtain 1000 g (2.2 lb) of opium, from which about 100 g of morphine

---

[12] *Confessions of an English Opium-Eater.*

or heroin can be produced. For this reason, poppies are only cultivated where labor is relatively inexpensive and abundant.

Opium contains over 20 alkaloids; the two alkaloids of major relevance to us are morphine (10%) and codeine (0.5%). It is of interest to note that these alkaloids are not present as such in the fresh plant but are formed as the result of oxidation reactions in the juice that exudes from the capsule. Noscapine and papaverine, other important naturally occurring opium alkaloids (6% and 1%, respectively), are chemically unrelated to morphine or codeine. These compounds have no analgesic activity nor abuse potential. The primary pharmacological effect of noscapine is to suppress cough, while papaverine, a nonspecific smooth muscle relaxant, was formerly used to dilate (widen the lumen of) blood vessels.

MORPHINE

Pharmacological Actions

Morphine's major pharmacological effects can be attributed to the actions of this drug on the central nervous system and on the gastrointestinal tract. Its actions on the central nervous system are responsible for analgesia, behavioral changes, respiratory depression, and suppression of cough (antitussive effect); the constipating effects of this drug are useful for the treatment of diarrhea. We shall discuss antitussive and antidiarrheal agents in Chapters 27 and 26, respectively.

Analgesia

No drug has been developed that is more effective than morphine for the relief of *severe pain*. In this regard, morphine is useful for the alleviation of almost all types of pain, regardless of its site of origin. It has been clinically observed that this drug is more effective against dull, constant pain than in relieving pain of a sharp and stabbing nature. Whereas it is generally agreed that morphine produces analgesia by virtue of an action in the central nervous system, the precise site of action and the underlying mechanism have not to date been ascertained. Doses of morphine that effectively relieve moderate-to-severe pain do not produce a general depression of the central nervous system.

The predominant contemporary theory attributes morphine's analgesic effects to a *modification of the patient's subjective awareness of pain* rather than an elevation of the pain threshold. Although patients continue to perceive pain, their reaction or response to this aversive sensation is altered. The anxiety and stress associated with pain are markedly reduced. Patients report that they still feel the pain and continue to be aware of its existence, but it no longer bothers them.

Behavioral Effects

The general behavioral effects produced by morphine differ depending upon whether the subject is pain-free or experiencing pain. Administration of a therapeutic dose (10 mg) of morphine to a patient suffering from pain and anxiety results in a dissipation of the distressing aspects of pain as well as relief from the coexisting anxiety. Some individuals feel euphoric, although this is not always the case. By contrast, in the absence of pain, mental distress or dysphoria is commonly experienced. This dysphoric state is characterized by nervousness, fear, and nausea. Moreover, central nervous system depression often occurs leaving the drug user mentally and physically lethargic for many hours.

Respiration

Morphine depresses the respiratory centers located in the medulla, a structure located in the brainstem (Chapter 9). Large doses of this drug reduce the rate of breathing as well as its depth. Indeed, *respiratory failure is the cause of death after an overdose of morphine.* What is the basis of morphine's action? Elevated carbon dioxide levels in the blood serve as a natural medullary stimulant for increasing the rate of respiration; morphine depresses the sensitivity of the respiratory centers to elevated concentrations of carbon dioxide. Just as tolerance develops to the euphoric and analgesic effects of morphine, the respiratory centers also become more resistant to the depressant action of the opiates. For this reason, the addict is able to survive doses of heroin and morphine that would produce respiratory failure and death in the nontolerant individual.

Other Actions in the Central Nervous System

The opiates cause constriction of the pupils, an effect to which the addict does not become tolerant; some degree of constriction is even present in total darkness. The pinpoint pupil is one of the cardinal signs of morphine poisoning. A far more distressing effect of the narcotic analgesics, experienced by a large percentage of patients taking these drugs for the relief of pain, is nausea and vomiting. This results from a drug-induced activation of the chemoreceptive trigger zone (CTZ), which is capable of stimulating the vomiting center. Apomorphine, a close chemical derivative of morphine, is the most potent chemical stimulant of the CTZ and is a clinically useful emetic agent for the treatment of poisoning.

Gastrointestinal Tract

For over 1000 years, opium has been used for the treatment of diarrhea. Even today, many parents employ paregoric (camphorated opium tincture) when their children are afflicted with diarrhea. Morphine produces constipation by increasing smooth muscle tone and/or by reducing the propulsive peristaltic movements of the gastrointestinal tract thereby slowing the passage of contents down the tract. Tolerance does not develop to the constipating effects of the narcotic agents.

Therapeutic Uses

Morphine is slowly and irregularly absorbed from the gastrointestinal tract, and it is, therefore, rarely administered orally for the relief of pain. By contrast, it is rapidly absorbed into the bloodstream after injection.

Pain

The most common therapeutic use of morphine and its derivatives is for the relief of **severe pain.** The narcotic analgesics are widely employed for the easement of postoperative pain, pain arising from acute traumatic injuries, heart attacks, and terminal cancer. Because of its addiction potential, narcotics are generally reserved for use in severe pain, and not for the mild-to-moderate pain amenable to relief by such nonnarcotic analgesics as aspirin (Chapter 14).

Sedation

The narcotic agents are sometimes employed when a patient is suffering from pain and is unable to sleep. The sedative properties of the opiates are also of value for the reduction of preoperative anxiety. In the absence of pain, barbiturate or nonbarbiturate sedative-hypnotics are a more reasonable therapeutic alternative.

Acute Opiate Poisoning

By far the most important toxic effect associated with opiate overdosage is **respiratory depression.** For the patient taking morphine to relieve pain, this is not a common occurrence. We may observe that there is a wide range between the therapeutic dose of morphine (about 8–15 mg) and a toxic dose (100–300 mg). About 250–500 mg constitutes a lethal dose for the nontolerant individual. As we shall discuss in a later section of this chapter, very marked tolerance develops to the toxic effects of morphine. The addict is capable of taking a dose of morphine that is 10–20 times the normal lethal dose, thus reflecting the great adaptation of the respiratory system.

Unlike medical patients who are assured of the exact dosage they are receiving in a prescription, the addict injects an impure compound containing an inexact amount of opiate. Doses even modestly in excess of the addict's normal "fix" may rapidly prove fatal, as evidenced by the postmortem discovery of such victims having hypodermic needles still lodged in their veins.

Acute poisoning by morphine produces a stuporous state or coma and a very substantial reduction in the rate of respiration. In addition, the individual exhibits the characteristic pinpoint pupils. The narcotic antagonists (see below) specifically and dramatically reverse opiate-induced respiratory depression, often within minutes after their administration. Because antagonists such as nalorphine or naloxone are capable of precipitating an abstinence syndrome in addicted individuals, these drugs must be employed with caution.

Medical Complications of Opiate Abuse

For individuals who are able to obtain their supply of narcotics through legal channels (thereby insuring their purity) and who maintain a normal diet, long-term dependence does not compromise their health. There is no evidence demonstrating that chronic use of opiates produces physical damage to the central nervous system or to the other organs of the body.

The situation is very different for street addicts who must illicitly obtain their drugs from pushers and who inject heroin using unsterile equipment. Addicts often share a needle with their confederates, thus increasing the likelihood of contracting hepatitis and other liver disorders, and as well as a bacterially induced inflammation of the membranes lining the inner surface of the heart (endocarditis). Tetanus and skin abscesses are also common complications resulting from unsterile equipment.

During the late 1930s extensive outbreaks of malaria were observed among addicts. The parasite causing malaria was transmitted from the diseased individual to the blood of a nondiseased addict who used the same needle. When malaria was eradicated in the United States, this complication of addiction also vanished. In 1971 the problem reappeared when addicted Vietnam veterans harboring this parasite began sharing their needles with nonveterans.

CODEINE

Codeine or methylmorphine is the second most important alkaloid derived from the opium poppy. This compound is very widely used as an analgesic and cough-suppressing agent. Its analgesic potency is considerably weaker than morphine; 120 mg of injected codeine produces the same degree of analgesia as 10 mg of morphine. When taken orally, 32 mg of codeine produce the same analgesic effect as two aspirin tablets. These two drugs are often used in combination, with the analgesic effect obtained exceeding that produced by the individual components. This suggests that aspirin and codeine act by different mechanisms to relieve pain.

We may generally summarize codeine's pharmacological effects by stating that they closely resemble morphine, but to a lesser extent. Codeine is a less effective analgesic and cough suppressant than morphine; it produces less sedation and is far less prone to be abused, and, finally, tolerance develops far less rapidly. Codeine is metabolized to morphine in humans, and it has been suggested that codeine's pharmacological effects may be attributed to this active metabolite.[13]

OTHER NARCOTIC ANALGESICS

Many semisynthetic derivatives of morphine and synthetic narcotic analgesic agents (opioids) have been investigated in search of a substitute for morphine. Although some of these compounds have proved to be more potent than morphine when equianalgesic doses are employed, these drugs produce equivalent respiratory depression and possess the same abuse liability. Pentazocine and other recently introduced drugs possessing weak antagonist activity appear to have a lower abuse potential than morphine.

Heroin

Heroin, or diacetylmorphine, a semisynthetic derivative of morphine, was introduced in 1898, and was purported to be a nonaddicting analgesic agent that did not cause respiratory depression. Moreover, this drug was even advocated for the treatment of morphine addiction. Within less than a decade, heroin's abuse potential was well recognized, and today its importation and manufacture are illegal in the United States. The beneficial properties of this compound are greatly outweighed by its dangerous abuse liability.

It is believed that the very rapid onset of heroin's action after intravenous administration accounts for its overwhelming endorsement by opiate addicts, who consider heroin to be the drug of first choice. Heroin crosses the blood-brain barrier more rapidly than morphine and, when given in equivalent doses, produces greater euphoric effects than the latter. Once in the brain, heroin is hydrolyzed to morphine, the compound believed to be responsible for heroin's activity. We shall return to a discussion of the behavioral effects elicited by the intravenous administration of heroin when we consider opiate dependence in this chapter.

Heroin is a very potent analgesic agent, approximately three times as active as morphine. Do you think that the therapeutic use of heroin is justified to relieve the severe pain and brighten the spirits of a patient suffering from terminal cancer? Do the benefits of such medication counterbalance the virtual absolute certainty that the patient will rapidly become dependent upon heroin?

[13] J. W. A. Findlay, E. C. Jones, R. F. Butz, and R. M. Welch, "Plasma Codeine and Morphine Concentrations after Therapeutic Oral Doses of Codeine-Containing Analgesics," *Clinical Pharmacology and Therapeutics* **24**: 60–68 (1978).

Meperidine (Demerol)

Meperidine or pethidine, as this drug is more commonly called outside the United States, was fortuitously discovered in 1939 as the result of a search for atropine-like agents possessing antispasmodic activity. This compound was the first totally synthetic narcotic analgesic agent. Notwithstanding some early claims to the contrary, meperidine possesses the same abuse potential as morphine, and it produces the same degree of respiratory depression. Physicians and nurses who are dependent upon opiates often abuse this drug, perhaps because they erroneously believe meperidine to be less likely to produce drug dependence.

Among the most extensively employed narcotic analgesic agents for the relief of severe pain, meperidine differs from morphine in several major respects: meperidine has a shorter duration of action and requires ten times the dose (100 mg) to produce equivalent analgesia; it is less constipating and may produce a widening of the pupils rather than constriction; meperidine has no antitussive properties. Unlike morphine, meperidine provides effective, reliable analgesia after oral administration.

Methadone (Dolophine)

Methadone has the same general pharmacological properties as morphine and has been employed for over two decades as a highly effective analgesic agent. Contemporary interest in this compound is predicated upon its use for the treatment of narcotic dependence. Although methadone is itself addicting, the withdrawal symptoms appear more slowly (after 24 to 48 hours), are of lesser intensity but of longer duration than are the symptoms associated with morphine abstinence. Oral administration of methadone prevents the heroin abstinence syndrome as a consequence of cross-dependence between these drugs. We shall evaluate the use of methadone for the treatment of opiate dependence in a subsequent section of this chapter.

Propoxyphene (Darvon)

Since its clinical introduction in 1957, propoxyphene (alone or in combination with the nonnarcotic analgesics aspirin or acetaminophen) has remained among the most frequently prescribed drugs in the United States. Notwithstanding the overwhelming commercial success of this drug, generated to no small extent by a highly effective promotional program, carefully controlled studies fail to demonstrate that low doses of propoxyphene possess greater analgesic activity than a placebo.[14]

[14] R. R. Miller, A. Feingold, and J. Paxinos, "Propoxyphene Hydrochloride: A Critical Review," *Journal of the American Medical Association* **213**: 996–1006 (1970).

This synthetic drug, chemically related to methadone, is promoted for oral use as an alternative to codeine (a considerably less effective alternative) for the relief of mild-to-moderate pain. Propoxyphene[15] is most frequently used in combination with aspirin (Darvon Compound, Darvon with A.S.A.) or acetaminophen (Darvocet) and, when so employed, possesses some reasonable degree of analgesic activity exceeding that provided by the nonnarcotic analgesics when they are taken in the absence of propoxyphene. These propoxyphene combinations are generally considered to be rational, since they combine the use of a peripherally acting nonnarcotic with a centrally acting narcotic. Propoxyphene-induced side effects include nausea, mild euphoria, sedation, and dizziness or light-headedness.

While the *abuse potential* of propoxyphene is not perceived to be great, cases of abuse are well documented. Physical dependence and tolerance do not appear to develop when the drug is taken at the normal therapeutic doses. At higher doses, the euphoric effects become more pronounced increasing the risk of nonmedical use. Abrupt withdrawal after the chronic administration of high doses has been associated with a relatively mild opiate withdrawal syndrome (see below).

Fatalities resulting from the intentional or accidental overdosage of propoxyphene have become an issue of increasing concern and alarm in recent years. This risk is significantly enhanced when propoxyphene is taken in combination with alcohol, sedative-hypnotics, antianxiety and antipsychotic agents, antidepressants, antihistamines, and other central nervous system depressants. Symptoms of acute drug overdosage include weakness, confusion, respiratory depression, coma, convulsions, and death. Since approximately 20 percent of all fatalities have been reported to occur within one hour after drug ingestion, emergency treatment (that is, the administration of narcotic antagonists) should be rendered as rapidly as possible.

Pentazocine and Related Drugs

Pentazocine (Talwin) is one of a new series of compounds that provides effective analgesia with little or no potential for abuse. Drugs with these desirable attributes possess both narcotic agonistic and narcotic antagonistic activities. Unlike almost all older narcotic analgesics, pentazocine will neither prevent nor lessen the intensity of the opiate abstinence syndrome. By contrast, when administered at high doses, it will precipitate a mild withdrawal syndrome in narcotic-dependent individuals. Pentazocine abuse has been documented when taken by injection, but not by mouth. Intravenous self-administration of this narcotic in combination with tripelennamine (Pyribenzamine) has been

---

[15] Propoxyphene is commercially available as the hydrochloride (Darvon) and the less soluble napsylate (Darvon-N) salts; because of differences in molecular weight, 100 mg of the napsylate are equivalent to 65 mg of the hydrochloride. The only clearly established advantage of the newer napsylate is for the manufacturer who maintains a monopoly on the distribution of this salt thereby compensating for the loss of the hydrochloride whose patent has expired.

reported; the latter drug, an antihistamine, appears to possess no psychoactive activity (except drowsiness), and the pharmacological rationale for this combination is obscure.

Side effects induced by high doses of pentazocine differ from morphine and include respiratory depression, associated with a rise in blood pressure and an increase in heart rate, and nalorphine-like behavioral aberrations (see below) such as irritability, disturbing dreams, and hallucinations.

Butorphanol (Stadol) has a spectrum of pharmacological activities that are similar to pentazocine but causes a lower incidence of adverse effects on behavior. This highly potent analgesic (three to five times more active than morphine) is available for use only by injection and is, therefore, more suited for the relief of acute, rather than chronic, pain. Abuse of butorphanol has not been reported to date.

Nalbuphine (Nubain) is another new and potent analgesic that possesses weak antagonistic activity and a relatively low abuse potential. Sedation is the most common side effect observed at therapeutic doses. At doses that produce the same degree of analgesia as morphine, nalbuphine depresses respiration to an equivalent extent. In marked contrast to morphine, however, the degree of respiratory depression is not substantially increased when higher doses are administered.

NARCOTIC ANTAGONISTS

Nalorphine (Nalline), a chemical derivative of morphine (Figure 13-2), was the first clinically developed narcotic antagonist. This compound causes many morphine-like effects, including effective analgesia, respiratory depression, and constriction of the pupils. In addition, nalorphine is capable of causing highly undesirable changes in behavior, such as irritability, frightening dreams, delusions, and hallucinations. In 1978, nalorphine was withdrawn from the U. S. market and replaced by naloxone.

Naloxone (Narcan) is a pure narcotic antagonist and is totally devoid of morphine-like activity. Unlike nalorphine, it does not cause respiratory depression, sedation, or adverse behavioral effects. Naloxone is the drug of choice for the treatment of poisoning by narcotic agents, and it reverses most of morphine's effects. In particular, small doses are able to rapidly antagonize the sedation and respiratory depression observed in cases of acute morphine poisoning. This antagonist is clinically employed as an antidote for opiate overdosage, regardless of whether the narcotic is a natural, semisynthetic, or synthetic analgesic. It has been hypothesized that the antagonists act by displacing agonist narcotic agents from their receptor sites in the central nervous system. Naloxone has a duration of action of about two hours, which is less than most narcotics. Hence, repeated doses may be required for the successful treatment of narcotic poisoning. By contrast, these antagonists are ineffective in reversing depression induced by barbiturate or nonbarbiturate sedative-hypnotics or alcohol.

When naloxone is administered to opiate-dependent individuals, it *precipitates an abstinence syndrome*. These effects are identical to those observed after abrupt cessation of opiates; however, the time course of these effects is markedly compressed. A naloxone-induced abstinence syndrome begins within minutes after injection of the antagonist, reaches its peak intensity in less than one hour, and lasts for a total of two hours. Naloxone has been used in this manner as a diagnostic test to determine whether an individual is physically dependent upon the opiates.

Naltrexone is another new narcotic antagonist, currently undergoing clinical trials for the treatment of opiate dependence. As we have already noted for other antagonists, when naltrexone is administered to an opiate-dependent individual, it precipitates an abstinence syndrome. However, when given prior to heroin, the antagonist prevents heroin's normal euphoric effects, as well as the development of physical dependence upon the opiates. Naltrexone's actions have been attributed to a long-lasting blockade of morphine receptor sites in the central nervous system.

NARCOTIC ABUSE AND TREATMENT

Let us now consider the abuse of narcotic analgesic agents. In this section, we shall consider the pharmacological characteristics of narcotic dependence (psychological dependence, tolerance, and physical dependence), as well as the patterns of abuse and its treatment with methadone.

Pharmacological Characteristics of Dependence

Psychological Dependence

Repeated frequent administration of heroin inevitably leads to a *compulsive* desire to take this drug in order to maintain a state of well-being. That is, the heroin user feels "normal" while under the drug's influence and physically and mentally ill ("sick") in its absence.

Addicts continue their heroin habit to obtain both the euphoric effects obtained from the use of the drug and to escape from their inner anxieties and frustrations. Another although less compelling force is the addict's desire to avoid the abstinence syndrome. These factors are by no means a complete explanation of the extreme psychological dependence produced by the opiates. They do not shed light on why an individual who has not taken opiates for several months or years very often rapidly returns to the opiate habit. What behavioral effects does an opiate-dependent individual experience after intravenous self-administration of heroin?

Within seconds after the drug has entered the blood, the face of the addict becomes flushed, the pupils become constricted, and a tingling sensation, which has been likened to a sexual orgasm, is felt in the abdomen. There is a feeling of contentment and being at ease or "fixed." For the next few hours, the user goes on the "nod," a condition in which he or she is drowsy, awakens, and then drifts off again into a dreamy state. Many literary scholars believe that *Kubla Khan* was inspired during an opium-mediated dream. In this regard, Sir Leslie Stephen has noted, "to tell the story of Coleridge without the opium is to tell the story of Hamlet without mentioning the Ghost."

While under the influence of narcotic agents, addicts are not the violent "dope fiends" often envisioned by the public. Rather they are more often totally disinterested in the outside world and its activities. Heroin does not cause criminal behavior; it is the attempt by addicts to get money to support their addiction that compels them to engage in such activities.

Tolerance

After repeated administration of the opiates, tolerance rapidly develops to the analgesic, euphoric, and respiratory depressing effects, but not to pupillary constriction or to constipation. The speed with which tolerance is acquired is dependent upon the specific opiate abused, its dosage, the interval between doses, and the setting in which the drug is taken, for example, a hospital or a street alley. Addicts have been reported to take up to 5000 mg intravenously in 24 hours, amounts far in excess of the normally toxic doses (250–500 mg) for nontolerant individuals.

After drug abstinence, opiate tolerance is lost or markedly reduced within several weeks. Addicts often voluntarily stop taking heroin several times per year. In this way, they partially lose their acquired tolerance to the euphoric effects, and consequently reduce their drug requirement when its cost outstrips available financial resources. When drug usage is resumed, the pleasurable effects can be derived from smaller doses. Overdosage and death from acute morphine poisoning is very often the consequence of addicts inadvertently taking amounts of opiates in excess of their level of tolerance.

The basic mechanism underlying morphine tolerance is not as yet known. The use of one narcotic agent confers cross-tolerance to all others; that is, one agent can be substituted for any other and thereby prevent the symptoms of withdrawal. When heroin is not available, the addict can use morphine, methadone, hydromorphone, paregoric, or codeine as substitutes.[16] Opiate cross-tolerance does not extend to barbiturates, alcohol, or amphetamine, and these drugs do not prevent or suppress the narcotic abstinence syndrome.

[16] *Pentazocine* (Talwin) is a moderately effective narcotic analgesic agent that also possesses weak narcotic antagonistic properties. Contrary to early impressions and claims, this drug has abuse potential especially when administered by injection. If taken within twelve hours after the last dose by a narcotic-dependent individual, the weak antagonist pentazocine might precipitate a mild withdrawal syndrome. At times thereafter, it would prove only slightly effective in relieving the symptoms associated with narcotic withdrawal.

Physical Dependence and the Abstinence Syndrome

Chronic administration of the opiates leads to the rapid development of physical dependence on these drugs. Unequivocal proof of physical dependence can be observed in the abstinence symptoms occurring after the abrupt stoppage of narcotic administration and their almost immediate termination after a narcotic agent is taken. The intensity of the abstinence syndrome varies with the relative degree of physical dependence, which, in turn, is dependent upon the dosage generally used at the time of drug withdrawal.

Symptoms begin within 8 to 12 hours after the last dose and resemble those signs encountered during a bout with influenza. The addict experiences tearing, a running nose, sweating, yawning, and difficulty in sleeping. This restless sleep is commonly referred to as the "yen." At about 20 hours, goose flesh (hence the term "cold turkey"), widened pupils, and tremors appear. At the peak intensity of withdrawal (about 48 to 72 hours), the addict suffers from insomnia, weakness, muscle spasms in the legs, chills, intestinal cramps, nausea, vomiting, diarrhea, fever, and an elevated blood pressure; in very severe cases, addicts may suffer from hallucinations and become delirious. These symptoms abate within one week, even in the absence of treatment, and at this time most of the addict's tolerance to opiates has been lost; unfortunately, the psychological dependence (craving) persists. Administration of a narcotic agent at any time during the abstinence syndrome will immediately terminate these symptoms and restore the addict to "normal." Although acute opiate withdrawal is thought to be a very dangerous and often fatal process, there is no evidence to support this belief. To date, the medical literature has failed to document any deaths directly attributable to withdrawal per se.

Opiate Dependence of the Newborn

Heroin and related opiates cross the placental barrier just as these drugs traverse the blood-brain barrier. Thus, as might be anticipated, the fetus is exposed to the opiates taken by the mother. In a comprehensive study,[17] observations were made on 384 infants born to heroin-dependent mothers. Of these infants, 259 (67%) manifested signs of narcotic withdrawal the first four days of life; 178 of these babies required drug treatment in order to suppress the abstinence syndrome. The severity of the symptoms, their time of onset, and the duration of these signs were observed to correlate with the maternal dose of heroin, the duration of maternal addiction, and the time the last dose of opiate was taken with relation to the time of birth. The withdrawal syndrome in the infants was characterized by irritability, hyperactivity, tremors, vomiting, a high-pitched cry, sneezing, and respiratory distress. The incidence of congenital abnormalities and infant mortality was no higher than that observed in infants born of non-opiate-dependent mothers, although the incidence of low birth

---

[17] C. Zelson, E. Rubio, and E. Wasserman, "Neonatal Narcotic Addiction: Ten Year Observation," *Pediatrics* **48**:178–89 (1971).

weights and slower rates of weight gain have been observed. While the national incidence of low birth weight (less than 2500 g or 5.5 lbs) is between 8 and 10 percent, the incidence is about five times higher in infants born of narcotic-dependent mothers.

Some 85 percent of opiate-dependent women are in the childbearing age of 15 to 40 and many are enrolled in methadone maintenance programs. A methadone withdrawal syndrome has been reported in newborns that occurs with greater frequency and intensity than heroin withdrawal and is of longer duration. Many view such problems to be balanced by the benefits of the program to the mother and infant, which include regular medical supervision of pregnancy, decreased usage of impure street drugs, and a normalization of the maternal life-style during pregnancy.

Patterns of Abuse

It is estimated that there are between 300,000 and 600,000 narcotic addicts in the United States. Recent years have witnessed new trends in the nature of the narcotic user. The "typical" addict in the past was a poor urban black or Chicano. We now see narcotic dependence migrating to the suburbs and into the homes of the white middle class. These white youths use opiates in an attempt to relieve their feelings of dissatisfaction, frustration, and disaffiliation with society. In other instances, drug use has been initiated in search of a new "kick" or out of curiosity. A far more disquieting trend is the use of heroin among teenagers. In a 1971 survey conducted in the state of New York, 15.6 percent of the heroin users were 14–17 years of age, and 50 percent were in the 18-to-24 age bracket.

Most addicts have experimented with other drugs (tobacco, alcohol, marijuana, amphetamine, and barbiturates) prior to their use of narcotics. In some instances, heroin dependence is a direct consequence of the use of other drugs. To come down from a "speed run" or counteract the extreme excitement produced by cocaine, heroin is often employed. Frequent use of heroin in this manner may result in a dependent state.

Considerable concern was voiced about veterans returning from Southeast Asia as heroin addicts. A large number of causative factors have been attributed to their use of this drug, including participation in an unpopular war, boredom while confined to base, and inability to procure *Cannabis*. Heroin was very inexpensive in Southeast Asia, of high quality (95 percent pure), and readily available. Some men mistakenly believed that dependence did not develop if heroin was smoked or sniffed. Early (overestimated) reports issued in 1971 revealed that 10 to 15 percent of the American troops stationed in Vietnam were heroin-dependent. To combat this problem, education, treatment, and rehabilitation programs were instituted, as well as mandatory urine analysis for troops leaving this area and a liberalization of previously restricted Veterans Administration benefits for narcotic-dependent individuals. The widely proclaimed "heroin plague," carried by returning servicemen, never materialized.

Treatment of Narcotic Dependence

Withdrawal is only the first and least important stop in the treatment of narcotic addiction.

—H. Isbell and V. H. Vogel (1948)

As discussed in Chapter 10, three elements contribute to the initial use and subsequent psychological dependence upon drugs. These elements are the drug, the individual, and the setting or environment. It is not possible at this time to assess the relative contribution each plays in the opiate-dependent state. Moreover, it appears unlikely that a single formula will be derived that will be applicable for all persons dependent on these drugs.

Experience has shown that curing narcotic dependence entails far more than removing the source of heroin from the addict for weeks or even months. We know that many addicts come, in a drug-free state, from a hospital or prison and become readdicted shortly after the return to a familiar environment. Attempts have been made to explain this *relapse* in terms of biochemical or physiological changes in the central nervous system, as well as by psychological (learning) mechanisms. Many believe that a better understanding of why relapse occurs holds the key to solving the opiate dependency problem.

Prior to the last decade, the outlook for the successful treatment of the narcotic addict was indeed bleak. Individuals were hospitalized or incarcerated, but soon after their release the large majority were soon readdicted. Today we are still faced with a monumental heroin addiction problem, but many believe that the "heroin epidemic" has been contained. Two basic treatment approaches have been introduced in the intervening years that have proved to be far more successful than previous methods. One of these approaches is psychosocial and the other is pharmacological in nature. Both methods attempt to encourage discontinuation of the use of the narcotic agent and to simultaneously rehabilitate the addict.

Psychosocial Approach

Psychosocial groups, such as Synanon, provide a community wherein former addicts live and work together. Like Alcoholics Anonymous, Synanon believes that the dependent individual will never be cured and will suffer relapses periodically. An essential part of this program is group therapy sessions in which the addict attempts to readjust to a drug-free life-style. Other programs have been instituted to serve as half-way houses, seeking to facilitate and ease the harsh transition from hospital or prison to society and the easy path to readdiction.

Pharmacological Approach

The major pharmacological approach to the treatment of opiate dependence involves the use of **methadone**. In 1976 there were about 90,000 addicts participating in a methadone maintenance program in their local communities throughout the United States. Notwithstanding the modest success of this program, there are individuals who are highly critical of its underlying philosophy and operation. Prior to examining these controversial issues, let us first briefly review pertinent aspects of methadone's pharmacology with respect to its use for the treatment of heroin dependence.

Heroin is most active intravenously and has a duration of action of 4 to 6 hours. Thereafter withdrawal effects begin, signaling the need for another injection. By contrast, methadone is highly active orally (obviating the need for an injection), and it acts for 24 hours after a single dose. Methadone has three effects: It prevents the heroin abstinence syndrome; it reduces or eliminates the desire or craving for heroin; and it blocks the pleasurable effects normally derived from an intravenous heroin injection. The absence of this euphoric effect eventually results in a discontinuation or marked reduction in the sporadic use of heroin. It should be noted that if sufficiently large doses of heroin are injected, the methadone blockade of euphoria can be overcome.

Careful adjustment of the dosage of methadone is important. If the dose is raised too rapidly during the early stages of therapy, the addict will experience a "high," although not of the intense magnitude obtained after intravenous heroin. Conversely, if the dose of methadone is reduced too quickly, the addict will suffer a mild abstinence syndrome.[18]

Reliable statistics on the success of methadone maintenance programs and their relative effectiveness when compared with other treatment modalities are difficult, if not virtually impossible, to obtain. One of the major obstacles has arisen from a lack of general agreement as to what criteria should be included when attempting to quantify treatment effectiveness. Common treatment goals might include a reduction (or for others, elimination) of alcohol and illicit drug use and criminal activities associated with such drug usage, and rehabilitative outcomes including gainful employment, school attendance, or homemaking.

A major argument against the existence of this program is that methadone addiction is merely substituted for heroin addiction, a state that could conceivably continue for the remainder of the addict's life.[19] Moreover, since methadone does not cure the addictive state, it is said to be a "cop-out" for the weak-willed who lack the fortitude to undergo simple abstinence. There is little

---

[18] Clonidine, a centrally acting α-adrenergic receptor blocking agent, is currently undergoing chemical trials for use in the treatment of narcotic dependence. This drug effectively suppresses the abstinence syndrome caused by methadone and other narcotics (Chapter 21).

[19] A conflict exists among workers in this field as to whether *abstinence* represents an attainable goal for all addicts, or whether, in many cases, it may be so unrealistic as to create unnecessary frustrations for both health care workers and addicts. Within two years after their termination from methadone maintenance programs in New York City, about 90 percent of 202 persons were again using narcotics, or were using alcohol or other drugs to their detriment, or were arrested, or had died (V. P. Dole and H. Joseph, "Methadone Maintenance. Outcome After Termination," *New York State Journal of Medicine* 77: 1409-12, 1977). Of those who completed detoxification from methadone maintenance programs, as many as 35 percent were narcotic-free and generally doing well up to six years later (B. Stimmel et al., "Ability to Remain Abstinent After Methadone Detoxification: A Six-Year Study," *Journal of the American Medical Association* 237: 1216–20, 1977).

doubt that the use of methadone leads to a dependent state, that is, methadone addiction. This author believes that the benefits to the individual (in terms of improved health and the return to a productive life) and to society far outweigh the moral disadvantages. Methadone for the addict has been likened to insulin for the diabetic or phenytoin (Dilantin) for the epileptic. That is, the drug permits a normal way of life.

Detractors of the program are not convinced that methadone effectively blocks heroin-induced euphoria and point to several published studies wherein heroin has been detected in the urine of a very high percentage of those persons participating in the program. Carelessly administered programs have led to the street usage of methadone; some cities have had a marked increase in the number of deaths attributed to methadone overdosage. Further, as some addicts "turn off" heroin, they "turn on" to alcohol, barbiturates, and amphetamine. In some communities, methadone therapy is viewed as a panacea for the heroin problem, with little effort directed toward determining the underlying motivating factors initially leading to the use of heroin; psychological, social, and vocational rehabilitation are also often neglected.

In summary, even the staunchest advocates of the methadone program do not view this drug as the final solution to the problem of heroin dependence. This author believes that methadone represents the best treatment currently available.[20] For this program to be successful, methadone can only be considered to be a part of the treatment regimen. An equally important element involves the rehabilitation of the addict which will enable this individual to return to society with dignity. The long-range objective must continue to be a search for the motivating factors that cause such individuals to seek a chemical escape from society.

SUMMARY

Even in this age of wonder drugs, it is easy to appreciate why morphine has been termed "God's own medicine." Recent advances in the biomedical sciences have made available compounds that are as effective as morphine for the relief of intense pain, the treatment of potentially life-threatening diarrhea, and the suppression of cough. However, none of these newer drugs have been shown to be clinically superior to the naturally occurring alkaloid morphine.

Although pain is a very real sensation, finding a lucid, concrete definition proves to be a difficult task. The emotional aspects of pain clearly modify our

---

[20] *Levo-alpha-acetylmethadol* (LAAM or methadyl acetate) is currently undergoing clinical trials as a substitute for methadone to which it is closely related. This orally active drug is reported to be as safe and effective as methadone and has a duration of action about three times as long; a single dose of LAAM can suppress the opiate abstinence syndrome for up to 72 hours, thus reducing the number of clinic visits from seven to three per week. (W. Ling, C. Charuvastra, S. C. Kaim, and J. Klett, "Methadyl Acetate and Methadone as Maintenance Treatment for Heroin Addicts," *Archives of General Psychiatry* **33**: 709–20, 1976.)

ability to speak of it in objective terms. We have all observed children fall and yet not complain about their injuries until they observe the bruised area bleeding. Clinical evaluation of analgesic agents is complicated by these psychic factors, as well as wide variation among individuals in their threshold perception of pain.

Morphine is thought to produce its potent analgesic effects by interfering with the patient's subjective appreciation of the emotional aspects of pain. The analgesic and behavioral effects of narcotic analgesics are thought to result from their interaction with opiate receptors, receptors normally activated by endogenous opiates (endorphins, enkephalins). These peptides are believed to inhibit the transmission of sensory information, for example, that resulting from a painful stimulus. Recent evidence suggests that placebo-induced analgesia and acupuncture analgesia may result from the release of these endogenous opiates.

Therapeutic doses of morphine produce a wide range of undesirable side effects, some of which include nausea, drowsiness, behavioral disturbances, and constipation. Higher doses cause respiratory depression by virtue of a direct drug action on the respiratory centers located in the medulla. Toxic amounts of the opiates may produce a potentially fatal cessation of respiration, a condition effectively reversed by prompt administration of narcotic antagonists (naloxone).

The major objection to the chronic administration of the narcotic agents is their proclivity to abuse. In the minds of many individuals, drug addiction is synonymous with narcotic dependence. Chronic use of the opiates results in psychological dependence; marked, but selective tolerance (tolerance to analgesia, euphoria, and respiratory depression, but not to constipation or pupillary constriction); and physical dependence. Abrupt withdrawal of the opiates or the acute administration of a narcotic antagonist precipitates an abstinence syndrome.

Extensive pharmacological research has been conducted over the years and will continue to be carried out in the future in an attempt to find an analgesic agent that relieves pain as effectively as morphine, is active after oral administration, causes no major adverse effects, and most importantly does not produce dependence with repeated usage.

Members of the opiate family possess a spectrum of pharmacological activities ranging from drugs that are pure agonists (morphine) to those that are pure antagonists (naloxone). Human and animal studies reveal that pure agonists are potent analgesics with high abuse potential, while pure antagonists are devoid of analgesic properties and abuse liability. A third group of opiates contains a mixture of varying proportions of agonistic and antagonistic properties; nalorphine, for example, is an antagonist with some agonist activity. In theory, an appropriately balanced mixed agonist-antagonist, with predominantly agonistic properties, should be capable of producing effective analgesia and yet have considerably less abuse potential than pure agonists. Clinical experience shows that pentazocine, butorphanol, and nulbuphine approach this objective. Narcotic agents of the future will undoubtedly be mixed agonist-antagonists. This spectrum of opiate properties can be readily predicted by evaluating a test compound in the opiate receptor-binding assay in the presence and absence of sodium.[21]

Successful treatment of narcotic dependence involves the discontinuation of drug usage and the rehabilitation of the addict to enable this individual to adequately adjust to society. Methadone is now widely used for the pharmacological treatment of narcotic dependence; it prevents heroin withdrawal effects and craving, and it blocks the euphoria produced by an intravenous injection of this illicit narcotic.

SUPPLEMENTARY READINGS

Beaumont, A., and J. Hughes, "Biology of Opioid Peptides," *Annual Review of Pharmacology and Toxicology* **19**: 245–67 (1979).

Beers, R. F., Jr., and E. G. Bassett, eds., *Mechanisms of Pain and Analgesic Compounds.* New York: Raven Press, 1979.

Costa, E., and M. Trabucchi, eds. *The Endorphins.* New York: Raven Press, 1978.

Dupont, R. I., A. Goldstein, and J. O'Donnell, eds., *Handbook on Drug Abuse.* Washington, D.C.: National Institute on Drug Abuse, 1979.

Eddy, N. B., and E. L. May, "The Search for a Better Analgesic," *Science* **181**: 407–14 (1973).

Goldstein, A., "Heroin Addiction. Sequential Treatment Employing Pharmacologic Supports," *Archives of General Psychiatry* **33**: 353–58 (1976).

Jaffe, J. H., and W. R. Martin, "Opioid Analgesics and Antagonists," in *Goodman and Gilman's The Pharmacological Basis of Therapeutics.* Edited by A. G. Gilman, L. S. Goodman, and A. Gilman. 6th ed., Chap. 22, pp. 494–534. New York: Macmillan, 1980.

Kosterlitz, H. W., H. O. J. Collier, and J. E. Villarreal, eds., *Agonist and Antagonistic Actions of Narcotic Analgesic Drugs.* Baltimore: University Park Press, 1973.

Lasagna, L., "The Clinical Effectiveness of Morphine and its Substitutes as Analgesics," *Pharmacological Reviews* **16**: 47–83 (1964).

Resnick, R. B., E. Schuyten-Resnick and A. M. Washton, "Assessment of Narcotic Antagonists in the Treatment of Opioid Dependence," *Annual Review of Pharmacology and Toxicology* **20**: 463–74 (1980).

Simon, E. J., and J. M. Hiller, "The Opiate Receptors," *Annual Review of Pharmacology and Toxicology* **18**: 371–94 (1978).

Snyder, S. H., and S. R. Childers, "Opiate Receptors and Opioid Peptides," *Annual Review of Neuroscience,* **2**: 35–64 (1979).

Villaverde, M. M., and C. W. MacMillan, *Pain: From Symptom to Treatment.* New York: Van Nostrand Reinhold, 1977.

[21] C. B. Pert and S. H. Snyder, "Opiate Receptor Binding of Agonists and Antagonists Affected Differentially by Sodium," *Molecular Pharmacology* **10**: 868–79 (1974).

14

Nonnarcotic Analgesic and Antipyretic Agents

Pain is a more terrible lord of mankind than even death himself.
—Albert Schweitzer (1875–1965)

From time to time, we are all victims of the minor pain associated with headaches, muscle cramps, and toothaches, to mention a few. It is easier to evaluate these pains in retrospect as "minor" rather than at the time of their occurrence. Your response is probably not unlike that of millions of other pain sufferers for the past several generations—you reach for one or two aspirin tablets or for an aspirin-containing product. In 1978, Americans spent $931 million on nonprescription internal analgesic (pain-relieving) agents. Of this total, over $570 million was expended to purchase aspirin alone and in combination with other ingredients and $217 million was spent for the purchase of acetaminophen (Datril, Tylenol).

This chapter will consider aspirin and related salicylates, para-aminophenol derivatives (acetaminophen), and anti-inflammatory agents such as phenylbutazone (Butazolidin). We shall observe that aspirin is far from being a simple pain reliever but, rather, possesses many other properties, some of which result from actions involving the prostaglandins.

HISTORICAL DEVELOPMENT

The **salicylates** are among the oldest class of drugs that still enjoy an unchallenged place in modern therapeutics. The medicinal properties of willow bark were well appreciated by the ancient Greek physicians. Willow bark was suggested as an inexpensive substitute for cinchona bark, which contains quinine, an effective antipyretic (fever-reducing) agent. In the early nineteenth century, salicin was extracted from the bark, and this compound was readily converted to salicylic acid.

The history of the clinical development of the classical analgesic-antipyretic agents may be likened to a student's correctly arriving at the right answer in a multiple choice test, notwithstanding a grossly inadequate and even incorrect understanding of the principle upon which the proper response is predicated.

In 1860, the German chemist Hermann Kolbe discovered that salicylic acid could be synthesized from carbolic acid (phenol). He observed that the salicylic acid, after standing for a time, would slowly decompose back to carbolic acid. Several years later, Lord Joseph Lister introduced carbolic acid into medicine as a germicide or antiseptic agent (Chapter 2). In 1873, Kolbe theorized that if salicylic acid could be converted to carbolic acid in his test tube, why could not this same reaction occur in the living body? Much to his delight, he observed that when salicylic acid was dusted on wounds, healing occurred and infection was absent. When this compound was administered to patients with typhoid fever, typhus, and pneumonia, in almost all cases the high fever was reduced; unfortunately, within several days, the patients were dead. Patients with rheumatism were more fortunate. Their fever subsided and their pain was reduced, but no one died from rheumatism.

Carbolic Acid   Salicylic Acid

The explanation underlying these observations finally emerged. Salicylic acid is not converted to carbolic acid in the body as was postulated, but rather is itself a germicidal agent when applied to wounds. Internal administration of this agent had no effect on the microorganisms responsible for typhoid fever, typhus, and pneumonia; the temporary improvement observed in these patients was merely the result of a marked reduction in temperature, as well as the alleviation of pain. In retrospect, the antipyretic activity of salicylic acid and similar effects elicited by the willow bark which contains salicin, a salicylate-like compound, were in agreement. In short, although salicylic acid was not found to be a useful germicide or antibacterial agent, it was shown to have antipyretic, analgesic and antirheumatic properties. Astute clinical observations, in the absence of a scientific basis, led to the discovery of the analgesic-antipyretic agent acetanilid in 1886.

At about the same time, the Bayer Company was faced with the dilemma of disposing of a vast surplus of para-aminophenol, a seemingly worthless byproduct in the manufacture of dyes. Appreciating its chemical similarity to acetanilid, this byproduct was converted to ethoxyacetanilid or *phenacetin*. Almost a century later, phenacetin is still employed as an effective but potentially dangerous analgesic-antipyretic agent. It is the "P" in APC (aspirin-phenacetin-caffeine) tablets. In 1899, the Bayer Company sought to develop a better antipyretic agent than salicylic acid. The product of these endeavors was acetylsalicylic acid (in German, a*cetyl* **Spir***säure*), known worldwide as *aspirin*.

In the short span of one-quarter of a century (1873–1899) the symptomatic treatment of pain, fever, and rheumatism was totally revolutionized. Let us now consider the salicylates.

EXTERNAL SALICYLATES

The salicylates are the most important class of analgesic-antipyretic agents. There are three compounds worthy of consideration in the salicylate class and all are familiar to the general reader, namely, salicylic acid, methyl salicylate (externally applied drugs), and acetylsalicylic acid.

Salicylic Acid   ·

This compound is far too irritating for internal use but, rather, is applied to the skin. It is the most widely used ingredient in nonprescription combination products (liquids, creams, ointments, and pads) intended for the treatment of corns, calluses, and warts (Dr. Scholl's products, Freezone Corn and Callus Remover). Salicylic acid is termed a *keratolytic agent,* a compound capable of dissolving the epidermal layers of skin and causing their peeling. This same compound is often used in combination with sulfur and/or resorcinol in *antiacne* preparations (Acnomel, Clearasil, Dry and Clear, Komed).

Methyl Salicylate

Methyl salicylate or *oil of wintergreen* is a colorless or light yellow liquid with a very characteristic odor and taste of wintergreen. It is the most commonly used external analgesic and counterirritant for the relief of aching pain from sore muscles and joints. When rubbed on the skin in the form of a liniment or lotion, it stimulates the flow of blood to the localized area (*rubefacient effect*), producing warmth and the relief of pain (Ben-Gay, Counterpain Rub, Heet, Musterole, Sloan's Liniment, Zemo). Other common ingredients used as external analgesic and counterirritants, often in combination with methyl salicylate, include menthol, camphor, thymol, turpentine oil, and chloroform.

Oil of wintergreen is frequently used alone as a liniment and as such is a common product found in the family medicine chest. Children are attracted to it because of its unique aroma. It is a toxic compound and the ingestion of as little as one teaspoonful (5 ml) has been know to cause fatalities in children.

ASPIRIN (ACETYLSALICYLIC ACID)

The very extensive use of aspirin and its ready accessibility to the public have perhaps diminished this drug's esteem in the mind of the public; perhaps this compound best exemplifies the old adage, "familiarity breeds contempt." Notwithstanding some of the potential dangers and adverse side effects associated with aspirin, it is among the safest drugs and is fully worthy of the designation "wonder drug."

Before we attempt to justify these accolades, a word about its chemical stability is in order. Aspirin is stable in dry air, but when exposed to warm moist air slowly hydrolyzes to salicylic and acetic acids. The presence of this latter acid accounts for the vinegar-like odor often detected in opened bottles of aspirin that have resided on your medicine shelf cabinet for some time. The pharmacological significance of this observation has yet to be determined.

| Aspirin | Salicylic acid | Acetic acid (vinegar odor) |

Pharmacologic Actions

Aspirin and sodium salicylate are readily biotransformed to salicylic acid in the body. Since both drugs have similar pharmacological properties, we shall use the terms *aspirin and salicylate* interchangeably. Aspirin has analgesic, antipyretic, and anti-inflammatory–antirheumatic actions, in addition to many other widely diverse minor actions in the body.

Many diverse and unrelated theories have been postulated to explain the mechanisms underlying the disparate effects of aspirin and related drugs. Pioneering research activities by John Vane and his co-workers in England led to the discovery in the early 1970s that many aspirin-induced effects result from inhibition of *prostaglandin* synthesis.[1] Since aspirin and the prostaglandins are inextricably linked, and because the very broad spectrum of biological effects and potential clinical uses of the prostaglandins have attracted considerable attention in recent years, it is appropriate that we at least introduce the reader to these extremely exciting compounds.

[1] J. R. Vane, "Inhibition of Prostaglandin Synthesis as a Mechanism of Action of Aspirin-Like Drugs," *Nature [New Biology]* **231**:232–35 (1971).

Prostaglandins

The prostaglandins are a family of approximately fifteen naturally occurring fatty acids (Figure 14–1). Although they have since been shown to be present in most tissues of the body, their name is derived from the initial discovery of these compounds in human and sheep seminal vesicles.

Prostaglandins are hormone-like substances believed to play important roles in regulating cellular metabolism and function. They may be classified as local or tissue hormones because they exert their actions in the immediate area in which they are released. Classical hormones, such as insulin, thyroid hormone, and estrogen, by contrast, are released from ductless (endocrine) glands into the general circulation wherein they are carried to and act at distant sites. No storage pool of prostaglandins exists in tissues; rather, they are synthesized to meet the immediate needs of the organism. Synthesis, controlled by the enzyme system *prostaglandin synthetase,* starts and shuts off within seconds.

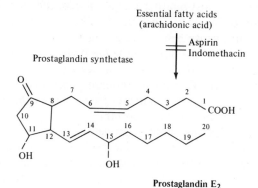

Prostaglandin E$_2$

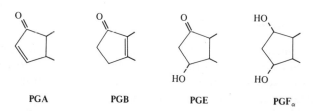

FIGURE 14–1. Abbreviated Biosynthesis and Basic Ring Structures of the Prostaglandins. Prostaglandins are biosynthesized from essential fatty acids such as arachidonic acid via several intermediate compounds. Prostaglandin synthetase, the primary enzyme controlling synthesis, is inhibited by aspirin, indomethacin, and other selected anti-inflammatory agents. Prostaglandins (PG) are designated according to the position of the carbon-to-carbon double bond and presence of ketone (C $=$ O) and hydroxyl (—OH) groups in the basic five-membered ring. The numbered subscript refers to the number of double bonds outside the ring; for example, PGE$_2$ refers to a prostaglandin of the E series with two double bonds.

No simple generalizations can be made with respect to the biological properties of the prostaglandins. Differences in activity, sometimes even in opposite directions, may exist among these derivatives in a given animal species; for example, PGE_1 inhibits and PGE_2 enhances the aggregation of blood platelets, thus retarding and promoting blood coagulation, respectively. Moreover, a single prostaglandin derivative may produce opposite effects in different animal species; for example, while PGF_2 causes vasoconstriction in dogs and rats, it produces vasodilation in cats and rabbits. The spectrum of some of the extremely diverse pharmacological effects elicited by very low doses of natural and synthetic prostaglandin derivatives and the potential clinical significance of such effects are summarized in Table 14–1.

Analgesic Actions of Salicylates

While morphine and related narcotics produce analgesia by their actions in the central nervous system, most pharmacologists accept the view that aspirin has a peripheral site of analgesic action. Unlike morphine, aspirin in therapeutic doses does not cause behavioral changes.

It has been suggested that the polypeptide *bradykinin* is the chemical mediator of pain in the periphery and initiates a pain message by stimulating a pain receptor. Prostaglandins of the E series are thought to sensitize pain receptors to bradykinin activation. The analgesic effects of aspirin are generally believed to result, at least in part, from its ability to inhibit prostaglandin synthesis.

Aspirin effectively alleviates mild-to-moderate pain, while morphine relieves pain of all intensities. Unlike morphine, aspirin has no abuse potential. That is, chronic aspirin administration does not lead to psychic or physical dependence. Moreover, tolerance does not develop to the analgesic effects of aspirin. Generally, an increase in salicylate dosage reflects a progression of the disease state and not drug tolerance.

Fever and Antipyresis

Aspirin reduces the body temperature in the presence of fever but does not modify normal temperature at the usual therapeutic doses. Before we examine the mechanism underlying aspirin's antipyretic action, let us briefly examine the normal regulation of temperature in the body.

Sites in the hypothalamus carefully control the production and loss of body heat in order to maintain our bodies at an optimal temperature of 98.6° F (37° C). When the temperature of the blood rises, cells in the anterior hypothalamus send nerve impulses to the periphery that cause sweating and vasodilation of the blood vessels in the skin. This results in a loss of body heat and a reduction in body temperature. Conversely, cells in the posterior hypothalamus are responsible for the production and conservation of body heat. These cells inhibit sweating and cause vasoconstriction of the blood vessels in the skin. We may liken the hypothalamus to the thermostat in our homes. *Fever* is the result of an alteration in the normal heat regulating mechanisms of the body by a mechanism thought to involve the prostaglandins of the E series. In effect, in fever the body's thermostat is set at a higher than normal level, and aspirin resets the thermostat.

Aspirin, in therapeutic doses, has no effect on heat production but does increase heat loss from the body by its action on the thermoregulatory centers in the hypothalamus. This is accomplished by causing marked dilation of the small blood vessels of the skin and by increased sweating. We are all familiar with the profuse sweating that occurs after one takes several aspirin tablets, and this may be thought to be an absolute requirement for the reduction of fever. Although there is little doubt that sweating is associated with the action of antipyretics and does promote the reduction in fever, it is by no means essential.

Salicylates are *nonspecific* antipyretic agents. That is, these drugs do not modify the underlying cause of fever, such as a bacterial or a viral infection; they only affect the symptom associated with these disorders, namely, fever.

Anti-Inflammatory and Antirheumatic Actions

In the past two decades, several classes of drugs (cortisone, phenylbutazone) have appeared which are capable of dramatically alleviating the symptoms of rheumatic and inflammatory diseases. Many individuals thought that aspirin might be relegated to a position of mere historical interest for the treatment of these disorders. However, with a better appreciation of the potential dangers associated with these newer compounds, this early enthusiasm has been markedly tempered. For many physicians, aspirin remains the first drug to be employed for most inflammatory and rheumatic diseases.

Inflammation is a local tissue response to injury caused by chemical or physical agents. Its cardinal symptoms are redness, heat at the site of inflammation, swelling, pain, and loss of motion. How can we explain these symptoms? Capillary dilation occurs at the site of injury, resulting in the increased flow of fluids into tissue spaces. This fluid transfer causes edema (swelling) and produces pressure on nerve endings; pain ensues. The increased blood supply underlies the heat at the site of inflammation. For many years, scientists have sought to determine whether injuries of all types caused the local release of a "mediator" substance that may be responsible for the increased capillary permeability. Among the many candidates nominated for this mediator role in inflammation are histamine, serotonin, bradykinin, and the prostaglandins.

Prostaglandins of the E series are believed to be the most important chemical mediators of the inflammatory response, and it is thought that aspirin-like compounds may produce their anti-inflammatory effects by inhibiting prostaglandin synthesis in the body.

Salicylates are very effective in reducing fever and the painful swelling of the joints associated with rheumatic fever. Many theories have been postulated to explain these beneficial effects, but none have met with universal approval. Aspirin may act by antagonizing prostaglandins or other mediator substances or may act rather nonspecifically to reduce the capillary permeability, edema, and pain.

TABLE 14-1. REPRESENTATIVE EFFECTS OF PROSTAGLANDINS AND THEIR POTENTIAL CLINICAL SIGNIFICANCE

System or Tissue, Physiological Effect	PG-Induced Effect*	Potential Clinical Significance
Cardiovascular system		
Blood pressure	Increased or decreased	Development of drugs for the treatment of hypertension, peripheral vascular disease, and circulatory shock.
Peripheral vascular resistance	Decreased	
Norepinephrine release	Inhibited	
Sodium excretion	Increased	
Blood platelet aggregation	Increased	Thromboxanes (PG-related) appear to play a physiological role in clot formation.
	Decreased	Development of anticoagulant drugs (prostacyclin) that prevent the formation of blood clots associated with heart attacks and stroke.
Respiratory system		
Bronchial smooth muscle	Relaxation	Development of antiasthmatic drugs.
	Contraction	Possible role in asthmatic attacks.
Nasal passages	Shrinkage	Shrinkage of swollen passages may lead to development of nasal decongestants.
Endocrine system		
Uterine smooth muscle	Contraction	Induction of abortion and initiation of labor at term. Clinically available drugs: dinoprost ($PGF_{2\alpha}$) and dinoprostone (PGE_2).

Luteinizing hormone release	Increased	Enhanced ovulation–development of drugs for correction of female and male infertility. Also potential male and female contraceptives.
Stomach		
Gastric acid secretion	Inhibition	Development of drugs for peptic ulcer disease.
Ulcer formation potential	Increased	Aspirin, indomethacin, and related inhibitors of PG biosynthesis may cause gastric erosions.
Miscellaneous effects		
Inflammatory response	Increased	PGE_2 is involved in chemical mediation of inflammation. Anti-inflammatory effects of aspirin, indomethacin, ibuprofen, and others (Table 14-2) result from inhibition of PG biosynthesis.
Pain sensation	Increased	PGs are thought to play a role in pain and fever. PGE enhances bradykinin-induced pain and acts as a chemical mediator of fever. The inhibition of PG synthesis by aspirin and acetaminophen serves as the basis for their analgesic and antipyretic properties.
Thermoregulation	Fever	
Intraocular pressure	Decreased	PGs reduce intraocular pressure which may lead to development of antiglaucoma drugs.

*PG-induced effects may differ according to the specific prostaglandin derivative, the dose or concentration, and the animal species tested. Not all these effects may prove to be relevant in human health and disease.

Toxicology of Salicylates

Salicylates are relatively nontoxic drugs; yet in the United States each year several hundred persons die as the result of acute overdosage, and this class of drugs has been consistently among the most frequently ingested by children under 5 years of age. The relative incidence of ingestions of baby aspirins to adult aspirins was 7.5–10 to 1 from the years 1965–1970. Parents have been notoriously careless in leaving medicines—baby aspirins, in particular—within the reach of their young children. They have compounded this problem by frequently persuading their children to take orange-flavored "candies." The potential dangers associated with this practice are all too obvious. Extensive and intensive campaigns by the government and private organizations publicizing the dangers associated with accidental aspirin ingestion by children have paid large dividends. From 1965 to 1974 there was an 83 percent decrease in fatal aspirin and salicylate poisoning in children less than 5 years old. Other factors responsible for this progressive decline in aspirin poisonings have been attributed to a reduction in the maximum number of baby aspirin tablets (1 ¼ grain or 81 mg) to 36 per bottle, and the use of safety tops designed to prevent 80 percent of children under 5 years old from opening the bottle.

Acute Toxicity

Shortly after ingestion of high doses of aspirin, we observe rapid and deep breathing, resulting from the drug's direct stimulating effects on the respiratory center in the medulla. Nausea, gastric irritation, sweating, fever, tinnitus (ringing in the ears), dizziness, mental confusion, hallucinations, coma, and an inability to urinate ensue. Life-threatening complex changes occur in the acid-base balance of the body. The more rapidly the child receives medical care, the better the prognosis for recovery. Death may occur within several hours or up to a few days. A single dose of 20–30 g (60–100 adult aspirin tablets) is the usual lethal dose for adults.

An immediate first aid measure is to attempt to induce vomiting by placing a finger in the throat or by administering a tablespoonful of syrup of ipecac. Emesis will remove the unabsorbed aspirin. Treatment at a hospital involves reduction of fever and the replacement of fluids and essential salts in order to prevent dehydration and restore the normal acid-base balance of the body. In more severe cases, an artificial kidney or peritoneal dialysis is employed to remove the salicylate from the body.

Salicylism

This term is used to describe a group of bothersome, but not particularly dangerous, symptoms that generally result from the ingestion of large therapeutic doses of salicylates such as are employed for the treatment of rheumatic fever, arthritis, or similar diseases. Daily doses of greater than 2 g (seven tablets) of aspirin frequently induce nausea, vomiting, tinnitus, hearing loss (which is reversible after discontinuation of therapy), headache, and mental confusion.

Aspirin Allergy

It has been conservatively estimated that 0.2 percent of the general population, or two per thousand, are allergic to aspirin. In relative terms, this figure is rather low. However, when we consider the number of individuals in the United States taking this drug and the absence of restrictions for obtaining it, the absolute number of persons—about 300,000–400,000—who might potentially be allergic to aspirin is significant. Signs of allergy include skin rashes, swelling of the eyelids, face, and lips, and asthmatic-like symptoms, which could prove fatal. Up to 20 percent of individuals suffering from allergic disorders, especially asthma or chronic hives, are most likely to be allergic to aspirin. Some allergists have even advocated that aspirin become a prescription drug.

Gastrointestinal Bleeding and Upset

You might now ask what are the adverse side effects confronting the average individual who only occasionally takes one or two aspirin tablets for minor aches and pains or for a headache and who is not allergic to aspirin?

Advertisements for buffered aspirin imply that *gastrointestinal upset* is a major problem frequently encountered with plain aspirin. In reality, only 5 percent of all persons suffer from dyspepsia (indigestion), nausea, and vomiting. Controlled studies have failed to demonstrate that gastric upset is prevented with buffered aspirin. These problems may be reduced by taking aspirin with food, milk, or a full glass of water, but not with an alcoholic beverage (see below).

Approximately 70 percent of all persons taking even one or two aspirin tablets suffer a *blood loss* of 2–6 ml (0.5–1 tsp). This results from irritation and ulceration of the gastric mucosa by insoluble salicylate crystals. For those of us who only take aspirin occasionally, this loss of blood is of little practical significance. This bleeding is painless and not necessarily correlated with gastric upset. However, blood loss may assume great significance for the senior citizen taking salicylates in high doses for long periods of time, for individuals with peptic ulcers, for those prone to anemia, or for menstruating women. In Chapter 12 we observed that high concentrations of alcohol are also capable of damaging the gastric mucosa. Aspirin is probably effective in relieving a hangover "the morning after," but it has been shown to enhance alcohol's destructive effects on the mucosa when both drugs are taken together.

Aspirin and Pregnancy

Recent evidence suggests that the use of aspirin during pregnancy may have adverse effects on both the mother and her fetus. The regular use of aspirin during pregnancy prolongs the periods of pregnancy and labor and increases maternal blood losses prior to and after delivery. These effects have been attributed to aspirin-induced inhibition of prostaglandin synthesis, blood platelet aggregation, and prothrombin synthesis, the latter actions increasing bleeding tendencies. Other human studies suggest that maternal aspirin use increases the frequency of anemia during pregnancy, the incidence of complicated deliveries, and the newborn mortality rate, and decreases the birth weight of the newborn. Interpretation of the influence of aspirin on the mortality rate and body weight of newborns remains controversial at present. It is strongly advised that aspirin-containing products not be used during the last three months of pregnancy except under the advice and supervision of a physician.

Aspirin-Drug Interactions

If we were to ask many people whether they had taken any drugs in the past 30 days, their response would probably be an emphatic "No." We could then pursue the questioning by asking if they had taken aspirin. The reply might be, "Oh, yes, but that does not count. I haven't taken any *real* drugs." Aspirin is a *real* drug. In Chapter 3 we indicated that the effects of one drug may be modified by the prior or concurrent administration of another drug. Let us now briefly survey some aspirin-drug and aspirin–diagnostic test interactions.

High doses of aspirin, about 5 g, have a uricosuric action; that is, these doses increase the urinary excretion of uric acid. Paradoxically, low doses, about 1 g or three tablets, inhibit uric acid excretion by the kidney tubules. Hence, low doses of aspirin should not be used to relieve the pain of gout with such uricosuric agents as probenecid (Benemid), sulfinpyrazone (Anturan), or phenylbutazone (Butazolidin). Acetaminophen may be used in such cases as an analgesic agent.

Diuretics promote the excretion of sodium, chloride, and water. Three to six tablets of aspirin have been shown to reduce excretion of salt by 50 percent. This antagonism may lead to increased edema in patients taking moderate doses of aspirin.

Aspirin is about 70 percent bound to plasma proteins (Chapter 3). Tolbutamide (Orinase), a compound used orally to reduce blood sugar in diabetes and coumarin-type anticoagulants are also protein-bound. Salicylates are capable of displacing tolbutamide from their protein binding sites, thereby increasing the amount of unbound, pharmacologically active tolbutamide in the plasma. The unfortunate consequences for the diabetic may be a precipitous drop in blood sugar with subsequent coma. Displacement of coumarin anticoagulants from protein binding sites may result in internal bleeding, and, if not treated, death may ensue.

Finally, it has been observed that aspirin may interfere with the protein-bound iodide (PBI) diagnostic test for thyroid function. This does not result from an aspirin-induced interference with normal thyroid function; rather, aspirin prevents the thyroid hormone (thyroxin) from normally binding to plasma proteins.

Therapeutic Uses of Aspirin

Analgesia

What is the unnamed mysterious "ingredient that doctors recommend most for pain?" Yes, aspirin is the drug of choice for the relief of mild-to-moderate pain. It has been shown to be far more effective for the treatment of headache, neuralgia (pain radiating from a nerve), myalgia or muscle pain, and arthralgia (pain from joints) than for deep-seated visceral pain (intestinal cramps and colic, for example). Aspirin is widely used for pain arising from muscles or bones, such as sprains, arthritic pain, and toothaches. Morphine and related narcotic analgesics are used for severe pain, regardless of their site of origin. (Table 14–2 compares the pharmacological properties of aspirin and morphine.)

What dose-response parameters are associated with aspirin as an analgesic agent? Stated in other words, how many 325 mg (5 grain) tablets must you take to demonstrate therapeutic effects that are greater than those seen with a placebo, and, if two tablets are good, will six tablets be three times better? Clinical studies comparing the effectiveness of one aspirin tablet with a placebo have yielded conflicting results. By contrast, it is generally agreed that two aspirins are definitely more effective than placebo medication. Maximum relief of pain is obtained with three or four tablets. Increased adverse effects may be anticipated by increasing the dosage.

TABLE 14-2. COMPARATIVE PHARMACOLOGICAL
PROPERTIES OF MORPHINE AND ASPIRIN

Pharmacological Properties	Morphine	Aspirin
Analgesic activity		
Analgesic classification	Narcotic	Nonnarcotic
Severity of pain	Severe	Mild-to-moderate
Origin of pain	All sites	Muscle and bone
Site of drug action	Central	Peripheral
Antipyretic activity	Absent	Present
Anti-inflammatory activity	Absent	Present
Anticoagulant activity	Absent	Present
Cough suppression	Present	Absent
Antidiarrheal activity	Present	Absent
Abuse potential	Marked	Absent
Psychological dependence	Yes	None or mild
Tolerance	Yes	No
Physical dependence	Yes	No

Antipyresis

For the reduction of fever, aspirin is the safest and most effective drug available. However, as we have previously indicated, aspirin provides only symptomatic reduction in fever without modifying the underlying cause.

Anti-Inflammatory and Antirheumatic Effects

In high daily doses of 5 to 6 g (15–20 tablets), aspirin relieves the pain, lowers the temperature, and reduces the inflammation in such diseases as rheumatoid arthritis and rheumatic fever. Although providing considerable symptomatic relief for these and related conditions, there is no evidence supporting the supposition that salicylates alter the ultimate course of the disease or modify the lesions of the heart.

Inhibition of Thrombosis

Excessive aggregation of blood platelets, with subsequent thrombus (clot in a blood vessel) formation, may be of great significance in the etiology of cerebrovascular accidents (stroke) and myocardial infarction (heart attack) and postoperative complications after cardiovascular surgery. Inhibition of the synthesis of prostaglandins and thromboxane (a prostaglandin-related endogenous compound) in platelets markedly reduces such intravascular clotting.

In a number of early clinical trials, the administration of low doses of aspirin has been shown to reduce the incidence of thrombosis postoperatively. The ability of aspirin to decrease the death rate in patients susceptible to or who have previously experienced strokes and heart attacks remains controversial. Similar controversy surrounds the antigout drug sulfinpyrazone (Anturane), also an inhibitor of prostaglandin synthesis, claimed by some to reduce the incidence of myocardial infarction in patients who have previously experienced one such episode. The future role of aspirin and other inhibitors of prostaglandin synthesis in the prevention of thrombosis remains to be determined.

PARA-AMINOPHENOL DERIVATIVES

Although aspirin is the drug of first choice for most individuals, those persons suffering from extreme gastrointestinal upset or those who are allergic to aspirin require an alternative drug. Some of these will now be discussed.

Phenacetin and its active metabolite, *acetaminophen,* are the major members of this class. Experimental evidence indicates that although phenacetin is an antipyretic agent in its own right, its analgesic activity may, in part, result from its biological product, acetaminophen.

Phenacetin → Acetaminophen
(N-acetyl-p-aminophenol)

These drugs have approximately the same analgesic and antipyretic potency as aspirin and are thought to act by the same mechanisms of action. Unfortunately, neither of these p-aminophenol derivatives have anti-inflammatory or antirheumatic activities. Compounds in this class are useful substitutes for patients who are allergic to aspirin or for those prone to severe gastrointestinal upset, irritation, or bleeding.

Phenacetin and APC

Phenacetin is rarely used alone but is most often found in combination products, such as APC, with aspirin and caffeine. Since phenacetin lacks anti-inflammatory activity, it should be anticipated that APC is less effective than plain aspirin for the treatment of diseases associated with inflammation, such as arthritis and rheumatism. There appears to be no rational justification for the inclusion of caffeine, since this compound possesses no analgesic, antipyretic, or anti-inflammatory activity, and caffeine does not enhance these aspirin-induced activities. Moreover, the amount of caffeine in these tablets, about 30 mg, or approximately one-quarter cup of coffee, is inadequate to produce central nervous system stimulation.

Phenacetin may cause *hemolytic anemia* in persons having a genetic deficiency of the enzyme glucose-6-phosphate dehydrogenase (Chapter 31). Drug-induced hemolytic anemia very rarely occurs in Caucasians but afflicts about 10 to 15 percent of American blacks. This idiosyncratic condition results from a shortened life span of red blood cells; these cells hemolyze or break down, liberating hemoglobin into the plasma. Phenacetin, when used in high doses over long periods of time, has been reported to cause kidney damage and may be subject to abuse.

Acetaminophen (Datril, Tylenol)

Acetaminophen (known in the United Kingdom as paracetamol) is the second most commonly used nonprescription analgesic and antipyretic and, when aspirin cannot be taken, is the safest and most effective aspirin substitute. It relieves pain and reduces fever by aspirin-like mechanisms, and both drugs possess approximately equivalent effectiveness and potency. Like phenacetin, acetaminophen lacks anti-inflammatory properties and does not alter platelet aggregation or blood clotting.

In recent years, acetaminophen has been gaining favor as a common household drug product. Unfortunately, there is a lack of general appreciation that, while this drug causes few adverse effects at normal therapeutic doses, acute overdosage may cause liver damage and failure (*hepatic necrosis*). Symptoms of acute toxicity may occur after the ingestion of about 7 g (approximately 22 325 mg tablets), while 15–25 g cause severe liver toxicity and may potentially represent a lethal dose. Death may occur at any time from two to seven days after drug ingestion.

Effective treatment of acetaminophen poisoning is far from entirely satisfactory and remains to be perfected. Many poison centers are now employing orally administered acetylcysteine (Mucomyst) to prevent hepatic necrosis.

OTHER DRUGS OF CONTEMPORARY INTEREST

Thus far, we have considered analgesic-antipyretic drugs that are available without a physician's prescription. Phenylbutazone and ibuprofen, two commonly employed prescription drugs of interest, will be discussed below. Table 14-3 summarizes the properties of commonly employed analgesic-antipyretic-anti-inflammatory agents.

Phenylbutazone (Azolid, Butazolidin)

Phenylbutazone is a potent anti-inflammatory agent with analgesic and antipyretic properties, but, because of its adverse side effects, its therapeutic applications are almost exclusively restricted to inflammatory conditions. The analgesic and antipyretic actions of phenylbutazone are probably mediated by a salicylate-like mechanism. Suppression of the inflammatory response is thought to occur by a decrease in capillary permeability. One of phenylbutazone's major metabolites in the body is a hydroxylated product, *oxyphenbutazone* (Tandearil), which retains the pharmacological effects of the parent and is also employed therapeutically.

Phenylbutazone is a potentially dangerous drug with many severe undesirable side effects developing in 10 to 45 percent of all patients employing this drug. Some of these toxic effects include *gastrointestinal symptoms* (nausea, vomiting, activation of peptic ulcers), skin rashes, and disorders of the liver. Edema formation and weight gain result from the retention of salt and water. A variety of serious blood disorders have been observed, some of which have proved fatal. The most dangerous of these is *agranulocytosis,* resulting from a disappearance of granulocytic white blood cells or leukocytes. The absence of these leukocytes eliminates one of the body's primary natural defenders against infections.

This drug has been found to be an effective agent for the treatment of acute gout, rheumatoid arthritis, and related disorders. In acute gout this compound usually produces rapid and dramatic relief of pain and inflammation of the joints. Far safer drugs are used for the prophylactic management of gout, that is, to prevent recurring attacks of acute gout. This agent is also employed to reduce the swelling, pain, and inflammation associated with rheumatoid arthritis; it also increases the patient's ability to move the affected joints. Phenylbutazone is not employed for trivial disorders that respond to safer drugs such as the salicylates. Patients using this drug should be under the direct supervision of a physician and should receive periodic blood examinations. The patient should be exceedingly vigilant for the sudden appearance of fever, sore throat, skin rashes, jaundice, weight gain, or black stools, all of which are the earliest signs of toxicity.

Ibuprofen (Motrin) and Related Drugs

While aspirin and phenylbutazone are effective anti-inflammatory agents, their clinical utility is limited by the high incidence of *adverse gastrointestinal symptoms* associated with their use in high doses. Ibuprofen (Motrin) and the chemically related fenoprofen (Nalfon) and naproxen (Naprosyn) are newly developed nonsteroidal anti-inflammatory agents with analgesic and antipyretic activities.

These prostaglandin synthesis inhibitors are useful for the treatment of rheumatoid arthritis and osteoarthritis. At doses that are therapeutically equivalent to aspirin, these promising drugs appear to cause somewhat less gastrointestinal bleeding and upset than aspirin.

SUMMARY ───

Drugs intended for the relief of pain and inflammation and for the reduction of fever are among the most commonly used drugs in therapeutics. Aspirin, the most widely used therapeutic agent in the world, is an effective peripherally acting analgesic agent for the relief of mild-to-moderate pain, especially that originating from muscles and bones. Contemporary scientific evidence suggests that many aspirin-induced effects result from drug-induced inhibition of prostaglandin synthesis. Prostaglandins, endogenous long-chain fatty acids, are postulated to sensitize pain receptors to bradykinin, the chemical mediator of pain. Whereas salicylates do not modify normal body temperature, these drugs are the most effective agents for the reduction of fever. Salicylates cause a loss of heat by a marked widening of the blood vessels of the

TABLE 14-3. REPRESENTATIVE ANALGESIC-ANTIPYRETIC-ANTI-INFLAMMATORY AGENTS

Generic Name (Trade Name) [Synonym]	Analgesic-Antipyretic*	Anti-Inflammatory*	Common Therepeutic Uses†	Remarks
Aspirin [ASA; acetyl-salicylic acid]	Marked	Marked	P-F, RA, ARF	Extremely effective drug. Adverse effects—gastrointestinal upset, bleeding; blood coagulation impairment; allergic disorders.
Acetaminophen (Datril, Tylenol) [paracetamol]	=ASA	None	P-F	Most widely used aspirin substitute for relief of mild to moderate pain and suppression of fever. No ASA-like adverse effects. Liver toxicity in high doses.
Phenacetin	=ASA	None	P-F	Effective but subject to abuse; causes kidney toxicity in high doses. Rarely used in United States.
Mefenamic acid (Ponstel)	=ASA	<ASA	P	Use limited to seven days and patients over 14 years of age. Gastrointestinal tract upset common.
Phenylbutazone (Butazolidin Azolid)	=ASA	=ASA	RA, OA, AG, AS	Potentially severe toxicity limits use in long-term therapy. Adverse effects—gastrointestinal intolerance, skin rashes, blood disorders.

Drug	Analgesic/Anti-inflammatory potency	Uses	Comments
Oxyphenbutazone (Oxalid, Tandearil)	=ASA	RA, OA, AG, AS	Active metabolite of phenylbutazone, same therapeutic uses and adverse effects; less gastro-intestinal upset.
Indomethacin (Indocin)	=ASA	RA, OA, AG, AS	High incidence of adverse effects limits usefulness –gastrointestinal intolerance; CNS effects, including headache and behavioral disorders; blood disorders.
Sulindac (Clinoril)	=ASA	RA, OA, AS	Indomethacin-like properties but lower incidence of adverse effects.
Tolmetin (Tolectin)	=ASA	RA, JRA	Effective anti-inflammatory agent. Adverse gastrointestinal effects. May be better tolerated than ASA.
Ibuprofen (Motrin) Fenoprofen (Nalfon) Naproxen (Naprosyn)	=ASA	RA, JRA, OA, AS	Ibuprofen, fenoprofen, and naproxen are chemically related (propionic acid derivatives), share common pharmacological properties, and cause similar adverse effects. Better tolerated than ASA or indomethacin. Gastrointestinal upset most common adverse effect.

*=ASA: approximately equivalent to aspirin; <ASA: less than aspirin.

†Abbreviations: AG = acute gout; ARF = acute rheumatic fever; AS = ankylosing spondylitis (inflammation and ossification of the spinal column); JRA = juvenile rheumatoid arthritis; P = mild to moderate pain; P-F = pain and fever; RA = rheumatoid arthritis.

skin and by sweating; however, sweating is not essential for this nonspecific reduction in body temperature. Salicylates are also highly effective in alleviating the pain, redness, swelling, and loss of motion associated with inflammatory and rheumatic diseases.

Although aspirin is a relatively nontoxic drug, high therapeutic doses invariably cause a group of characteristic adverse side effects, collectively termed salicylism. Accidental ingestion of very large concentrations, most frequently by young children, causes several hundred poisonings annually. Some individuals are unable to tolerate aspirin because of allergy or gastrointestinal upset, irritation, and bleeding. Recent evidence suggests that use of aspirin during pregnancy may cause adverse effects to both the mother and her fetus. This reinforces the general admonition regarding the prohibition of the use of all but essential drugs during pregnancy.

For most individuals, plain unbuffered aspirin, not in combination with other ingredients, remains the best single choice for the relief of moderate pain and inflammation and the reduction of fever. This choice is predicated upon its analgesic, antipyretic, and anti-inflammatory–antirheumatic activities, proven effectivensss, wide range of safety, low incidence of severe adverse side effects, and very inexpensive price.

When aspirin cannot be used, many experts consider acetaminophen to be the second best analgesic-antipyretic choice for the medicine chest. While acetaminophen causes relatively few adverse effects when taken at normal therapeutic doses, acute poisoning by this drug may cause severe liver toxicity which is potentially lethal.

SUPPLEMENTARY READINGS

Beaver, W. T., "Mild Analgesics: A Review of Their Clinical Pharmacology," *American Journal of the Medical Sciences* 250: 577–604 (1965); 251: 576–99 (1966).

Ferreira, S. H., and J. R. Vane, "New Aspects of the Mode of Action of Nonsteroid Anti-Inflammatory Drugs," *Annual Review of Pharmacology* 14: 57–73 (1974).

Flower, R. J., S. Moncada, and J. R. Vane, "Analgesic-Antipyretics, and Anti-Inflammatory Agents; Drugs Employed in the Treatment of Gout," in *Goodman and Gilman's The Pharmacological Basis of Therapeutics*. Edited by A.G. Gilman, L. S. Goodman, and A. Gilman, 6th ed., Chap. 29, pp. 682–728. New York: Macmillan, 1980.

Horrobin, D. F., *Prostaglandins. Physiology, Pharmacology and Clinical Significance.* Montreal: Eden Press, 1978.

Murray, T., and M. Goldberg, "Analgesic Abuse and Renal Disease," *Annual Review of Medicine* 26: 537–50 (1975).

Roe, R. L., "Drug Therapy in Rheumatic Diseases," *Medical Clinics of North America* 61: 405–18 (1977).

Smith, M. J. H., and P. K. Smith, eds., *The Salicylates: A Critical Biographic Review.* New York: John Wiley, 1966.

Van Tyle, W. K., "International Analgesic Products," in *Handbook of Nonprescription Products.* 6th ed., pp. 125–40. Washington, D.C.: American Pharmaceutical Association, 1979.

Villaverde, M. M., and C. W. Macmillan, *Fever: From Symptom to Treatment.* New York: Van Nostrand Reinhold, 1978.

Wilson, D. E., ed., "Symposium on Prostaglandins," *Archives of Internal Medicine* **133**: 29–146 (1974).

15

Central Nervous System Stimulants and Appetite Suppressants

Cocaine is capable of alleviating the serious withdrawal symptoms observed in subjects who are abstaining from morphine and of suppressing their craving for morphine. . . . On the basis of my experiences with the effects of cocaine, I have no hesitation in recommending the administration of cocaine, for such withdrawal cures.

—Sigmund Freud (1885)

At periodic intervals during our day-to-day living, we all seek some type of mental and physical uplifting. Perhaps you did not get enough sleep last night and are now faced with an arduous day at school or work; maybe the semester is rapidly drawing to a close but you are now obliged to write two term papers and cram for three final examinations in the next four days; possibly you are a truck driver who will receive a generous bonus if you can drive your cargo from New York to Los Angeles in the next 72 hours.

The employment of **central nervous system stimulants** to allay fatigue and prevent sleep may be construed as *use* or *misuse* depending upon the particular circumstances underlying the employment of these drugs. When viewed in comparison with the "speed freak," those persons merely seeking to forestall sleep for a few hours are strictly minor leaguers.

Central nervous system stimulants have been traditionally classified on the basis of their primary site of action. Adopting such a classical approach, we may categorize strychnine as a spinal cord stimulant; pentylenetetrazol (Metrazol), picrotoxin, and nikethamide (Coramine) as midbrain or brainstem stimulants; and caffeine, cocaine, amphetamine, and methylphenidate (Ritalin) as cerebral stimulants. Contemporary interest primarily focuses on the last class of drugs.

Because strychnine no longer finds a place in modern therapeutics, our interest in this compound is predicated upon toxicological considerations, for example, when a strychnine-containing rat poison is accidentally ingested by a child or favorite pet. For many decades, the *midbrain stimulants* were extensively employed to counteract the respiratory depression produced by overdoses of barbiturate and nonbarbiturate sedative-hypnotics, narcotics, and alcohol. These so-called *analeptic agents* have now been almost completely replaced by mechanical respirators, which are far safer and more effective.

In this chapter we shall discuss four stimulants of the central nervous system. Strychnine, caffeine, cocaine, and amphetamine have been chosen for consideration because of their contemporary use and/or general interest. In the last section, appetite suppressants will be examined.

STRYCHNINE

Strychnine is an alkaloid obtained from the seeds of *Strychnos nux vomica,* a tree indigenous to India. Nux vomica first made its appearance in Europe in the sixteenth century for use as a poison for rats and other unwelcome animals. About 60 years ago, strychnine was still extensively used as a bitter tonic to enhance the appetite, as a laxative, and as a respiratory and heart stimulant in opiate and barbiturate poisoning.

At present, we only encounter this compound as a rat poison and as an alleged adulterant in substandard street LSD. It has lost favor as a rodenticide because of the common accidental ingestion and poisoning of young children and household pets. Apart from this relatively limited use, strychnine's most faithful admirers are neurophysiologists and neuropharmacologists who employ this drug as a tool to learn more about neurotransmission in the central nervous system, particularly in the spinal cord. Our primary interest in this compound is as a convulsive poison, whether resulting from a child's ingestion of rat poison or an "acid head" getting a toxic amount of strychnine.

The putative neurotransmitter *glycine,* released from Renshaw cells, exerts an inhibitory influence on the flow of nerve impulses along motor neurons in the spinal cord. This negative feedback system serves as a brake to prevent overcontraction of skeletal muscles resulting from excessive activation by the motor neuron. Strychnine produces *convulsions* by blocking the inhibitory influence of glycine on the motor neurons. With this braking system inoperable, the motor nerve overactivates the skeletal muscles, leading to convulsions.

Symptoms of strychnine poisoning include feelings of stiffness in the muscles of the neck and face, twitching in the face and limbs, followed by violent tonic convulsions of the entire body which are characterized by a continuous state of muscle contraction. Death results from respiratory failure and asphyxia or exhaustion after a series of convulsions. The muscles of the face and jaw of the victim are generally contracted, giving the appearance of a grin; this has been aptly termed *risus sardonicus.* Poisoning is symptomatically treated with barbiturates, administered intravenously. The patient is generally kept in a cool, quiet room, insulated from jarring, noises, or other convulsion-provoking stimuli.

CAFFEINE

What accounts for the worldwide popularity of coffee, tea, cocoa, and cola-containing soft drinks? Undoubtedly, we drink these beverages, consciously or unconsciously, for the "lift" they provide. These stimulating properties are attributed to *caffeine,* a naturally occurring alkaloid (Table 15–1). Coffee's popularity may be documented by simply pointing out that 3 billion pounds are consumed annually in the United States.

The history surrounding the discovery of coffee is shrouded in legend. We are told that one Kaldi, an Arabian shepherd, observed his goats merrily running about instead of sleeping after feeding on the berries of a coffee plant. These goats were the property of a convent. A holy man astutely appreciated a practical application for this discovery, suggesting that a beverage be made from the berries and given to the members of the convent to permit them to remain awake during their protracted prayers. This practice continues to the present; at examination time, we never find students far from a coffee pot.

Caffeine and the chemically related *xanthines,* theophylline and theobromine, are stimulants of the central nervous system. In addition, they are capable of stimulating skeletal and cardiac muscle, relaxing the smooth muscle of the bronchioles, and increasing respiration and producing diuresis.[1]

Xanthine

Caffeine
(Trimethylxanthine)

[1] Xanthines inhibit phosphodiesterase, the enzyme responsible for the inactivation of cyclic adenosine-3', 5'-monophosphate (cyclic AMP—see Chapter 22). Catecholamines (such as epinephrine) and the xanthines produce similar effects on the heart and bronchial smooth muscle. In part this may be explained by noting that while the catecholamines promote the formation of cyclic AMP, the xanthines inhibit its breakdown.

TABLE 15-1. CAFFEINE CONTENT OF POPULAR BEVERAGES AND THEIR NATURAL SOURCES

Beverage	mg Caffeine	Natural Source	% Caffeine
Coffee		*Coffea arabica* (coffee bean)	1–2
Regular	100–150 per cup		
Instant	60–80 per cup		
Decaffeinated	2–4 per cup		
Tea	25–75 per cup	*Thea sinensis* (tea leaf)	2
Cocoa	up to 50 per cup	*Theobroma cocoa* (cocoa seed)	0.1–0.4
Cola beverages			
(Coca-Cola, Pepsi-Cola)	30–50 per 12 oz	*Cola acuminata* (kola nut)	2

Pharmacological Effects

Caffeine is a potent central nervous stimulant, which, with progressively increasing concentrations, activates the cortex, then the medulla, and in toxic doses, the spinal cord. When administered in doses of 50 to 200 mg, the equivalent of one-half to two cups of coffee, we note enhanced mental alertness with a reduction in drowsiness and fatigue. Whereas caffeine does not increase intelligence, it does lengthen the attention span. The performance of simple tasks adversely affected by boredom and fatigue is improved, but these findings are complicated by highly subjective factors such as motivation. Increasing the dosage of caffeine above 200 mg does not further increase mental and physical performance but rather has a detrimental influence because of such adverse effects as nervousness, irritability, tremors, and headache. Infrequent coffee drinkers suffer from insomnia, although this effect is not observed by the heavy drinker.

Caffeine is capable of strengthening the force of contraction of voluntary muscle, as well as reducing the ability of such muscle to become fatigued. Laboratory experiments with human subjects have demonstrated that caffeine permits an individual to carry out physically exhausting work for longer periods of time. The relative contribution of this compound's effects on the central nervous system and on skeletal muscle has not been determined to date.

Heavy coffee drinkers become psychically dependent upon caffeinated beverages. Such individuals generally require one or two cups of coffee in the morning before they can exhibit their normally agreeable dispositions. If for some reason coffee is withheld, a clearly demonstrable abstinence syndrome is observed. The withdrawal symptoms are relatively mild and are characterized by irritability, nervousness, and a headache. The question of the development of *tolerance* to caffeine's stimulating effects has long been of personal interest to the author, an intemperate coffee drinker. Whereas the author can easily consume four or five mugs of coffee after ten o'clock at night, my colleague claims that if he has a single cup after four o'clock in the afternoon he is doomed to suffer from insomnia that evening. This anecdotal evidence has been substantiated by scientific experimentation; 150 mg of caffeine added to decaffeinated coffee disrupted the normal sleep patterns of nondrinkers, whereas it was without effect in habitual coffee drinkers. Similarly, the chronic use of caffeine-containing products reduces the ability of these compounds to enhance alertness.

Toxicity and Adverse Effects

Caffeine is generally considered to be a relatively nontoxic compound. One fatality has been reported after an intravenous dose of 3.2 g, and it has been estimated that 10 g of caffeine would have to be taken orally to produce death.[2] Doses larger than 1 g produce excessive stimulation of the central nervous system resulting in irritability, insomnia, excitement, muscle twitching, and convulsions. The heart beats more rapidly, and the patient experiences palpitations. The stimulatory effects on the central nervous system can be readily managed with short-acting barbiturates. Children are more sensitive to the central excitatory effects of caffeine than adults and, therefore, it is probably wise to omit cola soft drinks, coffee, tea, and even cocoa from their diets.

Patients with peptic ulcers and heart disease are often admonished by their physicians to limit their consumption of coffee and other caffeine-containing beverages. Caffeine is a stimulant of gastric acid secretion in the stomach which impairs ulcer healing. Patients with high blood pressure should also restrict their consumption of these beverages because of caffeine's stimulatory effects on the heart muscle and the nervous system.

Clinical Uses

The xanthines, theophylline in particular, have proved to be valuable drugs for the treatment of such respiratory diseases as asthma, bronchitis, and emphysema. These drugs are able to relax the smooth muscles of the bronchi, thereby relieving the wheezing and other breathing difficulties associated with these diseases. These agents, by virtue of their direct stimulatory effects on the heart muscle, have been employed for the treatment of heart failure. In mild cases of central nervous depression resulting from fatigue or a modest overdose of sedative-hypnotics, tranquilizers, or antihistamines, several cups of strong, black coffee have beneficial stimulatory effects. When the patient is severely depressed, yet conscious, coffee is merely useful as a stop-gap measure until the patient can receive proper medical treatment.

---

[2] This author is unaware of any suicide attempts by individuals taking an overdose of coffee. However, toxicity resulting from the accidental or intentional ingestion of a large number of caffeine-containing "stay-awake" products is clearly within the realm of possibility.

Amphetamine is among the most effective antifatigue drugs, yet as we shall discuss in the next section, this agent has great abuse potential, and it can only be legally procured with a physician's prescription. To fill the need of those attempting to combat sleep and fatigue, over 25 different nonprescription stimulatory products are available. One of these products contains an active constituent that is advertised as a "non-habit forming stimulant that would give . . . a quick lift." As you might predict, this compound is caffeine, and it is available in quantities ranging from 65–200 mg per tablet. These quantities are equivalent to one-half to two cups of coffee, a fact omitted from the promotional material.

COCAINE

Coca leaves were chewed in ancient Peru before the arrival of the Incas. When the Spanish conquistadors arrived in 1532, the chewing of these leaves was restricted to the Incan aristocracy for use during religious and official ceremonies. Within a short time after the Spanish conquest, the peasants began to emulate the example set by the aristocrats and began chewing coca leaves. When chewed, coca reduced feelings of hunger, permitted the natives to endure long hours of forced hard labor in the mines, and erased feelings of inferiority after their defeat at the hands of the Spaniards.[3]

Cocaine was extracted from the coca leaf, *Erythroxylon coca,* in the middle of the nineteenth century and, by 1880, reports of its miraculous pharmacological properties abounded. It was alleged to cure morphine and alcohol addiction, tuberculosis, indigestion, and a stubborn case of impotency. In 1885, the Parke, Davis Company published a monograph describing its potential therapeutic applications:

[Coca is] a drug which through its stimulant properties, can supply the place of food, make the coward brave, the silent eloquent, free the victims of alcohol and opium habit from their bondage, and, as an anaesthetic render the sufferer insensitive to pain, and make attainable to the surgeon heights of what may be termed "aesthetic surgery" never reached before.

Ah, if only these claims proved true, with but a single drug, hunger could be eradicated; a nation could field an army composed only of heroes; the benefits of a complete Dale Carnegie course could be obtained for the price of a few leaves or a cocaine capsule; and the scourge of alcoholism and narcotic addiction might cease to exist! (In all fairness, we should note that cocaine *is* an effective local anesthetic agent.)

---

[3] Several million individuals in Peru and Bolivia reportedly chew coca leaves or smoke coca paste (60 to 80 percent cocaine sulfate).

At about this time, a young Viennese physician, Sigmund Freud, became obsessed with the idea that cocaine was able to cure individuals of morphine dependence. Notwithstanding reports describing the dangers of cocaine abuse, Freud continued to propound this concept for many years.

This author was totally disillusioned when he learned that his childhood hero Sherlock Holmes may have been a cocaine abuser. Although some faithful Holmes devotees vehemently deny the possibility, we find Dr. Watson frequently alluding to his colleague's habit in many of his accounts of the adventures of the world-renowned detective: Holmes was "alternating from week to week between cocaine and ambition"; he was a "self-poisoner by cocaine and tobacco"; "save for the occasional use of cocaine, [he] had no vices."

The nonmedical use of cocaine declined substantially in the United States after the passage of the 1914 Harrison Act which restricted its sale and distribution outside medical channels. In the late 1960s cocaine returned to the streets, and by 1977 the Director of the National Institute of Drug Abuse estimated that over 8 million Americans had used cocaine as a recreational drug (see below).

Therapeutic Use

In 1884, Carl Koller, an associate of Freud's, discovered cocaine's very potent *local anesthetic* properties on the eye. This finding was of extreme medical importance because it permitted, for the first time, operations on the eye while the patient was fully conscious. Although cocaine is still used to a limited extent today to anesthetize the ears, nose, and throat, it has been largely replaced by synthetic local anesthetics that possess lower toxicity and that are devoid of abuse potential.

Cocaine

Behavioral Effects, Abuse, and Toxicity

When employed for recreational purposes, cocaine is diluted (cut or "stepped on") and sold to the consumer at 25-50 percent purity at a retail cost of $75 to $100 per gram (1/30 oz). The drug may be self-administered by intravenous injection, oral administration (swallowing), inhalation (smoking), or application to the mucous membranes of the mouth. The most common method is by "sniffing" or "snorting." Finely divided cocaine is placed in a line—about 0.3 cm (1/8 in) wide and 2.5 cm (1 in) long—and snorted into the nostril through a plastic straw or rolled banknote; some users employ special spoons and other paraphernalia. Several minutes later additional drug is snorted into the other nostril. It had been commonly believed that orally ingested cocaine is hydrolyzed and inactivated by enzymes in the gastrointestinal tract. Recent studies have shown, however, that significant "high" feelings are obtained after oral administration, although the time required for the maximum "high" is longer than after "snorting" (45–90 minutes versus 15–60 minutes).[4]

The "high" produced by intranasal administration of cocaine is similar to that caused by a large dose of amphetamine (see below). Unlike amphetamine, which has a duration of action of several hours after a single injection, cocaine's effects dissipate within five to fifteen minutes necessitating a second dose. Intravenous injection (a route that has not gained widespread popularity among the contemporary upper socioeconomic class users), is reported to produce an intense feeling of euphoric excitement, coupled with total self-confidence of mental and physical capabilities. The user ceases to be hungry and loses the sensation of pain. "Coke," "snow," or "Charlie" is reported to be the most effective antifatigue agent known, and sexual performance is reported to be markedly enhanced (an effect apparently unappreciated by Sherlock Holmes).

High-dose use or long-term administration of cocaine may result in paranoid feelings of persecution and excitability that may cause the user to perpetrate extreme acts of violence. Cocaine-induced hallucinations may involve all five senses, with visual phenomena the most common and first to occur. The most unique false sensory perceptions after chronic cocaine usage are *tactile hallucinations* which are likened to feeling small animals moving in the skin. The following is a classic description of these so-called "cocaine bugs" or formication in patients suffering from chronic cocainism:

> The characteristic of their hallucinations of general perception is to arouse the sensation of a foreign body under the skin. The first [patient], scraping his tongue, imagines that he sees small black worms come out of it. . . The [second patient] tears off his skin and again, looking in the bottom of the wound, pulls out the microbes with his fingernails or with the point of a pin. The third . . . occupies himself looking for crystals of cocaine under the skin.[5]

Although cocaine is perceived by many to be a relatively "benign" stimulant, in addition to its adverse behavioral effects, toxic doses may increase heart rate with palpitations, and cause fever, abdominal pain, convulsions, and

---

[4] C. Van Dyke et al., "Oral Cocaine: Plasma Concentrations and Central Effects," *Science* **200**: 211–13 (1978).

[5] Translated from Magnan and Saury's French paper which appeared in 1889, by R. K. Siegel, "Cocaine Hallucinations," *American Journal of Psychiatry* **135**: 309–310 (1978).

death resulting from respiratory failure. A recent report on cocaine-related deaths documents these potential dangers.[6]

Cocaine's stimulatory effects on the central nervous system and the heart have been attributed to this drug's ability to potentiate norepinephrine's action at the adrenergic synapse, by preventing the re-uptake of norepinephrine by the postganglionic sympathetic nerve ending. We recall from Chapter 6 (Figure 6–2) that re-uptake is the major mechanism by which the action of norepinephrine is terminated at the adrenergic receptor site. When this process is inhibited, the neurotransmitter substance is able to stimulate the receptor more intensely for protracted periods of time.

There is no substantial evidence to suggest that psychological dependence develops after the occasional recreational use of cocaine. Unlike virtually all other major drugs of abuse, tolerance has not been shown to develop to cocaine; physical dependence has not been demonstrated either. Notwithstanding these saving graces, the behavioral and physiological risks associated with its use strongly argue that street beliefs regarding its safety require revision.

AMPHETAMINE

Amphetamine is a collective term referring to *dextro*amphetamine (Dexedrine), *levo*amphetamine, racemic amphetamine (Benzedrine), and methamphetamine (meth, speed). *Dextro-* and *levo*amphetamine are optical isomers and, therefore, they have identical chemical and physical properties. Their major difference is based upon the ability of these compounds to rotate polarized light in opposite directions; this difference is a direct consequence of a subtle dissimilarity in their *three-dimensional structures.* The chemist would say that the amphetamine isomers are mirror images of one another (Chapter 13). Of what pharmacological significance is this? It has been observed that the *dextro*-isomer is several times more potent than the *levo*-isomer as a central nervous system stimulant; the latter isomer, by contrast, possesses slightly greater peripheral adrenergic activating effects, such as elevating blood pressure.

Racemic amphetamine contains equal amounts of the *dextro*- and *levo*-isomers, and, therefore, on a milligram-for-milligram basis it produces less central nervous stimulation than the *dextro*-isomer. Methamphetamine is the *N*-methylated derivative of amphetamine, and its central stimulatory properties are equal to *dextro*-amphetamine. The hard-core amphetamine abuser prefers "meth" because it has fewer peripheral effects. For the purposes of our discussion, we shall simply refer to this group of compounds as "amphetamine," unless otherwise stated.

    [6] C. V. Wetli and R. K. Wright, "Death Caused by Recreational Cocaine Use," *Journal of the American Medical Association* **241**: 2519–22 (1979).

H

⬡—CH₂—CH—N⟨H⟩   (boxed H)
        |
       CH₃

Amphetamine

H

⬡—CH₂CH—N⟨H⟩   (boxed CH₃)
        |
       CH₃

Methamphetamine

The effects of amphetamine on the central nervous system have been attributed to its interactions with the catecholamines norepinephrine and dopamine (Chapter 6). Amphetamine stimulates the release of these neurotransmitters and inhibits their re-uptake by the presynaptic neurons from which they were released. Both actions result in increased amounts of neurotransmitter available to interact at their respective receptor sites.

We shall now consider the effects of amphetamine on human performance and then examine the medical uses and abuse potential of amphetamine. Since amphetamine-like drugs are the most important class of appetite suppressants, we shall include a discussion of this class of drugs at the end of this chapter.

Effects on Human Performance

Therapeutic doses of amphetamine elevate the mood, reduce feelings of fatigue and hunger, facilitate powers of concentration, and increase the desire and capacity to carry out work. Amphetamine's central stimulatory effects have been attributed to its actions on two brain systems, namely, the reticular activating system (RAS) and the reward system (Chapter 9). Stimulation of the RAS results in an enhanced state of arousal to environmental stimuli, heightening the level of physical and mental activity, and "rose-coloring" the individual's subjective appraisal of the world. The "flash" or explosive euphoric effect experienced after an intravenous injection of amphetamine may be the result of a profound stimulation of the reward system. The actions of these systems are thought to be mediated by a stimulation of adrenergic receptor sites located in the brain. The postulated mechanisms of action by which amphetamine interacts with adrenergic receptors to produce such effects are summarized in Figure 6-2.

Let us now consider amphetamine's effects on different parameters of human performance, including physical endurance and performance, attention span, the ability to perform simple and complex tasks, and its relationship to learning and the subjective feelings of mood. When applicable information is available, amphetamine and caffeine will be compared.

Physical Endurance and Performance

During World War II, it was reported that the German forces were employing methamphetamine to enhance the endurance of their troops. Such a drug, when employed in certain military situations, could spell the difference between victory or defeat, life or death. Experiments were conducted by the Allies to investigate the validity of these intelligence reports. The results of these experiments demonstrated that amphetamine-treated subjects were less sleepy and exhibited superior performance with respect to their motor coordination and physical endurance than did their buddies who were given placebos. Over the years many different observers have verified these results. It should be emphasized that amphetamine delays the need for sleep, but does not replace it.

Amphetamine administration has also been found to enhance the athletic performance of expert college swimmers, as well as track-and-fielders. These studies, conducted at Harvard by Smith and Beecher, demonstrated small but significant improvements in trained athletes with amphetamine. Drug effects were more obviously manifested in rested subjects than in those that were fatigued. With respect to the small changes (1.16%) detected, Weiss and Laties note that "one percent of a 4-minute mile is 2.4 seconds—the difference between fame and oblivion."

Periodically we read about the illicit use of amphetamine in athletic competition, where athletes hope to improve their performance beyond their normal capabilities (Chapter 10). Bicycle racing is among the most energy-sapping of all competitive sports, and this may account for the alleged extensive use of amphetamine to reduce fatigue and increase the stamina of cyclists. During the second half of the 1960s, amphetamine played a prominent role in the disqualification, forfeiture of victory, and death of many cyclists throughout Europe. Amphetamine use among weight lifters is not unknown. At the world weight lifting championships in Columbus, Ohio, in 1971, holders of the top six positions were disqualified when analysis of their urine revealed the presence of dextroamphetamine.

Attention Span, Task Performance, and Learning

There are many tedious tasks in which an individual is obliged to maintain complete attention for long periods of time, sometimes in search of subtle changes in the environment. Consider radar operators looking for alien (terrestrial or extraterrestrial) aircraft on their screens or pilots or truck drivers who must drive their vehicles for long distances at night. As boredom sets in, the degree of vigilance begins to deteriorate. Amphetamine has been shown to be highly effective in maintaining an active state of alertness for long periods of time. Caffeine is useful but not as effective as amphetamine in maintaining the span of attention. Amphetamine and caffeine have been shown to increase the rate at which simple arithmetic and verbal tasks are carried out, for example, crossing out numbers, elementary mathematical manipulations, and the rate of typing. It is not clear whether these results indicate a drug-induced facilitation in performance, or whether the more favorable test scores are merely the reflection of a reduction in boredom or fatigue. There is no evidence to support the claim that amphetamine increases scores on intelligence tests or enables an individual to solve complex problems, as in calculus, more rapidly.

Most of us would find it desirable to use a drug that would enhance our ability to learn new information and retain it. Consider the familiar situation of the student who has two days before an examination to read, digest, and interpret all the nuances of *War and Peace* and *The Brothers Karamazov*. It would appear that amphetamine could facilitate the acquisition of information, at least on a short-term basis, especially if the subjects are mentally fatigued. Educators have long contended that their priceless gems of knowledge should be indelibly inscribed in their students' gray matter and not transferred from the students' brains to their examination papers. Unfortunately, amphetamine has not been shown to cause permanent changes in our memory bank.

Mood

What subjective feelings does amphetamine produce? What changes in mood are reported by subjects after the administration of this drug? Smith and Beecher asked a group of athletes to check adjectives that best described their feelings after being given amphetamine in doses of 14 mg per 154 lb (some were given half or twice this dose). The results are summarized by the author:

> The increased feeling of mental and physical activation was the most definite amphetamine effect . . . there was more checking of such words as active, vigorous, and energetic on amphetamine than on placebo days; less checking of sluggish, weak, drowsy, and tired; more checking of alert and clearheaded; less checking of mentally slow; more checking of efficient, ambitious, industrious, and effective; and more checking of excited, on edge, anticipative, tense, jittery, and restless on amphetamine than on placebo days. The second most definite amphetamine effect was increased elation. There was more checking of elated, exhilarated, happy, cheerful, and overjoyed and less checking of depressed and moody. A third positive effect was increased boldness. The subjects checked bold, boastful, cocky, self-confident, playful, and domineering more, and insecure less, on amphetamine days than on placebo days. The fourth definite effect was greater friendliness, as indicated by more checking of friendly, talkative, good-natured, obliging, and trustful and less checking of grouchy, unsociable, and sarcastic.[7]

In summary, we are led to the inescapable conclusion that amphetamine, when administered in therapeutic doses, is capable of enhancing the performance of a great number of behavioral tasks (Table 15–2). This improvement in performance is subject to two possible interpretations. Many studies have demonstrated amphetamine's ability to enhance the performance of tasks when the performance is subject to depreciation as the result of fatigue or boredom. In these instances, amphetamine-induced enhancement of mood, industriousness, and vigor may be responsible for the restoration of adequate

[7] G. M. Smith, and H. K. Beecher, "Amphetamine, Secobarbital, and Athletic Performance. II. Subjective Evaluations of Performance, Mood, and Physical States," *Journal of American Medical Association* **172**:1509 (1960).

TABLE 15-2. COMPARISON OF THE BEHAVIORAL EFFECTS OF AMPHETAMINE AND CAFFEINE IN HUMAN SUBJECTS

Behavioral Dimension	Amphetamine*	Caffeine*
Approximate doses for equivalent CNS stimulation	5 mg (racemic)	150 mg
Physical performance and endurance	+	+
Reaction time	+	0
Hand steadiness	+	-
Motor coordination	+	?
Attention span	+	+
Simple task performance	+	+
Complex task performance	0	0
Learning	?	?
Mood	+	+
Mental alertness	+	+
Abuse potential	Great	Little
Psychological dependence	+	+
Tolerance	+	+
Withdrawal effects after chronic usage	Depression	Headache

*Key to symbols: 0 = no effect; + = enhancement; – = impairment; ? = findings equivocal.

performance. However, the studies of Smith and Beecher with nonfatigued, nonbored, and interested athletes would suggest that amphetamine is truly able to facilitate performance.

Medical Uses of Amphetamines

Dextroamphetamine and related drugs are extensively used in the United States and in many countries throughout the world. There are three medically approved uses of amphetamines in the United States, namely, for the treatment of narcolepsy, of hyperkinetic disorders in children, and for the short-term management of obesity. In 1979 an estimated 80 percent of the legal use of these drugs was for appetite suppression; the rationale underlying the use of these drugs as appetite suppressants has been challenged by some experts.

Narcolepsy

Amphetamine's effectiveness for the treatment of certain types of narcolepsy has been documented since 1935. This neurological disorder is characterized by recurrent attacks of sleep and by weakness in the extremities. These attacks are generally initiated by emotional excitement, such as hearty laughter or sudden anger. Amphetamine in rather large doses (30–50 mg, even up to 100 mg per day) prevents such attacks of sleep in virtually all patients.

Hyperkinetic Disorders in Children

The hyperkinetic child is characterized by extreme hyperactivity or motor restlessness, a poor attention span, and impulsive and often disorderly behavior. This disorder (variously referred to as the hyperkinetic or hyperactive child syndrome, minimal brain dysfunction, and minimal brain damage) is estimated to afflict 4–10 percent of American children in the 5- to 11-year-old range; its incidence is between five and nine times more common in boys than girls. It is generally believed that no single cause is responsible for this condition. The postulated etiologies include brain damage (caused by injury or infection), genetic influences, biochemical abnormalities (thought to involve brain catecholamines), and environmental factors (lead, food additives).

Carefully controlled studies reveal that *dextroamphetamine* and the related central nervous system stimulant *methylphenidate* (Ritalin) are the most effective drugs for the acute management of this disorder; approximately two-thirds of the children treated obtain a favorable response. Among the benefits derived from drug therapy are a reduction in aggressive and impulsive behavior, greater goal-directed behavior, and improvement in sustaining attention. Unlike the activating effects observed in adults, amphetamine and methylphenidate do not produce a state of euphoria or overstimulation in hyperkinetic children, nor do they slow down these children or suppress their initiative. Parents and teachers report that drug-treated children present fewer behavioral problems and, moreover, objective tests have demonstrated advances in academic performance. (At present it is not well understood why a stimulant should produce such a paradoxical calming effect in children.) On the basis of these highly favorable results, generally derived from short-term drug studies of three to six weeks in duration, an estimated 600,000 "hyperkinetic" American school children were receiving amphetamine-like drugs and other psychoactive agents in 1972.

To date only a limited number of studies have attempted to assess the benefits derived from the long-term drug administration. In one such study, children treated with methylphenidate for three to five years showed little improvement when compared with a matched group of hyperkinetic children who had received no treatment. Additional studies must be performed to examine the validity of these negative results.

At the start of therapy, children generally exhibit a reduced appetite and weight loss, but, with continued drug administration, tolerance develops to these undesirable side effects. Some studies have suggested that chronic administration of dextroamphetamine and, to a lesser extent, methylphenidate may suppress growth in weight and stature. Discontinuation of therapy often produces a growth spurt. Drug-induced increases in heart rate and blood pressure have been reported and concern has been expressed about whether these changes will have an adverse effect on the subsequent health of the child. Long-term studies do not suggest that the administration of amphetamine to the preadolescent child leads to an increased nonmedical use of drugs in later life. While the etiology of hyperkinetic disorders remains obscure, and the benefits derived from chronic stimulant therapy remain uncertain, it should be clearly stated that the diagnosis of this disorder should be based upon medical criteria and not merely the opinions of harassed parents, teachers, or principals.

Appetite Suppression

The *long-term* administration of amphetamine and related drugs for appetite suppression has been universally decried by responsible health professionals. It has been argued, however, that their use may be justified for limited periods of time—*weeks*—during the initial phase of dieting. We shall further examine the use of amphetamine and related drugs as appetite suppressants in the final section of this chapter.

Misuse and Abuse

The misuse and abuse of amphetamine transcends socioeconomic barriers, varying only with respect to the dosage, route of administration, and setting in which the drug is taken. The desired mood-elevating effects sought only differ with respect to the magnitude of their intensity. Misusers of amphetamine generally pass unnoticed as respectable members of our family, our friends, and neighbors. They include the homemaker who, for many years, has been taking diet pills to shed those few extra pounds; the rising young business executive wishing to radiate enthusiasm and seeking a vibrant, self-confident, yet aggressive personality; the serious student who is cramming all night to prepare for a final examination; or the truck driver who requires a supply of "Bennies" in order to drive nonstop coast-to-coast. By contrast, the true amphetamine *abuser* is not an esteemed member of society. "Speed freaks" are often totally unkempt individuals, without gainful employment, who may reside in a commune on the fringe of a college campus, although not students themselves.

Although misuse of amphetamine has been documented for over 40 years, only recently has the gravity and extent of the problem been fully appreciated and responded to in unequivocal terms. One source noted that in 1966 sufficient quantities of amphetamine were legally manufactured to provide every man, woman, and child with 35 tablets. This same author claimed that one-half of these amphetamines entered illegal channels of distribution. In 1971, the equivalent of fourteen 5 mg amphetamine tablets per person were produced. The following year the Bureau of Narcotics and Dangerous Drugs placed amphetamine and related drugs in Schedule II, thereby requiring the same legal controls over this drug class as for the opiate narcotics.

In 1979 an official publication of the Food and Drug Administration noted that

> ... stimulants account for more abuse than any other category of prescription drugs, and [the] nonmedical use of stimulants is increasing among 18- to 25-year-olds. In addition, within the class of anorectic [appetite suppressing] drugs, amphetamines have abuse rates relative to prescription sales on the order of 10 times those of other drugs. . . . High volume prescribers and dispensers of the drug for the treatment of obesity account for a substantial amount of the abuse.[8]

Amphetamine Abuse around the World

Prior to discussing the patterns of amphetamine abuse and its consequences to the abuser, let us first briefly review the abuse of this drug in the United States and abroad.

United States.   The first clinical application of amphetamine was its use as a nasal decongestant. The Benzedrine inhaler containing 325 mg of racemic amphetamine was a heavily promoted nonprescription product in 1932. Soon thereafter, the inhaler's contents of amphetamine were taken orally for their stimulatory effects. In 1937, amphetamine tablets were introduced for the treatment of narcolepsy, but their use was rapidly expanded to include emotional depression, obesity, chronic alcoholism, fatigue, and hyperkinetic disorders in children. In the same year, psychology students at the University of Minnesota observed the highly beneficial antifatigue effects of amphetamine and the information was soon disseminated throughout the nation.

Japan.   In an attempt to maintain motivation and enhance efficiency, toward the end of World War II amphetamines were extensively used by the armed forces and factory workers of Japan. "Elimination of drowsiness and repletion of the spirit" was the catchy phrase used by the drug companies in their efforts to deplete stockpiled stores of amphetamine after the war. These advertisements were so effective that by 1954 the Japan Pharmaceutical Association estimated that 1.5 million persons were abusing this drug, several hundred thousand of whom were classified as "addicts." In that year the government launched an all-out effort to correct this problem by means of education, psychiatric treatment and rehabilitation, and very strict legal penalties. By 1956, amphetamine abuse in Japan was largely brought under control.

Sweden. Sweden was formerly confronted with the world's most serious amphetamine abuse problem. It had more amphetamine abusers than any other country in Europe, with estimates ranging from 10,000 to 12,000 throughout the nation, with about half this total number in Stockholm, the undisputed

[8]*FDA Drug Bulletin* 9 (4): 24 (1979).

"amphetamine capital of the world." In the middle of the 1940s, oral amphetamine usage became fashionable among artists, actors, writers, musicians, and Bohemians. Several years later, its use spread to the asocial and criminal elements who started using these drugs intravenously. Phenmetrazine (Preludin) swept the market after its introduction to Sweden in 1955. This drug, employed medically as an appetite suppressant, continues to be the abused drug of choice in Sweden but has some limited competition from amphetamine, methamphetamine, diethylpropion (Tenuate and Tepanil, widely used appetite suppressants in the United States), and methylphenidate. During the late 1960s, one out of every three Swedish males arrested for any reason was a drug abuser.

Patterns of Amphetamine Abuse

The nature and extent of amphetamine abuse varies widely among individuals. At one end of the spectrum, we observe persons who only take this drug once or twice, "to see what it does." Others use this drug several times per week, usually on weekends. The respectable middle-aged person feels that amphetamine is essential for the normal performance of daily activities and regularly takes several tablets daily by mouth. Finally, at the other extreme, we witness the "speed freak" who uses massive doses of amphetamine intravenously on a continual basis for months or years.

Following an intravenous injection of methamphetamine, there is a sudden, generalized, overwhelmingly pleasurable euphoric feeling termed a "flash," which has been described as a "full body orgasm." There is an intense fascination with all thoughts and activities, with the pursuit of purposeful activity at first, followed later by more compulsive and ultimately disorganized acts. This is illustrated by individuals taking apart and repairing radios continuously for hours, although the radios were in perfect working order at the outset; others may spend an entire day shining shoes. Subjectively, the user claims that the drug enhances performance, whereas objective evaluation has actually shown a deterioration of performance.

Some users, while under the influence of amphetamine, have reported a considerable interest and improvement in the participation of sexual activities. Orgasm is delayed for both sexes, thus permitting marathon sexual relations. When orgasm is finally achieved, it is reported to be more powerful and pleasurable than in the absence of the drug. These reports have not been documented scientifically, however.

Adverse Effects

Tolerance rapidly develops to amphetamine and methamphetamine ("speed"), and the user finds it necessary to employ very large doses to obtain pleasurable effects. Veteran "speed freaks" are reported to inject up to 1000 mg every two hours continuously for three to six days. At the end of a "run," the user generally sleeps for twelve to eighteen hours prior to the start of a new round of drug administration. While users are taking the drug, amphetamine's very potent appetite-suppressing effects may result in weight losses of 20 pounds; cognizant of this fact, experienced users force themselves to eat. Pharmacologically there is a very good reason to eat, since food deprivation reduces the duration of drug action. The acidic urine resulting from starvation enhances the rapid excretion of amphetamine, thus necessitating frequent, high doses of the drug to maintain the euphoric state.

Apart from an obvious neglect of personal appearance, the amphetamine abuser suffers from many medical problems. Malnutrition makes such an individual more prone to infection. Injections, administered under less than operating room standards for asepsis, result in a high incidence of skin abscesses and ulcers, as well as hepatitis. Notwithstanding the ominous slogans "Meth is Death" and "Speed Kills," the acute toxicity of amphetamine is relatively low. Signs of toxicity include an elevation in blood pressure, heart palpitations, flushing of the skin, widening of the pupils, and convulsions. In isolated cases, death resulting directly from an overdosage of amphetamine has been demonstrated and is caused by a stroke. More often death has been attributed to secondary causes such as infectious disorders, hepatitis in particular, as well as suicides arising from rebound depression during periods of drug withdrawal or abstinence. The behavioral consequences are the most serious commonly encountered hazard associated with high dose amphetamine abuse.

Amphetamine Psychosis

Although tolerance rapidly develops to the peripheral effects of amphetamine, particularly effects on the cardiovascular system, this adaptation phenomenon does not protect the user from an **amphetamine-induced psychosis,** the most dramatic consequence resulting from the abuse of this drug. Many investigators find the clinical symptoms associated with this condition indistinguishable from non-drug-induced paranoid schizophrenia. Only a urine test, wherein the presence of amphetamine is detected, can discriminate the difference; there are no unique physical signs characteristic of amphetamine intoxication.

While the specific findings of investigators vary, Kalant has summarized the relative incidence of symptoms associated with amphetamine psychosis in 94 reported cases: delusions of persecution (83%), visual hallucinations (54%), auditory hallucinations (40%), tactile and olfactory hallucinations (18%), and excitation (41%). Unlike many other drug-induced psychoses, the amphetamine abuser is generally able to think clearly and have a good recollection of relevant and extraneous facts during the period of the psychotic episode.

Almost all individuals taking high doses of amphetamine become suspicious and somewhat paranoid. In the early stages, such individuals may suspect their family and friends of plotting against them. Later, they think they are being followed or pursued by the FBI, CIA, or members of organized crime who are "out to get them." In very advanced stages, patients think that their activities are being monitored or manipulated by radio or television transmitters or by unknown power sources. Similarly, visual hallucinations begin as fleeting shadows, and eventually progress to fully formed, clearly recognizable figures. Starting as simple noises, auditory hallucinations develop to the stage where the user participates in long conversations with his or her "persecutors."

Users are generally aware of the causal relationship between their use of amphetamine and the development of the psychotic state. Some users have found that heroin or other narcotic agents are able to reduce or abolish the anxiety and paranoia. Regular use of these narcotic agents frequently leads to physical dependence upon them. Most individuals who develop an amphetamine psychosis have been shown to have preexisting abnormal and unstable personalities. However, these reactions have been shown to occur in "normal, well-adjusted individuals" as well.

The amphetamine psychosis often subsides after the termination of drug administration; however, in many instances, the mental aberrations persist for days, weeks, and even months after the last dose. There are reports of impairment of memory and the inability to concentrate after the chronic administration of high doses of amphetamine. Studies to date have not as yet ascertained whether permanent brain damage or mental impairment does indeed occur.

Amphetamine Dependence

Unlike narcotic-dependent individuals who develop a compulsive desire to get their supply of heroin, amphetamine users have a *need* or "desire" to continue to take the drug, but the magnitude of this need does not reach overwhelming or compulsive proportions. After the continuous use of amphetamine, a profound degree of *tolerance* is acquired to the peripheral effects of this drug, as well as to the central stimulatory effects that are responsible for excitation and euphoria. Five to 10 mg are an average oral therapeutic dose; by contrast, the abuser is capable of tolerating intravenous doses of 500 to 1000 mg every two or three hours.

After the abrupt cessation of amphetamine, the user does not manifest any grossly discernible effects such as vomiting, violent tremors, or convulsions. The absence of such effects has raised the question as to whether, indeed, continuous use of amphetamine does cause *physical dependence*. This question has not been resolved. After the termination of a "speed run," the user is greatly fatigued, depressed, and very hungry. Are these effects, and those characterizing the amphetamine psychosis, the result of sleep deprivation? This question requires additional study. Finally, changes in the electrical activity of the brain have been observed during sleep after sudden amphetamine withdrawal, changes that are reversed after the administration of amphetamine. Such findings suggest that these alterations in brain patterns are a symptom of a withdrawal state.

In summary, we have observed in recent years a marked change in attitudes toward the dangers associated with amphetamine abuse. In 1957, an authoritative textbook of pharmacology stated, "As there is no acquired tolerance and no violent craving, tremor or 'physical dependence,' the drug is relatively easily withdrawn."[9] Moreover, at that time, amphetamine was generally considered to be a safe drug, possessing a wide range of useful therapeutic applications.

The abuse potential associated with this drug has now been well-documented in Japan, Sweden, and, more recently, in the United States. Rehabilitation of amphetamine abusers has proved to be a difficult task, with most investigators noting that the relapse rate approaches that observed with narcotic users. The valid therapeutic indications for this agent have also been subject to reevaluation, with many authorities now advocating that its medical uses be restricted to hyperkinetic disorders in children and narcolepsy.

APPETITE SUPPRESSANTS

> *There are various recommendations which a doctor gives to his patients, and which are very hard to get carried out. One of those is work for those who will not take it; another, rest for those who cannot get it; yet another is restraint of the appetites.*
>
> —Sir Thomas Lauder Brunton (1844–1916)

For cultural, social, and medical reasons, we feel obliged to curb our normally voracious appetites and maintain our weight in proportion to our height and body frame. As summer approaches, many observe, to their horror, an accumulation of winter fat that can no longer be easily camouflaged by a ski sweater and will prove all too obvious in a bathing suit. Entrepreneurs have enthusiastically responded by stressing the need to exercise (home exercise devices, membership in the neighborhood health spa) and by providing dietary aids (liquid diets, chewing gums, candies). In addition, great pressures have been exerted on the family physician to prescribe "that same drug that helped my neighbor, Miss Bones."

In recent years, a number of physicians have engaged exclusively in the very lucrative business ("practice" is far too charitable a word) of weight reduction. Not wishing to detain their customers by taking medical histories or by giving physical examinations, they indiscriminately dispense their own appetite suppressants along with a substantial bill for services. These products are living proof that polypharmacy is not merely of historical interest; not infrequently, such products contained amphetamine, thyroid, a laxative, a barbiturate, an atropine-like agent, digitalis, and a diuretic. Several deaths and national exposure have restricted, but not eliminated, this prostitution of medical practice.

[9] T. Sollmann, *A Manual of Pharmacology,* 8th ed. (Philadelphia: Saunders, 1957), pp. 508–9.

Concepts of Feeding and Obesity

Traditionally, obesity has been viewed as the inability of obese persons to control their food intake. In this regard, it has been stated that 90 percent of all cases of obesity arise from a caloric intake in excess of normal energy requirements. More recent work suggests that obesity is a disease having social, behavioral, and physiological determinants.

Studies with animals have shown the presence of two centers in the hypothalamus concerned with the normal control of feeding. These have been termed the feeding center and the satiety center. Chemical stimulation of the feeding center with norepinephrine induces food intake in rats who are food satiated; conversely, destruction of this site produces aphagia, that is, the animal refuses to eat and must be force-fed to survive. If the feeding center is viewed as an accelerator that is active at all times, the satiety center may be seen as a brake that inhibits the feeding center. Catecholamines (in particular, norepinephrine) containing neurons are present in the hypothalamus and have been postulated to be involved in the central control of feeding. Chemical or surgical destruction of the satiety center produces uncontrollable eating (hyperphagia). It is assumed that these feeding and satiety centers also function in humans.

The precise triggering mechanism responsible for stimulating the satiety center is not known with certainty. A **glucostatic** theory hypothesizes that "glucoreceptors" are present in the satiety center which respond to changes in blood glucose (sugar) metabolism. When glucose utilization by these cells is low, such as prior to a meal, the activity of the cells is reduced. This decreases the inhibitory influence of the satiety center, and promotes the desire to eat. When glucose utilization is high, as is observed after a meal, the cells have increased activity, activate the satiety center, and suppress additional food ingestion. At this time it is not clear how signals are transmitted between the gastrointestinal tract and the hypothalamus.

Drugs and Appetite Suppression

Anorexia (the depression of appetite) is a common side effect of many drugs. However, the truly effective appetite suppressant or **anorexiant** does not merely depress appetite *per se,* but rather causes the individual to lose interest, without discomfort, in food. Such an ideal anorexiant would cause the individual to eat less, regardless of the tantalizing aroma, enticing presentation, and quantity of food served. These same effects are observed after overindulgence in alcoholic beverages. Before the dieter lifts a glass to toast this newly discovered anorexiant, it should be noted that alcohol, itself, is very high in calories (7 kilocalories per gram).

At present, the ideal appetite suppressant does not exist, since the dieter must consciously restrict food intake while taking these drugs. We shall now

TABLE 15-3. APPETITE SUPPRESSANTS

Generic Name	Selected Trade Names
*Amphetamine-like agents**	
Dextroamphetamine	Dexedrine
Racemic (*dl*-) amphetamine resin	Biphetamine
Chlorphentermine	Pre-Sate
Diethylpropion	Tenuate; Tepanil
Fenfluramine	Pondimin
Mazindol	Sanorex
Methamphetamine	Desoxyn
Phendimetrazine	Plegine
Phenmetrazine	Preludin
Phenylpropanolamine (PPA)†	Appedrine, Dexatrim, Diet-Trim, Prolamine
*Amphetamine + Sedative**	Dexamyl
	Eskatrol
Bulk producers†	
Methylcellulose, carboxymethylcellulose	Melozets
Benzocaine-containing agents†	Slim-Line Gum
Glucose-containing agents†	Ayds

*Available only on the prescription of a physician.
†Nonprescription products.

consider some of the more common classes of appetite suppressants: amphetamine-like drugs, bulk producers, and benzocaine- and glucose-containing products. Representative examples of each class are presented in Table 15–3.

Amphetamine-Like Adrenergic Agents

Amphetamine-like adrenergic agents are by far the most important and widely used class of appetite suppressants currently available. Notwithstanding claims to the contrary in the promotional literature and the lack of similarity in the generic names (to make these compounds sound non-amphetamine-like), simple inspection of the chemistry of these drugs reveals the characteristic amphetamine skeleton. The abuse potential of amphetamine makes it promotionally prudent to keep this skeleton in the closet. Since these compounds are all noncatecholamine sympathomimetic compounds, it should be anticipated that they will have very similar properties. With one exception, they all produce some degree of central nervous system stimulation and, in high doses, cause abnormal cardiovascular changes.

Amphetamine skeleton

Phenylpropanolamine is a nonprescription sympathomimetic agent that pharmacologically resembles ephedrine and amphetamine. It is a less potent central nervous system stimulant than ephedrine, and both compounds have proved to be useful nasal decongestants. Less well established, however, are the appetite suppressing effects of phenylpropanolamine at the recommended dosage of 25 mg. Higher doses do produce anorexia but may also increase blood pressure and cause nervousness and insomnia.

The *mechanism(s)* responsible for suppression of appetite are not known. Amphetamine depresses the sense of taste for sugar as well as the sense of smell. We have all experienced a loss of appetite during a head cold when these senses are obtunded, and amphetamine's effects may be partially mediated by such an action. In rats, amphetamine has been shown to depress the appetite even after destruction of the satiety center. It has been suggested that these drugs may act by inhibiting the feeding center. Other investigators have argued that the observed reduction in food intake may be by a rather nonspecific "distracting" mechanism. That is, amphetamine produces a euphoric stimulating effect, giving the patient a "lift," which distracts from the normal desire to eat. Although this hypothesis appears quite tenable, a newer appetite suppressant, fenfluramine (Pondimin), causes drowsiness rather than the stimulation observed with all other amphetamine-like drugs.

Is amphetamine-induced activation a desirable or undesirable secondary effect? If distraction does play a part in turning the attention of dieters away from food, and psychological stimulation keeps their spirits elevated even when they are away from the dinner table, then this activation is desirable. However, amphetamine taken too close to bedtime produces insomnia, and the temptation of bedtime snacks is especially strong for many dieters. In an attempt to reduce the excessive stimulatory properties of amphetamine, often manifested by anxiety and nervousness, barbiturates and mild tranquilizers have been used in combination with amphetamine. The wisdom of such combinations has been questioned. An undesirable consequence of stimulation and euphoria is that it may lead to psychological dependence and abuse.

Clinically, it has been observed that amphetamine produces the greatest weight losses within the first three or four weeks of therapy. Thereafter, **tolerance** develops to the appetite suppressing effects, which commonly results in the patient increasing the dosage without medical supervision. Increased dosage often produces peripheral cardiovascular side effects, as well as irritability and nervousness. Patients often continue taking these drugs faithfully, even in the absence of additional weight loss. Ostensibly, they are seriously dieting, whereas subconsciously many individuals are continuing to take their medication for the euphoric effects. This has led to very widespread misuse of amphetamine among members of the "respectable" middle class. Persons with unstable personalities or a history of dependence on other drugs or alcohol are particularly susceptible to such abuse. Physicians are now aware of these inherent dangers, and, in recent years, most of them have markedly reduced prescribing these drugs for long courses of therapy.

Bulk-Producing Agents

Bulk-producing agents contain nondigestible, noncaloric gums that absorb water. When taken with water, methylcellulose, carboxymethylcellulose, and related compounds exert a "filling effect" by swelling in the stomach and providing a full feeling. In general, these agents are not effective since most obese individuals want real food rather than an unappetizing wafer or powder. These drugs are also employed as laxatives (Chapter 26).

Benzocaine-Containing Products

Benzocaine is a local anesthetic that acts by producing a numbing sensation in the mouth, thus diminishing one's taste for food. There are very few studies documenting the effectiveness of this approach to appetite suppression.

Glucose-Containing Products

Widely advertised glucose-containing products, such as Ayds, are claimed to be effective because they elevate the glucose levels in the body. Recalling the glucostatic hypothesis, it might be suggested that they act by stimulating the glucoreceptors in the satiety center and in so doing inhibit the feeding center. The amount of glucose in these products is relatively low and probably insufficient to produce the desired effects. If glucose-containing products were truly effective, a person might derive similar benefits from one teaspoonful of corn syrup (the active ingredient in Ayds), one-half hour prior to meals.

Thyroid Preparations

Persons with depressed thyroid activity have a low rate of metabolism and are generally sluggish and overweight. Thyroid-containing products are often useful in such hypothyroid individuals to stimulate their rate of metabolism and to burn fat. Unfortunately, in patients with normal thyroid function, these products do not contain enough thyroid to produce such effects; elevating the dosage of these thyroid drugs increases the incidence of undesirable cardiovascular side effects. Moreover, administration of thyroid to such individuals inhibits their normal production of this hormone; as a result, the net amount of available thyroid remains unchanged. Thyroid should not be used to promote weight reduction in patients with normal thyroid activity.

Outlook for Drugs in the Treatment of Obesity

The drugs discussed are no cure for obesity but rather serve as a crutch in the initial period during which the patient must adjust to dietary restrictions. Because of the rapid development of tolerance to amphetamines, these drugs should only be used for a relatively short period of time, if at all. Most non-amphetamine drugs have not been subjected to careful clinical evaluation to substantiate their promotional claims. The ideal drug, yet to be developed, will truly act on the appetite centers of the hypothalamus so that the patient will not eat too much even in the presence and availability of food.

SUMMARY

Of the central nervous system stimulants that were formerly of therapeutic importance or extensively employed for nonmedical purposes, only the cerebral stimulants continue to be of contemporary importance. Caffeine is the most frequently employed central nervous stimulant throughout the world, and it is the active ingredient in coffee, tea, and cola beverages. The use of coffee serves a beneficial purpose by providing mild mental and physical activation. Whereas the compulsive imbibing of this drink should not be encouraged, especially by young persons, the hazards associated with intemperance by healthy individuals remain controversial.

After remaining relatively dormant for about half a century, cocaine assumed increasing importance as an illicit recreational drug in the late 1960s, with the incidence of its usage increasing at this time. This euphoriant, generally self-administered by "snorting," is capable of producing hallucinations when taken in high doses or on a chronic basis, as well as antisocial paranoid behavior; cocaine-induced deaths have been recently documented.

Amphetamine has been shown to enhance human performance when administered in low doses. There are many useful applications for the temporary mental and physical stimulating effects of this drug, for example, in military operations when fatigue can prove disastrous to the individual combatant and to the success of the operation. Far more controversial, however, is its use to enhance competitive athletic performance by artificially elevating an individual's naturally acquired physical attributes.

Amphetamine abuse is no longer considered to be a minor problem. The greatest dangers associated with the high-dose, long-term administration of amphetamine are the behavioral changes. Amphetamine psychosis cannot be differentiated from paranoid schizophrenia, even by the trained observer. After continuous use of amphetamine, psychic dependence occurs and a marked degree of tolerance develops. At present, experts are debating whether physical dependence develops to this stimulant.

Amphetamine and methylphenidate have been found to be useful for the management of hyperkinetic disorders in children and for their alerting properties in narcolepsy. While amphetamine and related drugs are effective for the short-term management of appetite suppression, the development of tolerance and the potential of abuse limit their value. In general, most nonprescription appetite suppressants have not been subjected to critical clinical evaluation. At present, pushing aside a dinner plate heavily laden with high-caloric foods remains the most effective method of controlling weight.

SUPPLEMENTARY READINGS

Andrews, G., and D. Solomon, eds., *The Coca Leaf and Cocaine Papers.* New York: Harcourt Brace Jovanovich, 1975.

Cantwell, E., ed., *The Hyperkinetic Child: Diagnosis, Management, and Current Research.* New York: John Wiley, 1975.

Connell, P. H., *Amphetamine Psychosis.* Maudsley Monographs, No. 5. London: Oxford University Press, 1958.

Ellinwood, E. H., and M. M. Kilbey, eds., *Cocaine and Other Stimulants.* New York: Plenum Press, 1976.

Gilbert, B., "Drugs in Sports," *Sports Illustrated,* June 30, 1969, pp. 30–42.

Hoebel, R. G., "Pharmacological Control of Feeding," *Annual Review of Pharmacology and Toxicology* 17: 605–21 (1977).

Kalant, O. J., *The Amphetamines: Toxicity and Addiction.* 2nd ed. Springfield, Ill.: Charles C Thomas, 1973.

Mulé, S. J., ed., *Cocaine: Chemical, Biological, Clinical, Social and Treatment Aspects.* Cleveland: CRC Press, 1976.

Reichman, F., ed., "Hunger and Satiety in Health and Disease," *Advances in Psychosomatic Medicine* 7: 1–336 (1972).

Sjoqvist, F., and M. Tottie, eds., *Abuse of Central Stimulants.* New York: Raven Press, 1969.

Smith, D. E., ed., *Amphetamine Use, Misuse, and Abuse.* Boston: G. K. Hall, 1979.

Wang, S. C., and J. W. Ward, "Analeptics," *Pharmacology and Therapeutics [B]:* 3:123-65 (1977).

Weiss, B., and V. G. Laties, "Enhancement of Human Performance by Caffeine and the Amphetamines," *Pharmacological Reviews* 14: 1–36 (1962).

Weiss, G., and L. Hechtman, "The Hyperactive Child Syndrome," *Science* 205: 1348–54 (1979).

16

Drugs Used for the Treatment of Mental Disorders

I consider the etiology of schizophrenia to be a dual one, namely, up to a certain extent psychology is indispensable to explain the nature and the causes of the initial emotions, which give rise to metabolic alterations. These emotions seem to be accompanied by chemical processes causing specific temporary or chronic disturbances or destructions.

—Carl Jung (1957)

As a result of drugs introduced within the past ten years, the treatment of psychiatric patients has been completely and permanently altered. . . . The importance of psychopharmaceutical treatment . . . cannot be exaggerated.

—Nathan S. Kline (1966)

Over the ages, individuals suffering from mental illness have not received the benevolent sympathy generally shown to persons afflicted with a physical malady. In 1972, we witnessed an example of such prejudice toward an individual with a history of mental illness in the political arena. An otherwise qualified individual was dropped as a vice-presidential candidate when it was learned that he had been hospitalized for depression several years before. The widespread bias concerning mental diseases is surprising when we consider the frequency of these diseases. It has been estimated that one out of every two hospital beds in the United States is occupied by an individual suffering from a psychiatric disorder. Although we no longer believe that such persons are possessed by demons, we still may harbor conscious or subconscious fears about our safety in their presence.

In this chapter we shall discuss the different types of mental illnesses, theories relating to their causes, and the drugs used to modify abnormal behavior. These drugs are broadly classified as **psychoactive or psychotropic agents.** We shall consider drugs used for the treatment of psychoses (the antipsychotic agents, neuroleptics, or "major tranquilizers"), the mood disorders of depression and mania (antidepressants and antimanic agents), and the neuroses (antianxiety agents, anxiolytics, or "minor tranquilizers").

MENTAL ILLNESS: AN OVERVIEW

Mental illnesses many manifest themselves in many ways and with varying degrees of subtlety. In some instances the symptoms may be so slight that psychiatrists are unable to agree as to whether or not the individual is "normal." At the other end of the spectrum, we observe persons whose behavior is clearly abnormal, based upon contemporary standards of normalcy. Individuals claiming to be the Messiah, or those who sit alone in their rooms, weeping, proclaiming their worthlessness, and openly discussing their plans of suicide are suffering from some form of mental disorder. At times it is a difficult task to draw the line between a person who may be somewhat eccentric or strange and another who is in need of psychiatric help. Rudyard Kipling once observed that, "Every one is more or less mad on one point." In a recent provocative paper, Rosenhan argues that a psychiatric diagnosis may be biased by the patient's environment, for example, hospitalization in a mental institution:

> At its heart, the question of whether the sane can be distinguished from the insane (and whether degrees of insanity can be distinguished from each other) is a simple matter: do the salient characteristics that lead to diagnoses reside in the patients themselves or in the environments and contexts in which observers find them? . . .[1]

What are some of the typical symptoms that constitute **abnormal behavior?** *Perceptual* aberrations are observed in individuals suffering from psychoses. Such individuals may experience illusions, a misinterpretation of actual stimuli, or hallucinations, which are false perceptions not based upon reality. Both illusions and hallucinations may involve one or more of the senses. Intelligence, memory, and *thought processes* may be impaired. In neuroses, the content of thinking may be disturbed, giving rise to obsessions or phobias. Delusions or false beliefs inconsistent with the patient's background are seen in paranoid disorders; such delusions may be of grandeur or of persecution. Extreme *emotional swings* are characteristic of manic-depressive disorders or of other conditions in which the individual manifests totally inappropriate feelings based upon the occasion. Finally, *verbal or motor behavior* may be disturbed, as illustrated by persons who are unable or refuse to speak or by others who talk excessively or repeat words or sentences. Tremors, stupor, or mechanical movements continuously performed are examples of impaired motor behavior. A given symp-

---

[1] D. L. Rosenhan, "On Being Sane in Insane Places," *Science* **179**: 251 (1973).

tom may appear in more than one behavioral disorder, and, therefore, it is not a single sign but rather the entire array of symptoms that are evaluated collectively to determine the appropriate psychiatric diagnosis.

The specific cause of the mental disorder may or may not be known. **Organic disorders** arise from some physical or chemical injury to the brain. These disorders may be characterized by an impairment in environmental orientation, memory, judgment, and intellectual function and are often manifested by abnormal behavior, such as illusions, hallucinations, and delusions; in some instances, seizures may also be observed. **Functional disorders** do not have a clearly recognizable physical cause. We may anticipate that the etiology of these disorders will be better understood with future advances in the pathophysiology and biochemistry of mental disease. Based upon the specific nature of the symptoms and the degree to which they are manifested, functional disorders are classified as being neuroses, psychoses, or affective disorders.

Mental deficiency is a legal designation that is not meaningful in a clinical context. It does not help to define the cause of the intellectual impairment, nor does it suggest which treatment is most appropriate. The terms "idiot," "imbecile," or "moron" merely suggest the potential mental resources and the likely degree of educability.

Neuroses and Psychoses

In **neurotic disorders,** most commonly marked by anxiety and tension, the emotions and reactions of the patient are an intensification of those exhibited by normal individuals. *Anxiety* is a state characterized by extreme apprehension, irritability, and greater than normal hypersensitivity. *Tension* is manifested by such physical symptoms as a rapid heart beat, widening of the pupils, perspiration, flushing, and cold extremities. These symptoms are reminiscent of sympathetic stimulation. Although thinking and judgment may be impaired, the disturbances observed in neuroses are milder than those observed in psychotic conditions. There is a minimum loss of contact with reality, and the patient generally appreciates that he or she is ill.

The **psychotic** patient lives in a private world, having only a marginal appreciation of what is real. Thought processes are so impaired that they markedly interfere with the patient's ability to successfully interact with other members of society. Such an individual frequently experiences illusions, hallucinations, and delusions and may also suffer from impairments of perception, intellectual capabilities, mood, motivation, and behavior.

At this point, you may ask, "What proportion of the American people are mentally ill?" Two problems immediately arise when answering this complex question: (1) What do we consider to constitute mental illness? and (2) What criteria should we employ for making this head count? Let us put aside the first problem and focus our attention on the second. If we consider admission to a mental hospital to be evidence of mental illness, we can say that 15 to 20 percent of the population fall into this category. By contrast, research workers attempting to detect some degree of psychopathology in persons living at home in New York City estimated that 80 percent were mentally ill based upon their criteria.

EVOLUTION OF THE TREATMENT OF MENTAL ILLNESS

Whereas today we generally consider mental illness to be a fabric composed of psychological, sociocultural, and biochemical threads, in earlier times mystical causes were generally thought to be responsible for its etiology. During the Stone Age, diseases, as well as life itself, were all thought to be influenced by *spiritual* forces. The concept that evil spirits or demons were the mediating forces underlying disease even existed among the Hebrews, Egyptians, Chinese, and early Greeks. The treatment was entirely logical: Drive the spirit from the body of the afflicted wretch. This was generally accomplished by trephining or exorcism. Exorcism, or the driving out of the demon, took many forms. If the demon failed to respond to such subtle persuasion as prayers, incantations, loud noises, or obnoxious odors, other more drastic measures were employed to save the mentally ill person. These involved whipping, starvation, or torture—all with the best interests of the patient in mind.

After meticulous observation, Hippocrates (*c.* 460–377 B.C.) reached the conclusion that mental disorders did not arise as the consequence of the invasion of spirits, but rather that it was the result of injury or disease of the brain, or from "disturbances in the humors of the brain." Thinking regressed during the Middle Ages, as witnessed by a revival of demonology, but it was now strongly influenced by theological overtones. Increasingly harsh treatments were justified on the basis that the demons within the patient had to be punished, as well as the mortal harboring these spirits. Witches were viewed as the earthly partners of the devil and were thought to be empowered with supernatural powers capable of causing disease, famine, and drought for the innocent people of the time. This philosophy prevailed until the middle of the eighteenth century.

By the eighteenth century, asylums for the mentally ill were established; however, patient treatment continued to remain abysmal. Patients were crowded like cattle into dark cells, food was grossly inadequate, and beatings were employed to calm the more violent persons. A major revolution occurred in 1792 when Pinel removed the chains from the inmates at a Paris asylum. Moreover, he substituted kindness, concern, and sympathetic understanding for beatings. His "Moral Treatment" was remarkably successful; many patients, whom society had long given up as lost, were "cured" and released.

Enlightenment concerning the treatment of the mentally ill took many more years to reach the New World. Dorothea Dix was enraged at the conditions she observed in the 1840s. She noted a gross inadequacy in the quantity and quality of existing treatment facilities. In the available facilities, the mentally ill were housed together with the indigent, the mentally retarded, and criminals. Her efforts were principally responsible for arousing the public's awareness to the problem of behavioral diseases and led to the construction of new mental hospitals. Large overcrowded hospitals with inadequate staffs, both in number and training, inadvertently resulted in the repudiation of Pinel's "Moral Treatment," and a reduction in the discharge rate.

In the first half of this century, while the population of the United States doubled, the number of patients in state mental hospitals quadrupled. After a progressive increase in the hospital population in the post–World War II years, the trend was dramatically reversed in 1955. In 1955, there were 558,900 patients in state and local government hospitals in the United States; by 1970, this number was reduced by 40 percent to 338,600, and by 70 percent in 1976 when the hospital population had declined to 170,700. Do these figures merely reflect a reduction in the number of patients admitted to mental hospitals? Quite the contrary; whereas 178,000 patients were admitted in 1955, 330,000 entered in 1966, and 435,000 in 1976. The reduction in the population of these hospitals may be explained by comparing the average duration of hospitalization: six months in 1955, two months in 1966, and only 26 days in 1975.

One of the major factors responsible for the decrease in psychiatric hospital populations and in the reduction in the duration of hospitalization was the introduction of effective psychoactive drugs in the mid-1950s that proved useful for the treatment of psychoses, neuroses, and affective disorders. After outlining the theories concerning the causes of mental disease, we shall discuss the properties of these therapeutic agents.

THEORIES CONCERNING CAUSES OF MENTAL ILLNESS

While we are able to specifically pinpoint the cause of organic brain disorders, we can only hypothesize what factors are responsible for functional disorders. We shall categorize these theories into three major groups: psychological, sociocultural, and biochemical. The first two categories will be discussed together.

Psychological and Sociocultural Theories

Many psychological theories of mental illness view these disorders as the product of adverse past experiences, often having their roots during childhood. As a defense mechanism against conflict, threats, frustration, deprivation, and uncertainty, the patient *learns* to establish protective or defensive behavioral responses, which when carried into later life are considered to be abnormal. Proponents of psychological theories advocate a treatment regimen involving the reshaping of the patient's behavior. The patient is taught to refrain from manifesting the old abnormal behavioral response and, instead, to substitute a new, socially acceptable response.

A stressful environment, be it in a work situation, family, neighborhood, ethnic group, or nation has been shown to adversely affect behavior. There is evidence to suggest that both functional and organic disorders can be unfavorably influenced by *sociocultural* factors. Whereas some behavioral disorders may be unique for a given culture, others are observed universally. Family instability and disintegration, as well as war and unemployment, have a detrimental effect on behavior.

Biochemical Theories

For many years it has been recognized that a relationship exists between the biochemical reactions occurring within the body and the manifested behavior. This interrelationship may be studied in one of two ways. We may alter the normal biochemical reactions and study changes in behavior, or conversely, we may modify the behavior of the organism and seek biochemical correlates that may help us to better understand the basis for the behavioral changes.

$$\text{Behavioral Changes} \rightleftharpoons \text{Biochemical Changes}$$

The concept that biochemical factors may underlie mental illnesses has been succinctly stated by Ralph Gerard: "Behind every crooked thought there lies a crooked molecule."

Theories ascribing biochemical causes to mental illness fall into three general categories: (1) those in which a chemical or biochemical agent is introduced into the body from external sources; (2) those in which a behaviorally toxic compound is manufactured within the body; and (3) those in which the illness arises as a result of a genetic defect. Let us briefly examine each of these theories.

The first category is most familiar to us. The psychotomimetics (hallucinogens) such as LSD or mescaline produce profound alterations in behavior, as do alcohol and amphetamine (amphetamine psychosis). Farm workers exposed to toxic concentrations of organophosphate insecticides have been reported to become disoriented and experience hallucinations. Advanced symptoms of lead poisoning in children are often characterized by confusion and delirium.

Over 2000 years ago, Hippocrates first introduced the concept that toxic compounds are manufactured by the body. This idea was reintroduced in 1884 by Thudichum, the father of modern neurochemistry:

Many forms of insanity are unquestionably the external manifestations of the effects upon the brain substance of poisons fermented within the body, just as mental aberrations accompanying chronic alcoholic intoxication are the accumulated effects of a relatively simple poison fermented out of the body. These poisons we shall, I have no doubt, be able to isolate after we know the normal chemistry of its uttermost detail. And then will come in their turn the crowning discoveries to which our efforts must ultimately be directed, namely, the discoveries of the antidotes to the poisons and to the fermenting causes and processes which produce them.[2]

The present-day search for such biochemical factors has been predicated upon Thudichum's statement. We no longer speak of poisons but, rather, now talk about neurotransmitter substances or abnormal proteins. Normal behavior, moods, emotions, and thought processes are significantly influenced by, and perhaps even directly controlled by, neurotransmitter substances in the brain. Psychiatric aberrations may be the consequence of a qualitative or quantitative abnormality in these naturally occurring compounds in a discrete area of the brain. Several contemporary biochemical theories will be presented below.

Evidence has been accumulated in recent years that tends to support the provocative hypothesis that there is a *genetic predisposition* to certain forms of mental illness. It might be suggested that a biochemical defect is inherited. The most meaningful studies have sought to compare the concordance rates of mental disease in monozygotic (identical) and dizygotic (fraternal) twins. Whereas fraternal twins show a concordance rate of about 10 to 15 percent, the incidence of schizophrenia in identical twins is as high as 60 to 85 percent. The rate observed in dizygotic twins does not differ significantly from that seen in siblings. One may argue, with justification, "Well, what about the influence of environmental factors?" Environmental influences are of great importance and can only be properly evaluated when concordance rates are compared in identical twins separated at birth. At present, observers see a greater genetic component influencing mental deficiency, schizophrenia, and manic-depression than has been found for neuroses.

DRUG TREATMENT OF MENTAL ILLNESS

The search for effective methods of treating mental diseases has been a long one. Many drugs and physical treatment measures have been employed; some of these methods received only limited acceptance by the medical practitioners of the time, while others were adopted as the treatment of choice for many years. During the 30-year period after World War I, schizophrenia was treated by malaria-induced fever, and by convulsions and coma induced by insulin, chemicals such as pentylenetetrazol (Metrazol), and electroshock. A highly im-

---

[2] J. W. L. Thudichum, *A Treatise on the Chemical Constitution of the Brain* (London: Balliere, Tindall and Cox, 1884).

aginative (although quite irrational and somewhat random) assortment of drugs were also employed. The nineteenth century saw the use of digitalis, ipecac, calomel (mercurous chloride), and quinine—drugs which have no major action on the central nervous system in therapeutic doses. In the middle of the last century, the bromides, belladonna, *Cannabis* (marijuana), and chloral hydrate were employed, in addition to the time-honored standards, alcohol and opium; the barbiturates were also used for many decades during this century. Insulin-induced coma and convulsive therapy were once in vogue for the treatment of schizophrenia. The years 1949 to 1957 witnessed a violent revolution in the treatment of mental illness. Drugs were developed for the management of psychoses, neuroses, mania, and depression, and virtually all other previously employed drug treatments became obsolete.

Rauwolfia serpentina, the Indian snakeroot, is a shrub indigenous to India and other countries of Southeast Asia. For centuries, preparations of this root had been used by Indian physicians for the treatment of a wide variety of disorders including high blood pressure (hypertension) and mental diseases; these reports were first verified scientifically in 1931. However, over twenty years elapsed before *Rauwolfia* and its active constituent *reserpine* were clinically used in Western medicine as antihypertensive and antipsychotic agents. We shall discuss reserpine's antihypertensive properties in Chapter 21. The high incidence of adverse side effects of reserpine and its unequivocal inferiority to chlorpromazine as an antipsychotic agent (see below) led to the almost total demise of its use in the treatment of mental illness. However, reserpine has proved to be an invaluable chemical tool providing us with a better understanding of the influence of monoamines (norepinephrine and serotonin) on brain function. In particular, the behavioral consequences of reserpine-induced depletion of these amines from nerve endings in the central nervous system have served as the basis of theories relating to the etiology of psychosis and depression, as well as explanations concerning the mechanisms by which psychoactive drugs act.

ANTIPSYCHOTIC AGENTS: PHENOTHIAZINES

The phenothiazine derivatives are among the most extensively used classes of drugs in all of medical practice. Chlorpromazine (Thorazine), the most commonly employed phenothiazine, was given to more than 50 million patients from 1955 to 1965, and it has been the subject of more than 10,000 publications. In addition, we find that several dozen phenothiazine derivatives are employed for psychiatric disorders; some of these are listed in Table 16–1. Prior to the introduction of chlorpromazine, violent patients were physically restrained or heavily sedated. By contrast, the phenothiazines calm the patient without producing incoordination or a clouding of consciousness, thus permitting them to meaningfully participate in psychotherapy sessions.

TABLE 16-1. REPRESENTATIVE ANTIPSYCHOTIC PHENOTHIAZINE DERIVATIVES

Generic Name	Selected Trade Names	Relative Potency	General Class Properties		
			Extrapyramidal Effects	Nonextrapyramidal Effects	

A. Aliphatic side chain

$R=CH_2CH_2CH_2N\overset{CH_3}{\underset{CH_3}{}}$

Generic Name	Selected Trade Names	Relative Potency	Extrapyramidal Effects	Nonextrapyramidal Effects
Chlorpromazine Triflupromazine	Thorazine Vesprin	Low	Moderate	Sedation Hypotension Liver jaundice Blood disorders

B. Piperidine side chain

$R=CH_2CH_2-$

Generic Name	Selected Trade Names	Relative Potency	Extrapyramidal Effects	Nonextrapyramidal Effects
Mesoridazine Piperacetazine Thioridazine	Serentil Quide Mellaril	Intermediate	Low	Fewest side effects

C. Piperazine side chain

$R=CH_2CH_2CH_2N\overline{}N-Z$

Generic Name	Selected Trade Names	Relative Potency	Extrapyramidal Effects	Nonextrapyramidal Effects
Acetophenazine Butaperazine Carphenazine Fluphenazine Perphenazine Prochlorperazine Trifluoperazine	Tindal Repoise Proketazine Prolixin; Permitil Trilafon Compazine Stelazine	High	High	Lower incidence

Phenothiazine, chlorpromazine's parent molecule, was synthesized in 1883, and it was subsequently observed to be useful as a urinary antiseptic and anthelmintic (antiworm) agent. In 1952, the recently synthesized chlorpromazine was used to induce a state of artificial hibernation during surgery in an attempt to reduce the incidence of shock. During the process of artificial hibernation, consciousness was retained, and it was observed that patients were calm and relaxed and noticeably indifferent to the normal anxieties associated with surgery. The potential applications of chlorpromazine for the treatment of mentally ill patients were recognized and tested. Chlorpromazine was shown to calm psychotic patients exhibiting agitation, excitement, and hostile behavior.

Pharmacological Actions

Prior to discussing the use of chlorpromazine for the treatment of psychiatric disorders, we shall briefly review some of the pharmacological actions of this drug. Chlorpromazine is among the most protean of all drugs, and even a simple catalog of its actions and effects represents a lengthy compilation. For example, it can block norepinephrine, dopamine, serotonin, acetylcholine, and histamine receptor sites. Apart from its profound influence on behavior, chlorpromazine has extensive actions on the endocrine glands; for example, it interferes with several phases of the human female reproductive cycle.

There is a considerable body of indirect evidence (supplemented with a very modest amount of direct information) suggesting that schizophrenia may result from a defect in the dopaminergic system, more specifically, from a functional increase in **dopaminergic activity** in the limbic system. The antipsychotic activity of the phenothiazines, thioxanthenes, butyrophenones, and other clinically active drugs appears to be related to their ability to bind to and block dopamine receptor sites. (As will be noted below, many antipsychotic agents cause adverse effects involving the extrapyramidal system; these neurological effects have also been attributed to blockade of central dopamine receptors).

Another contemporary hypothesis suggests that chlorpromazine's major site of antipsychotic action is the reticular activating system. You will recall from Chapter 9 that the reticular activating system (RAS) receives sensory stimuli, and, after appropriate filtration has taken place, alerting impulses are transmitted up to the cerebrum. It has been postulated that chlorpromazine either depresses the collaterals entering the RAS, or directly depresses the RAS (a less likely possibility), or perhaps increases the ability of the RAS to filter the sensory inputs traveling to the cerebrum. The stimuli that are successfully filtered might be those responsible for the abnormal thought processes and hallucinations experienced by the psychotic patient.

Therapeutic Uses

Psychoses

Although chlorpromazine is incapable of curing psychotic disorders, it has radically altered the outlook for mentally ill patients. Many patients totally unresponsive to other treatments and individuals long maintained on the back wards of psychiatric hospitals have become amenable to psychotherapy. Other patients who, in the pre-chlorpromazine era, would have spent months and years in hospitals prior to release are now being treated on an outpatient basis. Let us briefly examine the spectrum of chlorpromazine's antipsychotic effects.

The phenothiazine tranquilizers have been demonstrated to be effective in alleviating many of the symptoms associated with schizophrenia. Violent and overly active patients become quiet, calm, and cooperative with their therapists. Thought disturbances, hallucinations, and illusions gradually subside. Unlike the barbiturates that produce general depression, chlorpromazine does not produce a clouding of consciousness in therapeutic doses. Apathetic and retarded patients have also been shown to return to normal as well.

Although the phenothiazines have been demonstrated to be useful in managing many of the clinical manifestations of acute and chronic schizophrenia, not all symptoms of psychosis improve to an equivalent extent. For example, insight, judgment, memory, and orientation are less markedly improved than are combativeness, tension, hostility, hyperactivity, or hallucinations. Apparently, the more grossly manifested symptoms improve to a greater extent with phenothiazine therapy; a satisfactory explanation for these observations is not available at present.

Cooperative studies conducted by the Veterans Administration and the National Institute of Mental Health demonstrated that two-thirds of the acutely ill, hospitalized schizophrenics were improved after receiving phenothiazine treatment, while improvement was observed in only 25 percent of those given placebo medication. Moreover, whereas 50 percent of the patients given a placebo were rated as showing "no improvement" or "worse," only 10 percent of those given a phenothiazine drug were so rated. We observe great variation in the time required for the improvement to be observed clinically. Some patients show signs of getting better within a few days or weeks after phenothiazine treatment, while others show a gradual improvement over several years. The average patient manifests the greatest therapeutic gains within the first six weeks, although additional benefit from drug therapy is often observed over the subsequent three to six months.

After a psychotic patient has been shown to improve following a course of treatment with the phenothiazines, what are the consequences of drug withdrawal? Unfortunately, a very high relapse rate is observed among patients who have discontinued taking medication and in those whose dosage has been substantially reduced. A series of independently conducted studies has shown relapse rates of about 35 to 45 percent within four to six months. That such regressions occur even when the patient is maintained on placebo medication further reinforces the view that the phenothiazines are highly effective clinically.

You may ask how long patients must be maintained on these antipsychotic agents after they have been successfully treated. The phenothiazines do not cure psychoses, and, as we shall soon observe, these drugs have undesirable adverse effects. Some physicians maintain that patients should continue to take their medication for the remainder of their lives, just as diabetics are obliged to take insulin. Other clinical investigators prefer to gradually withdraw these drugs, while maintaining both close psychiatric supervision and strict vigilance for signs of regressions in behavior.

What is the eventual prognosis for the schizophrenic patient? That is, does such an individual ever become normal? At present, the results are rather disheartening. Estimates suggest that only about 10 to 15 percent of these patients ever function normally.[3] The remaining patients retain varying degrees of psychopathology, with many requiring periodic rehospitalization. These facts emphasize the importance of developing psychoactive drugs that are capable of *curing* psychotic illnesses.

Mania

Chlorpromazine and other phenothiazine derivatives with sedative properties are highly useful for rapidly controlling manic patients. Lithium carbonate, which is administered simultaneously with the phenothiazine, has a slower onset of antimanic activity. Once the manic symptoms are brought under control, the phenothiazine is discontinued and chronic lithium therapy maintained (see below).

Nausea and Vomiting

Selected phenothiazines (chlorpromazine, prochlorperazine [Compazine]) are employed at nonsedative doses to prevent the nausea and vomiting caused by various diseases and by radiation sickness, as well as by certain drugs, such as anticancer agents. Among the phenothiazines lacking antipsychotic activity that are used for their antiemetic effects are promazine (Sparine), promethazine (Phenergan), and thiethylperazine (Torecan). Unlike chlorpromazine, promethazine has been found to be highly effective in preventing motion sickness.

Adverse Effects

Thus far we have emphasized only the positive aspects associated with phenothiazine therapy. Although several serious adverse effects result from the use of these drugs, the phenothiazines have a very wide margin of safety. In a recent review, 186 cases of chlorpromazine poisoning were tabulated; 78 were in

---

[3] You may wish to consider these statistics in light of Rosenhan's paper. See footnote 1.

children and 108 in adults. Of these poisonings, four proved fatal in children and three in adults, thus attesting to the low acute toxicity of these drugs. Unlike the barbiturates and antianxiety agents, chronic administration of the phenothiazines does not produce drug dependence.

The very extensive pharmacological actions of the phenothiazines are also reflected by the wide diversity of side effects associated with their use. These include neurological effects, hypotension, liver and blood disorders, rashes, and photosensitivity of the skin.

Neurological Effects

The most frequently observed phenothiazine side effects, seen in about 40 percent of the patients, are **extrapyramidal symptoms.** These symptoms are characterized by a parkinsonian disease state in which the patient experiences difficulty in walking, has a shuffling gait, muscle rigidity, and tremors of the limbs. In addition, many patients exhibit abnormal facial movements, are restless, and exhibit incoordinated jerkiness. For many years, it was believed that these extrapyramidal symptoms were a necessary prerequisite for antipsychotic activity. This view is no longer generally accepted. Some of these effects are reduced by the coadministration of anticholinergic anti-Parkinson drugs (Table 8–1).

The most serious complication associated with the chronic administration of antipsychotic agents is **tardive dyskinesia,** a syndrome which may be seen in 10 percent to up to 35–40 percent of patients receiving these drugs. Symptoms of this neurological disorder include involuntary movements of the lips, tongue, and jaw, and purposeless, quick darting movements of the extremities. Tardive dyskinesia occurs only after long-term drug administration or after chronic high doses are abruptly reduced or withdrawn. These symptoms often persist and may become more intense after the termination of therapy. Since at present no effective treatment exists to reverse this problem, considerable attention has been directed toward preventing its occurrence. Such preventive measures include the institution of drug-free holidays and the imposition of limits on the duration of high-dose therapy.

The biochemical basis for these neurological side effects has been the subject of considerable speculation and investigation. Clinicians have been long puzzled by the observation that while some antipsychotic agents cause a high incidence of extrapyramidal effects, other drugs produce very few. The extrapyramidal system of the brain is concerned with the control and coordination of motor functions. Normal function is modulated by a balance between the excitatory influence of the cholinergic system and the opposing inhibitory influence of the dopaminergic system. Thus, inhibition of one system permits the relative predominance of the other. As noted above, all commonly employed antipsychotic agents are effective dopamine antagonists; many of these same drugs also possess varying degrees of anticholinergic (antimuscarinic or atropine-like) activity. For example, while the piperazine phenothiazines (trifluoperazine) and the butyrophenone haloperidol possess rather modest anticholinergic activity, the piperidine phenothiazines (thioridazine) have relatively potent anticholinergic activity; chlorpromazine has intermediate activity. As you might predict, the incidence of adverse extrapyramidal effects is highest in those drugs that cause greatest disruption in the delicate cholinergic-dopaminergic balance (namely, trifluoperazine and haloperidol) and lowest in drugs that minimally alter this balance (thioridazine).

It has been hypothesized that tardive dyskinesia results from prolonged blockade of the dopamine receptors. In an attempt to overcome this postsynaptic block and restore the normal homeostatic balance, there is both an increased synthesis of dopamine and an increase in the sensitivity and/or number of dopamine receptor sites. These changes promote the predominance of the dopaminergic system—and are even more exaggerated if administration of the antipsychotic agent is terminated. Clinically these neuropharmacological changes are manifested by the appearance of the symptoms of tardive dyskinesia.

Nonneurological Effects

During the first few days that patients receive chlorpromazine, they often experience a sudden drop in blood pressure and may feel faint upon assuming an erect position after lying down. This condition, termed *orthostatic hypotension,* has been attributed to chlorpromazine's actions on both the peripheral blood vessels and the hypothalamus, resulting in an interference with the body's ability to maintain adequate circulatory adjustments in the blood flow to the brain.

Among the most dramatic side effects associated with phenothiazine therapy are the allergic reactions, which include liver jaundice and the blood disorder agranulocytosis. Liver jaundice, seen in about one out of every 200 patients, begins within the early weeks of therapy. The patient first experiences flu-like symptoms—weaknesses, abdominal pain, fever, diarrhea, nausea, and vomiting—with subsequent liver abnormalities. Agranulocytosis (a disease characterized by a marked drop in certain white blood cells) is relatively rare, seen in about one patient in 3000, but is associated with a mortality rate of 30 to 50 percent. Photosensitivity, a state resembling a severe sunburn of the skin, is another allergic reaction. Some patients, after receiving phenothiazines for long periods of time, experience color changes of the skin characterized by a blue-gray metallic discoloration over areas normally exposed to sunlight.

Antipsychotic Agents: An Overview

The antipsychotic agents, although incapable of curing psychotic disorders, are able to reduce the disease symptoms in about two-thirds to three-fourths of the patients. As a direct consequence, mental hospitals have been able to become more therapeutically oriented rather than serving merely a custodial function. Since the clinical introduction of these drugs in 1954, state mental hospital populations have been markedly reduced, mainly by virtue of the decrease in the average duration of patient hospitalization and a return to home with treatment continued on an outpatient basis.

In the opinion of experts, there appears to be little difference in the overall clinical effectiveness of the commonly employed phenothiazine antipsychotic agents listed in Table 16–1, but there are differences in the relative incidence of adverse side effects. Table 16–2 lists some nonphenothiazine antipsychotic agents currently employed. Their use in the United States is considerably more limited than the relative use of the phenothiazines.

ANTIDEPRESSANT AND ANTIMANIC AGENTS

> *He . . . a short tale to make*
> *Fell into a sadness, then into a fast,*
> *Thence to a watch, thence into a weakness,*
> *Thence to a lightness, and by this declension,*
> *Into the madness wherein he now raves*
> *And all we mourn for.*[4]
>
> —William Shakespeare (c. 1602)

As the old spiritual song aptly tells us—"I'm sometimes up and I'm sometimes down"—fluctuations in mood are a very normal behavioral pattern in life. The **affective disorders,** *depression* and *mania,* are characterized by extreme changes in mood and differ from normal fluctuations in mood in their intensity, duration, and the nature of the symptoms exhibited. In this section, we shall consider the treatment of depression (extreme sadness) and mania (excessive elevations of the mood).

Depression

We have all experienced varying degrees of depression. These are generally temporary and nondisabling and may be precipitated by personal, social, and economic stresses, frustrations, failures, and losses. After being "down in the dumps" for some time, we usually spring back and return to normal, even in the absence of medical treatment. Consider, by contrast, those individuals who, for long periods of time, feel hopeless, helpless, and worthless. Such persons usually have long episodes of crying, suffer from a loss of appetite, and have insomnia. Pleasure and satisfaction may no longer be derived from their family, friends, and work. They may experience delusions and other impairments of thought processes. The situation may seem so bleak that such patients develop suicidal thoughts which may even be set into positive action.

---

[4] *Hamlet,* act 2, scene 2.

TABLE 16-2. SELECTED NONPHENOTHIAZINE ANTIPSYCHOTIC AGENTS OF CONTEMPORARY INTEREST

Class	Representative Structure	Generic Name	Selected Brand Name(s)	Remarks
Thioxanthenes		Chloprothixene Thiothixene	Taractan Navane	Chemically and pharmacologically similar to phenothiazines. Slightly less active than phenothiazines with similar structures.
Butyrophenones		Haloperidol	Haldol	Effective for mania and hyperactive psychoses. Effective in schizophrenia. Butyrophenones block CNS dopamine receptor sites.
Dibenzoxazepines		Loxapine	Daxolin, Loxitane	Phenothiazine-like properties with high incidence of extrapyramidal effects.
Dihydroindolones		Molindone	Lidone, Moban	Pharmacological actions similar to piperazine phenothiazines (Table 16-1).

This latter type of depression is deemed a variety of mental illness. It has been estimated that during the course of a lifetime, about 8 percent of men and 16 percent of women will experience a depressive illness, although not all of these are sufficiently severe to warrant hospitalization. Because of the self-limiting nature of depression, about half the hospitalized patients will spontaneously recover, even in the absence of drug therapy or such physical treatment as electroconvulsive therapy (ECT).

Depressive illnesses may be classified on the basis of their presumed etiology. *Reactive* or *exogenous depressions* result from environmental or emotional stresses, frustrations, or losses. Certain drugs, including the oral contraceptives, reserpine, and high doses of cortisone-like drugs have been observed to cause depression in some patients. By contrast, *endogenous depressions* are of unknown etiology and are thought to have a biochemical basis. Affective disorders are often classified as being *unipolar*, characterized by episodes of only depression or mania, or *bipolar*, characterized by alternating periods of depression and mania. There appears to be a genetic predisposition for bipolar manic-depressive illnesses.

One contemporary hypothesis attributes affective disorders to alterations in the normal concentrations of norepinephrine in the brain. This hypothesis argues that mania is the result of excessive amounts of norepinephrine interacting with selected receptor sites in the brain. Conversely, deficient amounts of norepinephrine produce *depression*. These key receptor sites may be located in the reward system of the medial forebrain bundle. This "catecholamine hypothesis of affective disorders," albeit based upon indirect evidence and not accepted by all investigators in the area, is very useful to us in understanding the postulated mechanisms by which mood altering drugs are thought to act (Figure 16–1). At this point, you might find it helpful to review the section concerning "Adrenergic Transmission" in Chapter 6.

Electroconvulsive Therapy

Depression may be treated with drugs, namely, the tricyclic derivatives and the monoamine oxidase inhibitors, and by electroconvulsive therapy (ECT). Let us first briefly consider the advantages and disadvantages of ECT prior to considering chemical agents.

ECT provides the most rapid and effective method of treating endogenous depression, with about 70 to 90 percent of the patients showing clinical improvement. In this procedure, electrodes are attached to the patient's temples and an electric current of about 100 volts is passed through the cortex for about one-half second; patients lose consciousness before they can feel any pain. After a very brief period during which patients experience seizures, they become quiet and regain consciousness in about 30 minutes, at which time they are generally drowsy, confused, and disoriented. A course of therapy may consist of three such treatments per week. Dramatic improvement is generally observed after six sessions, with several additional treatments administered to prolong the remission of symptoms.

In addition to the high rate of success with ECT, the rapidity with which depression is alleviated is often of great importance when the patient is a potential suicide risk. The precise mechanism responsible for the beneficial effects observed in ECT is not known. Increased synthesis and release of norepinephrine and other neurotransmitters in the brain have been noted in animals after ECT. The increased concentrations of norepinephrine at crucial receptor sites in the brain could account for the reversal of depression. When proper precautions are taken, ECT is a relatively safe procedure, and yet, as might be anticipated, there are some very unpleasant aspects associated with its use. Some of the major disadvantages include patient apprehension associated with the induction of seizures, as well as confusion, and temporary amnesia after a series of treatments; bone fractures occasionally occur. The reversal of depression is not permanent, with relapses often occurring.

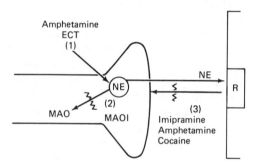

FIGURE 16–1. Site and Mechanism of Antidepressant Agents. The catecholamine hypothesis of affective disorders postulates that depression results from a deficiency in the effective concentration of norepinephrine (NE) available to interact at adrenergic receptor sites in the brain. Mechanisms that increase this effective concentration at the receptor site (R) should alleviate depression.

(1) *Stimulate the release of NE from nerve endings.* Amphetamine and electroconvulsive therapy (ECT) act by this mechanism. ECT is the most rapid and effective method currently available for the treatment of depression.

(2) *Prevent the inactivation of NE.* Monoamine oxidase inhibitors (MAOI) are thought to act as antidepressant agents in part by preventing the breakdown of NE by the intraneuronal enzyme monoamine oxidase (MAO). MAOI have fallen out of clinical favor in recent years because of their questionable effectiveness and relatively high incidence of toxicity.

(3) *Prevent the re-uptake of NE.* The action of NE at the adrenergic receptor site is primarily terminated by the re-uptake of NE by the presynaptic neuron from which it was originally released. The tricyclic antidepressants, imipramine for one, the most effective drugs presently available for the treatment of depression, act by this mechanism. Amphetamine and cocaine, an extreme euphoriant, also act in this manner. (While both amphetamine and cocaine elevate the mood, neither drug is clinically useful as an antidepressant.)

Monoamine Oxidase Inhibitors

The modern chemical treatment of depression began on a tuberculosis ward in 1951. In that year, **iproniazid** was being evaluated as an antituberculosis agent. This compound is a close chemical relative of isoniazid (INH), a highly useful drug for the treatment of this disease. At this time tuberculosis wards were melancholy places, with patients usually manifesting attitudes of despair and often resignation to a hopeless outcome. Much to their delight, physicians were amazed to observe that after the administration of iproniazid, patients— even terminal patients—were extremely cheerful and were highly optimistic about the future. Examination of the x-rays demonstrated no major regression of the pathological lesions of the lungs, and the improvement was attributed to a change in their psychological behavior. Because of the pronounced central stimulatory effects, trials with iproniazid for the treatment of tuberculosis were terminated. In 1952, iproniazid was observed to be a monoamine oxidase (MAO) inhibitor. Major clinical interest in this compound died for five years until 1957, when Kline and co-workers reported its highly beneficial effectiveness in the treatment of depression.

Subsequent years have witnessed the development and clinical introduction of many other MAO inhibitors for the treatment of depression. Half of these agents have been withdrawn from the market because of their toxicity to the eyes, blood, or liver. Considerable controversy exists regarding the therapeutic merits of the MAO inhibitors, with many studies failing to show their superiority over placebo medication. For this reason, and their well-documented adverse side effects, the surviving MAO inhibitors (Table 16–3) are now being used only when depressed patients fail to respond to the tricyclic antidepressants. It should be mentioned that the relative ability of a drug to inhibit MAO has not been correlated with its therapeutic effectiveness. This strongly suggests that an additional mechanism may be responsible for the action of this class of drugs.

Tricyclic Antidepressants

Imipramine (Tofranil) was developed as a potential antipsychotic agent, which is not surprising in view of its close similarity to chlorpromazine. However, when tested in 1958, imipramine was observed to be a highly effective antidepressant agent. The ensuing widespread clinical acceptance of this drug and the other members of this class has been attributed to its greater efficacy

Chlorpromazine (Thorazine)
(A phenothiazine derivative)

Imipramine (Tofranil)
(A dibenzazepine derivative)

and lower toxicity than the MAO inhibitors; in addition, there is greater ease of administration and patient acceptability when compared with ECT. Let us now consider the pharmacology of imipramine and the related tricyclic anti-depressants (Table 16-3).

Unlike iproniazid, imipramine does not produce central nervous stimulation or euphoria. When given to nondepressed patients, imipramine produces feelings of fatigue. Depressed patients, by contrast, respond with an elevation of the mood, increased physical activity, and mental alertness, and with improvement in appetite and the ability to sleep.

The effects of the tricyclic antidepressant agents have been attributed to their ability to prevent the re-uptake of norepinephrine after its release from the adrenergic neuron and interaction at the receptor sites (Figure 16-1). Thus, norepinephrine is available to activate the receptor site for longer periods of time with enhanced intensity. Some clinically effective tricyclic antidepressants are potent inhibitors of *serotonin* uptake, suggesting that this central neurotransmitter may play a role in depression and in the mechanism of action of these drugs. This class of drugs does not inhibit MAO.

TABLE 16-3 ANTIDEPRESSANT AGENTS OF CONTEMPORARY IMPORTANCE

Generic Name	Selected Trade Names	Remarks
Monoamine oxidase inhibitors		
Isocarboxazid	Marplan	These two compounds are chemically
Phenelzine	Nardil	classified as hydrazine MAO inhibitors. Among the many disadvantages are questionable effectiveness, slow onset of action, liver toxicity, and CNS disturbances.
Tranylcypromine	Parnate	This drug, a nonhydrazine, is among the most frequently employed MAO inhibitors. Tranylcypromine has an amphetamine-like action and possesses few hydrazine-like side effects. Severe hypertension may occur when this drug is taken with certain cheeses and wines.
Tricyclic antidepressants		
Amitriptyline	Elavil, Endep	This class of drugs is the most effective
Desipramine	Norpramin Pertofrane	currently available for the treatment of depression. Unlike the MAO inhibitors,
Doxepin	Adapin Sinequan	these drugs do not produce CNS stimulation. Tricyclic antidepressants pro-
Imipramine	Imavate Janimine Presamine SK-Pramine Tofranil	duce atropine-like side effects such as dryness of the mouth, constipation, and difficulty in focusing the eyes.
Nortriptyline	Aventyl	
Protriptyline	Vivactil	
Trimipramine	Surmontil	

Controlled studies have shown that the effectiveness of the tricyclic antidepressants comes close to ECT, with about 60 to 70 percent of depressed patients showing improvement. Although variation is observed in the onset of antidepressant actions among the various tricyclic compounds, favorable signs appear within one to two weeks, with maximal effects in four to six weeks. It would be of great practical and theoretical significance to be able to predict in advance which of the one-in-three patients will not favorably respond to the tricyclics.

In Chapter 3 we observed that marked differences may exist in the rate of drug metabolism among members of the same species. While we can account for some of these differences on the basis of the influence of previously or concurrently administered drugs (for example, resulting from enzyme induction), in other instances genetically predetermined factors are responsible for intraspecies variation (pharmacogenetics). In very recent years, it has been demonstrated that after an identical oral dose of a given tricyclic antidepressant agent, the variation in the blood concentration of the pharmacologically active drug may vary as much as 10- to 40-fold in different human subjects! These extreme variations in the blood concentration of drugs has been attributed to both pharmacogenetic factors and enzyme induction, and is now thought to provide a plausible explanation why, after the same dose of an antidepressant, one patient obtains a favorable therapeutic response, another suffers from a high incidence of adverse side effects, and a third manifests no clinical improvement.

Mania

Mania is characterized by *extreme euphoria* or irritability and some of the following symptoms: extreme physical activity, apparent lack of fatigue, reduced periods of sleep, and distractability, with many projects initiated but rapidly abandoned prior to their completion. In the absence of appropriate treatment, a manic episode may persist for an average of three months. It has been estimated that the incidence of depression is ten times higher than that of mania.

Treatment of Mania: Antipsychotics and Lithium

Acute episodes of mania are effectively controlled with the phenothiazine (chlorpromazine) or butyrophenone (haloperidol) class of antipsychotic agents or with lithium carbonate.

In normal individuals, therapeutic doses of **lithium carbonate** (Eskalith, Lithonate, Lithane) produce no behavioral effects, and, in this respect, it differs from all other psychotherapeutic agents. This inorganic salt normalizes the extreme mood and motor activity, permitting the manic patient "to come down" in the absence of a "drugged" or tranquilized feeling. Since the full antimanic effects of this drug are only apparent after its administration for seven to ten days, lithium is commonly given with an antipsychotic agent. The latter class of drugs is effective within three to five days; after the patient has been stabilized, the antipsychotic drug is withdrawn and lithium therapy maintained. Chronic administration of lithium has been shown to effectively prevent recurrent episodes of bipolar affective disorders.

The mechanism by which lithium produces its antimanic effects is not well understood. Many of the diverse effects of lithium may be attributed to its ability to alter the movement of sodium across cell membranes.[5] Lithium is thought to reduce the functional excess of norepinephrine that is presumed to be involved in mania. Such actions include an inhibition of norepinephrine release and a reduction in the sensitivity of the receptor site to this neurotransmitter.

Optimum therapeutic effects are obtained when plasma lithium concentrations are maintained between 0.8 and 1.5 milliequivalents per liter. Lower plasma levels are generally associated with a less than optimal response, while exceeding the upper plasma concentration limit increases the incidence of toxicity. Toxic doses of lithium can cause muscle rigidity, convulsions, and coma.

ANTIANXIETY AGENTS: THE "MINOR TRANQUILIZERS"

The irretrievably ingrained term "minor tranquilizer" is most unfortunate because it implies that these agents act like major tranquilizers but to a lesser extent; one might expect large doses of the minor tranquilizers to have approximately the same clinical effects as small doses of the major tranquilizers and to be effective in the same range of clinical conditions. Actually, this is not the case; the minor tranquilizers more closely resemble sedative-hypnotic drugs such as the barbiturates than major tranquilizers such as the phenothiazines.[6]

—D. F. Klein and J. M. Davis (1969)

Neuroses are probably the most common of all disorders afflicting man. Since anxiety is the major symptom characterizing neuroses, perhaps it is not inappropriate to term our era the "age of anxiety" as some investigators have suggested. It has been estimated that about 50 percent of the patients who visit physicians have emotional illnesses rather than the physical disorders of which they complain. We can, thus, appreciate the great therapeutic successes obtained with placebo medication (Chapter 3).

In Chapter 11, we considered the use of the barbiturate and nonbarbiturate sedative-hypnotic drugs and their employment in low doses as antianxiety

---

[5] During the 1940s, lithium chloride was employed as a salt substitute for cardiac patients being maintained on a low salt diet. Lithium proved to be an unfortunate choice. Since it cannot be excreted as easily as sodium ions, with repeated use lithium levels became elevated and a number of patients died as the result of poisoning by this ion. While lithium was being routinely used in Europe as an antimanic agent by the mid-1960s, it was not approved for this use in the United States until some five years later.

[6] *Diagnosis and Drug Treatment of Psychiatric Disorders* (Baltimore: Williams & Wilkins), p. 342.

agents. We shall now discuss meprobamate and the benzodiazepine derivatives, compounds very extensively employed for the treatment of neuroses. Representative antianxiety (anxiolytic) agents are listed in Table 16–4.

Meprobamate

The discovery of meprobamate, the first modern antianxiety agent, dates back to 1945. During the course of a search for an antimicrobial agent that would be effective against bacteria that were resistant to penicillin, one test compound was observed to produce profound muscle relaxation and a calming effect in rats. This compound, *mephenesin carbamate* (Tolseram) was marketed in 1946 as a skeletal muscle relaxant. Although a relatively effective drug, mephenesin had a very short duration of action thus necessitating repeated drug administration at frequent intervals. **Meprobamate,** introduced in 1955 as Miltown and Equanil, was not only a longer acting muscle relaxant than its parent compound mephenesin, but also possessed antianxiety activity.

Notwithstanding the immediate and overwhelming acceptance of meprobamate by the general public and lay press, medical investigators have been divided in their evaluation of the therapeutic merits of this agent. The anti-meprobamate forces ascribe the success of meprobamate to extremely effective and successful advertising, highly favorable early clinical reports, and the introduction of the drug at precisely the right time. This "right time" coincided with the early days of chlorpromazine, when the medical world was extremely enthusiastic about the wonders of tranquilizers and their potential benefits for the treatment of mental illness. Subsequent double-blind studies have been less laudatory in their praise of meprobamate as an antianxiety agent. While most, although by no means all, studies have shown meprobamate to be more effective than a placebo, this drug has rarely been shown to be superior to the barbiturates for the relief of anxiety.

$$
\begin{array}{c}
\quad\quad\quad\quad\quad\quad \overset{\displaystyle O}{\underset{\displaystyle\|}{}} \\
\quad\quad\quad\quad CH_2\,O\overset{\|}{C}-NH_2 \\
\quad\quad\quad\quad\quad | \\
CH_3CH_2CH_2\,\overset{|}{\underset{|}{C}}-CH_3 \\
\quad\quad\quad\quad CH_2\,O\overset{\|}{C}-NH_2 \\
\quad\quad\quad\quad\quad\quad\underset{\displaystyle O}{\|}
\end{array}
$$

Meprobamate (Miltown, Equanil)

Meprobamate possesses sedative, muscle relaxant, and anticonvulsant properties. The precise mechanisms of action responsible for meprobamate's antianxiety effects have not been determined. It is suggested that this drug achieves its calming effects by producing depression at the level of the thalamus, thereby reducing the sensitivity of the thalamus to receive sensory inputs from the limbic system and ascending reticular activating system. The muscle relax-

TABLE 16-4. SELECTED ANTIANXIETY AGENTS

Class	Generic Name	Selected Trade Name(s)	Remarks
Propanediols	Meprobamate	Equanil Miltown	Modest antianxiety effects, mild sedation, muscle relaxation. Abuse potential documented.
	Tybamate	Tybatran	Meprobamate-like properties, with shorter duration of action.
Benzodiazepines	Chlordiazepoxide	Librium	First benzodiazepine. Antianxiety, muscle relaxing effects. Used for treatment of anxiety, musculoskeletal disorders, chronic alcohol withdrawal.
	Diazepam	Valium	Most widely prescribed drug in U.S. Antianxiety agent; more effective for treatment of muscle spasms than chlordiazepoxide; valuable for controlling status epilepticus.
	Oxazepam	Serax	Antianxiety agent with sedative effects. Rapid onset, short duration of action.
	Clorazepate	Azene Tranxene	Antianxiety agent. Long duration of action.
	Lorazepam	Ativan	Rapid onset
	Prazepam	Verstran	Long duration of action
Miscellaneous	Hydroxyzine	Atarax Vistaril	Antianxiety agent with antihistaminic, sedative, and antiemetic effects.

ant properties have been attributed to a depression of nerve impulses at the association neurons, the neurons connecting sensory and motor nerves.

In recent years, meprobamate, the barbiturates, and related drugs have been less frequently used and have been largely supplanted by diazepam and other benzodiazepines (see below). Meprobamate is less effective clinically, has a smaller margin of safety between therapeutic and lethal doses, and possesses greater abuse potential than the benzodiazepines. When meprobamate is taken in relatively high doses of about 3200 mg or eight tablets on a daily basis for several months, physical dependence has been shown to develop. Abrupt withdrawal of drug administration produces an abstinence syndrome similar to that observed with the barbiturate and nonbarbiturate sedative-hypnotic agents (Chapter 11). These symptoms include tremors, convulsions, hallucinations, and other signs of psychotic behavior.

Benzodiazepines

Benzodiazepine-like compounds were initially synthesized in the early 1930s, with evaluation of their biological activity to come over twenty years later. One of the compounds in this series, **chlordiazepoxide,** aroused considerable interest when it was observed to abolish aggression in animals at dosage levels considerably below those that impair normal activity. These "taming" effects, originally noted in the naturally vicious macaque monkey, were later observed in such diverse mammalian species as the baboon, sea lion, kangaroo, deer, and marmoset.

The benzodiazepines are the most commonly used class of antianxiety agents and include chlordiazepoxide (Librium) and **diazepam** (Valium); other members of this class are listed and compared in Table 16-4. Since 1972, Valium has been the most widely prescribed drug in the United States. In 1977, 54 million prescriptions were written for diazepam, 13 million for chlordiazepoxide, and 13.6 million for the benzodiazepine hypnotic flurazepam (Dalmane). It has been conservatively estimated that 8000 tons of the benzodiazepines were consumed in the United States in 1977.

Chlordiazepoxide
(Librium)

Diazepam
(Valium)

Although the benzodiazepines have not been clearly demonstrated to be superior to the barbiturates for the treatment of anxiety, these drugs possess a number of distinct advantages that undoubtedly contribute to their widespread popularity among clinicians. (1) The most important advantage of the benzodiazepines is their very wide margin of safety when taken in high doses. In the absence of their use with other drugs (in particular, alcohol and other central nervous system depressants), they are virtually "suicide-proof." (2) Unlike the barbiturates, these drugs do not cause significant stimulation of liver microsomal drug-metabolizing enzymes; that is, they are not enzyme inducers (Chapter 3). Hence, tolerance is less likely to develop to their antianxiety properties when they are taken over prolonged periods of time. Moreover, they do not increase the rate of metabolism of other drugs that the patient may be taking. (3) Relief of anxiety and tension is accomplished in the absence of marked impairment of physical and/or mental function. (4) The abuse potential of the benzodiazepines is relatively low compared to the barbiturates and meprobamate. While physical dependence has been clearly demonstrated to develop after chronic administration of high and even therapeutic doses, the benzodiazepine withdrawal syndrome (with alcohol and barbiturate-like signs), is generally of mild intensity. The growing appreciation that these drugs cause psychological dependence has led to increased concern over their use.

Therapeutic Uses, Actions, and Adverse Effects

Therapeutic uses. The benzodiazepines are the most commonly employed drug class for the treatment of anxiety. The primary difference among the members of this class is their duration of action (Table 16–4). Chlordiazepoxide is among the most extensively used drugs for preventing the abstinence syndrome associated with chronic alcohol ingestion and for suppressing the syndrome (characterized by tremors, seizures, delirium) after its onset (Chapter 12).

Diazepam is the drug of choice for the emergency treatment of status epilepticus (Chapter 11). This drug has also been found to be useful in controlling the spasticity associated with multiple sclerosis, cerebral palsy, and traumatic spinal cord lesions. It is commonly prescribed for the treatment of common musculoskeletal disorders including back strain and "slipped disc."

Actions. Evidence obtained from behavioral, electrophysiological, pharmacological, and biochemical studies suggests that the therapeutic effects of the benzodiazepines in the treatment of anxiety, seizures, and muscle relaxation may result from a common mechanism.[7] These results suggest that the benzodiazepines act by potentiating the actions of *GABA* (gamma-aminobutyric acid), a putative inhibitory neurotransmitter in the mammalian central nervous system. More specifically, it has been postulated that the benzodiazepines

---

[7] J. F. Tallman, S. M. Paul, P. Skolnick, and D. W. Gallager, "Receptors for the Age of Anxiety: Pharmacology of the Benzodiazepines," *Science* **207**: 274–81 (1980).

produce their therapeutic effects by interacting with receptor sites, and that these activated benzodiazepine receptors interact with GABA receptors resulting in an enhancement in the inhibitory effects of GABA.

Adverse effects.   The most common undesirable side effects associated with benzodiazepine administration are drowsiness, dizziness, and muscle weakness. Several studies have presented evidence suggesting that there is an increased risk of birth defects such as cleft palate in babies whose mothers have taken antianxiety agents (diazepam, meprobamate) during the first three months of pregnancy. Although the evidence is by no means conclusive, the use of benzodiazepines by pregnant women should be restricted to cases of essential need.

SUMMARY

In less than three decades, psychoactive drugs have had a profound impact on society. Specifically, they have markedly altered the prognosis for many patients suffering from mental illness. In earlier times, these illnesses proved so incapacitating that the patient was faced with the prospect of spending many years in a psychiatric hospital, or, if permitted to remain at home, becoming a completely unproductive member of society. The consequences were an emotional and financial drain on the family and society. Psychoactive drugs, in particular the antipsychotic agents, have substantially reduced the period of hospitalization, as well as enabled these patients to be effectively treated on an outpatient basis.

Mental disorders are generally classified as being neuroses, psychoses, and affective disorders (mania, depression). Anxiety and tension characterize neuroses, while disturbances in normal thought processes are seen in psychoses, and extreme mood swings are manifested in affective disorders. Some mental illnesses have clearly defined etiologies (organic), while others arise from unknown causes (functional). Psychological and sociocultural and biochemical theories have been postulated to explain the etiology of functional disorders. Many of the contemporary biochemical hypotheses are predicated upon qualitative and quantitative changes in the neurotransmitters in the brain or by the presence of abnormal protein factors. No single theory has proved totally satisfactory to all investigators.

The antipsychotic phenothiazine derivatives have been shown to be clinically effective beyond any reasonable doubt and are among the most widely used drugs in medicine. This may be more readily appreciated when we realize the high incidence of mental disease in society; about 50 percent of all patients in psychiatric hospitals are diagnosed as being schizophrenic. The phenothiazines, as chlorpromazine, and other neuroleptics are incapable of curing psychoses but are effective in reducing the symptoms associated with abnormal behavior. Contemporary research findings attribute the antipsychotic effects of these drugs to blockade of dopamine receptor sites in the limbic system. Hyperactive patients become calm, and disordered thought processes become more normal. As a result, therapists are able to effectively communicate with their patients, providing them with insight into the nature of their behavioral disorders. Unfortunately, schizophrenic patients often relapse after the cessation of drug therapy, and even the large majority of those continuing to take medication never again become fully "normal." Although there are a large number of undesirable side effects associated with the use of the phenothiazines, among the most important of which is tardive dyskinesia, their benefits to the individual are generally far in excess of the risks.

Fluctuations of mood are normal, except when these mood swings become excessive and the individual becomes disabled and unable to function effectively. The tricyclic antidepressants such as imipramine have proved to be a very useful alternative to electroconvulsive therapy. Although we have not attempted to differentiate the many faces of depression, it should be pointed out that antidepressive agents are not uniformly successful in all the variations of this disorder. Lithium has been demonstrated to be highly effective in the control of acute manic episodes and for the attenuation of the wide moods associated with chronic manic-depressive (bipolar) disorders.

Drugs employed for the treatment of neuroses are commonly, but inappropriately, termed minor tranquilizers. These drugs include the use of low doses of barbiturate and nonbarbiturate sedative-hypnotic agents (Chapter 11), meprobamate, and the benzodiazepines. There is some doubt regarding the relative effectiveness of meprobamate and the benzodiazepines. The latter group of drugs, including diazepam, are preferred because of their relative safety when taken in overdose, their low abuse potential, the absence of marked impairment of mental and physical function, and their relative inability to act as enzyme inducers.

At present there are a large number of psychoactive drugs available for the physician to prescribe. Some are a bit more effective or a little less toxic than others. Although currently available drugs provide relatively effective symptomatic relief, patients are not cured of their mental disorders. When scientists are able to determine the specific biological causes of the various mental illnesses, specific drugs can be designed that will have a definite bull's-eye to zero in on. Drugs producing a cure will be a reality.

SUPPLEMENTARY READINGS

Barchas, J. D., P. A. Berger, R. D. Ciaranello, and G. R. Elliott, eds., *Psychopharmacology—From Theory to Practice.* New York: Oxford University Press, 1977.

Clark, W. G., and J. del Giudice, eds., *Principles of Psychopharmacology.* 2nd ed. New York: Academic Press, 1978.

Cole, J. O., A. M. Freedman, and A. J. Friedhoff, eds., *Psychopathology and Psychophar-macology.* Baltimore: Johns Hopkins Press, 1973.

Costa, E., and P. Greengard, eds., *Mechanism of Action of Benzodiazepines.* New York: Raven Press, 1975.

DiMascio, A., and R. I. Shader, eds., *Clinical Handbook of Psychopharmacology.* New York: Science House, 1970.

Frazer, A., and A. Winokur, eds., *Biological Bases of Psychiatric Disorders.* New York: Spectrum Publications, 1977.

Glick, S. D., and J. Goldfarb, eds., *Behavioral Pharmacology.* St. Louis: C. V. Mosby, 1976.

Hollister, L. E., *Clinical Pharmacology of Psychotherapeutic Drugs.* New York: Churchill Livingstone, 1978.

Iversen, S. D., and L. L. Iversen, *Behavioral Pharmacology.* New York: Oxford University Press, 1975.

Iversen, L. L., S. D. Iversen, and S. H. Snyder, eds., *Handbook of Psychopharmacology,* 14 vols. New York: Plenum Press, 1976-78.

Lipton, M. A., A. DiMascio, and K. F. Killam, eds., *Psychopharmacology: A Generation of Progress.* New York: Raven Press, 1978.

Seiden, L. S., and L. A. Dykstra, *Psychopharmacology—A Biochemical and Behavioral Approach.* New York: Van Nostrand Reinhold, 1977.

Shader, R. I., and A. DiMascio, *Psychotropic Drug Side Effects: Clinical and Theoretical Perspectives.* Baltimore: Williams & Wilkins, 1970.

Simpson, L. L., ed., *Drug Treatment of Mental Disorders.* New York: Raven Press, 1976.

Usdin, E., D. A. Hamburg, and J. D. Barchas, eds., *Neuroregulators and Psychiatric Disorders.* New York: Oxford University Press, 1977.

17

Psychotomimetic Agents

The psychedelic experience involves then, . . . a number of elements, and you can say that what is involved is a magnification, distortion, and alteration of conscious experience—conscious experience because the drug produces the effect on how one feels and what one is aware of.

—Allan Y. Cohen (1970)

The senses become extraordinarily acute and fine. The eyes pierce Infinity. The ear perceives the most imperceptible in the midst of the sharpest noises. Hallucinations begin. External objects take on monstrous appearances and reveal themselves under forms hitherto unknown. . . . Sounds have odor and colors are musical.[1]

—Charles Baudelaire (1860)

In the previous chapter we discussed drugs capable of modifying the abnormal behavior of psychotic patients and/or causing a reduction or elimination in hallucinations, illusions, and aberrations in thought processes. By contrast, in the next two chapters we shall consider compounds that alter normal behavior, producing changes in the perception of visual and auditory stimuli and expanding the range of consciousness to broad new horizons and dimensions. These same drugs can also instill feelings of panic and impending disaster in the mind of the drug user.

Rational evaluation of the effects produced by these compounds is often colored by the orientation and prejudices of the writer. The literature arising from members of the drug-using culture has described vivid sensory experiences and dynamic transcendental sensations, events normally far beyond the grasp

[1] *The Artificial Paradise* (hashish).

of mere mortals; bad trips and potential drug hazards are usually minimized or totally neglected. In contraposition are the writings of those representing the establishment, wherein we witness a total rejection of pseudotranscendental experiences and a condemnation of members of the drug cults; emphasis in these writings is directed toward the real and imagined dangers associated with the use of these compounds. No doubt, a more realistic evaluation of these drugs and their effects lies somewhere between these widely separate positions.

In this chapter we shall be discussing **psychotomimetic agents**—drugs capable of producing hallucinations, sensory illusions, and bizarre thoughts. But toxic doses of the bromides, cortisone-like steroids, narcotic antagonists, alcohol, lead, amphetamine, and cocaine may produce similar behavioral effects, and yet we do not classify these drugs as psychotomimetic agents. We reserve the designation *psychotomimetic* for those compounds that consistently alter thought processes and sensory perceptions. Moreover, the induction of these psychic changes constitutes the primary effect of these drugs in moderate doses and not simply one of a great number of other, more clearly manifested central or peripheral responses to the drug. We should point out that the inclusion of certain drugs within this particular category, for example marijuana, is not immune to challenge.

Having decided what general criteria will be employed to determine whether a drug is appropriately classified as a psychotomimetic agent, we should note in passing that not even our designation *psychotomimetic* is secure! Drugs in this same category are also termed *hallucinogens, psychedelics, psychotogens, psychodysleptics,* and so forth, with each term denoting a subtle difference in its meaning from the others. This author shall not attempt to justify his choice of "psychotomimetic" upon some profound, erudite semantic consideration, but simply point out that this term has gained wide acceptance in the scientific and lay literature.

HISTORICAL OVERVIEW AND PERSPECTIVES

Psychotomimetic plants have been long known to members of such diverse cultures as those residing south of the Rio Grande to Argentina, on islands located in the South Pacific, and in Siberia, India, and South Africa.

Primitive cultures, where sickness and death are usually ascribed to a supernatural cause, have long accorded psychoactive plants a high, even sacred, rank in their magic, medical and religious practices, because their ethnopharmacology often values the psychic effects of "medicine" more than the physiological.[2]

[2] R. E. Schultes, "Hallucinogens of Plant Origin," *Science* **163**:245 (1969).

Literary and popular first-hand descriptions of the mind-expanding properties of the psychotomimetic agents appear in the writings of the illustrious members of the mid-nineteenth-century Parisian *Le Club des Hachichins* (hashish), including such individuals as Victor Hugo, Honoré de Balzac, Théophile Gautier, Alexandre Dumas *père,* and Charles Baudelaire; in accounts of peyote (mescaline) from the pens of Havelock Ellis and Aldous Huxley; and in Timothy Leary's accounts of "religious experiences" with LSD.

The discovery of LSD is of particular importance to us because of the profound influence it had in arousing public awareness of psychotomimetic agents. It was also a major contributory factor in generating considerable research on brain function and mental disease.

In 1938, the Swiss chemist Albert Hofmann was preparing synthetic compounds similar to the alkaloids of ergot. One compound in the series was **lysergic acid diethylamide (LSD)** shown in Figure 17.1, which, he hoped, would possess pharmacological properties similar to nikethamide (Coramine), a central nervous system stimulant or analeptic agent (Chapter 15) then commonly used for the treatment of respiratory depression caused by barbiturates. Five years later, Hofmann accidentally ingested an unknown quantity of LSD and made the following observations in his notebook:

> Last Friday, April 16, 1943, I was forced to stop my work in the laboratory in the middle of the afternoon, and to go home, as I was seized by a peculiar restlessness associated with a sensation of dizziness. Having reached home, I lay down and sank in a kind of drunkenness which was not unpleasant and which was characterized by extreme activity of imagination. As I lay in a dazed condition with my eyes closed (I experienced daylight disagreeably bright), there surged upon me an uninterrupted stream of fantastic images of extraordinary plasticity and vividness and accompanied by an intense, kaleidoscope-like play of colors. This condition gradually passed off after about two hours.[3]

Hofmann astutely appreciated that these strange behavioral sensations were the consequence of LSD ingestion. To further explore the phenomenon, he took a very modest dose of LSD, 0.25 mg; six hours later he was still experiencing visual hallucinations. We now know that this apparently "modest" dose is about five times the amount required to produce behavioral changes.

Four years later, based upon his studies in Zurich, Stoll published the first report on the effects of LSD in human subjects. Scientific interest in LSD skyrocketed for several reasons. Extremely small absolute doses (0.050 mg or 1/600,000 oz)[4] produced profound alterations in behavior, with little or no

---

[3] A. Hofmann, "Psychotomimetic Agents," in *Drugs Affecting the Central Nervous System,* ed., A. Burger (New York: Marcel Dekker, 1968), Vol. 2: 184–85.
[4] One oz. of LSD could send 600,000 people on a trip!

TRYPTAMINE DERIVATIVES

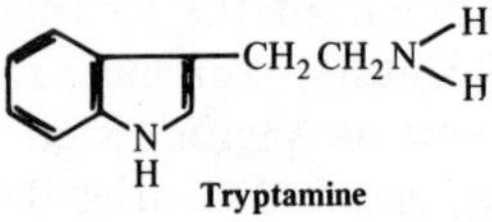

Tryptamine

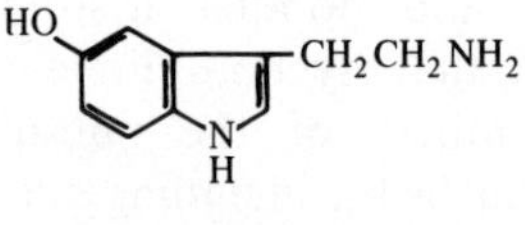

Serotonin (5-Hydroxytryptamine)

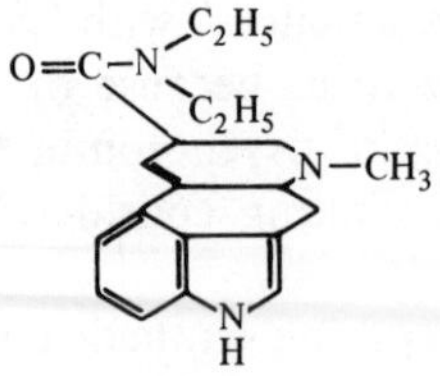

LSD

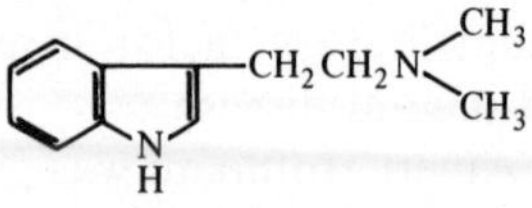

DMT (N, N-Dimethyltryptamine)

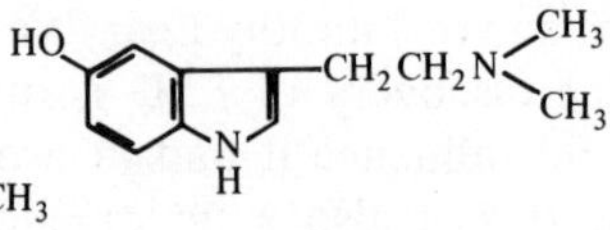

Bufotenin

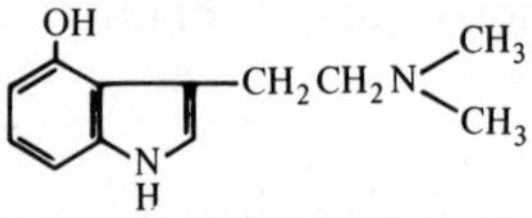

Psilocin

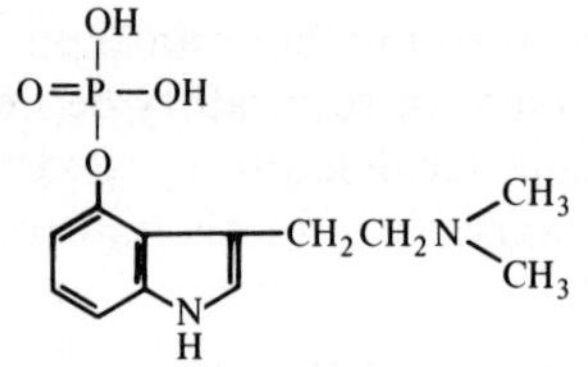

Psilocybin

β-PHENYLETHYLAMINE DERIVATIVES

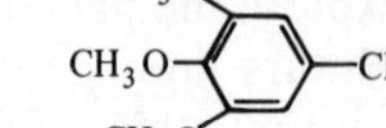

β-Phenylethylamine

Dopamine

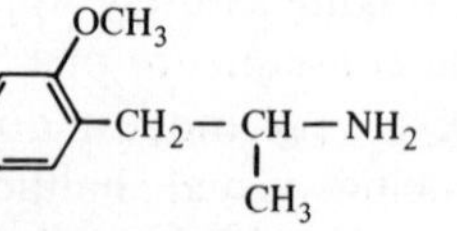

Norepinephrine

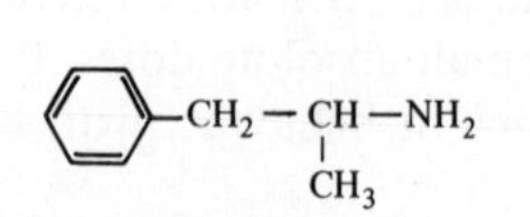

Mescaline

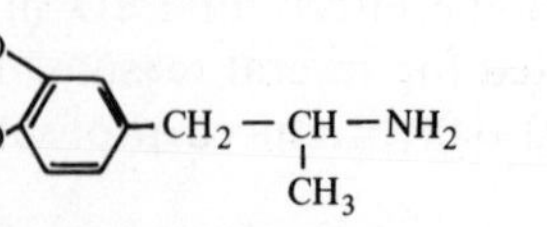

DOM (STP)
(2, 5-Dimethoxy-
4-methylamphetamine)

Amphetamine

MDA (Methylenedioxyamphetamine)

FIGURE 17–1. Aminergic Psychotomimetic Agents.

effects on other organ systems. These drug effects, in several respects, possessed some similarity to the aberrations observed in psychotic patients, and it appeared at the time that LSD might be a useful tool for inducing an artificial psychotic state which could serve as a model for determining the biochemical or physiological cause(s) of schizophrenia. After determining the etiology of schizophrenia, the medicinal chemists could be dispatched to their laboratories and shortly thereafter emerge with the appropriate drug capable of effecting a cure. Our understanding of the biochemistry and neurophysiology of the central nervous system has advanced significantly in the past three decades, but we have yet to determine the specific causes of mental illness or develop a curative drug.

Apart from their use as tools to uncover the mysterious events occurring within the brains of schizophrenic patients, the psychotomimetic agents are themselves the focal point of much research. In expert hands, these agents may have diagnostic and therapeutic applications for the treatment of the mentally ill. In addition, we wish to gain a better understanding about the consequences of the nonmedical use of marijuana and other psychotomimetic agents currently employed by a large proportion of our population. Studies are presently being conducted in many laboratories to determine whether these agents are capable of producing subtle adverse psychological and physiological damage that may only manifest itself after continuous administration for long periods of time.

CLASSIFICATION

It is convenient for us to divide the psychotomimetic agents into four subcategories, namely, aminergic, anticholinergic and miscellaneous psychotomimetics, and marijuana (Table 17–1). This system is predicated in part on the chemical structures of these compounds, as well as their presumed mechanism of action in the central nervous system. As you will observe, many similar psychic effects are produced by compounds of the different classes.

Pharmacological and chemical considerations preclude placing marijuana[5] in the first two categories, and in good conscience this author cannot relegate this drug to a miscellaneous class. Because of the great impact marijuana has had on our contemporary society, as well as its unique pharmacological properties, we have decided to consider this drug in a separate chapter. Others may prefer to view Chapter 18 as merely a continuation of this chapter.

---

[5] Considerable controversy surrounds marijuana today. This controversy even extends to the spelling of the name of this drug, for example, marijuana or marihuana. This author has adopted the former spelling.

TABLE 17-1. PSYCHOTOMIMETIC AGENTS

Name	Street Name	Source	Route of Administration	Effects Sought
Aminergic agents				
LSD (lysergic acid diethylamide)	Acid, Cubes, Sugar	Semisynthetic from ergot alkaloids	Oral	Insight, exhilaration, sensory distortion
Lysergic acid amide	Heavenly blue, Pearly gates	*Ipomoea violacea* (morning glory seeds)	Oral	Same as LSD
DMT (dimethyl-tryptamine)	Businessman's special	Synthetic	Injected	Same as LSD, shorter duration of action (1-2 hr)
Bufotenin		Cohoba snuff, glands of frog	Injected	Same as LSD
Psilocybin Psilocin		*Psilocybe mexicana* (Mexican magic mushroom)	Oral	Same as LSD
Mescaline	Mesc	*Lophophora williamsii* (peyote cactus)	Oral	Same as LSD
Amphetamines (Benzedrine) Dextroamphetamine (Dexedrine) Methamphetamine (Desoxyn)	Bennies, Peaches, Splash Dexies, Oranges, Co-Pilots Meth, Speed, Crystal	Synthetic	Oral or injected	Euphoria, increased mental and physical activity
DOM (dimethoxy-methylamphetamine)	STP (serenity, tranquility, peace)	Synthetic	Oral	Same as LSD, action up to 72 hr
MDA (methylene-dioxyamphetamine)	Love pill	Synthetic	Oral	Same as LSD, but milder, amphetamine-like euphoria

Drug	Source	Street names	Route	Effects
Anticholinergic agents				
Stramonium (Asthmador)	*Datura stramonium* (jimson weed)		Inhaled	Sensory changes
Ditran	Synthetic		Oral	Sensory changes
Miscellaneous agents				
Nutmeg	*Myristica fragrans* (nutmeg tree)		Oral	Euphoria, dream-like state
Phencyclidine (Sernyl)	Synthetic	PCP, Hog, Peace pill, Angel dust	Oral, inhaled, or snorted	Euphoria, antianxiety effects
Cannabis				
THC (tetrahydro-cannabinol)	*Cannabis sativa* (hemp) or synthetic		Inhaled or oral	Euphoria, dream-like state, increased perception
Marijuana	*Cannabis*	Grass, Weed, Pot, Dope, Hemp; *Cigarette*—Joint, Reefer	Inhaled or oral	Same as THC
Hashish	*Cannabis*	Hash	Inhaled or oral	Same as THC, more pronounced than marijuana

AMINERGIC PSYCHOTOMIMETIC AGENTS

Compounds in the aminergic class include LSD and other *tryptamine derivatives* (such as DMT, bufotenin, psilocin and psilocybin), and mescaline and the *β-phenylethylamine derivatives* (amphetamine, DOM or STP, and MDA) (Figure 17-1). Other authors have classified the aminergics as *sympathomimetic psychotomimetics,* which denotes an interaction with the catecholamines (norepinephrine, epinephrine, and dopamine). Some of these compounds, LSD in particular, are thought to interact with receptor sites whose neurotransmitter is 5-hydroxytryptamine or serotonin (thus, serotonergic receptors). Hence, we have preferred to employ the more general term *aminergic,* which denotes both sympathetic (adrenergic) and serotonergic receptor interactions.

The best known and most extensively studied aminergic psychotomimetic agent is LSD, and, therefore, we shall treat this compound most comprehensively.

Lysergic Acid Diethylamide (LSD)

LSD is the most potent psychotomimetic agent presently available, producing clearly demonstrable behavioral effects in adult human subjects given oral doses of 0.025–0.050 mg. By contrast, mescaline is among the least potent agents in this class and must be given in amounts that are 5000 times higher than LSD!

After oral administration, LSD is rapidly absorbed into the blood and distributed throughout the body. Virtually all its pharmacological effects are attributed to actions in the central nervous system, with only negligible effects in other parts of the body. Since the brain does not selectively concentrate LSD, the absolute amount of this psychotomimetic agent in the brain is extremely low, further demonstrating the exquisite susceptibility of the central nervous system to this compound.

Pharmacological Effects

The ability of LSD to alter behavior is not only observed in humans. LSD has been demonstrated to interfere with the ability of spiders to spin their webs in organized patterns; it makes cats fearful of mice; and fish maintain a vertical nose-up position and swim backward after administration of LSD. Let us now outline some of the effects observed in humans after moderate amounts are orally ingested.

Physiological. Within 20 to 60 minutes after ingestion, marked sympathetic stimulation occurs, effects thought to be mediated by LSD's actions on the central nervous system. The more commonly observed effects include a widening of the pupils, sweating, an increase in heart rate, salivation, and a rise in body temperature. Fluctuations in mood are seen, sometimes euphoric and, at other times during the same drug trip, distressful or dysphoric; hilarious laughter may be immediately followed by extreme anxiety, fits of crying, and panic.

Psychological. The most dramatic effects produced by LSD are those concerned with sensory perceptions, mainly those involving color, as recorded above by Hofmann. *Colors* become more intense and pulsate, with sudden bursts of kaleidoscopic color or rainbows often reported. Although hallucinations are rare after moderate doses of LSD, illusions, mistaking a spot on the wall for a face, for example, occur frequently. Enhanced sensitivity to touch, odor, and taste have been noted, but these sensory changes are of small magnitude; auditory hallucinations are quite rare. By contrast, auditory hallucinations are quite common in paranoid schizophrenia.

Significant alterations in *thought processes* take place. Subjects often describe that they are participating in a unique experience. They believe that this experience is transcendental and that they now possess great insight into the world and its problems; they are outside their own bodies and able to view themselves from a distance. Freedman describes this *depersonalization* induced by LSD:

> It is the intense experience without clouded consciousness—the heightened "spectator ego" witnessing the excitement, which is characteristic for these drugs in usual dosages. There is a split of the self—a portion of which is a relatively passive monitor rather than an active focusing, and initiating force, and a portion of which "received" vivid experiences.[6]

Highly laudatory lay reports have appeared describing the beneficial effects of LSD on intelligence, sensory perception, and creativity. What do the results of studies, objectively measuring the performance of these parameters, reveal? Moderate doses of LSD severely impair most intellectual functions, such as short-term memory and problem solving. However, interpretation of the results of these tests are often complicated by the lack of subject motivation. Distortions of *time and space* are common, causing some subjects to think that time is passing more slowly than usual, while other individuals perceive the reverse. The size and distance of objects are poorly approximated.

Subjective reports of enhanced *creativity* while under the influence of LSD have not been substantiated. Dramatic changes in artistic work have been noted after LSD, with more abstract forms depicted; poetry and musical composition have not been observed to possess greater quality of expression. This is not surprising because there is a reduction in attention span.

The behavioral changes produced by LSD usually last for six to eight hours and are often followed by insomnia, but by the following day recovery is

[6] D. X. Freedman, "On the Use and Abuse of LSD," *Archives of General Psychiatry* **18**:332 (1968).

generally complete. A "good trip" provides an incentive for continued usage of this drug.

Tolerance and Cross-Tolerance

Repeated administration of LSD produces tolerance to the psychic effects of this drug within four days; a similar drug-free period is required for the loss of tolerance. Cross-tolerance has been demonstrated between LSD and mescaline, psilocybin, and psilocin, but this phenomenon has not been observed to occur between LSD and marijuana or amphetamine.

LSD and mescaline are chemically different (Figure 17-1), and yet these two psychotomimetic agents produce similar effects on behavioral and autonomic functions. It may be argued that these pharmacological similarities are fortuitous and are merely the consequence of two separate and distinct mechanisms of action. However, when cross-tolerance is observed, it suggests, although by no means conclusively establishes, that the compounds share a common cellular site of action.

Mechanism of Action of LSD

The precise mechanism responsible for the psychic effects produced by LSD is not known at this time. Research attempts have been complicated by the very wide range of neurophysiological and biochemical changes produced by this psychotomimetic agent.

There is a large body of evidence that links LSD's actions to its effects at *serotonin* receptor sites in the central nervous system (Table 9-2). Serotonin generally functions as an inhibitory neurotransmitter. Many of the areas inner-vated by serotonergic neurons are associated with the visual and limbic systems and are involved in the control of sensation, mood, and attention. As might be anticipated, if LSD were to modify the activity of these systems, it would have profound effects on behavior. It is currently believed that, while LSD is capable of inhibiting both receptors on presynaptic serotonergic cell bodies and post-synaptic serotonergic receptors, the cell bodies are far more sensitive to LSD. These serotonergic raphé cells normally exert an inhibitory influence on their postsynaptic sites. LSD-induced inhibition would, therefore, free such post-synaptic sites from this inhibition and permit them to become more active (Figure 17-2). This unmodulated activity could account for the behavioral effects of LSD.

On the basis of neurophysiological studies, it has been hypothesized that the visual hallucinations induced by LSD result from an excessive amount of sensory input reaching the cerebral cortex. This leads to a bombardment of the highest centers of the brain, and visual hallucinations result. As the regulatory systems controlling the flow of sensory input become progressively more dis-rupted, subjects' appreciation of the "real world" becomes diminished and their behavior more bizarre.

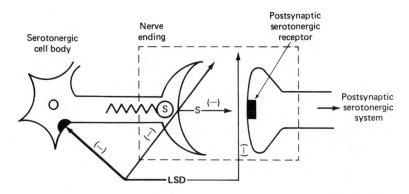

FIGURE 17-2. Postulated Mechanism of Action of LSD on Serotonergic Systems in the Brain. In the absence of LSD, a nerve impulse activates the release of serotonin (Ⓢ) from the endings of serotonergic nerves. Serotonin, an inhibitory neurotransmitter, interacts with postsynaptic receptors resulting in a decrease in the activity of the postsynaptic serotonergic system. LSD inhibits both the presynaptic serotonergic (raphé) cell body and the postsynaptic serotonergic receptor; receptors on the former site are far more sensitive to LSD. Inhibition of the presynaptic receptors decreases the activity and inhibitory influence of the serotonergic neuron on the postsynaptic system. This permits the conduction of unmodulated excitatory influences that activate higher brain centers and possibly accounts for the behaviorally disrupting effects of this compound. Other psychotomimetics, such as psilocybin and dimethyltryptamine, may produce their effects by a similar mechanism. (The nerve ending and postsynaptic receptor areas are depicted greatly enlarged.)

Psychological and Physical Hazards

LSD is a relatively nontoxic compound in humans, and no deaths have been specifically attributed to the direct effects of this compound. Moreover, chronic administration of this psychotomimetic agent does not produce physical dependence. What factors then were responsible for the drug cult "turning off" LSD after 1968?

The clear dangers of LSD are psychological and social: These are the high risk or the lack of certainty as to the outcome of a drug trip, and the availability or attractiveness of such drugs to the unwary and unprepared. The risk is enhanced when taken by the wrong people at the wrong time for the wrong motive; e.g., young people in a personal "hangup" attempting to short-cut personal growth and decisions in a search for their "real" selves. LSD is tempting in this real search for the "true self"; somewhere inside is the mirror which will reveal the fairest one of all. Unfortunately, looking inside one's self under the drug simply further removes the subject from those anchors to reality which provide necessary guidelines for judgment.[7]

[7] D. X. Freedman, "The Psychopharmacology of Hallucinogenic Agents," *Annual Review of Medicine* **20:**414 (1969).

In his writings during the 1960s, Leary emphasized the mystical insights and other pleasurable sensations associated with a good trip. However, during the late 1960s it became quite clear that *bad trips* could also occur, and, indeed, did occur with alarming frequency. These adverse reactions include confusion, extreme anxiety and panic, and marked psychotic states. During an acute psychotic episode, accidental or intentional suicide attempts (stopping freeway traffic or testing one's innate aerodynamic abilities from a sixth floor window) and violent acts have been reported. For most, the effects of a bad trip terminate within 24 hours; however, some individuals become totally absorbed in mystical experiences and drop out of the straight society, losing all interest in worldly activities and pursuits.

Flashbacks, a trip in the absence of a drug, have also contributed to disenchantment with LSD. Weeks or months after the last dose of LSD, the user unpredictably experiences hallucinations, often resulting in loss of control and panic. The mechanism underlying this phenomenon has yet to be determined, but we know that LSD has long been removed from the body. This suggests some long-lasting influence of the psychotomimetic agent upon the neuronal circuitry or biochemistry of the brain.

Probably the most devastating blow to LSD's popularity were studies suggesting that this compound causes *chromosomal damage.* The early studies demonstrating these chromosomal breaks were reevaluated when it was also shown that alcohol, aspirin, caffeine, and ergonovine (an ergot alkaloid) have similar effects. Most scientists believe that there is no strong evidence linking LSD, in moderate doses, with chromosomal breaks or congenital abnormalities in humans; some investigators have suggested that impurities in street samples of LSD are responsible for the observed chromosomal breaks.

In summary, LSD's prominence on the drug scene has been substantially reduced because of reports of bad trips, flashbacks, and the possibility of chromosomal aberrations. Just as the fashion cult rejects last year's clothing designs, the drug cult is very perfidious with respect to their choice of drugs. Whereas LSD was in vogue in the 1960s, marijuana was far more fashionable in the 1970s.

Morning Glory Seeds

When the Spanish arrived in Mexico in the sixteenth century, they observed that the Aztecs employed ololiuqui seeds in their religious ceremonies to facilitate communication with the gods. This plant, *Ipomoea violacea,* is better known to the gardener and abuser as *morning glory.*

The active psychotomimetic principle in the morning glory seeds is *lysergic acid amide,* a close chemical relative of LSD but about one-tenth as potent. After chewing several hundred seeds, the subject becomes drowsy, with changes in perception, confusion, hallucinations, nausea, and vomiting frequently experienced.

Psilocybin and Psilocin

The "sacred mushroom," Teonanacatl, was worshiped by the Indians of Central America over 3000 years ago. "Mushroom stones," depicting the head or entire figure of a god and bearing a mushroom on top if its head, have been found in Guatemala and date back to this period.

> Teonanacatl was not only ingested at social, festive occasions but also by the priest-doctors and the soothsayers: these became endowed by the mushroom god—with clairvoyant properties which enabled them besides other things to identify the causes of disease and indicate the way in which they could be treated.[8]

In the late 1930s, the mushroom cult of southern Mexico was rediscovered by the outside world. In 1958, Hofmann (of LSD fame) isolated psilocybin and psilocin from *Psilocybe mexicana,* the magic mushroom. Psilocybin is converted to psilocin in the body, the latter compound having behavioral activity.

Although a certain amount of "folk knowledge" abounds about psilocybin, its effects are very similar to those produced by LSD, but LSD is about 100 times more active. After oral administration of psilocybin, psychic effects are observed within 30 to 60 minutes and are totally dissipated within three to five hours.

Mescaline

Among the plants the Spanish conquistadors observed to be worshiped by the Mexican natives was the peyote cactus (*Lophophora williamsii*). The missionaries on these early expeditions were highly successful in converting the natives to Christianity but encountered great resistance in their attempts to prohibit the worship of the "flesh of the gods." In fact, the ritualistic use of the sacred cactus or "mescal buttons" expanded north and was adopted by many Indian tribes living in the southwestern United States, who later formed the Peyote Religion.

> The Peyote Religion, or the Native American Church of North America, as it is more formally designated, and having a current membership of about 250,000, is a Christian, pan-Indian religion identifying the Christian Trinity with the Great Spirit of Indian religion and believing in the necessity of worship of God and brotherhood and charity toward all mankind. Strict abstinence from alcohol is advocated. The place of peyote is central since it is believed that God made a special

---

[8] A. Hofmann, "Chemical, Pharmacological and Medical Aspects of Psychotomimetics," *Journal of Experimental Medical Science* 5:40 (1961).

gift of this sacrament to the natives of this continent in order that they might commune more directly with him.[9]

Notwithstanding the strictly religious nature of the meetings at which peyote was consumed, concern was expressed by the "white man" in his legislative and judicial chambers that Indians must be protected against such evils as peyote for it "had immoral effects; it is demoralizing and excites baser passions," noted Congressman Carl Hayden in his 1918 address in the House of Representatives. Laws forbidding the use of peyote by members of this church were declared unconstitutional in 1964. The court stated in their opinion that "To remove the use of peyote is to remove the theological heart of peyotism."

Pharmacological Effects

Mescaline, a β-phenylethylamine derivative (Figure 17–1) is responsible for the pharmacological effects of peyote. Although mescaline is the least active of the commonly used psychotomimetic agents, many have been attracted to its use because of the very vivid and intense visual hallucinations and psychic effects it produces. An oral dose produces a hallucinatory state lasting from five to twelve hours. Consider Aldous Huxley's description of mescaline's effects:

> Though the intellect remains unimpaired and though perception is enormously improved, the will suffers a profound change for the worse. The mescaline taker sees no reason for doing anything in particular and finds most of the causes for which, at ordinary times, he was prepared to act and suffer, profoundly uninteresting. He can't be bothered with them, for the good reason that he has better things to think about.[10]

Huxley proceeds to describe the visual effects in a later section:

> How significant is the enormous heightening of the perception of colour! . . . Mescalin raises all colour to a higher power and makes the percipient aware of innumerable fine shades of difference, to which, at ordinary times, he is completely blind.[11]

The behavioral changes produced by mescaline are very similar to those caused by LSD and both drugs are thought to share a common mechanism of action. The major differences are dosage (LSD is about 5000 times more active), and mescaline is said to produce greater hallucinogenic and lesser depersonalizing effects. As with LSD, mescaline produces such autonomic changes as an increase in pupil size, faster heart rate, nausea, tremors, and a rise in blood pressure. Complex discrimination tasks, problem solving, and short-term

---

[9] R. L. Bergman, "Navajo Peyote Use: Its Apparent Safety," *American Journal of Psychiatry* **128**:51 (1971).

[10] A. Huxley, *The Doors of Perception* (New York: Harper and Row, 1954), p. 572.

[11] Ibid.

memory are impaired after mescaline, but this may be the result of a lack of subject motivation while under the influence of this drug.

Mescaline is among the most sought after street drugs, but at this time it is almost impossible to procure. Laboratory analysis of purported "mescaline" generally reveals the presence of other compounds such as LSD, STP, or PCP (phencyclidine).

Amphetamine-Mescaline Derivatives

In Chapter 15, we considered the amphetamine psychosis and its distinguishing characteristics. Amphetamine is not cross-tolerant with LSD, mescaline, and psilocybin, thus suggesting a different mechanism of action.

DOM and MDA are more recent additions to the drug scene. As you will observe from Figure 17-1, they are chemically related to amphetamine and mescaline, but these derivatives are more potent than the former compounds.

DOM (STP)

DOM is 2, 5-dimethoxy-4-methylamphetamine to the chemist and STP (serenity, tranquility, and peace) to the drug user. This compound produces euphoric and hallucinogenic effects at doses of 5 mg, making it about 50 to 100 times more active than mescaline. After oral administration, initial effects are noted within 90 minutes, peak effects occur at about 3 to 4 hours, with hallucinations terminating in about 6 to 24 hours. High doses of DOM have been reported to produce hallucinogenic episodes for as long as 72 hours. The relatively high incidence of "bad trips," panic reactions, for example, associated with DOM have earned this compound a notorious reputation among drug users.

MDA

MDA (methylenedioxyamphetamine) is about twice as active as mescaline. This compound is said to produce psychotomimetic effects in the absence of marked perceptual distortions, mystical overtones, or changes of colors; these effects are in sharp contrast to those produced by mescaline.

ANTICHOLINERGIC PSYCHOTOMIMETIC AGENTS

In Chapter 8 we noted that high doses of the anticholinergic agents (atropine, scopolamine) are capable of producing confusion, delirium, disorientation, and hallucinations. Many nonprescription sleep aids, for example, Sominex, Sleep-Eze, Sure-Sleep, and Compoz, formerly contained scopolamine or related belladonna alkaloids; the behavioral aberrations resulting from the intentional or accidental overdosage of these proprietary products have been attributed to the anticholinergic ingredients. Asthmador cigarettes intended for the relief of asthmatic symptoms, have been subject to abuse. This product contains the belladonna alkaloid stramonium, which consists of atropine and scopolamine.

Ditran and related piperidyl glycolates with pronounced anticholinergic properties produce visual and auditory hallucinations, sometimes accompanied by paranoid delusions. Subjects report unpleasant feelings and even terror, but never euphoria. These drugs impair intellect, cause confusion, and interfere with normal locomotor activities. Drugs in this class have been investigated by the military services as "disabling compounds" under the code "BZ."

Little tolerance develops to the psychic effects produced by these anticholinergic drugs after repeated usage. Cross-tolerance has not been demonstrated between the anticholinergic and aminergic psychotomimetic agents, suggesting a different mode of action. The behavioral changes observed can be only partially explained on the basis of a blockade of cholinergic receptor sites in the central nervous system, and an additional mechanism, as yet unidentified, is probably involved.

PHENCYCLIDINE

> *Lots of my kids have tried PCP and liked it, but they don't like its "chemical" feel. . . . Here they are, getting blitzed out of their brains, and they're worried about the experience being an "organic" one.*
>
> *They were like animals, screaming and hallucinating wildly—they had to be mechanically restrained.*
>
> *I wouldn't ever use that stuff again. It's a chemical lobotomy.*[12]
>
> —M. Dolan (1978)

Phencyclidine, one of the most widely publicized and notorious street drugs of the second half of the 1970s, is variously referred to as PCP, "angel dust," "animal tranquilizer," "hog," "peace pill," and "killer weed." It has been clinically marketed as Sernyn and Sernylan.

PCP was synthesized in 1957 and employed in human clinical trials evaluating it as a short-acting, intravenously administered general anesthetic agent possessing analgesic activity. Clinical trials were terminated eight years later when it became clear that a very large percentage of patients receiving this drug awakened from anesthesia experiencing excitement, delusions, and hallucinations. Subjects often reported that this drug produced unpleasant and extremely frightening effects, such as feelings of impending doom and disturbances in the perception of the size of their hands or feet. In 1967, now bearing the trade name Sernylan, PCP was introduced as a primate anesthetic agent and continued to be used in veterinary medicine until 1979.

---

[12] Quotations from "PCP—A Plague Whose Time Has Come," *American Pharmacy* NS18: 70–77.

The nonmedical use of PCP was initiated in the Haight-Ashbury district of San Francisco in 1967, but was soon to disappear because of the widely publicized "bad trips" associated with its use. In the 1970s, PCP made its reappearance often being sold to unsuspecting drug takers as mescaline, LSD, THC (tetrahydrocannabinol, the primary ingredient in marijuana), cocaine, and other white powders having psychoactive properties. Hundreds of street deaths were attributed to PCP use during the late 1970s. PCP-related deaths are usually indirect: suicides resulting from severe depression; drownings caused by sedation and detachment from reality; self-inflicted wounds associated with hallucinations; and violence and murder resulting from extreme paranoia and delusions of superhuman strength.

Little of the illicitly used PCP has been diverted from medical channels of distribution. It is generally prepared by amateur chemists who find its synthesis to be simple and inexpensively performed from readily obtainable starting materials.

Phencyclidine
[1–(1–phenylcyclohexyl) piperidine]

PCP can be smoked (often sprayed as a liquid or dusted on dried parsley or an inferior grade of marijuana), snorted, or orally ingested. Effects are observed two to five minutes after smoking and fifteen to twenty minutes after oral ingestion or snorting. The "high" persists for 4 to 6 hours after which the user gradually "comes down" over the next 12 to 24 hours. The intensity and duration of the drug-induced effects are dose-related; low and moderate doses are 5–10 and 10–20 mg, respectively. Symptoms associated with good trips include euphoria, which provides a satisfying escape from anxieties, depression, or external pressures and frustrations. Adverse behavioral effects caused by low to moderate doses of PCP include agitation, confusion, and disorientation. High doses (in excess of 20 mg) cause marked elevation in blood pressure and other cardiovascular complications, muscle rigidity, seizures, and prolonged periods of coma which may last for several days. Recovery to "normal" may require several weeks.

SUMMARY

Psychotomimetic agents, also commonly termed hallucinogens and psychedelics, are compounds capable of altering thought processes and sensory perceptions as primary effects, and in nontoxic doses that do not significantly modify the function of other systems. Many of these compounds are constituents of plants that have been employed for centuries by various cultures as an integral part of their medical practice and religious ceremonies.

In this chapter we have chosen to subdivide these psychoactive compounds into aminergic, anticholinergic, and miscellaneous psychotomimetic agents; marijuana will be discussed in detail in the next chapter. Pertinent information on representative members of each class is summarized in Table 17-1.

LSD, the prototype member of the aminergic class, is the most potent psychotomimetic agent currently available. After oral administration, LSD causes profound behavioral changes manifested by altered sensory perceptions, marked changes in thought processes, and distortions in time and distance perception. The mechanism(s) underlying these dramatic psychic effects are thought to involve interactions with brain serotonin receptor sites. Adverse behavioral effects may include bad trips (characterized by extreme panic), acute psychotic reactions, and flashbacks.

Other aminergic compounds of abuse include morning glory seeds, psilocybin, psilocin, DOM (STP), MDA, and mescaline. Of these, mescaline has been the most actively sought after because of the unusual vivid images and other psychic changes it produces.

The anticholinergic and miscellaneous psychotomimetic agents have been far less widely used than the aminergic agents. Hallucinations and behavioral aberrations have been noted after high doses of proprietary sleep aids containing scopolamine and other anticholinergic belladonna alkaloids. Lack of cross-tolerance between the aminergic and anticholinergic agents suggests a different mechanism of action.

Phencyclidine (PCP), formerly employed as a primate anesthetic agent, is capable of producing extremely unpleasant and frightening effects, paranoia, and delusions of excessive strength. This compound has a low margin of safety and produces elevated blood pressure and coma of prolonged duration in elevated doses. Many hundreds of deaths have been associated with the use of PCP, resulting primarily from alterations in normal behavior.

SUPPLEMENTARY READINGS

Abood, L. G., "The Psychotomimetic Glycolate Esters," in *Drugs Affecting the Central Nervous System.* Edited by A. Burger, Vol. 2: 127–67. New York: Marcel Dekker, 1968.

Brown, F. C., *The Hallucinogenic Drugs.* Springfield, Ill.: Charles C Thomas, 1972.

Efron, D. H., B. Holmstedt, and N. S. Kline, eds., *Ethnopharmacologic Search for Psychoactive Drugs.* Washington, D.C.: U.S. Government Printing Office, 1967.

Hoffer, A., "D-Lysergic Acid Diethylamide (LSD): A Review of Its Present Status," *Clinical Pharmacology and Therapeutics* 6:183–255 (1965).

Hoffer, A., and H. Osmond, *The Hallucinogens.* New York: Academic Press, 1967.

Hofmann, A., "Psychotomimetic Agents," in *Drugs Affecting the Central Nervous System.* Edited by A. Burger, Vol. 2: 169–235. New York: Marcel Dekker, 1968.

Hollister, L. E., *Chemical Psychoses.* Springfield, Ill.: Charles C Thomas, 1968.

Lewin, L., *Phantastica: Narcotic and Stimulating Drugs; Their Use and Abuse.* New York: E. P. Dutton, 1931.

Long, S. A., "Does LSD Induce Chromosomal Damage and Malformations? A Review of the Literature," *Teratology* **6**:75–90 (1972).

Martin, W. R., ed., *Drug Addiction II: Amphetamine, Psychotogen, and Marihuana Dependence. Handbook of Experimental Pharmacology.* Vol. 45, Pt. 2. Berlin: Springer-Verlag, 1977.

Petersen, R. C., and R. C. Stillman, eds., *Phencyclidine (PCP) Abuse: An Appraisal.* NIDA Research Monograph 21. Washington, D.C.: U.S. Government Printing Office, 1977.

Schultes, R. E., and A. Hofmann, *The Botany and Chemistry of Hallucinogens.* 2nd ed. Springfield, Ill.: Charles C Thomas, 1979.

Sioris, L. J., and E. P. Krenzelok, "Phencyclidine Intoxication: A Literature Review," *American Journal of Hospital Pharmacy* **35**: 1362–67 (1978).

Stillman, R. C., and R. E. Willette, eds., *The Psychopharmacology of Hallucinogens.* New York: Pergamon Press, 1978.

18

Marijuana

> *Marihuana has been used as an intoxicant in various parts of the world for centuries and in this country for 75 years. Yet, use of the drug has been regarded as a problem of major proportions for less than a decade. We shall not find the reasons for contemporary social concern in pharmacology texts or previous government reports, for we are dealing with two separate realities: a drug with certain pharmacological properties and determinable, although variable, effects on man; and a pattern of human behavior, individual and group, which has, as a behavior, created fear, anger, confusion and uncertainty among a large segment of the contemporary American public. The marihuana behavior pattern is the source of the marihuana controversy.[1]*
>
> —National Commission on Drug Abuse (1972)

Many questions are being hotly debated today by all segments of our society, issues upon which very reasonable people disagree. One such issue involves the desirability of legalizing marijuana. Not since the prohibition of alcohol has a drug aroused such contention and debate, creating a sharp polarization of sides. Whereas many of the arguments advanced to support a position, pro or con, are rational and based upon a foundation of solid fact, we have also witnessed rhetoric generated by emotions and misconceptions. We shall now attempt to summarize the current pertinent information concerning marijuana, first considering *Cannabis,* the natural source of this drug.

CANNABIS: AN OVERVIEW

Cannabis sativa, the hemp plant, is an annual weed that grows freely in most parts of the world, including the entire United States. Parts of this plant have

---

[1] *Marihuana: A Signal of Misunderstanding,* First Report of the National Commission on Marihuana and Drug Abuse (Washington, D.C.: U.S. Government Printing Office, 1972), p. 6. We shall henceforth refer to this source as the Commission. As indicated in the preceding chapter, this author prefers the spelling "marijuana" rather than "marihuana."

been used to make rope and paint, while its seeds were formerly an important ingredient in bird foods.

We know that some sources of *Cannabis* possess great psychoactive potency, while others cause little or no behavioral changes. These differences have been attributed to varying concentrations of the naturally occurring substance **delta-9-tetrahydrocannabinol**, which is simply abbreviated Δ^9-THC, or, for our purposes, **THC**. We shall discuss some aspects of *Cannabis* chemistry in a later section.

The concentration of THC in *Cannabis* is influenced by the climate, soil, cultivation, and method of preparation of the plant. Perhaps the single most important factor is the hereditary characteristics or particular variant of *Cannabis*. Experienced users consider that at least 2 percent THC is essential for the product to be of good quality. Most of the marijuana imported into this country comes from Mexico: this plant variant contains over 1 percent THC. By contrast, *Cannabis* from India contains 5–12 percent THC. The indigenous American variety is clearly of inferior quality. Finally, THC is subject to deterioration upon standing. This problem has been proved to be of importance for street users as well as for scientists who wish a standard concentration of THC to properly conduct their experiments.

Three grades of *Cannabis* are available and are generally referred to by their Indian names. Bhang, the least active, is obtained from the leaves and stems of the uncultivated plant. Marijuana is of this grade, and it is the type most frequently smoked in the United States. Ganja is a product of intermediate potency and contains higher concentrations of THC. This product, used exclusively in India, is obtained from the flowering tops and leaves of cultivated *Cannabis*. Charas, or **hashish**, as it is more commonly known in this country, possesses 5 to 10 times the potency of the commonly available marijuana. "Hash oil," a preparation containing up to 60 percent THC, is prepared by boiling hashish in a solvent and then filtering and retaining the concentrated matter. To prepare hashish, the resin is scraped from the leaves near the flowering tops of the plant, pressed into firm blocks and then smoked. Although inhalation by smoking is the most common route of administration of *Cannabis* in the United States, these plant products are frequently incorporated into candies, baked into cookies (often as a party prank), or drunk, in India.

Historical Background

The pharmacological properties of *Cannabis* have been recognized for several thousand years and have been described by both medical and literary writers. In earlier times as today, the benefits and hazards associated with the use of this plant have been the focus of controversy. Some ancient Chinese writers viewed *Cannabis* as a "delight giver"; others felt it to be a "liberator of sin." The Hindus of India employed this compound to transfix their attention to prayer.

We are told the word "assassin" may be derived from hashish or Hasan. Hasan, an eleventh century Arabian, attracted a following of young men who, while under the influence of hashish, were reported to carry out murders to further their leader's political objectives. References to hashish also appear in the *Arabian Nights.*

After Napoleon's ill-fated military expedition to Egypt in 1798, many of his soldiers returned to France with a taste for hashish, notwithstanding their general's protestations forbidding its use. During the 1840s, some of the most distinguished French writers of the day gathered together to enjoy the pleasures of hashish (which was cooked in a sweet meat delicacy) during meetings of *Le Club des Hachichins.* In the book of the same name, Gautier describes the effects of this drug.

> All around me I heard the shattering and crumbling of jewels of all colors, songs renewed themselves without ceasing, as in the play of a kaleidoscope. At certain moments, I saw my comrades, but disfigured and grotesque, half men, half plants.
>
> A half-hour had scarcely passed when I fell again under the power of the Hashish. This time the vision was much more complicated and extraordinary. Thousands of millions of butterflies, with their wings rustling like fans, perpetually swarmed in an atmosphere which was faintly luminous. ... My hearing was prodigiously developed; I heard the sound of colors; green, red, blue, and yellow sounds came to me in distinct waves. ... There was something particular in the intoxication of Hashish, that is, it is not continuous, it takes you and it leaves you, you mount to Heaven and you fall back to Earth without transition—as in insanity there are lucid moments.[2]

The effects described by Gautier, notwithstanding some literary exaggerations, were obtained with hashish. Hallucinations and delusions of this magnitude would not be expected to occur with the marijuana that is generally smoked in the United States.

During the early years of this century, marijuana made its way into this country carried by Mexican laborers. By the 1920s and 1930s the major users were Mexican-Americans, as well as the black population of New Orleans. The general public became aware of the use of this drug in 1926 when a New Orleans newspaper published a series of articles linking marijuana use with the city's crime problem. In 1931 only sixteen states had antimarijuana laws, with limited effort expended by the authorities to insure their enforcement. The following year witnessed an "educational" campaign by Harry Anslinger, Commissioner of the Federal Bureau of Narcotics, the leading advocate of antimarijuana laws. In his testimony before a congressional committee in 1937, Anslinger stated: "But here we have a drug that is not like opium. Opium has all of the good of Doctor Jekyll and the evil of Mr. Hyde. This drug [marijuana] is entirely the monster Hyde, the harmful effect of which cannot be measured."

---

[2] T. Gautier, *Le Club des Hachichins* (Paris: Feuilleton de la Presse, 1943). (Published first in 1843.)

Assisting Commissioner Anslinger in this battle was the World Defense Association who warned the unsuspecting public about the evils of marijuana:

> While the marihuana habit leads to physical wreckage and mental decay, its effect upon character and morality are even more devastating. The victim frequently undergoes such moral degeneracy that he will lie and steal without scruple; he becomes utterly untrustworthy and often drifts into the underworld where, with his degenerate companions, he commits high crimes and misdemeanors. Marihuana sometimes gives a man the lust to kill, unreasonably and without motive. Many cases of assault, rape, robbery and murder are traced to the use of marihuana.[3]

Testimony given before the 1937 House Committee studying the desirability of a federal antimarijuana law was weighted heavily in favor of the proponents of such a measure. *The Marijuana Tax Act* was easily enacted into law that year and placed marijuana in the same class as the opiates (heroin, morphine) and cocaine. From this time forth, the possession and use of marijuana was illegal in the United States.

The major impediment to rational discussions concerning the legalization of marijuana has its roots in the evils perceived to exist in 1937. Certainly, the classification of marijuana as a "narcotic" (which is totally incorrect pharmacologically and chemically) creates bias in the minds of many persons. In 1937, as today, a large segment of the population view marijuana as a threat to public safety (crime), public health (mental and physical deterioration, addiction liability, escalation to "hard" drugs), and social order (lack of motivation, sexual promiscuity). We shall attempt to discuss the evidence supporting or refuting these threats during the course of this chapter.

Chemistry

Cannabis contains a group of closely related compounds that are collectively termed *cannabinoids*. There is an unusual feature about the chemistry of the cannabinoids which we have not observed with any of the other psychotomimetic agents, with the exception of myristicin derived from nutmeg. These compounds do not contain a nitrogen atom and, therefore, are not alkaloids (Figure 18–1).

The major natural psychoactive compound in *Cannabis* is Δ^9-THC; Δ^8-THC also possesses biological activity.[4] In only the past decade have these compounds been isolated in pure form from the plant, synthesized in the laboratory, and subjected to biological testing. Recent studies in man and animals have demonstrated that Δ^9-THC is converted to 11-hydroxy-Δ^9-THC. It has been postulated that this metabolite, and perhaps others, are responsible for the physiological and psychic effects produced by marijuana, and more specifically

---

[3] Reprinted in A. Mather, ed., *Treatises on Narcotics* (Chicago, 1946), p. 39.

[4] As noted on Figure 18–1, Δ^1-THC is the same compound also designated as Δ^9-THC.

NUMBERING SYSTEMS

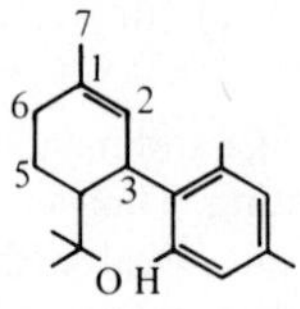

Monoterpenoid system (MS) 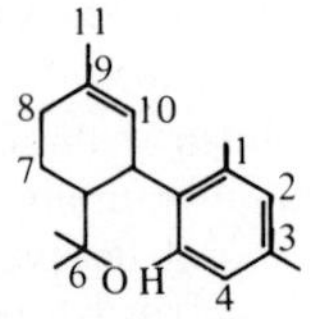   Formal system (FS)

CANNABINOIDS

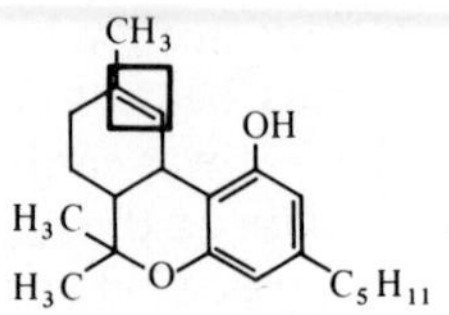

Δ^1 – THC (MS)
Δ^9 – THC (FS)
(Natural product)

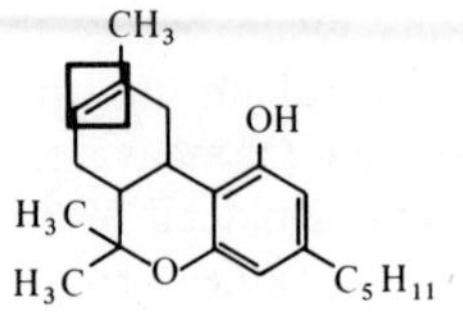

$\Delta^{1(6)}$ – THC (MS)
$\Delta^{(8)}$ – THC (FS)
(Natural product)

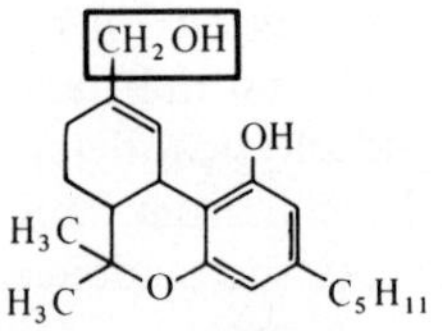

7-Hydroxy-Δ^1-THC (MS)
11-Hydroxy-Δ^9-THC (FS)
(Active metabolite)

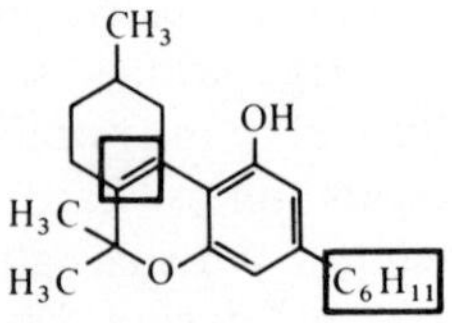

Synhexyl

(Synthetic derivative)

FIGURE 18–1. Chemical Structures of Key Cannabinoids. Two different numbering systems are currently employed in the scientific literature for the designation of the tetrahydrocannabinols; namely, the formal system (used in this book) and the monoterpenoid system. Delta (Δ) refers to the position of the carbon-to-carbon double bond

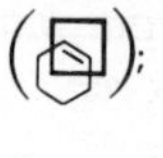

; for example, Δ^1 indicates that a double bond is present between carbons 1 and 2.

by Δ^9-THC. These observations may provide a basis for the "reverse-tolerance" some regular users of marijuana report. We shall consider this phenomenon in greater detail when we discuss tolerance to marijuana.

PHARMACOLOGICAL EFFECTS OF MARIJUANA

Attempts to force marijuana into one of the standard pharmacological pigeon holes are doomed to be fruitless. It should be regarded as unique.

—Leo Hollister (1971)

372

For purposes of convenience we have chosen to classify marijuana in this book as a psychotomimetic agent. This is actually an oversimplification when we consider the pharmacological properties of this complex drug. Marijuana causes hallucinations in high doses. It enhances the excitatory effects of amphetamine, prolongs barbiturate sleep time, reduces blood pressure, and possesses analgesic activity.

Factors Modifying the Marijuana Response

In Chapter 3 we discussed at length the factors that modify our response to drugs. We find these factors to be of particular importance when evaluating a drug such as marijuana that possesses low potency and causes minimal physical and mental effects in the commonly employed doses. Among the variables that modify the marijuana response are dosage, route of administration, set, and setting.

Dosage

In only recent years have both reliable methods for the quantitative determination of THC in *Cannabis* samples and chemically pure synthetic THC become available. We have previously alluded to the difficulties encountered when there is considerable batch-to-batch variation in the THC content of *Cannabis* samples, resulting from innate variant differences or deterioration. Pure THC, of known concentration, permits accurate dose-response relationships to be determined.

Route of Administration

Differences exist in the pharmacological response obtained after the oral administration of THC and smoking this compound or marijuana. Some of these differences may be, in part, attributed to dosage. There is a rapid onset of drug action after smoking, within seconds to minutes; these effects rarely last for more than two hours. Different inhalation techniques and the variable escape of smoke in the air complicate evaluating dose-response relationships. After the oral ingestion of THC, initial effects may not occur for 30 to 120 minutes, but then continue for five to seven hours. Oral administration of THC produces less intense effects than are obtained after smoking.

Set and Setting

The *set* refers to the "internal environment" of the subject and is influenced by personality, life-style, previous experience with marijuana and other drugs, as well as by expectations of the anticipated effects of the drug and mood at the time of drug administration. By contrast, the *setting* refers to the "external environment," that is, whether marijuana is administered in the company of drug-using "heads" in a psychedelic pad while enjoying the "vibes" of a rock band, or in sterile laboratory surroundings. In this regard, Jones makes the following observations concerning the "effects" of placebo (noncannabinoid) cigarettes:

> Most of the subjects anticipated that they would get high even though they were told that an inactive substance might be given. The typical marihuana user in San Francisco is exposed to a wide range of potencies and tends to set broad limits for what he is willing to call marihuana.
>
> The criteria he must use to set those limits are confounded by a host of psychological and social variables in addition to the THC content of the plant. The experienced user comes to the laboratory with an over-learned set of expectations. The overt and convert advertising in the media and in the marihuana . . . culture is a potent force. Prior experience with a drug is an important determinant of the placebo effect. It may be that smoking of a material that smells and tastes like marihuana may serve as a signal that produces an internal state that is interpreted by the subject as being high.[5]

Let us now consider the effects of marijuana or THC, either after smoking or oral ingestion, on physiological, behavioral, and mental functions.

Physiological Effects

Low to moderate doses of marijuana produce minimal physiological changes. Virtually all investigators have observed an increase in pulse rate and a reddening of the conjunctiva, giving the eyes a bloodshot appearance; these effects temporally coincide with the onset and duration of the behavioral changes. Slight changes in blood pressure and pupil size, as well as fine hand tremors and a modest reduction in maximum muscle strength, have been also noted.

Behavioral Effects

After low "social" doses of marijuana, the subject continues to appear normal to the observer. It has been reported that this drug, in low doses, has a biphasic action, that is, a brief stimulatory phase followed by sedation. During the initial phase, subjects are anxious and restless, experience *euphoria,* and have *enhanced perceptions of the five senses.* In a comprehensive questionnaire prepared by Tart, some of the most common sensory perceptual responses reported were:

> I can see patterns, form, figures, meaningful designs in visual material that do not have any particular form when I'm straight, that is, just a meaningless series of lines or shapes when I'm straight. . . . I can see new colors or more subtle shades of color. . . . I can hear more subtle changes in sounds, for example, the notes of music are

[5] R. T. Jones, "Marihuana-Induced 'High': Influence of Expectation, Setting and Previous Drug Experience," *Pharmacological Reviews* 23:363 (1971).

purer and more distinct, the rhythm stands out more. . . . My sense of touch is more exciting, more sensual. . . . Touch, taste and smell sensations take on new qualities. . . . I enjoy eating very much and eat a lot.[6]

The *sedative phase* lasts for a longer period of time. Consciousness is altered, and the individual passes in and out of a *dream-like state* in which there is a constant and uncontrolled flow of ideas, often bearing no causal relationship to one another; long-forgotten thoughts reappear. Moderate doses intensify these psychic effects producing rapid fluctuations in emotions, more pronounced sensory images, a shortened attention span, and fragmentation of thoughts and expressions. Moderate doses of marijuana also markedly alter the appreciation of *time and distance.* The "internal clock" slows, with time intervals estimated to be twice as long as in actuality. Similarly, objects are perceived to be further away than in reality.

Marijuana, in high doses, produces a loss of personal identity, fantasies, sensory and mental illusions, disordered thought processes, and hallucinations. In a later section, we shall consider panic and acute psychotic reactions which occur during "bad trips."

Many anecdotal references have been made to the alleged aphrodisiac properties of marijuana. Careful analysis of these reports reveals that this drug does not promote sexual desires but rather enhances the drug user's perception of his or her partner. The subject may report being in closer mental contact with the partner; there is a union of the souls as well as their bodies. The potential adverse effects of marijuana on sexual function are discussed below.

Mental and Physical Performance

While under the influence of marijuana, the *memory span* is shortened. The user often forgets the essence of a conversation while it is still in progress or even forgets what was said at the beginning of a sentence by the time the sentence has concluded. These reports suggest a drug-induced impairment of short-term memory. Whereas simple and familiar tasks are minimally impaired, complex behavioral tasks such as complicated mathematical operations, comprehension of difficult reading passages, and counting in reverse by algebraic regressions are poorly performed. The degree of impairment is dependent upon the dosage of marijuana employed. Apparently, the regular marijuana user is better able to compensate for these deficits than the novice, for the veteran shows less impairment in the performance of such tasks. Whether this effect is the consequence of drug tolerance or greater subject effort remains to be determined.

You may now pose the very relevant question. What influence does the use of marijuana have on the safe operation of an automobile? Studies conducted under simulated driving conditions after the subject received low doses of mari-

[6] C. T. Tart, "Work with Marijuana: II. Sensations," *Psychology Today,* May 1971, p. 43.

juana indicate that this drug may impair certain motor and mental abilities (time and distance perceptual distortions, slowed reflexes) required for safe driving. An approximately equivalent amount of alcohol, sufficient to produce a "socially high" state, caused a far greater deterioration of "driving." Nevertheless, this author sees little likelihood in the prospect that the National Safety Council will endorse the use of marijuana for drivers seeking to unwind during the evening rush hour traffic.

In passing we should note that recent studies suggest that even heavy marijuana users have difficulty in distinguishing the effects of *Cannabis* from those produced by alcohol. Both drugs inhibit the restraints imposed by influences of the highest brain centers (Chapter 12).

ADVERSE EFFECTS AND POTENTIAL DANGERS

In the early 1970s, it was estimated that 24 million Americans had used marijuana at least once, that 8.3 million were current users, and that 30 to 40 percent of all individuals 18 to 25 years of age had tried this drug. National Institute on Drug Abuse estimates in 1977 revealed a sharp increase in drug usage; 43 million Americans had tried it on at least one occasion, the number of current users had almost doubled to 16 million, and approximately 60 percent of all 18 to 25-year-olds had tried marijuana, including 28 percent of all college graduates.

Of far greater concern is evidence that young people are using marijuana at an earlier age, more often, and in greater numbers than was previously observed. In 1977, one out of every nine high school seniors was smoking marijuana on a daily basis (almost twice the percentage of daily users of 1975), with 28 percent of high school seniors reporting to have used it prior to the tenth grade. In a 1977 study, 29 percent of eighth and ninth graders had smoked marijuana on at least one occasion and 15 percent had used the drug in the preceding month. For sixth and seventh graders, the comparable incidence of usage was 8 and 4 percent.

Is smoking pot a harmless fad devoid of danger to user and society, or does the use of this drug result in physical, mental, and moral deterioration when used for longer periods of time? Perhaps the most cogent argument in support of the present antimarijuana laws is that we simply do not have the definitive answers at this time. We shall now discuss the current available information concerning these questions with the full realization that in five or ten years new information may markedly alter the facts presented here.

Acute Toxicity

Countless investigators have replicated the 1839 observations of O'Shaughnessy that *Cannabis* has a very low level of toxicity. One report estimated the therapeutic index (lethal dose/effective dose) of THC to be

40,000. In that same study, the therapeutic indexes of alcohol and secobarbital (Seconal) were ten! To date, no documented report has been able to demonstrate lethality resulting from an overdosage of *Cannabis* in humans.

Adverse Behavioral Reactions

In moderate and even high doses, marijuana produces few significant physiological changes. What about adverse behavioral effects?

> Most of the millions of persons who use marijuana appear to suffer no adverse reactions therefrom. Indeed, most users report reinforcing feelings of pleasure and relaxation and a welcome diminution of aggression when smoking pot. However, despite this apparent innocuousness, clinical findings suggest that there are some rare individuals who under certain conditions react to marijuana with an acute psychotic syndrome.[7]

The *acute psychotic reaction* associated with the smoking of marijuana is characterized by disorganized thinking, paranoia, loss of personal identity, and hallucinations. As yet, no direct causal relationship has been demonstrated between this drug and these behavioral aberrations. Whereas this psychotic state is more likely to occur in persons with a history of psychiatric instability, it has also been observed in psychologically healthy individuals. It has not been determined whether marijuana speeds up the occurrence of such behavior which, in the absence of the drug, would have taken place spontaneously at some future date. This psychotic reaction is effectively controlled with chlorpromazine.

A far more common adverse behavioral effect associated with the use of marijuana is the *panic reaction.* Some *Cannabis* users become apprehensive, nervous, and panic-stricken and harbor the fear that they are losing their minds. This condition, more frequently experienced by first-time users, responds more favorably to friendly reassurance than to medication or hospitalization. "Flashbacks" are a clearly established phenomenon associated with the use of LSD. Only a few such reports of flashbacks have been observed with marijuana users, and these have been generally mild and of a pleasurable nature.

Abuse Potential

Since many individuals consider marijuana to be a "narcotic," in their minds it logically follows that this drug should have the same abuse potential as the narcotic agents such as heroin. Let us examine the facts with respect to the development of psychological dependence, physical dependence, and tolerance to marijuana.

[7] H. S. Kaplan, "Psychosis Associated with Marijuana," *New York State Journal of Medicine* **71**:434 (1971).

The magnitude of *psychological dependence* to marijuana rests upon the frequency of its use; it ranges from little or no dependence by the intermittent user (up to ten times per month) to very strong or even compulsive drug-seeking behavior by the "pot head" or very heavy user (Table 18–1). As we shall discuss in a later section of this chapter, the heavy user, one who uses marijuana several times per day, comprises about 2 to 4 percent of all *Cannabis* users in the United States. In contrast to the habitual narcotic user, individuals apparently do not become *physically dependent* upon marijuana when it is taken in relatively small amounts for recreational purposes in a social setting. Physical dependence, as evidenced by a withdrawal syndrome, has been demonstrated in an experimental setting when the subjects took very high doses on a regular basis, doses far in excess of those normally employed for recreation. Symptoms of withdrawal, beginning six to eight hours after the last dose, include restlessness, irritability, tremors, nausea, vomiting, diarrhea, and sleep disturbances.

Tolerance and "Reverse Tolerance"

Does *tolerance* develop to the effects of marijuana after continuous administration? Experimental evidence supports the conclusion that both tolerance and "reverse tolerance" may be observed. Explaining how or why an individual becomes more susceptible to the effects of a drug (reverse tolerance or sensitization) is a more puzzling task. Several hypotheses have been proposed. In low doses the behavioral effects of marijuana are very subtle. The drug "virgin" must "learn to get high," a perceptual accomplishment acquired only after repeated use of this drug. Experienced users recognize the unique smell and taste of marijuana smoke and prepare their "internal environment" for the anticipated high. A related postulate suggests that the neophyte must learn how to smoke a "joint" most effectively, namely, inhaling deeply and maintaining the inspiration 40 to 60 seconds.

The last explanation comes not from the experienced "head" but from a laboratory. We have previously indicated that 11-hydroxy-Δ^9-THC (also designated 7-hydroxy-Δ^1-THC) is a major metabolite of Δ^9-THC (or Δ^1-THC) and that it may be the biologically active compound responsible for the psychic effects observed after Δ^9-THC administration. Laboratory results indicate that Δ^9-THC disappears from the blood of regular marijuana users twice as rapidly as from the blood of nonusers. It has been suggested that the drug metabolizing enzyme systems (Chapter 3) of the users more efficiently form the active metabolite 11-hydroxy-Δ^9-THC, thus producing equivalent psychic effects at lower doses of Δ^9-THC. A biologically active metabolite of THC has been found to remain in the body for as long as eight days after drug administration. If marijuana were to be taken on a regular basis, the body levels of this compound would increase and less additional drug would be required to produce a behavioral "high."

Another practical point of interest comes from these same studies. Δ^9-THC is completely metabolized by humans, hence assaying the urine of a suspected

TABLE 18-1. SUMMARY OF THE POSSIBLE HAZARDS ASSOCIATED WITH THE VARIABLE FREQUENCY OF USE OF MARIJUANA

Classification of Usage	Frequency of Use	Psychological Dependence	Behavioral Changes	Physical Changes
Experimental or intermittent	Once only up to 10 times per month	Little or none	Highly variable, in general none	Not demonstrated
Moderate	More than 10 times per month, up to once per day	Moderate	Preexisting personality: Stable—minimal; Unstable—greater incidence of adverse behavioral changes	Little if any
Heavy (American "pothead")	Several times daily	Strong	Possible change in life style	Some impairment of breathing efficiency ("marijuana bronchitis")
Very heavy*	Many times daily	Almost compulsive	Lack of motivation and enthusiasm for work (Asia and Africa)	Greater breathing impairment Possible physical dependence

*Information concerning very heavy users has been obtained from Commission-sponsored studies in Jamaica and Greece and from the medical literature of India and Afghanistan. Such individuals generally employ hashish and have marked differences in nutrition and life-styles from those in the United States. These factors complicate interpretation of the available information.

marijuana user for the presence of THC would be a fruitless exercise. However, the urine does contain the metabolites of THC, which after suitable advancements in analytical methodology will probably be detected on a routine basis.

Long-Term Effects

In the past 90 years, three major studies have been conducted to ascertain the dangers associated with *Cannabis* usage. These were the Indian Hemp Commission (India, 1893–1894), Mayor LaGuardia's Report (New York City, 1944), and, most recently, the National Commission on Marihuana and Drug Abuse (United States, 1972). It is significant to point out that all three reports reached basically the same conclusions concerning the influence of *Cannabis* on the health of the user, the progression to "hard" drugs such as heroin, and the commission of crimes.

Health of the User

The two earlier reports observed that the regular but moderate use of *Cannabis* (be it charas or hashish in India, or marijuana on the sidewalks of New York) does not cause physical and mental deterioration or insanity. However, in the Sixth Annual Report on *Marihuana and Health* (1976), a number of areas of health concern were voiced.

Pulmonary effects. Since marijuana is most commonly self-administered by smoking, its adverse effects on the lung and on pulmonary function are of obvious interest. It has been experimentally observed that very heavy marijuana smoking by healthy young male subjects has been demonstrated to produce mild but statistically significant obstruction of the airways causing impairment of pulmonary function.

Immune response. The integrity of the normal immune response is essential as a critical defense mechanism against invasion by foreign infectious microorganisms to which we are constantly exposed. The results of human and animal studies published to date are contradictory and fail to provide a clear answer as to whether chronic marijuana use impairs the immune response and, even if it is impaired, whether this significantly interferes with the health of the user.

Endocrine effects. In a few studies but not in others marijuana use has been shown to decrease blood levels of the principal male sex hormone testosterone and reduce the sperm count in otherwise healthy young males.

Cardiovascular effects. Because of the ability of marijuana to increase the heart rate, it would appear prudent for patients with heart disease or impaired cardiac function to avoid the use of this drug. In this regard, elderly individuals may be at greater risk.

Brain damage.   Several widely publicized reports have claimed that heavy use of *Cannabis* in humans and monkeys causes physical damage to the brain. These highly controversial reports have not been confirmed and have been criticized based upon the experimental design and/or analysis employed. In view of the potential significance of these findings, the possibility of subtle brain damage after long-term, heavy marijuana use cannot be excluded.

Genetic changes.   THC has been shown to cross the placental barrier, and when administered to mice in very high doses causes fetal deaths and a reduction in fetal body weight. Chromosomal breaks have not been reported to occur in animals, nor have birth defects been observed in humans after regular usage of marijuana.

Amotivational syndrome.   Our society generally places great emphasis on the importance of hard work and achievement-oriented activities. Consequently, it is understandable that considerable concern has been expressed that

> ... regular marihuana use may contribute to the development of more passive, inward-turning, amotivational personality characteristics. ... [Such personality changes] include apathy, loss of effectiveness, and diminished capacity or willingness to carry out complex long-term plans, endure frustration, concentrate for long periods, follow routines, or successfully master new material.[8]

This so-called *amotivational syndrome* leads to an alteration in life-style and subtle changes in personality and modes of thinking. The 1972 Commission concluded that there was

> ... no evidence to date to demonstrate that marihuana use alone caused these behavioral changes either directly or indirectly. Many individuals reach the same point without prior marihuana use or only intermittent or moderate use; and many more individuals use marihuana as heavily but do not evidence these changes.[9]

Progression to "Hard" Drugs

One of the principal arguments advanced to support the strict antimarijuana laws is predicated upon the time-honored assumption that smoking marijuana leads to the use of more potent and dangerous drugs such as heroin, LSD, and cocaine. Both proponents and opponents of this thesis acknowledge that a high percentage of heroin-dependent persons first used marijuana. The recent Commission report has presented evidence showing that current marijuana users are twice as likely to use other illicit drugs (such as hashish, LSD, mescaline, methamphetamine, cocaine, and heroin) than former

---

[8] W. H. McGlothlin and L. J. West, "The Marihuana Problem: An Overview," *American Journal of Psychiatry* **125**:372 (1968).
[9] Commission Report, p. 62 (1972).

marijuana users. Opponents are quick to point out that these facts do not demonstrate a causal relationship. Virtually all scientific authorities agree that marijuana does not itself lead to other drugs of abuse. Perhaps we will better understand why some individuals freely experiment with drugs for curiosity and pleasure when we gain a greater insight into such an individual's innate personality traits.

Crime

Notwithstanding reports in the mass media condemning marijuana as the *cause* of violent acts, most notably the 1968 My Lai massacre in Vietnam, these reports have rarely withstood critical scrutiny. All three marijuana reports reach the same general conclusion.

> The weight of the evidence is that marihuana does not cause violent or aggressive behavior; if anything, marihuana generally serves to inhibit expression of such behavior. Marihuana-induced relaxation of inhibitions is not ordinarily accompanied by an exaggeration of aggressive tendencies.[10]

MARIJUANA USERS AND PATTERNS OF USE

As we have previously noted, in 1977 about 43 million Americans had tried marijuana at least once and 16 million were currently using this drug. What general information do we have concerning these people? In the past, twice as many males were marijuana users, but females are rapidly closing the gap. Most of the individuals reside in cities, towns, and in the suburbs, although rural users are not uncommon. Use is highest in the Northeast and Western parts of this country, with the lowest incidence in the South. Moreover, pot smokers are found among all occupations and vocations.

The incidence of marijuana use in the United States is compared for different age categories for the years 1971 and 1977 in Table 18–2. Inspection of these data reveals that both the percentage of individuals who have ever used marijuana and those who have used the drug in the past month (an indication of current use) have increased in all age categories from 12 to 34. The highest incidence of usage is among 16- to 25-year-olds. Use is age-related, with only 7 percent of those over 35 years old having ever tried marijuana. Dramatic increases in usage have been observed in 12- to 17-year-old youths, a trend that is continuing. From 1976 to 1977, there was a 25 percent increase in the total number of individuals in this age category who had ever tried marijuana and a 30 percent increase in current users.

---

[10] Commission Report, p. 73 (1972).

TABLE 18-2. MARIJUANA USE IN THE UNITED STATES: 1971 VERSUS 1977

Age	Percent Ever Used		Percent Used in Past Month (Current Users)	
	1971	1977	1971	1977
12-13	6	8	2	4
14-15	10	29	7	15
16-17	27	47	10	29
18-25	39	60	17	28
26-34	19	44	5	12
35 and over	7	7	0	1
All youth (12-17)	14	28	6	16
All adults (18+)	15	25	5	8

Source: Data from *Marihuana and Health,* Seventh Annual Report to the U.S. Congress (Washington, D.C.: U.S. Government Printing Office, 1977).

The User and Reasons for Use

We cannot insert various personality characteristics into a computer and from it get a printout of the "typical" marijuana user's profile. There are no "typical" users. The only dominant personality trait we can generally note is that the individual is willing to experiment with drugs, and, in particular, with an illicit drug. Although peer group pressures often lead to drug trials, the experimenter is usually a willing participant, who most often also smokes and drinks. Parental influence is also considered to be an important factor. Frequently, the user's parents are cigarette-smoking, liquor-drinking, and medicine-taking people. These medicines are most often tranquilizers, sedatives, and other psychoactive agents.

What people use marijuana, and what effects does its frequency of use have on their personality (Table 18–1)? *Experimenters,* individuals who use this drug once monthly or less, take it merely to share a social experience with friends. Their life-style, activities, academic performance, and goal-orientation remain normal. Such persons are conventional and rational in their behavior. *Intermittent users* employ this drug two to ten times per month, usually as part of socializing and recreational activities. They often belong to a close and intimate group that shares similar tastes with respect to music, art, and food. As with the experimenters, the intermittent users are conventional in most respects.

Moderate and heavy users differ from the preceding groups with respect to their basic personalities and their reasons for smoking marijuana. These individuals are generally more pessimistic, insecure, and irresponsible; they are nonconformists, who dislike routine and regimentation and seek pleasure. As might be anticipated, these people have unconventional life-styles, activities, and attitudes. In this group are individuals who smoke marijuana on a regular basis, from ten times per month to several times a day. Their reasons for the use of this drug include a desire for "kicks," a wish to "expand awareness and understanding," and to relieve anxiety and boredom. Although this group constitutes only about 8 percent of all adults who use marijuana, most of the generalizations expressed about this drug are based upon these individuals.

Why do individuals *discontinue* using marijuana after one or more trials? The most frequently expressed reason is simply a loss of interest or the lack of novelty in the experience. Less common reasons include fear of legal penalties, social pressures, and concern about the potential mental and physical dangers associated with the repeated use of this drug.

Potential Therapeutic Uses

In 1839, several years prior to the first meeting of *Le Club des Hachichins,* W. B. O'Shaughnessy, an Irish physician working in India, published the first medical report concerning *Cannabis.* He observed this drug to be devoid of toxicity in animals, and on the basis of his clinical experiments suggested it to be a useful anticonvulsant, muscle relaxant, and pain-killer. In 1912, a leading textbook of therapeutics spoke with praise about the value of *Cannabis* in cough mixtures, for the relief of pain, the prevention of migraine headaches, to lessen the tremors of Parkinson's disease, for sedation, and as a muscle relaxant in menstrual disorders. Other authors advocated *Cannabis* for the reduction of the withdrawal symptoms associated with chronic alcoholism and heroin dependence. Tincture of Cannabis was only deleted from the *United States Pharmacopoeia* in 1942.

Many factors contributed to the demise of *Cannabis* as a therapeutic agent. There was, and continues to be, marked variation in the THC content of *Cannabis* obtained from various sources, and therefore, the physician was unable to count upon a predictable therapeutic response. Insolubility in water precluded its use by injection. Finally, more potent and reliable drugs were introduced: aspirin and morphine for the relief of pain; the barbiturates and chloral hydrate for the induction of sleep; and phenytoin and phenobarbital for the management of convulsive disorders.

Because of the unusually low toxicity of marijuana and its derivatives, there has been a revival of interest in marijuana as a therapeutic agent. In particular, studies are currently underway evaluating its potential usefulness for the treatment of glaucoma, as an antiemetic agent for cancer patients, and for the management of asthma.

The observation that smoking marijuana causes *a reduction in the intraocular pressure* of individuals with normal pressure within the eyes, has lead to studies testing its potential effectiveness in the treatment of glaucoma, a major cause of blindness (Chapter 7). In 1975–1976 there was considerable lay interest in a patient with glaucoma who was arrested for growing marijuana on his back porch for medical purposes. Charges were dropped when his physicians certified that conventional therapy was ineffective and that his blindness could only be prevented by self-administration (smoking) marijuana. An eye drop preparation has been shown to be effective in animals; however, its safety and effectiveness in humans have not been established to date.

Pronounced nausea and vomiting is a common and highly debilitating adverse effect associated with the administration of chemotherapeutic agents for the treatment of cancer. While most of the available *antiemetic* agents have not proven to be effective, the results of preliminary clinical trials with marijuana in human subjects have been encouraging. Legislation has been enacted in many states permitting clinical trials evaluating marijuana for this purpose.

While marijuana smoke causes irritation of the lungs, it also produces a temporary increase in the size of the air conducting passages—that is, it is a *bronchodilator.* Administration of THC in an aerosol preparation does not produce irritation while retaining the beneficial bronchodilatory properties. Because it produces these effects by a mechanism that differs from other available preparations, THC or a synthetic derivative may prove to be a useful alternative agent for the treatment of asthma.

SUMMARY

Cannabis sativa, an ubiquitous weed, is the natural source of marijuana and hashish. The magnitude of the psychoactive effects of smoking hemp plant products have been attributed to their Δ^9-tetrahydrocannabinol (THC) content. The pharmacological effects produced are influenced by the dose and route of drug administration, as well as by the set ("internal environment" of the subject) and the setting ("external environment").

The major physiological effects associated with smoking marijuana are an increase in pulse rate and a bloodshot coloration of the eyes. These consistent observations follow the same time course as the behavioral effects. Psychic effects include euphoria, greater cognizance of the five senses, a dream-like state, and fluctuations in mood; short-term memory and time and distance perception are also impaired by this drug.

Marijuana is one of the least toxic known drugs; however "bad trips" characterized by panic are well recognized. In rare instances, an acute psychotic reaction occurs, most commonly in those persons having a preexisting unstable behavioral condition. Unfortunately, it may be these same individuals who are the heaviest users of marijuana. Psychic dependence develops in moderate and heavy users, and physical dependence has only been demonstrated under experimental conditions in which exceedingly high doses were employed. Both tolerance and "reverse tolerance" (sensitization) have been observed after repeated drug usage.

Opposition to the repeal of antimarijuana laws and legalizing (not just decriminalizing) this drug, is based upon the fear that its regular use poses a threat to the public health and safety and social order. Various Marihuana

Commission reports have not been able to demonstrate a causal relationship between the use of this drug and mental, physical, or moral deterioration; the progression to "hard" drugs, such as heroin; crimes; sexual promiscuity; or lack of motivation.

In 1977, it was estimated that 43 million Americans had used marijuana at least once, and that 16 million were regular users. Moreover, the use of this drug by 12- to 17-year-olds is increasing at what many consider to be an alarming rate. In view of its very extensive use in society, considerable concern has been expressed about its potential health dangers. While chronic marijuana use has been shown to impair pulmonary function, far more controversial are reports alleging that it causes adverse effects on the immune response, endocrine function, the cardiovascular system, the brain, and on chromosomes. Additional long-term studies must be objectively conducted and assessed to establish the validity of these reports.

While considerable controversy surrounds most aspects of marijuana usage, even its harshest critics concede that this drug possesses extremely low acute toxicity. At present, clinical trials are being conducted to evaluate marijuana and its derivatives for possible therapeutic uses. Potential medical applications include its use for the treatment of glaucoma and asthma, and, most promising, as an antiemetic agent for patients receiving cancer chemotherapy.

SUPPLEMENTARY READINGS

Braude, M. C., and S. Szara, eds., *Pharmacology of Marihuana,* Vols. 1 and 2. New York: Raven Press, 1976.

Cohen, S., and R. C. Stillman, eds., *The Therapeutic Potential of Marijuana.* New York: Raven Press, 1976.

Dornbush, R. L., A. M. Freedman, and M. Fink, eds., "Chronic Cannabis Use," *Annals of the New York Academy of Sciences* **282**: 1–430 (1976).

Lemberger, L., "Potential Therapeutic Usefulness of Marijuana," *Annual Review of Pharmacology and Toxicology* **20**: 151–72 (1980).

Marihuana and Health, Seventh Annual Report to the United States Congress From the Secretary of Health, Education, and Welfare. Washington, D.C.: U.S. Government Printing Office, 1977.

Marihuana: A Signal of Misunderstanding, First Report of the National Commission on Marihuana and Drug Abuse. Washington, D.C.: U.S. Government Printing Office, 1972.

Marijuana: Report of the Indian Hemp Drugs Commission, 1893–1894. Baltimore: Waverly Press, 1969 (original publication 1894).

Mayor's Committee on Marijuana: The Marijuana Problem in the City of New York. Lancaster, Penn.: Jacques Cattel Press, 1944.

Mechoulam, R., ed., *Marijuana: Chemistry, Pharmacology, Metabolism and Clinical Effects.* New York: Academic Press, 1973.

Singer, A. J., ed., "Marijuana: Chemistry, Pharmacology, and Patterns of Social Use," *Annals of the New York Academy of Sciences* **191**:1–269 (1971).

section four ─────────

Drugs Affecting the Cardiovascular System and Kidneys

19

Introduction to the Cardiovascular System

The blood is the life.
—Deuteronomy 12:23

A man is as old as his arteries.
—Thomas Sydenham (1624-1689)

All living cells require nutrients and oxygen to generate the energy necessary to carry out functions that insure their development, maintenance, and multiplication. In addition, cells also need a mechanism that will efficiently eliminate accumulated waste materials. For a single-celled (unicellular) organism such as the amoeba, these processes are accomplished simply. Food is ingested, and, after digestion has occurred within the food vacuoles, the nutrients are distributed throughout the cytoplasm of the cell by diffusion. That is, the material is transferred from a region containing a higher concentration of that substance to areas having lower concentrations. Similarly, as the unicellular organism depletes its oxygen supply, additional oxygen rapidly diffuses into the cell from the external environment. As wastes build up within the cell, these materials simply diffuse outward across the cell membrane.

As long as all the cells of an organism border the external environment, diffusion proves to be adequate for the exchange of materials between the environment and the cells. Complex multicellular organisms have cells far removed from the outside world and, therefore, require an efficient transport system to bring the essential materials of the environment to the cell. In essence this is the function of the circulatory system.

THE CARDIOVASCULAR SYSTEM: AN OVERVIEW

The **circulatory** or **cardiovascular system** consists of a pump and a closed set of tubes that are engineered to permit the transport of a carrier fluid to all the cells of the body. The *heart* is a muscular pump that propels the blood, a carrier fluid, through specialized tubes or blood vessels. The *blood* carries nutrients and oxygen to the cells and waste products away from cells for ultimate removal from the body. Enzymes, buffers, hormones, and other chemical mediators are transported in the blood and serve to modify the biochemical and physiological activities of cells, tissues, and organs, in a manner that best promotes the survival of the organism. The body's primary defenders against invading microbes are the antibodies and white blood cells, and they are carried to their bastions by the circulatory system. Body temperature is in part regulated by the loss of heat by the blood vessels lying near the surface of the skin.

There are three major types of *blood vessels* in the body: arteries, veins, and capillaries. The arteries carry blood away from the heart, while the veins lead the blood back to the heart; capillaries connect arteries and veins. Capillaries are of microscopic dimensions, about 1 mm long (1/25 of an inch) and 0.01 mm in diameter. If you were to place all the capillaries of the body end to end, their total length would circumscribe the earth 2.5 times! The exchange of materials between the blood and the cell takes place across the single-celled thick wall of the capillaries.

Many drugs have been developed to treat diseases of the cardiovascular system. Some of these drugs exert their primary action on the heart, modifying the rate and force of its contraction or correcting an abnormal heart beat; others are used to maintain an adequate blood supply to this organ. Agents acting directly or indirectly on the blood vessels are employed to treat high blood pressure and improve circulation to the extremities. Finally, drugs can increase or reduce the speed at which blood clots. In the next two chapters, we shall consider some of the more important drugs used to correct abnormal cardiovascular functions.

To permit an appreciation of these drug-induced effects, it is necessary for us first to consider the physiology of this system. You will readily appreciate that alterations in the normal activity of the heart directly influence the blood vessels and vice versa. This chapter will present an integrated overview of the mechanisms by which the heart and blood vessels work together to maintain the normal flow of blood throughout the body, and it will serve to provide a basic background for our discussion of drugs in the next two chapters. In Chapter 21 we shall consider the physiology of the kidneys and the pharmacology of diuretics, drugs that increase the excretion of urine.

THE HEART

Our earliest forebears appreciated the importance of the heart for the continuation of life. Poets and popular songwriters of all ages would be at a great loss without this organ. From the pens of great and inferior writers, references are made to broken, sad, heavy, weary, tender, kind, happy, and mighty hearts, as well as the displacement of this organ to the sleeve, throat, or boots; indeed, on occasion, this organ is even stolen. We shall not take the time here to question the physiological or anatomical validity of these references.

In the adult human, the heart is the size of a closed fist. This pump beats at an average of about 70 times per minute,[1] without rest, day and night, in excess of 2.5 billion times during the 70 average years of life. It is essential that the heart continuously function in this manner, because even after only several minutes of blood deprivation, irreversible changes occur that permanently impair brain function.

The heart consists of four chambers, two above and two below (Figure 19–1). The upper chambers are called *atria* (or auricles) and the lower ones

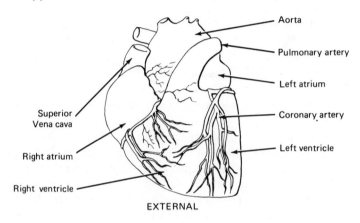

EXTERNAL

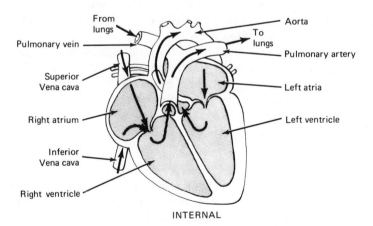

INTERNAL

FIGURE 19–1. External and Internal Views of the Heart.

[1] In general, heart rate is faster in small animals than in large animals of similar kinds. For example, the elephant or horse heart rate is 25 to 40 beats per minute; dog, 80; cat, 125; rabbit, 200; and mouse 300 to 500.

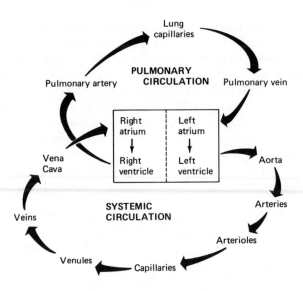

FIGURE 19-2. Schematic Representation of Pulmonary and Systemic Circulation.

ventricles, with blood flowing from the atria to the ventricles. The right and left sides of the heart actually function as two separate pumps. The chambers on the right side receive blood that has just completed its circuit around the body and pumps the blood to the lungs to pick up a fresh supply of oxygen and discharge carbon dioxide. The freshly oxygenated blood returns from the lungs and enters the left atrium and then the left ventricle. This latter muscular chamber propels the blood into arteries and throughout the body and then returns it to the right side of the heart in the veins. We may say then that the right chambers are concerned with *pulmonary circulation* and the left side with *systemic circulation* (Figure 19-2).

In this section we shall consider (1) the general properties of heart muscle; (2) the events that transpire during each contraction of the heart; (3) the rate at which the heart beats and the amount of blood it pumps with each contraction; and (4) the blood supply to the heart muscle itself.

Properties of Heart Muscle

If we were to electrically stimulate a muscle cell (fiber), we would observe that the excitation spreads to neighboring fibers; this spread of excitation is termed *conduction.* All muscles of the body, including the *myocardium* or heart (cardiac) muscle, are capable of responding to such stimuli by contracting, with both physical and chemical factors influencing the force of myocardial contraction. Physical factors, including the extent to which the myocardium is stretched by the volume of blood in the ventricles, modify contractile force. Autonomic influences provided by adrenergic and cholinergic nerves as well as the relative concentration of cations (potassium, sodium, calcium, magnesium) and hormones all may alter the rate and/or force of contraction of the heart.

Let us assume that we removed the skeletal (voluntary) muscle from the leg of a rat and this rodent's heart and suspended both in an oxygenated physiological salt solution. In the absence of stimulation, no activity would be exhibited by the skeletal leg muscle, while, by contrast, the heart would continue to beat spontaneously for many hours. Cardiac muscle possesses inherent *automaticity,* that is, the initiation of its contractions is not dependent upon an external source of stimulation. Let us now take a closer look at the events that occur when the heart beats and examine the basis for the intrinsic activity of cardiac tissue.

The Cardiac Cycle and the Heart Beat

Every minute the heart beats about 70 to 75 times, or approximately once every 0.8 seconds. During this rather short period of time, the following mechanical sequence of events occurs, which comprise the *cardiac cycle:* (1) both atria contract stimultaneously forcing the blood into the ventricles which are in a state of relaxation; (2) the blood-filled ventricles contract expelling the blood into the pulmonary or systemic circulation; and (3) the atria and ventricles relax. Contraction of the heart is termed *systole,* whereas the period of relaxation is referred to as *diastole.* When the heart rate is substantially hastened, there is a reduction in the time available for resting and complete refilling, which in time leads to such impairments of cardiac function as congestive heart failure (see below).

The **heart beat** originates in a small mass of specialized muscular tissue located in the right atrial wall near the mouth of the superior vena cava, the vein responsible for funneling blood from the head, neck, upper extremities, and chest back into the heart. This specialized tissue is the **sinoatrial node** or **S.A. node** (Figure 19–3), and it acts as the normal pacemaker of the heart. The S.A. node sets the pace for contractions of the heart by initiating electrical impulses that travel through the muscle fibers of the atria and ventricles. More specifically, this excitatory impulse travels from the S.A. node to the *atrioventricular node (A.V. node).* This latter node has right and left branches *(atrioventricular bundle)* which direct the impulse down each ventricle. Each A.V. bundle branch in turn subdivides into many smaller fibers (Purkinje fibers) which make contact with the muscle fibers of the ventricles.

An excitatory nerve impulse always precedes the mechanical contraction of the atria and ventricles, and these nerve impulses cause changes in electrical activity which can be detected on the surface of the body with the aid of an electrocardiogram or ECG (EKG). The ECG is an invaluable clinical tool for monitoring changes in heart rate or rhythm and is employed in diagnosing different cardiac disorders such as abnormal heart beats or arrhythmias as well as drug effects on the heart.

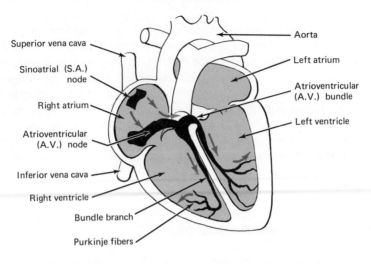

Aorta
Left atrium
Atrioventricular (A.V.) bundle
Left ventricle

Superior vena cava
Sinoatrial (S.A.) node
Right atrium
Atrioventricular (A.V.) node
Inferior vena cava
Right ventricle
Bundle branch
Purkinje fibers

FIGURE 19–3. The Conductive System of the Heart.

Cardiac Arrhythmias

The normal rhythm of the heart may be altered by disturbances in the pacemaker activity of the S.A. node or by another part of the heart usurping the pacemaker function. For example, the A.V. node or Purkinje fibers may begin to generate impulses more rapidly than the S.A. node and thereby set a new pace for the heart. As a result, the atria and ventricles contract independently and at different rates, disrupting normal cardiac rhythm and causing the heart to become a less efficient or even an inefficient pump. Some of these arrhythmias merely prove to be annoying to the patient, while others are capable of causing immediate death. We shall consider cardiac arrhythmias and their drug treatment in Chapter 20.

Heart Rate and Cardiac Output

Under resting conditions, the normal heart rate of an adult male is about 70 beats per minute. The well-conditioned athlete's heart beats less than 50 times per minute, which is indicative of a highly efficient pump. Strenuous exercise, fever, and high environmental temperatures, as well as emotional stresses, all increase this rate. Primarily by means of *nervous* control mechanisms, the body is able to maintain its resting heart rate and also quicken this rate to satisfy tissue requirements for a greater supply of blood.

Autonomic Mechanisms

The heart is innervated by sympathetic and parasympathetic nerves (Chapter 5) which modify its rate and force of contraction. Parasympathetic nerve fibers supply the S.A. and A.V. nodes, with some autonomic nerve fibers extending to the muscles of the atria. Sympathetic nerves are more extensively distributed throughout the heart muscle, both to the above listed areas and to ventricular muscle.

The *vagus* is the only parasympathetic nerve innervating the heart and its actions are mediated by the release of acetylcholine from the postganglionic parasympathetic (cholinergic) nerve endings. Activation of the vagus causes a slowing of the heart rate (bradycardia) and a reduction in the force of contraction. This *parasympathetic cardioinhibitory* effect has been attributed to acetylcholine-induced depression of the S.A. and A.V. nodes. Activation of the *sympathetic (accelerator)* nerves produces opposite effects, namely, an increase in heart rate (tachycardia) and a more powerful force of contraction. These actions are mediated by the release of norepinephrine from the sympathetic (adrenergic) nerve endings, and this neurotransmitter stimulates both the S.A. node and the heart muscle.

Thus our heart rate is influenced by a balance between the inhibitory effects of parasympathetic (vagus) activation and the stimulatory effects of sympathetic (accelerator) activation. Under normal resting conditions, the vagus nerve exerts the predominant influence. An increase in heart rate might be the consequence of a reduction in vagal activity and/or an increase in sympathetic stimulation.

Cardiac Output

The volume of blood pumped by the heart each minute is termed the **cardiac output;** it is dependent upon both the amount of blood expelled by each contraction or stroke of the left ventricle (*stroke volume*) and the *heart rate.* The normal cardiac output is 5.5 liters (5500 ml or 6 quarts) of blood per minute. Trained athletes can increase their cardiac output up to six times above resting levels during exercise. Since heart rate can only be effectively increased about three times above the resting level, the stroke volume must be doubled. One physiological mechanism by which stroke volume is enhanced involves sympathetic stimulation. This results in a more forceful ventricular contraction, more blood is ejected each time the heart beats, and the efficiency of the pumping action of the heart is increased.

Cardiac output	=	Stroke volume	×	Heart rate
(ml/min)		(ml/contraction)		(contractions/min)

In **congestive heart failure,** the heart beats very rapidly and weakly. This rapid rate prevents adequate ventricular filling during the diastolic (relaxation) phase, and the weak contraction does not completely expel the blood. Let us assume that you wish to fill a bicycle tire with a hand pump in a finite period of time. Consider the effort expended and efficiency realized if you made short, rapid strokes or, alternatively, slower, but complete strokes. In congestive heart failure, digitalis slows the heart rate, permitting more time for filling, and causes the heart to contract more forcefully and completely, thereby increasing the stroke volume and cardiac output.

Blood Supply to the Heart

To maintain the continuous activity of the heart, this organ requires an adequate supply of nutrients and oxygen. The *coronary arteries* (Figure 19–1) normally supply the heart with about 4 to 5 percent of the total cardiac output. During strenuous activity, the coronary blood flow may increase as much as four to six times above normal.

Let us see how coronary blood flow can be modified to meet the demands of the heart. With increased activity, either in the force or rate of contraction, the oxygen requirements of heart muscle are increased. It is currently believed that when the oxygen supply to heart muscle becomes deficient, a stimulus is generated which causes a widening or dilation of the coronary vessels, thereby increasing blood flow. Oxygen starvation of the myocardium results in angina (Chapter 20).

CIRCULATION AND BLOOD VESSELS

Let us now focus our attention upon blood vessels, and, in particular, their regulation of blood pressure. After left ventricular contraction, the blood travels from the aorta to the arteries to arterioles (finer subdivision of the arteries) to capillaries to venules to veins and back into the heart through the right atrium (Figure 19–2). Since our cells do not maintain constant energy requirements throughout the course of a day, adequate circulatory regulation necessitates a transfer of blood flow from inactive tissues to those that are active.

Blood Pressure

Circulation of blood around the body only occurs because of *gradients* or differences in blood pressure among the blood vessels. Blood flows from vessels having higher pressure into those vessels of lower pressure. The blood pressure in the aorta is 100 mm Hg; it falls to 60 mm Hg in the arterioles and to 30 mm Hg in the capillaries; as blood enters the veins it has a pressure of 10 mm Hg, and as it enters the right atrium, blood exerts essentially no pressure.

Arterial blood pressure fluctuates with each contraction of the heart. As blood is ejected from the left ventricle into the aorta, the blood pressure is suddenly increased as the blood enters and swells this elastic artery. This maximum arterial pressure resulting from ventricular contraction, or systole, is termed the *systolic pressure*. During the relaxation or diastolic phase of the cardiac cycle, arterial pressure falls, with a precipitous drop in pressure precluded by the nature of the elastic recoil of the arteries. This lower pressure is called the *diastolic pressure*. Blood pressure is recorded as the systolic over the diastolic pressure; the average normal blood pressure for a college-aged student is about 120/80. When blood pressure exceeds 145/90, the individual is said to have high blood pressure or *hypertension.* The approximate average of the diastolic and systolic pressures represents the *mean blood pressure,* with their difference referred to as *pulse pressure.*

Arterial blood pressure is directly influenced by the *cardiac output* and *peripheral resistance* (Figure 19–4). Within certain limits, we may say that the faster the heart rate and the greater the force of myocardial contraction, the higher will be the arterial pressure. The increase of one or both of these parameters tends to increase cardiac output, which increases the volume of blood within the arteries, which in turn increases the blood pressure.

Peripheral resistance refers to the opposition or resistance the walls of the blood vessels (mainly the arterioles) exert upon the flow of blood. This resistance to flow is inversely related to the diameter of the arterioles, that is, the smaller the diameter, the greater the resistance, and the higher the blood pressure. Why should this be the case? As the diameter of the arterioles becomes smaller, the resistance of these vessels to blood flow becomes greater, with less blood leaving the arteries to enter the arterioles. The increased volume of blood remaining in the arteries elevates the pressure within these blood vessels.

Nerve endings, primarily those arising from the sympathetic division of the autonomic nervous system, innervate all blood vessels except the capillaries. Under the direction of the vasomotor center located in the medulla, these sympathetic nerves are able to modify the activity of the smooth muscles in the arterioles which control the degree to which the arterioles are dilated or constricted. Hence, the sympathetic nervous system plays a major role in the regulation of blood flow as well as the control of blood pressure. To permit the normal maintenance of blood pressure, the sympathetic vasoconstrictor nerves are always active. Many antihypertensive agents, that is, drugs used to reduce high blood pressure, act by interfering with norepinephrine-mediated vasoconstriction of blood vessels. The induction of vasodilation reduces peripheral resistance and lowers arterial blood pressure. We shall return to our discussion of antihypertensive agents in Chapter 21.

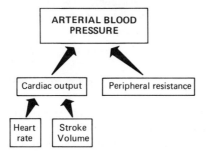

FIGURE 19–4. Major Factors Modifying Arterial Blood Pressure.

SUMMARY

The cardiovascular or circulatory system consists of the heart and blood vessels. Two separate circulatory systems operate simultaneously: The pulmonary circulation permits the exchange of oxygen and carbon dioxide between the blood and lungs, while the systemic circulation provides oxygen and nutrients to the cells of the body.

The cardiac cycle is initiated by nerve impulses arising within the heart itself (thus endowing the heart with the property of automaticity), in particular, at the sinoatrial node. A specialized conducting system carries these impulses throughout the artria or upper chambers of the heart to the myocardium of the ventricles, the lower chambers. Blood is pumped from the atria to the ventricles to the arteries to arterioles to capillaries to venules to veins and back into the heart. The heart rate is primarily controlled by the autonomic nervous system, the activity of which is mediated by the release of neurotransmitter substances. Parasympathetic or vagal activation slows the rate of contraction, whereas sympathetic activation increases the heart beat and strengthens the force of contraction. Cardiac output is determined by the heart rate, stroke volume (the amount of blood ejected by each heart beat), and the peripheral resistance in the arterioles. An increase in these factors enhances cardiac output and tends to elevate blood pressure.

The general concepts presented in this chapter will provide you with the basic background required for our consideration of drugs having their primary action on the heart (Chapter 20) and blood vessels (Chapter 21).

SUPPLEMENTARY READINGS

Andreoli, K. G., V. Hunn, D. P. Zipes, and A. G. Wallace, *Comprehensive Cardiac Care: A Text for Nurses and Other Health Professionals.* 3rd ed. St. Louis: C. V. Mosby, 1975.

Antonaccio, M., ed., *Cardiovascular Pharmacology.* New York: Raven Press, 1976.

Brater, D. C., and H. F. Morrelli, "Cardiovascular Drug Interactions," *Annual Review of Pharmacology and Toxicology* 17: 293–309 (1977).

Burch, G. E., and T. Winsor, *A Primer of Electrocardiography.* 6th ed. Philadelphia: Lea & Febiger, 1972.

Cranefield, P. F., *The Conduction of the Cardiac Impulse.* New York: Futura Publishing Co., 1975.

Guyton, A. C., C. E. Jones, and T. G. Coleman, *Circulatory Physiology: Cardiac Output and its Regulation.* 2nd ed. Philadelphia: Saunders, 1973.

Montcastle, V. B., ed., "The Circulation," in *Medical Physiology.* 13th ed., Vol. 2, Part 7. St. Louis: C. V. Mosby, 1974.

Scheinman, M. M., ed., "Symposium on Cardiac Emergencies," *Medical Clinics of North America* 63 (1): 1–299 (1979).

20

Drugs Affecting
the Heart

The heart of animals is the foundation of their life, the sovereign of everything within them, the sun of their microcosm, that upon which all growth depends, from which all power proceeds.

—William Harvey (1628)

In this chapter we shall discuss drugs that exert their primary action on the heart, modifying both the force of contraction and rhythm, and compounds that increase coronary blood flow. Three prototype drugs will be discussed: digitalis, quinidine, and nitroglycerin. *Digitalis* is a cardiotonic agent, that is, a drug that enhances the force of contraction of the failing heart; *quinidine,* an antiarrhythmic agent, corrects abnormal heart rhythms; and, *nitroglycerin,* a representative coronary vasodilator that enhances the flow of blood supplying the heart muscle that is used for the treatment of angina. All three of these drugs have been employed for the treatment of heart disorders for over 60 years, and, notwithstanding highly significant recent advances in the development of new drugs, they have retained their preeminent status in therapeutics.

DIGITALIS

After the physician has diagnosed congestive heart failure, only one class of drugs is employed—the digitalis glycosides. Prior to examining the pharmacological properties of digitalis, let us briefly review the historical background surrounding the use of this drug, as well as its source and chemistry.

Medical reports concerning the *foxglove* first appeared in Wales in the thirteenth century. About 300 years later, this plant was given the descriptive and scientific name *Digitalis purpurea,* a very appropriate designation since the flowers are purple and have the shape of fingers. The modern history of digitalis began in the late eighteenth century with the astute clinical observations of William Withering (1741–1799). Withering was not only an actively practicing physician but was also a well-recognized botanist, mineralogist, and chemist. As a member of the prestigious Lunar Society at Birmingham, Withering interacted with such famous English contemporaries as James Watt, inventor of the steam engine; Joseph Priestley, discoverer of oxygen; Erasmus Darwin, physician, scientist, and grandfather of Charles Darwin; and Josiah Wedgewood, pottery manufacturer.

Withering's great interest in the medicinal properties of plants caused him to investigate the reports of a curious folk remedy, which he describes:

> In the year 1775, my opinion was asked concerning a family recipe for the cure of dropsy [edema]. I was told that it had long been kept a secret by an old woman in Shropshire who had sometimes made cures after the more regular practitioners had failed. I was informed also that the effects produced were violent vomiting and purging; for the diuretic effects seemed to have been overlooked. This medicine was composed of twenty or more different herbs; but it was not very difficult for one conversant in these subjects to perceive that the active herb could be no other than foxglove.[1]

Over the next decade, Withering administered this drug to his "sick poor" patients, carefully observing its beneficial therapeutic effects as well as the early signs of digitalis toxicity; these were carefully outlined in the medical classic, *An Account of the Foxglove,* which was published in 1785. Although Withering recognized the powerful effects of this drug on the heart, he attributed its beneficial effects to be the consequence of a diuretic action; by 1800, the primary site of digitalis was correctly identified as the heart.

Notwithstanding the strong warnings Withering sounded about the appropriate therapeutic uses of digitalis and its inherent toxicity, this drug was carelessly employed during the nineteenth century, causing it to eventually fall into disfavor among the physicians of the day. Fortunately, digitalis was rescued from oblivion by the combined efforts of the famous English heart specialist, Sir James Mackenzie (1853–1925) and the equally distinguished Scottish pharmacologist, Arthur Cushny (1866–1926). Mackenzie and Cushny described the effects of digitalis on the heart and established guidelines for its rational therapeutic use in the treatment of such heart diseases as atrial fibrillation and congestive heart failure.

In strict terms, *digitalis* refers to the leaf or to selected chemicals derived from the leaves of *Digitalis purpurea* or purple foxglove. However, a great many

---

[1] W. Withering, *An Account of the Foxglove and Some of Its Medical Uses: With Practical Remarks on Dropsy, and Other Diseases* (London: C. G. J. & J. Robinson, 1785).

other natural sources contain chemically related steroid glycosides (see below), which possess the same desirable and toxic effects on the heart; some of these sources include such plants as the lily of the valley, the Christmas rose, oleander, and milkweed, as well as the salivary gland and skin of certain toads.

All of these cardioactive compounds are chemically classified as **glycosides.** A glycoside is a chemical which, when hydrolyzed, gives rise to a sugar and a nonsugar (aglycone or genin) as products. Digitalis glycosides consist of an aglycone fraction that has a steroid nucleus,[2] and it is this part of the molecule that is essential for the observed action on the heart. The attached sugar is not required for biological activity but does increase water solubility and the ability of these compounds to cross cell membranes.

(Digitoxose)$_3$ Steroid   Lactone
    Sugar   *Aglycone*

Digitoxin: A Cardiac Glycoside

Although all cardiac glycosides are generally believed to act on the heart by an identical mechanism, major differences among these drugs exist with respect to their relative degree of absorption after oral administration, as well as to their onset and duration of action (Table 20–1). Extensive studies conducted over the past three decades have elucidated structure-activity relationships

TABLE 20-1. RELATIVE PROPERTIES OF SELECTED CARDIAC GLYCOSIDES

Generic Name (Trade Name)	Source	Absorption (%)	Onset of Action*	Duration of Action
Digitalis, powdered whole leaf	*D. purpurea*	20	Medium	Long
Digitoxin (Crystodigin)	*D. purpurea*	100	Slow	Long
Digoxin (Lanoxin)	*D. lanata*	60	Fast	Medium
Deslanoside (Cedilanid D)	*D. lanata*	40	Fast	Medium
Ouabain (G-Strophanthin)	*Strophanthus gratus* and *S. Kombé*	100 (given only intravenously)	Rapid	Short

*All drugs but ouabain may be given orally.

[2] The steroid structure is present in such biologically diverse compounds as the male and female sex hormones, cortisol, vitamin D, and cholesterol.

among the digitalis glycosides; for example, the pharmacological activity is modified by chemical changes in the steroid nucleus and lactone ring as well as by the addition or removal of the attached sugar groups. Let us now consider the general pharmacological properties of the cardiac glycosides.

Pharmacological Actions

We may view the basic actions of digitalis on the heart to be twofold. First, this drug has a positive **inotropic effect;** that is, digitalis *stimulates the force of contraction of heart muscle.* Second, it modifies the spread of *electrical activity* in the myocardium which causes a *reduction in heart rate.* Let us examine each of these major actions and consider the resulting physiological consequences.

Inotropic Effects

By virtue of a direct action on the myocardium, digitalis causes the heart to contract more forcefully and completely and with greater efficiency; that is, this positive inotropic effect is accomplished without the consumption of additional nutrients or oxygen. As a consequence, we observe that patients with congestive heart failure have an increase in cardiac output to levels approaching normal. This positive inotropic effect is also observed in persons with normal hearts, but cardiac output is rarely increased. Epinephrine also enhances the force of myocardial contraction, but it increases heart rate and the expenditure of nutrients and oxygen. Hence, epinephrine is not useful for the treatment of heart failure.

The precise mechanism underlying the positive inotropic effects of digitalis remains a subject of controversy among investigators. One widely accepted theory suggests that digitalis interferes with the movement of sodium and potassium across the cell membrane of the heart (by inhibiting the enzyme [Na^+ + K^+]-adenosine triphosphatase) in a manner that facilitates the contraction of cardiac muscle in response to electrical excitation. This process of *excitation-contraction coupling* is thought to be enhanced by a digitalis-induced increase in the free concentration of calcium close to the myofibrils, the muscle fibers. Regardless of the ultimately determined mechanism of action, it is a well-established fact that selective alteration in the blood concentrations of these inorganic ions has a profound effect on the action of digitalis, increasing or decreasing the toxicity of this drug; a decrease in the concentration of potassium in the blood (hypokalemia) is the most common factor predisposing patients to digitalis toxicity.

Electrophysiological Effects

In addition to its positive inotropic effect, digitalis has several other complex effects on the heart. Therapeutic doses of the cardiac glycosides slow the heart rate, an effect attributed to both direct and indirect effects on the heart. Digitalis directly depresses the conducting tissues responsible for carrying the excitatory impulse from the S.A. node pacemaker. The indirect effect of this drug arises from an activation of the vagus nerve, which by virtue of its innervation of the S.A. node causes a slowing of the heart rate.

Therapeutic Effects

The most important therapeutic uses of digitalis are for the treatment of congestive heart failure and atrial fibrillation.

Heart Failure

A patient suffering from **congestive heart failure** has a feeble, but rapid, heart beat, a below-normal cardiac output, and impaired systemic circulation. Impaired blood flow to the kidneys reduces urine output and leads to edema or swelling. Incomplete emptying of blood from the heart during ventricular contraction eventually causes an enlargement of the heart and an increase in venous pressure. The beneficial effects produced by digitalis in congestive heart failure have been attributed primarily to this drug's positive inotropic effects in the absence of increased energy requirements. The greater force of contraction increases the expulsion of blood from the heart, increases cardiac output, and improves systemic circulation; venous pressure is decreased facilitating venous return of the blood. Enhanced urinary excretion is observed and edema is relieved. With the reduction in heart rate, more complete filling occurs during the phase of cardiac relaxation or diastole prior to each contraction. The size of the heart also decreases and begins to return to normal.

Atrial Fibrillation

Depression of conduction of the excitatory impulse, in particular at the A.V. node, serves as the basis for the therapeutic use of digitalis in the treatment of **atrial fibrillation.** In this cardiac arrhythmia, the atria contract many times more often than the ventricles, causing these lower heart chambers to be bombarded by impulses. The ventricles respond by weakly and inefficiently contracting. Digitalis depresses A.V. nodal conduction, slows the rate of ventricular contractions, and helps reestablish a synchronous and effective heart beat. This drug rarely cures atrial fibrillation; electric cardioversion or other drugs (propranolol) must be employed to reestablish a normal atrial rhythm.

Toxicity

Of all drugs in common usage, the therapeutic index of the cardiac glycosides is among the lowest (2 or possibly 3). Thus, the difference between an effective therapeutic dose and a toxic dose is very small, a fact fully appreciated by Withering about two centuries ago. Successful therapeutic use of digitalis to a large measure depends on the physician's ability to carefully adjust the dosage to best fit each patient's unique requirements, while minimizing toxicity.

Approximately one out of five patients receiving digitalis exhibits signs and symptoms associated with drug-induced toxicity. Noncardiac and cardiac symptoms are associated with digitalis overdosage and poisoning.

Loss of appetite, nausea, and vomiting usually herald the earliest signs of digitalis toxicity; stomach cramps with pain and diarrhea are other gastrointestinal symptoms that are often also present. Other noncardiac symptoms of toxicity include extreme fatigue, visual disturbances (the perception of colors, blurred vision), and behavioral aberrations such as nightmares, agitation, and hallucinations. In approximately one-half of all cases, these noncardiac symptoms make their appearance prior to those affecting the heart.

As you might anticipate, many of the toxic effects are an exaggeration of the normal pharmacological action of this drug on the heart. High doses cause partial or total heart block by preventing impulses arising in the S.A. node from reaching the ventricles. The automaticity, or inherent ability of the heart muscle to contract, may be enhanced by toxic amounts of digitalis. Ventricular tachycardia represents a particularly ominous sign because it may be followed by *ventricular fibrillation,* the most common cause of death caused by digitalis overdosage.

Reduction in the normal blood concentration of potassium (*hypokalemia*) predisposes patients (even those who were previously well-controlled) to digitalis toxicity. Drugs commonly cause excessive potassium loss from the body, in particular, diuretic agents (drugs that promote urine output) of the thiazide class (Chapter 21). Since potassium inhibits the excitability of the heart, subnormal serum or myocardial levels increase the risk of digitalis-promoted enhanced pacemaker activity, potentially resulting in arrhythmias. Treatment of overdosage may involve temporary withdrawal of digitalis administration, giving the patient an oral dose of potassium chloride, or, in severe cases of toxicity, administration of an antiarrhythmic agent.

Other Related Nontherapeutic Compounds

The biologically active secretions of the toad, which are chemically and pharmacologically related to digitalis, have been known to the people of various lands for many centuries. Roman women used the toad as a poison, albeit with limited success, to dispose of unfaithful husbands, while South American Indians employed the skin secretions as an arrow poison for game hunting and in warfare. The ancient Chinese and Europeans of the Middle Ages prepared medicines from both the venom and dried toad.

Venoms generally serve to protect animals against their enemies. Although toad poisons would prove lethal if introduced into the bloodstreams of their adversaries, the toad lacks teeth to bite and is incapable of accurately squirting the venom. In spite of the bitter taste of the skin secretions, some snakes and rats include toads as part of their diets. The process of venom regeneration is very slow, thus preventing these amphibia from manufacturing the poison repeatedly for defensive purposes. In short, although these venoms possess high toxicological activity, they apparently are of little value for the survival of the toad.

For over a century it has been known that the toad's heart is more resistant to the effects of its own cardioactive venoms and to digitalis and related cardiac glycosides than are frogs and other animals. The exact mechanism underlying this inherent or natural tolerance is unknown and remains one of the mysteries of pharmacology.

Let us explore a variation on this basic theme. The milkweed (*Asclepias curassavica*) of Costa Rica manufactures digitalis-like glycosides that are toxic to vertebrates, but not to certain insects. The monarch butterfly is able to safely feed on the poison glycoside-containing milkweed, but when this butterfly becomes a bird's prey, the predator bird becomes violently ill, manifested in part by vomiting. Once sensitized in such a manner, the bird would undoubtedly be judicious in eliminating the monarch butterfly from its menu. In addition, other types of butterflies that do not feed on milkweeds, but closely mimic the monarch in appearance, are also avoided by these birds, although such insects are in fact quite palatable. This type of mimicry provides an example of natural selection which promotes the survival of palatable butterflies as well as unpalatable ones.

QUINIDINE

Prior to considering the pharmacology of quinidine, the prototype drug in its class, we shall first briefly discuss the nature of cardiac arrhythmias.

Arrhythmias

As will be recalled from Chapter 19, electrical impulses normally arising in the cardiac pacemaker—the sinoatrial (S.A.) node—rapidly spread to the atria, to the atrioventricular (A.V.) node, along specialized conducting tissues, and culminate in the contraction of the ventricles. Most of the commonly encountered cardiac arrhythmias arise from disorders in the automaticity of the cardiac muscle or as the result of abnormalities in the normal conduction of nerve impulses.

Under certain conditions, sites in the cardiac muscle exhibit greater than normal *automaticity,* generating nervous impulses at a frequency exceeding that of the S.A. node, and thereby usurping the pacemaker function. These sites, referred to as abnormal or *ectopic pacemakers,* cause an abnormal sequence of contractions in different parts of the heart. Arrhythmias that are caused by disorders in impulse formation can be managed by drugs that depress the automaticity of the cardiac muscle (Table 20–2).

TABLE 20-2. COMPARATIVE PROPERTIES OF COMMONLY EMPLOYED ANTIARRHYTHMIC AGENTS

Generic Name (Synonyms) [Trade Name]	Automaticity	Conduction Velocity	Refractory Period	Therapeutic Uses*	Remarks
Digitalis glycosides (Table 20-1)	↑	↓	↑	AF, AFl, PAT	Does not cure AF.
Quinidine salts [Quinaglute]	↓	↓	↑	AF, AFl, PS, PST, VT	Caution in A.V. block. Not used to treat digitalis toxicity.
Procainamide [Pronestyl]	↓	↓	↑	Same as quinidine	Properties similar to quinidine but less effective for AF and AFl.
Lidocaine (lignocaine B.P.) [Xylocaine]	↓	0	→	VA	Local anesthetic used intravenously for emergency treatment of ventricular arrhythmias in heart surgery or myocardial infarction.
Phenytoin (diphenylhydantoin) [Dilantin]	↓	↑	→	PAT	Antiepileptic drug used for PAT associated with digitalis toxicity.
Propranolol [Inderal]	↓	↓	→	AF, AFl, PAT	β-adrenergic blocking agent produces marked reduction in heart rate.

*Key to abbreviations: AF = atrial fibrillations; AFl = atrial flutter; PAT = paroxysmal atrial tachycardia; PS = premature systoles; PST = paroxysmal supraventricular tachycardia; VA = ventricular arrhythmias; VT = ventricular tachycardia.

Certain arrhythmias, such as atrial fibrillation and atrial flutter, are thought to originate from disturbances in the normal *conduction of nerve impulses*. A *circus movement* is said to occur when an impulse originates at one site in the heart muscle, spreads in a circular (circus) pathway through the heart, and returns to restimulate the originally excited muscle in a continuous manner. Disorders of this type appear to be associated with a reduction in the conduction velocity of the nerve impulse and a greatly reduced refractory period (the time during which the heart muscle is nonresponsive to restimulation by an impulse). Drugs capable of modifying the conduction velocity and the refractory period are useful in abolishing circus movements.

Cardiac arrhythmias are not uncommon. Their incidence is estimated to be 10–25 percent in hospitalized patients during early phases of digitalis therapy, 20–50 percent in patients receiving general anesthetics, and 80–90 percent in patients with acute myocardial infarction (heart attack); ventricular arrhythmias are the primary cause of death after myocardial infarction.

The primary modes of treatment in arrhythmias include: electrical pacemakers and cardioversion (DC electroshock); drugs modifying autonomic function; and drugs that alter the properties of the cell membrane. The most commonly used antiarrhythmic agents (Table 20–2) act by this last mechanism.

Quinidine

Quinidine, an isomer of quinine, is a naturally occurring alkaloid contained in the bark of the cinchona tree. In 1914, a Dutch sea captain visited the Austrian cardiologist Wenckeback seeking treatment for his atrial fibrillation. The captain told this distinguished physician that the arrhythmia stopped whenever he took quinine during his business trips to countries having a malaria problem. Wenckeback, impressed by this story, prescribed quinine to other patients with similar heart disorders and obtained moderately successful results. Four years later, quinidine was tried and was found to be a far more useful antiarrhythmic agent than quinine. It is now among the most widely employed drugs for cardiac arrhythmias.

Quinidine

Antiarrhythmic Effects of Quinidine

Quinidine's depressing effects on the heart result from a decrease in myocardial excitability and the conduction velocity of the nerve impulse, as well as prolongation in the refractory period of the heart. Let us briefly consider each of these actions.

Decreased Excitability

For the heart's pacemaker to generate an impulse, this specialized tissue must first attain a certain threshold or minimum level of activation. Normally, the S.A. node is able to reach this minimum threshold level more readily than any other part of the heart, but in abnormal conditions pacemaker function arises in areas of the heart other than the S.A. node. Quinidine depresses the excitability of both normal and abnormal (ectopic) pacemakers, although the ectopic pacemakers are more sensitive to the drug's inhibitory action.

Decreased Conduction

Quinidine and related drugs depress or slow the velocity at which electrical excitation is spread throughout the myocardium, an effect attributed to a direct drug-induced action on the atria, A.V. node, and ventricles.

Prolonged Refractory Period

For a brief period of time after the heart has contracted in response to an excitatory stimulus, it is unresponsive or refractory to a second excitatory stimulus; this refractory period prevents fatigue of the cardiac muscle. Quinidine increases the interval between one contraction and the time when the myocardium is capable of responding to the next excitatory impulse. In this manner, the heart muscle does not contract with every impulse generated by the pacemaker. Quinidine is primarily used for the clinical treatment of atrial fibrillation and other cardiac arrhythmias.

NITROGLYCERIN

> *They are afflicted with it [angina pectoris], are seized while they are walking (more especially if it be uphill, and soon after eating) with a painful and most disagreeable sensation in the breast, which seems as if it would extinguish life, if it were to increase or to continue; but the moment they stand still, all this uneasiness vanishes.*
>
> —William Heberden (1710-1801)

Coronary artery disease, the major cause of death in Western nations, results from an inadequate blood supply to the heart muscle. **Angina pectoris** is a type of coronary artery disease that occurs when the oxygen requirements of the myocardium temporarily exceed the supply, such as during vigorous exercise. The oxygen deficiency produces an extreme crushing pain in the left arm and chest. Drugs used for the treatment of angina are thought to act by dilating the coronary vessels, thereby increasing coronary blood flow and/or also by reducing cardiac work and demand for oxygen. The major antianginal drugs are nitrates ($-O-NO_2$) and nitrites ($-NO_2$), and of these nitroglycerin is among the oldest and most useful. Propranolol, a β-adrenergic blocking agent, is being used with increasing frequency for the prevention of anginal attacks.

Antianginal Nitrates and Nitrites

Many nitrates and nitrites are capable of relaxing smooth muscle, with the muscles in the walls of the coronary arteries particularly sensitive. If we analyze the properties of the many available drugs in this therapeutic class, we observe that they primarily differ with respect to their route of administration (inhalation, oral ingestion, or sublingual, that is, under the tongue), rate of onset, and duration of action. We shall now discuss nitroglycerin, the prototype antiangina agent.

Nitroglycerin (Glyceryl Trinitrate)

Within one to two minutes after placing a 0.4 mg tablet of nitroglycerin under the tongue, the patient generally begins to obtain relief from the pain associated with an attack of angina. Moreover, when given prior to exercise, this medication makes the patient less susceptible to an attack, but unfortunately, this prophylactic effect lasts only for about one-half hour.

In the past, nitroglycerin's beneficial effects were ascribed exclusively to *coronary vasodilation.* By virtue of its ability to relax smooth muscle, nitroglycerin reduces the resistance exerted by the walls of the blood vessels and thereby increases coronary blood flow. In addition, nitroglycerin is now also thought to act by decreasing the amount of work done by the heart and, therefore, lowering the oxygen requirements of this organ. Both actions are believed to contribute to the ultimate antiangina effect, with the latter thought to be more important.

Tolerance.   One may ask why drugs in this class are not taken chronically to prevent the occurrence of angina. Long-acting nitrates, such as pentaerythritol tetranitrate (Peritrate) are employed as prophylactic agents, but their beneficial effects are limited by the development of *tolerance* which is observed within days to a few weeks after the initiation of drug therapy. Moreover, cross-tolerance to the effects of nitroglycerin may develop in patients taking long-acting nitrates, thus reducing the effectiveness of the former drug during an acute attack of angina.

For industrial workers, however, the development of tolerance to the nitrites and nitrates is highly desirable. Compounds such as nitroglycerin are used in the manufacture of explosives.[3] During their first days of employment, new workers in this industry often experience very severe headaches, as well as dizziness and a drop in blood pressure upon arising. Although tolerance is rapidly acquired to these nitrite-induced effects, tolerance is also quickly lost if the worker is not exposed to these compounds for even a few days, such as a long weekend; it has been termed the "Monday disease." To prevent this loss of tolerance, workers usually carry nitrites home with them, or rub these chemicals in their clothing.

Propranolol

Exercise enhances sympathetic nerve activity causing an increase in the force and rate of cardiac contractions. This leads to greater consumption of oxygen by the heart muscle and precipitation of an anginal attack in susceptible individuals. In recent years, β-adrenergic receptor blocking agents, in particular propranolol, have gained widespread acceptance in the treatment of angina.

Propranolol (Inderal) antagonizes these exercised-induced, sympathetically mediated positive inotropic (force) and chronotropic (rate) effects on the heart. While coronary blood flow is generally diminished after administration of propranolol, this is more than offset by a marked reduction in the oxygen requirements of the heart muscle. Chronic use of propranolol decreases the frequency of anginal attacks. Patients are generally advised to employ sublingual nitroglycerin to terminate acute attacks.

SUMMARY

The normal function of the cardiovascular system is dependent upon the ability of the heart to serve as an effective pump. If this pump is inefficient, either because it contracts feebly or nonsynchronously, the body's requirements for an adequate blood flow will not be achieved. In addition, the heart muscle itself needs a continuous supply of oxygen and nutrients to carry out its activities.

The steroid glycosides obtained from the foxglove plant, *Digitalis,* are among the most powerful stimulants of the force of myocardial contraction. This positive inotropic action enhances the cardiac output and improves the systemic circulation of blood, without the expenditure of additional oxygen or nutrients. Moreover, direct and indirect actions of digitalis slow the heart rate.

The various digitalis products available to the physician for the treatment of congestive heart failure and atrial fibrillation differ primarily with respect to their onset and duration of action. Although digitalis represents one of the most valuable therapeutic agents available, it possesses a very narrow margin of safety. As a consequence, a therapeutic dose borders upon a toxic dose.

---

[3] Pure nitroglycerin, a liquid, is used to prepare dynamite. However, when used medically, it is mixed with inert ingredients such as lactose to form safe, nonexplosive tablets.

Quinidine is an antiarrhythmic agent, that is, it corrects abnormal atrial or ventricular rhythmic contractions of the heart. These effects are accomplished by (1) a reduction in the excitability of the heart to impulses arising from normal and abnormal (ectopic) pacemakers; (2) a decrease in the speed of the conduction of the nerve impulse; and (3) a prolongation of the refractory period of the heart.

The pain or fear of pain arising from angina can be highly detrimental to the patient attempting to carry out normal day-to-day activities. This pain has been attributed to a state of myocardial oxygen deficiency. Antianginal nitrites and nitrates such as nitroglycerin are believed to act as coronary vasodilators by increasing the blood flow supplying the heart, as well as by reducing cardiac work and the oxygen requirements of this organ. Rapid tolerance develops to these effects which proves to be a marked disadvantage for the patient with angina, while an advantage for the industrial worker who is spared from nitrite-induced severe headaches. The antianginal properties of the β-adrenergic receptor blocking agent propranolol have been attributed to its ability to reduce the oxygen requirements of the heart muscle. These beneficial effects result from antagonism of exercise-promoted, sympathetically mediated increases in the force and rate of cardiac contractions.

SUPPLEMENTARY READINGS

Anderson, J. L., D. C. Harrison, P. J. Meffin, and R. A. Winkle, "Antiarrhythmic Drugs: Clinical Pharmacology and Therapeutic Uses," *Drugs* **15**: 271–309 (1978).

Brower, L. P., and S. C. Glazier, "Localization of Heart Poisons in the Monarch Butterfly," *Science* **188**: 19–25 (1975).

Charlier, R., *Antianginal Drugs.* New York: Springer-Verlag, 1971.

Doherty, J. E., and J. J. Kane, "Clinical Pharmacology of Digitalis Glycosides," *Annual Review of Medicine* **26**: 159–71 (1975).

Epstein, S. E., D. R. Redwood, et al., "Angina Pectoris: Pathophysiology, Evaluation, and Treatment," *Annals of Internal Medicine* **75**: 263–96 (1971).

Gensini, G. G., ed., *The Study of Systemic Coronary and Myocardial Effects of Nitrates.* Springfield, Ill.: Charles C Thomas, 1972.

Marks, B. H., and A. M. Weissler, eds., *Basic and Clinical Pharmacology of Digitalis.* Springfield, Ill.: Charles C Thomas, 1972.

Mason, D. T., "Digitalis Pharmacology and Therapeutics: Recent Advances," *Annals of Internal Medicine* **80**: 520–30 (1974).

Needleman, P., ed., *Organic Nitrates. Handbook of Experimental Pharmacology,* Vol. 40. Berlin: Springer-Verlag, 1975.

Resnekov, L., ed., "Symposium on Cardiac Rhythm Disturbances, I & II," *Medical Clinics of North America* **60**(1, 2): 1–386 (1976).

Smith, T. W, and E. Haber, "Digitalis," *New England Journal of Medicine* **289**: 945–52, 1010–15, 1063–72, 1125–29 (1973).

21

Antihypertensive and Diuretic Agents

The patient should develop "a way of life" compatible with the handicap which exists. . . . Drugs which are prescribed specifically for blood pressure reduction are of little value.

—Hugh J. Morgan (1943)

[P]henobarbital has long been the treatment of choice . . . [and] appears to be useful in most cases of hypertension. At least there does not seem to be any disagreement among clinicians with regard to the value of this single drug in the treatment of the disease.

—John C. Krantz, Jr., and C. Jelleff Carr (1951)

Great progress has been made in attempting to add to the armamentarium of the physician drugs based upon a correction of the basic etiological factors of hypertension. At present not any of these experiments has brought to the clinics a completely suitable drug useful in the treatment of the disease. Nevertheless great strides have been made.

—John C. Krantz, Jr., and C. Jelleff Carr (1958)

Albeit imperfect, empiric, and palliative, antihypertensive drug therapy, when effectively and judiciously administered, prevents or postpones cardiovascular and renal complications and prolongs useful life.

—Ray W. Gifford, Jr. (1972)

As can be readily appreciated from the chronology of these quotations, the development of effective and relatively nontoxic drugs for the management of hypertension represents a comparatively recent advance in therapeutics. In spite of the monumental progress that has been made in the past three decades, hypertension and its associated medical complications continue to represent a major cause of death in the United States and Western Europe. Diuretics, drugs that promote the excretion of electrolytes and water by the kidneys, are not only employed to treat edema (excessive accumulation of bodily fluids), but are the most extensively prescribed class of drugs for the treatment of hypertension. In this chapter we shall examine the major classes of antihypertensive and diuretic agents.

HYPERTENSION AND ANTIHYPERTENSIVE AGENTS

A large number of chemically unrelated drugs are now available that are capable of reducing elevated blood pressure by a variety of mechanisms. In the absence of a basic understanding of the cause or causes of primary or essential hypertension, drug therapy is largely empirical and merely serves to modify the symptoms of the disorder without correcting the underlying pathophysiological factors responsible for its occurrence. We shall begin by considering an overview of hypertension.

Hypertension

Hypertension or high blood pressure is the most common disease of the cardiovascular system; recent estimates indicate that about 23 million Americans have elevated blood pressure. Severe and persistent hypertension has far-reaching adverse effects on the body, affecting the heart, arteries, and kidneys. Hypertension increases the work load placed on the heart, eventually resulting in an increase in the size of this organ. Unfortunately, the coronary blood flow does not proportionately increase to meet the greater requirements for oxygen, and angina pectoris often ensues. Atherosclerosis progresses more rapidly in hypertensive individuals, thereby increasing the risk of coronary artery disease. The blood vessels in the kidneys and brain are weakened by chronic hypertension, which may, in time, lead to their rupture. Damage to the kidneys and impairment of renal function is a common consequence of hypertension. Stroke is a destruction of brain tissue resulting from the rupture and bleeding of a cerebral blood vessel.

About 85 to 90 percent of all cases of high blood pressure are of unknown etiology and are referred to as *primary* or *essential hypertension.* In such cases, we often observe extensive *constriction of the arterioles.* Although this arteriolar vasoconstriction has not been shown to result from aberrations in vasoconstrictor catecholamines, many of the effective antihypertensive agents currently employed prevent the synthesis or release of catecholamines or deplete their stores in nerve endings. It has also been postulated that primary hypertension may be caused by an imbalance of *sodium* in the smooth muscle of blood vessels. A sodium-restricted diet and the use of diuretic agents that promote the excretion of sodium both reduce hypertension.

In recent years, increasing interest has been focused upon the possible involvement of the *renin-angiotensin system* in some hypertensive disorders. A reduction in the arterial blood pressure or low levels of plasma sodium stimulate the secretion of the enzyme *renin* from the kidneys. This enzyme is involved in the formation of *angiotensin II,* the most potent vasoconstrictor and pressor compound known. In addition to increasing arterial blood pressure (by causing arteriolar vasoconstriction), angiotensin II promotes the release of aldosterone from the adrenal cortex. This hormone causes a reduction in the excretion of salt and water by the kidney leading to an increase in blood volume and blood pressure. Catecholamines have been shown to stimulate renin secretion by an interaction involving β-adrenergic receptors (Chapters 5 and 6). While it is generally accepted that the renin-angiotensin system plays a role in some hyertensive states, it remains to be determined how widespread and to what magnitude this system is involved in essential hypertension.

High blood pressure that is caused by an identifiable underlying disorder is referred to broadly as *secondary hypertension.* Often the underlying condition is one that involves the blood vessels (arteriosclerosis or "hardening of arteries") or kidneys. Whereas primary hypertension can be controlled, it cannot be cured. By contrast, secondary hypertension can often be cured by correcting the underlying cause.

MANAGEMENT OF HYPERTENSION: AN OVERVIEW

The primary therapeutic objective in hypertensive therapy is to maintain blood pressure within normal limits without reducing cardiac output or interfering with the circulation of blood to vital organs such as the brain, heart, and kidneys. Life expectancy is inversely related to blood pressures over a wide range. Long-term studies have established that holding blood pressure at or near normotensive levels decreases the morbidity and mortality generally associated with hypertension. Effective treatment significantly reduces the complications of congestive heart failure and damage to the kidneys, to a lesser extent reduces the frequency of stroke, but appears to confer little benefit in decreasing the incidence of coronary artery disease.

Antihypertensive therapy is highly individualized with respect to the selection of drugs and the dosage employed. Among the most important factors taken into consideration with respect to the choice of drug therapy is the coexistence of other medical disorders (kidney disease, diabetes, gout, asthma) and the severity of the hypertensive state. The latter is generally assessed by evaluating the patient for tissue damage to the heart, kidneys, and eyes, and by monitoring diastolic blood pressure. Hypertension is often asymptomatic and, therefore, may remain undiagnosed and untreated for extensive periods of time.

Physicians often use a combination of drugs for the management of hypertension. Smaller doses of several individual drugs may be prescribed to produce reductions in blood pressure of the same magnitude as might be achieved by employing a large dose of a single drug. Judicious combination therapy may retard the development of tolerance to the beneficial antihypertensive effects and reduce the incidence and/or severity of adverse side effects; for example, one drug may be used to antagonize or minimize the adverse effects caused by another antihypertensive agent.

Patient noncompliance is a major problem in the clinical management of hypertension. If asymptomatic or experiencing only minor discomfort from the hypertensive state, the patient may unilaterally conclude that the drug-induced side effects are more distressful[1] than the potential benefits to be derived from the prescribed drugs and fail to take the medication as directed, if at all.

Drug Treatment of Primary Hypertension

As we shall observe, with the possible exception of the diuretic agents, virtually all other hypertensive agents ultimately act by reducing sympathetically induced vasoconstriction of the arterioles. You will recall from Chapter 19 that arterial blood pressure is influenced by cardiac output and the peripheral vascular resistance exerted primarily in the arterioles. Vasoconstriction increases peripheral resistance, which causes an elevation in blood pressure; conversely, vasodilation of the arterioles reduces peripheral resistance and blood pressure. We shall return to this fundamental principle many times during our discussion of antihypertensive agents. From a therapeutic viewpoint, drugs that cause peripheral vasodilation should not reduce cardiac output or interfere with the circulation of blood to the vital organs of the body. That is, blood must continue to circulate adequately to and supply the nutritional requirements of the brain, heart, and kidneys.

We shall categorize antihypertensive agents according to their primary site of action (Figure 21-1) and shall consider the most important pharmacological properties of prototype members of each class. Although primary attention will be focused upon the major mechanisms responsible for the antihypertensive effects, it should be borne in mind that in many instances secondary actions contribute to the ultimately observed effects. Our discussion will include centrally acting drugs, ganglionic blocking agents, drugs acting at peripheral sympathetic nerves and adrenergic receptors, compounds causing arteriolar vasodilation, and diuretics. Table 21-1 lists representative drugs from each of these classes.

---

[1] Disturbances in sexual function, which may include decreased libido, inability to maintain an erection, and interference with ejaculation in men and the failure to achieve orgasm in women, may occur in 20 to 30 percent of patients receiving the antihypertensive agents clonidine, guanethidine, and methyldopa.

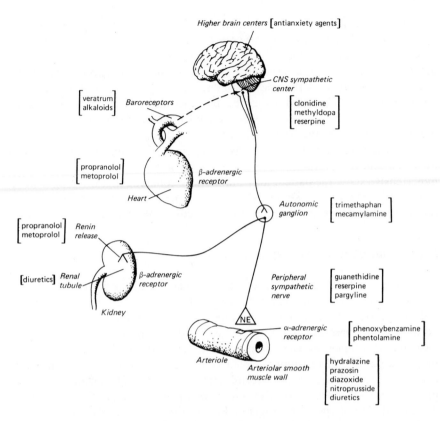

FIGURE 21-1. Sites of Action of Antihypertensive Agents.

Centrally Acting Drugs

The *vasomotor center,* located in the brainstem, transmits impulses through the spinal cord to sympathetic vasoconstrictor fibers which innervate all the blood vessels of the body. This center is normally active, and its impulses maintain a partial state of contraction in the smooth muscles of the blood vessels; this state is termed *vasomotor tone.* The level of activity of this system is controlled by central and peripheral influences.

Higher centers of the brain, including the hypothalamus and cerebral cortex, control the activity of the vasomotor center and, thereby, influence the degree of arteriolar vasoconstriction and arterial blood pressure. In the periphery, blood flow and arterial blood pressure are controlled by circulatory reflexes, the most important of which is the *baroreceptor reflex.* An increase in arterial blood pressure stretches the walls of the major arteries located in the chest and neck causing excitation of stretch receptors in the carotid sinus and aortic arch. Signals are transmitted from these receptors to the vasomotor center and reflex signals are sent back to the heart and blood vessels causing a slowing of the heart rate, dilation of the blood vessels, and a reduction in blood pressure to normal levels. A reduction in blood pressure below normal levels sets into motion the opposite effects.

Centrally acting drugs include the sedatives and drugs that reduce sympathetic function by their direct or indirect effects on the vasomotor center.

Antianxiety agents. The barbiturates (phenobarbital) and benzodiazepines (chlordiazepoxide, diazepam) do not possess specific antihypertensive properties. Their depressant effects on the higher brain centers produces a calming effect and relieves anxiety which may contribute to a mild hypertensive state in some patients.

Veratrum alkaloids. The veratrum alkaloids (obtained from the green and white hellebore) reduce heart rate and arterial blood pressure by reflexly inhibiting central sympathetic function. These drugs sensitize baroreceptors resulting in reflex inhibition of the vasomotor center in the brain stem. The veratrum alkaloids have a low margin of safety and are rarely used in modern medicine.

Methyldopa and clonidine are thought to lower blood pressure by mechanisms that result in depression of the central sympathetic center. Available evidence does not permit us to exclude the possibility that the peripheral actions of these drugs contributes to their antihypertensive effects.

Methyldopa. You will recall from Chapter 6 (Figure 6-1) that norepinephrine is formed in the body via the following synthetic pathway: tyrosine → dopa (dihydroxyphenylalanine) → dopamine → norepinephrine. When methyldopa (Aldomet) was shown to possess antihypertensive activity, it was initially postulated that this compound prevented the decarboxylation of dopa to form dopamine, and thereby inhibited the synthesis of norepinephrine. While such a peripheral action may contribute to the observed reduction in elevated blood pressure, more recent studies suggest that the primary site of action of methyldopa is in the central nervous system. It is now believed that methyldopa enters this synthetic pathway, and that it (rather than dopa) is preferentially decarboxylated to form α-*methylnorepinephrine* via the intermediate compound α-methyldopamine. The antihypertensive effects result from α-methylnorepinephrine-induced blockade of the central sympathetic centers. Compounds acting like α-methylnorepinephrine are termed *false neurotransmitters.*[2]

Methyldopa is a useful drug for the chronic treatment of hypertension and may also be administered intravenously for the emergency management of life-threatening hypertensive crises. Drowsiness, sedation, and weakness are common side effects associated with the use of this drug. Salt and water retention leading to edema and weight gain are common if a diuretic is not coadministered with methyldopa.

---

[2] The use of methyldopa to form a biologically less active neurotransmitter or false neurotransmitter bears some similarity to the chemotherapeutic use of *antimetabolites* to form abnormal products that cannot be effectively utilized by bacterial or cancer cells (Chapter 2).

TABLE 21-1. COMPARATIVE PROPERTIES OF ANTIHYPERTENSIVE AGENTS

Site of Action*	General Mechanism	Representative Examples Generic Name (Trade Name)	Remarks
Higher brain centers (cerebral cortex)	Antianxiety effects, mild sedation.	Phenobarbital Chlordiazepoxide (Librium)	Nonspecific antihypertensive effect; useful when anxiety causes mild hypertensive state.
Central sympathetic center (hypothalamus)	Decreases sympathetic tone in periphery.	Methyldopa (Aldomet) Clonidine (Catapres) Reserpine (Serpasil) ‡ Propranolol (Inderal) ‡	Effective drugs with a high incidence of CNS depression. *Methyldopa:* false neurotransmitter formation. *Clonidine:* also peripheral actions—inhibition of NE release from sympathetic nerve endings and renin from kidneys.
Baroreceptors (carotid sinus and aortic arch)	Sensitizes baroreceptors to BP changes resulting in reflex inhibition of vasomotor center (medulla).	Alkavervir (Veriloid) Cryptenamine (Unitensen)	Veratrum alkaloids (from hellebore plant) are effective antihypertensive agents but high incidence of adverse effects; rarely used.
Autonomic ganglia	Inhibits transmission of nerve impulses at autonomic ganglia.	Trimethaphan (Arfonad) Mecamylamine (Inversine)	Ganglionic blocking agents are effective but cause high incidence of adverse effects especially orthostatic hypotension and fainting; rarely used. *Trimethaphan:* used for hypertensive crisis.
Peripheral sympathetic nerves	(1) Depletes NE† from sympathetic nerve endings. (2) Blocks NE release and depletes NE. (3) Blocks NE release.	Reserpine (Serpasil) Guanethidine (Ismelin) Clonidine (Catapres) ‡ Pargyline (Eutonyl)	*Reserpine's* antihypertensive actions include: (1) depletion of peripheral NE stores, (2) depression of sympathetic centers in hypothalamus, (3) tranquilization. *Guanethidine:* used for severe hypertension; may cause orthostatic hypotension. *Pargyline:* monoamine oxidase inhibitor; mechanism underlying antihypertensive effects not well understood.
α-adrenergic receptors	Antagonizes NE-induced activation of α-adrenergic receptors pro-	Phenoxybenzamine (Dibenzyline) Phentolamine (Regitine)	High incidence of adverse cardiovascular effects; rarely used.

Site*	Mechanism of Action	Drug†	Comments
	ducing arteriolar vasoconstriction.		
β-adrenergic receptors	Antagonizes NE-induced activation of β-adrenergic receptors: (1) in the heart reducing cardiac output; (2) in the kidney blocking renin release, thereby inhibiting angiotensin II synthesis.	Propranolol (Inderal) Metoprolol (Lopressor) Nadolol (Corgard)	*Propranolol:* primarily used in combination with other drugs; inhibits reflex heart stimulation caused by hydralazine.
Arteriolar smooth muscle	(1) Direct vasodilation reducing peripheral vascular resistance. (2) Diuretics alter concentration of ions in smooth muscle causing vasodilation.	Hydralazine (Apresoline) Prazosin (Minipress) Minoxidil (Loniten) Diazoxide (Hyperstat I.V.) Sodium nitroprusside (Nipride) Diuretics Propranolol (Inderal)	*Hydralazine:* high incidence of adverse effects including reflex stimulation of heart rate and cardiac output. *Diazoxide:* thiazide devoid of diuretic properties; administered intravenously for hypertensive crisis; causes salt and water retention and an increase in blood sugar (hyperglycemia). *Nitroprusside:* administered intravenously for short-term management of hypertensive crisis.
Kidney	(1) Blocks renin release from kidney, inhibits angiotension synthesis. (2) Diuretics increase urine output, reduce plasma volume, decreasing cardiac output and blood pressure.	Chlorothiazide (Diuril) Furosemide (Lasix) Spironolactone (Aldactone)	*Diuretics:* only weak antihypertensive effect when used alone; very commonly employed in combination with other antihypertensive agents (Table 21-2).

*Sites depicted on Figure 21-1.

†NE = norepinephrine

‡Secondary actions thought to contribute to the antihypertensive effects.

Clonidine.　Clonidine, a recently introduced drug, is thought to produce hypotension and bradycardia primarily by a mechanism involving activation of central α-adrenergic receptors that cause inhibition of sympathetic nerve activity[3] in the vasomotor center. Clonidine (Catapres) has also been shown to act peripherally by inhibiting the release of norepinephrine from sympathetic nerves and renin from the kidneys. Very common side effects caused by clonidine include sedation, dry mouth, and orthostatic hypotension (see below).

Ganglionic Blocking Agents

Drugs capable of interrupting the transmission of the nerve impulse at the autonomic ganglia are among the most potent antihypertensive agents available, although, due to their lack of specificity of action, they are rarely used in modern therapeutics. In the autonomic nervous system messages are carried from the spinal cord along two motor nerve fibers, the second of which innervates an effector cell; these two neurons synapse at the *autonomic ganglion* (Chapter 5). *Ganglionic blocking agents* compete with acetylcholine for cholinergic receptor sites located at the synapse of the autonomic ganglia, thereby reducing the transmission of nerve impulses from preganglionic nerves to *both* sympathetic and parasympathetic postganglionic nerves.

Blockade of postganglionic sympathetic nerve transmission prevents arteriolar vasoconstriction resulting in a profound reduction in blood pressure; this is the desired therapeutic response. Normally when we stand after lying down, a sympathetically mediated vasoconstrictor reflex is activated which enables us to maintain adequate blood flow to the brain. Ganglionic blocking agents also prevent this compensatory vasoconstriction, causing a deficiency in the blood supply to the brain which results in fainting. This is termed *orthostatic hypotension* and is one of the undesirable side effects associated with many antihypertensive agents.

As you might predict, transmission of nerve impulses to postganglionic parasympathetic neurons is also suppressed, causing many undesirable side effects, including dry mouth, constipation, urinary retention, blurred vision, and an inability to accommodate the muscles of the eye for close vision. The ganglionic blocking agents are rarely used in the contemporary treatment of hypertension, having been replaced by safer, more specific, and equally effective drugs.

[3] In preliminary clinical trials, clonidine has been found to be highly effective in suppressing the withdrawal symptoms associated with dependence on methadone and other narcotics (Chapter 13). It has been hypothesized that after opiate abstinence, messages are sent to a brain stem nucleus (locus ceruleus) from opiate receptors, causing excessive firing of norepinephrine-containing nerves and resulting in the multiple mental and physical symptoms associated with withdrawal. Clonidine is thought to act by suppressing the excessive activity of these sympathetic neurons.

Drugs Acting at Peripheral Sympathetic Nerves

Antihypertensive agents having their primary site of action at sympathetic (adrenergic) nerve endings may act via several separate and distinct mechanisms; these include depletion of norepinephrine, blockade of the release of norepinephrine, and modification of the normal synthesis of norepinephrine. In all cases, we observe a reduction in the effective concentration of norepinephrine released by the sympathetic nerve endings in response to a nerve impulse, and, as a consequence, we see a reduction in sympathetically mediated vasoconstriction. Unlike the ganglionic blocking agents, these drugs do not interrupt the transmission of nerve impulses in postganglionic parasympathetic neurons and are, therefore, far more specific in their effects.

Depletion of norepinephrine: reserpine. In Chapter 16 we considered reserpine and its contribution to providing a better fundamental understanding of the biochemistry of mental illness and the mechanism of action of psychoactive drugs. Although reserpine is now rarely used as an antipsychotic agent, at present it is employed for the treatment of mild hypertension, very often in combination with a thiazide diuretic, such as chlorothiazide (see below).

Reserpine's hypotensive effects have been primarily ascribed to a depletion of norepinephrine from peripheral sympathetic nerve endings by altering the ability of the nerve ending storage granules to properly bind and concentrate norepinephrine. The improperly stored neurotransmitter is free to diffuse from these protective binding sites and is inactivated by enzymes inside the neuron. Depletion of norepinephrine from the nerve ending reduces the concentration of neurotransmitter available to be released and interact with the arterioles to cause vasoconstriction.

In addition to its peripheral effects, reserpine also exerts a marked action on the central nervous system. This compound has been shown to cause depletion of norepinephrine and serotonin from nerve endings located in the hypothalamus, and these effects are generally thought to be responsible for reserpine's tranquilizing or calming properties.

With reserpine-induced impairment of sympathetic activation, there is a disruption of the balance between opposing sympathetic and parasympathetic effects, resulting in a predominance of parasympathetic activity. This leads to a variety of undesirable side effects, including nasal congestion and stuffiness, visual disturbances, slowing of the heart rate, diarrhea, and an increase in gastric acid secretion, with possible ulcer formation. In addition, behavioral changes may occur, leading to drowsiness, apathy, and even severe depression.

Blockade of norepinephrine release: guanethidine. Guanethidine (Ismelin) is a potent drug used for the treatment of severe hypertension. This drug is believed to lower blood pressure by two different actions on norepinephrine in peripheral sympathetic nerves. One of these actions involves a gradual depletion of the stores of this catecholamine by a reserpine-like interference with its storage in vesicles in nerve endings. A second and far more important action involves the ability of guanethidine to effectively prevent the release of norepinephrine in response to a nerve impulse, an action produced by stabilization of the neuronal membrane. Drugs acting by this latter mechanism are referred to as *adrenergic neuron blocking agents.* While such drugs do not interfere with the action of direct-acting adrenergic agents, that is, drugs that themselves activate the adrenergic receptor site (phenylephrine), these drugs prevent the action of some indirect adrenergic agents (tyramine) that enter the neuron and stimulate the release of norepinephrine from nerve endings (Chapter 6).

The most frequently encountered adverse side effect caused by guanethidine is postural hypotension, which is generally manifested as dizziness when the patient arises from bed in the morning. Unlike reserpine, methyldopa, and clonidine, guanethidine does not cross the blood-brain barrier and, therefore, does not cause sedation or depression.

Adrenergic Receptor Blocking Agents

Alpha-adrenergic receptor blockers: phenoxybenzamine.   Norepinephrine-induced activation of α-adrenergic receptors causes arteriolar vasoconstriction. While it might be assumed that an α-adrenergic blocker, such as phenoxybenzamine (Dibenzyline) or phentolamine (Regitine), might be useful for the treatment of hypertension, the clinical results have been generally disappointing because of the high incidence of reflex tachycardia, palpitations of the heart, and orthostatic hypotension.

Beta-adrenergic   receptor   blockers: propranolol.   The β-adrenergic blockers propranolol (Inderal),[4] metoprolol (Lopressor), and nadolol (Corgard) have been recently approved for use as antihypertensive agents in the United States. These drugs are thought to produce their antihypertensive effects by one or more of the following mechanisms: (1) by competitively antagonizing catecholamines at peripheral sites (the heart), resulting in a reduction in cardiac output; (2) by a central action reducing the sympathetic outflow to the periphery; and (3) by blocking renin release from the kidneys and thereby inhibiting angiotensin II synthesis.

Propranolol is primarily employed in combination with other antihypertensive agents; it inhibits the reflex stimulation of the heart associated with the administration of hydralazine (see below). Propranolol and nadolol nonselectively block β_1- and β_2-adrenergic receptors (Chapter 6), the latter action resulting in pronounced bronchoconstriction in patients with bronchial asthma and other obstructive respiratory disorders. The blocking actions of metoprolol are relatively selective for the β_1-receptors in the heart.

---

[4] This was the second most commonly prescribed drug in the United States in 1979.

Direct Arteriolar Vasodilators

Arteriolar vasodilators act directly on the smooth muscle of the arteriolar wall causing vasodilation, a reduction in peripheral vascular resistance, and a decrease in blood pressure.

Hydralazine (Apresoline). In addition to its ability to reduce elevated blood pressure by vasodilation, hydralazine also causes reflex stimulation of heart rate and cardiac output. These latter effects, if not antagonized with propranolol, could negate the antihypertensive effects of this drug. Hydralazine's potential utility in the treatment of moderate-to-severe hypertension has been greatly limited by many adverse side effects, a number of which are potentially very serious.

Diazoxide (Hyperstat I.V.). Diazoxide is chemically related to the thiazides (see below), but lacks diuretic activity. Within five minutes after intravenous administration, there is a dramatic reduction in blood pressure that persists for from two to twelve hours. Diazoxide is among the most valuable drugs currently available for the treatment of *hypertensive crisis;* this medical emergency is characterized by diastolic blood pressures exceeding 140 mm Hg and, if not treated immediately, may cause moderate-to-severe tissue damage. The use of diazoxide is not generally required for more than four or five days at which time the patient's blood pressure is controlled with orally effective antihypertensive agents. Adverse side effects associated with diazoxide administration include salt and water retention and a rise in blood glucose levels (hyperglycemia).

Diuretics

Thiazides: chlorothiazide. In this section, we shall limit our discussion of diuretics to the thiazide class and their antihypertensive effects. In the second part of this chapter, we shall examine the physiology of the kidney and the general pharmacology and therapeutic applications of all major classes of diuretic agents.

Acting by a variety of mechanisms at different sites in the kidney (Figure 21–2), diuretic agents increase the excretion of salts and water. The *thiazides* are the most frequently employed class of diuretics (Table 21–2). *Chlorothiazide* (Diuril), the first member of this class introduced in 1957, remains the prototype thiazide.

Diuretic agents are among the most widely used group of drugs for the treatment of hypertension. When employed alone, the thiazides possess only weak antihypertensive properties and are only useful for the management of mild hypertension. Their main clinical utility is to augment the hypotensive effects of other coadministered antihypertensive agents, permitting a reduction in the dosage of these drugs and thereby decreasing the incidence of side effects associated with their use. Moreover, the thiazides antagonize the salt and water retaining properties of many antihypertensive agents.

Arterial blood pressure is strongly influenced by the cardiac output and volume of blood (plasma volume) contained in the arteries. During the early phases of chlorothiazide administration, we observe a reduction in plasma volume and, consequently, a decrease in cardiac output. After continuous drug administration for several weeks, plasma volume and cardiac output return to predrug levels, but peripheral resistance remains reduced and the hypotensive effects are maintained. Thus, the antihypertensive effects of the thiazides cannot be explained simply on the basis of a reduction in body fluid volumes. Although at present the basic antihypertensive mechanism of the thiazides is not known, it has been suggested that the observed arteriolar vasodilation may result from a direct drug action on the arteriolar smooth muscle, possibly by causing a favorable redistribution in the concentration of sodium and potassium in the muscle.

KIDNEY PHYSIOLOGY AND DIURETIC AGENTS

The urine of a man is one of the animal matters that have been the most examined by chemists, and of which the examination has at the same time furnished the most singular discoveries to chemistry, and the most useful application to physiology, as well as the art of healing. This liquid which commonly inspires men only with contempt and disgust, which is generally ranked amongst vile and repulsive matters, has become, in the hands of the chemists, a source of important discoveries.[5]

—Count Antoine François de Fourcroy (1755–1809)

It is no exaggeration to say that the composition of the blood is determined not by what the mouth takes in but by what the kidneys keep.
Superficially, it might be said that the function of the kidneys is to make urine; but in a more considered view one can say that the kidneys make the stuff of philosophy itself.[6]

—Homer W. Smith (1953)

In this section we shall discuss the various diuretic agents. First, however, we shall provide the reader with a foundation of those basic elements of kidney physiology required to understand the actions and effects of these drugs.

Kidney Physiology

The kidneys serve three primary physiological functions: (1) they are primarily responsible for the elimination of the end products of metabolism and

[5] *A General System of Chemical Knowledge, and Its Application to the Phenomena of Nature and Art,* in *Familar Medical Quotations,* ed. M. B. Strauss (Boston: Little, Brown, 1968) p. 648.
[6] *From Fish to Philosopher* (Boston: Little, Brown, 1953).

the retention and conservation of useful nutrients; (2) they maintain the electrolyte balance of body fluids which in turn controls the volume of the fluids of the body; and (3) they play a critical role in maintaining the acid-base balance of the body.

Each of our two kidneys contains over one million *nephrons,* each of which is capable of forming urine. The nephron (Figure 21–2), the fundamental unit of the kidney, consists of the *glomerulus,* from which the fluid is filtered, and a long *tubule*[7] in which the filtered fluid is converted to urine. We shall now examine these component parts and the function of the nephron in somewhat greater detail.

The rate of blood flow through both kidneys is about 20 percent of the total cardiac output. Blood enters the glomerulus through the afferent arteriole and exits via the efferent arteriole. The glomerulus consists of a network of capillaries. The pressure of blood in the glomerulus causes *filtration* of water, most of the essential components of the extracellular fluid, and the waste products of metabolism. The glomerular filtration rate in a healthy individual is 125 ml per minute. Proteins and protein-bound drugs and other substances are not filtered by the glomerulus.

The filtrate flows first into the *proximal tubules* and then into the *loop of Henle.* Ascending from the loop of Henle, the fluid passes into the *distal tubules* to the collecting duct; after emptying into the renal pelvis, the urine is transported to the bladder via the ureter. The nephron normally reabsorbs and thus returns to the blood 99 percent of the glomerular filtrate, with only 1 percent excreted as urine. The normal daily urine output is 1.5 liters.

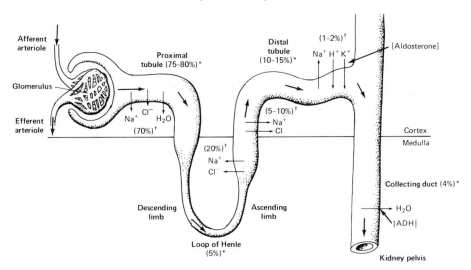

FIGURE 21–2. The Nephron with Sites of Electrolyte and Water Reabsorption. Key to symbols: * = percentage of water reabsorbed in each segment of the kidney tubule; † = percentage of sodium reabsorbed.

---

[7] The total length of all the tubules in both kidneys is about 112 km (70 miles).

Water and Electrolyte Reabsorption

Approximately 75–80 percent of the electrolytes and water filtered by the glomerulus is reabsorbed across the walls of the *proximal tubules* and returned to the blood. Sodium is actively reabsorbed, with chloride and water following by a passive process. Although you might assume that inhibition of salt and water reabsorption at the proximal tubules might represent a primary site of action of diuretic agents, experimental evidence does not support this prediction; inhibition of transport processes in the distal tubules results in a far more copious urine output.

As the filtrate enters the descending limb of the *loop of Henle,* water is reabsorbed and the remaining fluid becomes far more concentrated (hypertonic).[8] As the fluid passes up the ascending loop of Henle, about 20–30 percent of the sodium and chloride are reabsorbed. Since this segment of the kidney tubules does not permit the reabsorption of water, the fluid becomes more dilute (hypotonic).

In the *distal tubules,* under the influence of the hormone *aldosterone,* additional sodium and chloride are reabsorbed and potassium or hydrogen ions are added to the fluid. The exchange of sodium and hydrogen ions represents an important mechanism by which the kidneys carry out one of their critical functions, namely, maintenance of the acid-base balance of the body. Water reabsorption occurs in the *collecting duct,* a transport process mediated by *antidiuretic hormone* (ADH, vasopressin), a hormone released from the neurohypophysis (posterior pituitary gland, Chapter 22).

Diuretic Agents

Diuretic agents enhance urine output by one or more of the following mechanisms:

1. Enhancement of the rate of glomerular filtration (theophylline)
2. Inhibition of the reabsorption of sodium by a direct action on the kidney tubules (mercurials, thiazides, ethacrynic acid, furosemide)
3. Inhibition of sodium reabsorption by an osmotic action (mannitol)
4. Inhibition of the exchange of sodium ions for hydrogen ions (carbonic anhydrase inhibitors)
5. Inhibition of the ability of aldosterone to promote the reabsorption of sodium (spironolactone)
6. Inhibition of the release of antidiuretic hormone (ethyl alcohol)

[8] The process involved with the concentration of the glomerular filtrate, termed the *countercurrent mechanism,* is quite complex and beyond the scope of this text.

Pharmacological Properties

Diuretics are generally classified according to their chemistry or pharmacological actions; examples of the major classes of diuretics appear on Table 21-2. The sites of action of these drugs are depicted in Figure 21-3.

Organomercurials (mercurials). Mercury-containing compounds play a prominent role in the history of therapeutics. For 400 years after the arrival of Columbus in the New World, mercury ointment was the treatment of choice for syphilis. In the sixteenth century, Paracelsus promoted *calomel*[9] (mercurous chloride) as a cathartic and diuretic. During the last century, Guy's Hospital pills (containing calomel, squill, and digitalis) were a highly regarded diuretic preparation.

The modern age of organic mercurial diuretics began shortly after World War I when merbaphen (Novasurol), a chemotherapeutic agent used for the treatment of syphilis, was found to produce marked diuresis. The organomercurials were to remain unchallenged as diuretic agents for the next three decades. After the development of orally active, potent, effective, and less toxic diuretics in the 1950's, however, the popularity of the organomercurials plummeted, and they are now rarely used.

The mercurials promote the loss of salt and water by depressing tubular mechanisms responsible for the active reabsorption of sodium and chloride. The primary use of this class of drugs is for the treatment of edema caused by congestive heart failure, kidney disease, and cirrhosis of the liver. Within twelve hours after a single injection of an organomercurial agent, a loss of 2.5 percent of the body weight (in excess fluids) is considered to be an average therapeutic response.

---

[9] To combat the 1793 yellow fever epidemic in Philadelphia, the most illustrious physician of the postcolonial period, Dr. Benjamin Rush (1745–1813), ordered generous bloodletting and calomel for his patients. Space limitations preclude the author from mounting a defense on behalf of this patriot-Continental Congressman–signer of the Declaration of Independence–medical educator against the charges made by some fellow Philadelphia physicians accusing him of "killing more people [with his recommended cure] than the plague itself."

The use of calomel and bloodletting was a versatile treatment that enjoyed great favor with the physicians of the period and was generally thought to be a panacea for a wide variety of medical complaints. One pioneer physician is reported to have remarked that he could fill the steamboat *Andrew Jackson* with all the calomel that he had prescribed and float it on the blood he had drawn from his patients!

Mercurous chloride should not be confused with *mercuric* chloride (mercury bichloride, bichloride of mercury), a highly toxic compound that was widely employed in the past as an antiseptic for the unabraded skin and as a disinfectant of inanimate objects susceptible to damage if boiled. As a precaution against their inadvertent dispensing when mercurous chloride is requested, mercuric chloride tablets are required to be of a distinctive color (traditionally blue) and have an angular or irregular, not round, shape (commonly a coffin shape). Moreover, the law requires that if mercuric chloride tablets are to be dispensed in small quantities, their glass containers must be of a distinctive angular shape and have irregular or roughened edges or sides.

TABLE 21-2. REPRESENTATIVE DIURETIC AGENTS

Generic Name	Selected Trade Names	Properties of Class/Drugs
Organomercurial (mercurial) diuretics		Effective drugs replaced by orally active, potent, and less toxic diuretics; given intramuscularly; rarely used.
Mersalyl with theophylline	Mersalyn	
Mercaptomerin	Thiomerin	
Carbonic anhydrase inhibitors		Rarely used for diuresis because of low potency and rapid development of tolerance. Primarily employed for treatment of glaucoma.
Acetazolamide	Diamox	
Dichlorphenamide	Daranide, Oratrol	
Ethoxzolamide	Cardrase, Ethamide	
Methazolamide	Neptazane	
Thiazide (benzothiadiazide) diuretics		The most widely employed class of diuretics. Orally active, rapid onset of diuresis, absence of tolerance, relatively low toxicity. All thiazides produce approximately same degree of diuresis at equieffective doses; they differ with respect to potency and time course of action. Therapeutic uses: usually the first class of drugs used in hypertension, alone or in combination; treatment of edema associated with congestive heart failure, premenstrual tension, cirrhosis of liver, pregnancy, kidney disorders, and drug-induced edema. Most adverse effects result from electrolyte imbalances, in particular, decrease in blood potassium (hypokalemia).
Bendroflumethiazide	Naturetin	
Benzthiazide	Aquatag, Exna	
Chlorothiazide	Diuril	
Chlorthalidone	Hygroton	
Cyclothiazide	Anhydron	
Hydrochlorothiazide	Esidrix, HydroDiuril, Oretic	
Hydroflumethiazide	Saluron	
Methyclothiazide	Enduron	
Metolazone	Zaroxolyn	

Polythiazide
Quinethazone
Trichlormethiazide

Renese
Hydromox
Metahydrin, Naqua

"Loop" or "high-ceiling" diuretics
Ethacrynic acid
Furosemide

Edecrin
Lasix

Most powerful diuretics in common use. Rapid onset of action (1 hr) after oral administration. Therapeutic uses: treatment of edema associated with disorders of the heart, kidney, or liver. Most adverse effects are caused by excessive loss of fluid and electrolytes (hypokalemia); temporary hearing losses reported.

Potassium-sparing diuretics
Spironolactone
Triamterene

Aldactone
Dyrenium

Rarely used alone; these relatively weak diuretics are employed in combination with other diuretics to prevent excessive potassium depletion.

Osmotic diuretics
Mannitol
Urea

Osmitrol

Rarely used, intravenously administered diuretics.

Xanthine diuretics
Theophylline
Aminophylline (theophylline ethylenediamine)

Not very effective diuretics; rarely used.

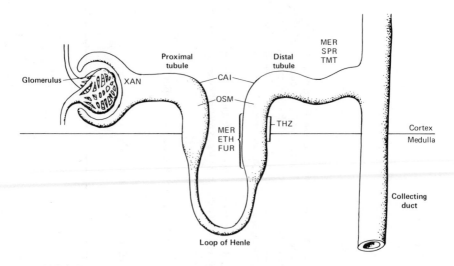

FIGURE 21-3. Sites of Diuretic Action in the Nephron. Key to abbreviations: CAI = carbonic anhydrase inhibitors; ETH = ethacrynic acid; FUR = furosemide; MER = mercurials; OSM = osmotic agents; SPR = spironolactone; THZ = thiazides; TMT = triamterene; XAN = xanthines.

Carbonic anhydrase inhibitors.   In 1937, shortly after the clinical introduction of sulfanilamide as an antibacterial agent (Chapter 28), it was recognized that this drug altered the electrolyte balance; in particular, it caused metabolic acidosis resulting from increased excretion of bicarbonate and turned the urine alkaline. This side effect was found to result from sulfanilamide-induced inhibition of the enzyme *carbonic anhydrase*. This enzyme catalyzes the hydration of dissolved carbon dioxide to form carbonic acid which in turn rapidly dissociates to yield hydrogen ions and bicarbonate.

$$CO_2 + H_2O \overset{\text{Carbonic anhydrase}}{\underset{\text{Acetazolamide}}{\rightleftharpoons}} H_2CO_3 \rightleftharpoons H^+ + HCO_3^-$$

Normally potassium and hydrogen ions exchange for sodium ions in the distal tubules; the exchange of potassium increases as the excretion of hydrogen ions decreases. After the administration of a carbonic anhydrase inhibitor, the urine contains greater than normal amounts of sodium and potassium ions in addition to bicarbonate and chloride ions. This additional excretion of salts is accompanied by the loss of a greater volume of water.

With the realization that sulfanilamide[10] was a relatively weak enzyme inhibitor, the search began for more active drugs with greater potential clinical

[10] The sulfonamide class provides interesting illustrations as to how new drugs are developed. Astute exploitation of the *side effects* of sulfanilamide and related drugs has led to the discovery and introduction of three classes of drugs: diuretics (acetazolamide, chlorothiazide), oral antidiabetic agents (chlorpropamide, tolbutamide) and antithyroid agents (propylthiouracil).

utility as diuretic agents. Among a series of new sulfonamide-like compounds developed in 1950, *acetazolamide* was found to be 300 times more active than sulfanilamide as a carbonic anhydrase inhibitor and, shortly thereafter, was made clinically available as an orally active diuretic agent.

Acetazolamide (Diamox) and other members of this class have not proven to be highly useful diuretic agents. Their therapeutic utility is limited by their relatively low potency and by rapid development of tolerance (refractoriness) to their diuretic effects.

The discoveries of the presence of carbonic anhydrase in the eye and of high concentrations of bicarbonate in the aqueous humor have led to speculation that this enzyme might play a physiological role in the formation or secretion of this fluid. Acetazolamide and related drugs (Table 21–2) decrease the rate of formation of aqueous humor and thereby reduce elevated intraocular pressure. These drugs have been found to be useful in the treatment of glaucoma (Chapter 7).

Thiazides (benzothiadiazides).   While searching for more potent carbonic anhydrase inhibitors, one promising member of a series of compounds being evaluated was found to be one-twentieth as active as acetazolamide in inhibiting carbonic anhydrase but five to ten times more effective in promoting the loss of sodium and chloride in the urine. This compound, *chlorothiazide* (Diuril), was the first thiazide diuretic made available for therapeutic use. While differences exist among the subsequently introduced thiazides (Table 21–2) with respect to their time course of action and potency, none of these drugs is safer nor produces significantly greater diuresis than chlorothiazide at equivalent therapeutic doses. In passing, it should be noted that it is possible to totally separate carbonic anhydrase inhibition from diuretic activity. Bendroflumethiazide possesses negligible enzyme inhibitory activity while producing the same degree of diuresis as chlorothiazide at one two-hundredth of the daily dose.

The thiazides increase the elimination of sodium, chloride, potassium, and water by inhibiting the active reabsorption of sodium and chloride ions at the distal tubules. They do not alter the acid-base balance and, unlike the organomercurials and carbonic anhydrase inhibitors, their diuretic effectiveness is not altered by changes in the pH of the urine.

The clinical popularity of the thiazides can be attributed to a number of significant factors: (1) They are capable of producing marked diuresis after oral administration; (2) they have a relatively rapid onset of action (2 hours) and long duration of action (12–24 hours); (3) they maintain the ability to produce effective diuresis even after extended periods of drug administration; and (4) while capable of producing potentially dangerous adverse effects resulting from electrolyte imbalances, these drugs possess a relatively low order of toxicity.

As noted above, the thiazides are most often the first class of drugs to be employed in the management of *hypertension,* and mild hypertensive states are often controlled with the sole use of these drugs. They are quite effective in the management of edema associated with congestive heart failure, cirrhosis of the liver, premenstrual tension, pregnancy, various types of kidney disorders, and of edema induced by drugs such as estrogens, glucocorticoids (cortisone-like steroids), and antihypertensive agents.

Chlorothiazide and related drugs produce a paradoxical *reduction* in urinary output (by as much as 30–50 percent) in patients with **diabetes insipidus,** a hormonal disorder resulting from a deficiency of antidiuretic hormone and characterized by extreme diuresis. While the normal 24-hour urinary output is 1.5 liters, in untreated diabetes insipidus 8–12 liters of highly dilute urine are excreted each day and up to 25–30 liters in severe cases. Thiazides are thought to produce their antidiuretic effect by decreasing the glomerular filtration rate and increasing the reabsorption of the filtrate by the proximal tubules.

Many of the *adverse effects* caused by the administration of thiazides and other diuretic agents result from *excessive losses of potassium* and sodium from the blood (hypokalemia and hyponatremia, respectively) or from a drop in blood pressure. Early signs of electrolyte abnormalities include dryness of the mouth, weakness, lethargy, muscle cramps, pain, or fatigue, marked reduction in urinary output (oliguria), and gastrointestinal disturbances. Hypokalemia predisposes patients to digitalis toxicity. To counteract potential depletion of this essential electrolyte, patients receiving diuretics are often advised to increase their intake of potassium-rich foods such as bananas, oranges, grapefruits, and apricots. Thiazides increase serum levels of uric acid (hyperuricemia) and, in susceptible individuals, may precipitate acute attacks of gout.

Ethacrynic acid and furosemide.   The most powerful diuretics in common use, ethacrynic acid (Edecrin) and furosemide (Lasix), produce a common spectrum of pharmacological effects and cause a rapid onset of diuresis after oral administration. These drugs inhibit sodium and chloride reabsorption in the ascending loop of Henle; hence, their designation *"loop" diuretics.*

These drugs are used for the treatment of edema caused by disorders of the heart, kidneys, and liver. They even cause marked diuresis in patients responding maximally to other diuretics, including the thiazides, and their routine use is generally reserved for those patients who fail to respond to the thiazides; these drugs are also referred to as "high-ceiling" diuretics. They are about two to three times more effective than the thiazides and about ten times more effective than spironolactone and triamterene in promoting the excretion of filtered sodium.

The primary adverse effects caused by these drugs result from the rapid and excessive loss of fluid and electrolytes, in particular, potassium. *Ototoxicity,* resulting in temporary hearing losses, has been reported after the administration of ethacrynic acid, with fewer cases after furosemide.

Potassium-sparing diuretics.   Spironolactone (Aldactone) and triamterene (Dyrenium), referred to as potassium-sparing diuretics, are most frequently administered in combination with other diuretic agents to prevent excessive potassium depletion; these relatively weak diuretics are rarely used alone.

Spironolactone is an *aldosterone antagonist* at the distal tubules. It antagonizes aldosterone-mediated sodium-potassium exchange resulting in a reduction in sodium reabsorption and the retention of potassium. Triamterene is not a true aldosterone antagonist but promotes sodium loss while conserving potassium.

Osmotic diuretics.   Mannitol and urea are readily absorbed by the glomerulus but are only reabsorbed by the kidney tubules to a very limited extent. When administered in large intravenous doses, these drugs are retained, promoting water retention in the tubules and elimination in the urine.

Mannitol is used to reduce intraocular pressure and cerebrospinal fluid pressure before, during, and after surgery. Urea is employed to reduce elevated intracranial pressure resulting from brain tumors and head injuries.

Xanthines.   In Chapter 15 we considered the central nervous stimulating properties of the xanthines. While caffeine is the most active central stimulant in this class, its diuretic properties are relatively modest. By contrast, of the xanthine derivatives, *theophylline* is the most potent diuretic.

Theophylline and aminophylline (theophylline ethylenediamine) increase cardiac output and renal plasma flow and thereby augment the rate of glomerular filtration. Additionally, they may have a direct effect on the kidney tubules reducing the reabsorption of sodium and chloride. These drugs are rarely employed as diuretic agents in contemporary medicine, but are used for the treatment of bronchial asthma (Chapter 27).

SUMMARY

The past three decades have witnessed the development of highly effective antihypertensive agents for the chronic management of essential (primary) hypertension. Notwithstanding the impressive progress that has been made, the development of even more effective and less toxic drugs for the treatment of this disorder continues to remain a major priority of contemporary pharmacological research. More effective approaches are required to educate the general population about the adverse health consequences associated with untreated hypertension and to achieve greater compliance among patients diagnosed as hypertensives but who are failing to take their medication as prescribed.

Most of the available antihypertensive agents act directly or indirectly to reduce norepinephrine's vasoconstrictor effects on the arterioles. Vasodilation of these small blood vessels reduces peripheral vascular resistance and lowers elevated arterial blood pressure.

Methyldopa and clonidine reduce blood pressure by mechanisms that depress the central sympathetic center, the activity of which controls the vasomotor center, which in turn reduces the degree of arteriolar vaso-constriction and arterial blood pressure. The action of methyldopa is mediated by the false neurotransmitter α-methylnorepinephrine. Veratrum alkaloids sensitize baroreceptors causing reflex inhibition of the vasomotor center.

Ganglionic blocking agents interfere with the transmission of nerve impulses from preganglionic nerves to both sympathetic and parasympathetic postganglionic nerves. More specific antihypertensive agents are available that, by a variety of mechanisms, reduce the norepinephrine released by sympathetic nerves in response to a nerve impulse. Reserpine and guanethidine deplete norepinephrine storage in nerve ending vesicles; guanethidine also inhibits the release of norepinephrine after nerve stimulation. The antihypertensive effects of β-adrenergic receptor blocking agents (propranolol) have been attributed to antagonism of catecholamine-induced effects on the heart, resulting in a reduction in cardiac output; to depression of the central sympathetic center; and/or to blockade of renin release thereby inhibiting the synthesis of the potent endogenous vasopressor agent angiotensin II.

Hydralazine and the thiazide diuretics (chlorothiazide) act on the smooth muscle wall of the arterioles. Hydralazine causes direct vasodilation, while antihypertensive diuretics may alter the concentration of sodium and potassium levels in the smooth muscles. The initial antihypertensive effects result from a reduction in plasma volume and cardiac output.

The functional units of the kidney consist of the glomerulus and the tubule. After filtration of protein-free plasma by the glomerulus, the filtrate passes from the distal tubules, to the loop of Henle, to the distal tubules, to the collecting duct. The nephron generally reabsorbs and returns to the blood 99 percent of the glomerular filtrate.

Diuretic agents are used for the treatment of hypertension as well as edema associated with disorders of the heart, kidneys, and liver. Organomercurials, xanthines, and carbonic anhydrase inhibitors (acetazolamide) have been replaced by potent, orally active, and less toxic diuretics, in particular the thiazides, the most extensively prescribed class of diuretics. The thiazides increase the excretion of electrolytes and water by inhibiting the reabsorption of sodium and chloride ions at the kidney tubules. The most common adverse effects associated with the use of the thiazides result from excessive depletion of blood potassium (hypokalemia); this problem can be minimized by increasing potassium intake or coadministering potassium-sparing diuretics (spironolactone, triamterene). Ethacrynic acid and furosemide ("loop" or "high-ceiling" diuretics), the most effective diuretics in common use, produce marked diuresis even after the use of maximally effective doses of the thiazides.

SUPPLEMENTARY READINGS

Antihypertensive Agents

Genest, J., E. Koiw, and O. Kuchel, eds., *Hypertension: Pathophysiology and Treatment.* New York: McGraw-Hill, 1977.

Kaplan, N. M., *Clinical Hypertension.* 2nd ed. Baltimore: Williams & Wilkins, 1978.

McMahon, F. G., *Management of Essential Hypertension.* Mount Kisco, N.Y.: Futura Publishing Co., 1978.

Perloff, D., ed., "Symposium on Hypertension," *Medical Clinics of North America* 61(3): 463–700 (1977).

Scriabine, A., and C. S. Sweet, eds., *New Antihypertensive Drugs.* New York: Spectrum Publications, 1976.

Wollam, G. L., R. W. Gifford, Jr., and R. C. Tarazi, "Antihypertensive Drugs: Clinical Pharmacology and Therapeutic Use," *Drugs* 14: 420–60 (1977).

Diuretic Agents

Jacobson, H. R., and J. P. Kokko, "Diuretics: Sites and Mechanisms of Action," *Annual Review of Pharmacology and Toxicology* 16: 201–14 (1976).

Mudge, G. H., "Diuretics and Other Agents Employed in the Mobilization of Edema Fluid," in *Goodman and Gilman's The Pharmacological Basis of Therapeutics.* Edited by A. G. Gilman, L. S. Goodman, and A. Gilman, 6th ed., Chap. 36, pp. 892–915. New York: Macmillan, 1980.

Reidenberg, M. M., *Renal Function and Drug Action.* Philadelphia: Saunders, 1971.

Renkin, E. M., and R. R. Robinson, "Glomerular Filtration," *New England Journal of Medicine* 290: 785–92 (1974).

Drugs Affecting the Endocrine System

22

Introduction to Hormones and the Endocrine System

[The endocrine system] may be compared to an orchestra, in which, when one instrument is out of tune, a perfect ensemble is impossible. . . . The leader of the glandular orchestra is the pituitary. It is not only the conductor of the orchestra, but it itself plays several important instruments in the ensemble, as well as acting as a link or mediator between soma and psyche. It is constantly monitoring the internal environment, and it is ideally situated to function in response to psychic stimuli.[1]

—William Boyd (1971)

Regulation and integration of the myriad functions carried out by the body are accomplished by the cooperative efforts of the nervous system and the endocrine system. The endocrine glands, via their chemical messengers, the **hormones**, act to maintain a constant internal body environment, or homeostasis, in spite of marked changes occurring in the external environment and within the organism. When, however, a deficient or excessive quantity of hormones is released by these glands, the internal environment of the body may become markedly disrupted.

Naturally occurring hormones or their synthetic analogs are employed therapeutically when a hormone deficiency exists; this is an example of *replacement therapy*. Conversely, when excessive amounts of hormones are released, drugs may be employed to reduce hormonal synthesis or release, or to antagonize their physiological effects. Moreover, certain hormones such as cortisol are used for the treatment of inflammatory diseases of nonendocrine etiology.

[1] *An Introduction to the Study of Disease* (Philadelphia: Lea & Febiger, 1971), p. 421.

This chapter is intended to provide an overview of the endocrine system and hormones. In particular, we shall consider the general physiological functions and actions of hormones and the mechanisms responsible for the control of their release. One of the primary controlling influences are the hormones of the pituitary gland. The general principles considered in this chapter will serve as a basis for the next two chapters, which will discuss the sex hormones and insulin in some detail.

For many centuries, observations were reported concerning the gross effects of castration and other disorders now known to be the consequence of endocrine dysfunction. However, only since the turn of this century have general concepts evolved concerning the physiological role of the endocrine glands. Among the first significant studies dealing with endocrine function were those of Berthold who, in 1849, castrated cockerels and was able to cause regrowth of their degenerated combs by grafting testicular tissue on the bird's body. On the basis of these experiments, Berthold concluded that the testes released some substance into the blood that was responsible for maintaining secondary sex characteristics and male behavior. Forty years later, Brown-Séquard, a distinguished 72-year-old scientist, attempted to regain his lost youth by injecting himself with testicular extracts obtained from young dogs and guinea pigs. His remarkable claims of rejuvenation have since been dismissed as a placebo effect or as a consequence of autosuggestion. In contrast to the unsuccessful experiments of Brown-Séquard, in another laboratory in 1891, extracts prepared from sheep thyroid were shown to be effective in treating human patients with decreased thyroid gland function.

The modern concept of hormones was finally crystallized in 1902 by Bayliss and Starling, when they demonstrated that a chemical secretion released from the upper segment of the small intestines, termed *secretin*, was able to activate the secretion of pancreatic juice. In 1905, Starling coined the word *hormone* (from a Greek word meaning setting into motion) to refer to secretin. Based upon our present concept of endocrine chemicals, this word is inappropriate, but it has nevertheless gained international acceptance.

Efforts in the twentieth century have been directed toward the isolation and identification of the hormones released from endocrine glands, and, in more recent years, scientists have been concerned with determining the mechanisms of hormonal release and action at a molecular level.

HORMONES

The glands of the body are of two general types, namely, those having connecting ducts and those without ducts. The *exocrine* glands, those responsible for the secretion of sweat, tears, saliva, gastric acid, digestive enzymes, as

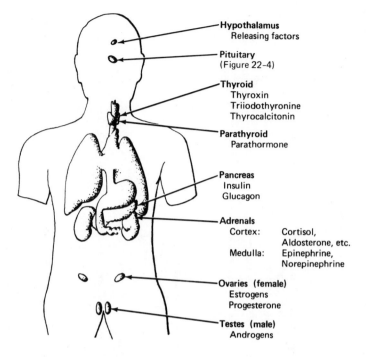

Hypothalamus
  Releasing factors

Pituitary
  (Figure 22-4)

Thyroid
  Thyroxin
  Triiodothyronine
  Thyrocalcitonin

Parathyroid
  Parathormone

Pancreas
  Insulin
  Glucagon

Adrenals
  Cortex: Cortisol,
             Aldosterone, etc.
  Medulla: Epinephrine,
             Norepinephrine

Ovaries (female)
  Estrogens
  Progesterone

Testes (male)
  Androgens

FIGURE 22-1. The Endocrine Glands.

well as a variety of other secretions, deliver their secretions through ducts. By contrast, the **endocrine** or **ductless glands** (Figure 22–1) release their secretions, the **hormones,** directly into the bloodstream for transport to other parts of the body where they exert their action. Whereas growth hormone and thyroid hormone are capable of influencing virtually all the cells of the body, most hormones act rather selectively on specific tissues referred to as *target tissues.* For example, antidiuretic hormone released from the pituitary gland acts on the kidney tubules to promote the conservation of body water, and the parathyroid hormone controls the metabolism of calcium and phosphorous in bones.

Physiological Functions of Hormones

We may group the physiological functions of hormones into three categories: regulation of metabolism; enhancement of growth and development; and, effects on the nervous system. While hormones are capable of modulating the rate of specific biochemical reactions or physiological functions, these compounds do not initiate their activity. Table 22–1 summarizes the primary functions of specific hormones.

TABLE 22-1. PRIMARY PHYSIOLOGICAL FUNCTIONS OF HORMONES

Endocrine Gland	Hormone	Primary Physiological Functions
Pituitary gland	(See Table 22-2)	
Adrenal gland		
Adrenal medulla	Epinephrine	Effects on smooth muscle and cardiovascular system Metabolic effects—carbohydrates and fats "Fight or flight" (Chapters 5, 6)
	Norepinephrine	Vasoconstriction—maintenance of blood pressure
Adrenal cortex	Glucocorticoids (Cortisol)	Metabolic effects—proteins, carbohydrates, and fats Resistance to stress
	Mineralocorticoids (Aldosterone)	Regulation of salt and water balance
Thyroid gland	Thyroxine and Triiodothyronine	Influence growth and development Metabolic effects—stimulates oxygen consumption
	Thyrocalcitonin	Reduces blood calcium levels
Parathyroid gland	Parathormone	Control of calcium and phosphate levels
Pancreas	Insulin	Reduces blood sugar; effects on carbohydrate, fat, and protein metabolism (Chapter 24)
	Glucagon	Elevates blood sugar
Ovaries	Estrogens Progesterone	Normal development, function, and maintenance of reproductive organs and secondary sex characteristics of female (Chapter 23)
Testes	Testosterone	Normal development, function, and maintenance of secondary sex characteristics of male (Chapter 23)

444

Metabolism

Many hormones serve the body by regulating the rate of metabolic reactions involving carbohydrates, proteins, fats, minerals, and water. Most of these reactions occur even in the absence of hormones but proceed at rates that are far too slow or too rapid to efficiently serve the immediate needs of the organism. In other instances, we observe that hormones modify the ability of electrolytes (sodium, potassium, chloride, calcium) and nutrients to move into or out of cells. Some of the pituitary hormones (tropic hormones, such as corticotropin, thyrotropin) regulate the development and secretory activity of endocrine glands located in the periphery, the latter in turn playing important roles in the regulation of metabolic functions.

Growth and Development

Metamorphosis, growth, maturation, reproduction and aging are all under hormonal control. The metamorphosis of the tadpole into a frog is directly influenced by thyroid hormone. Inadequate or excessive secretion of growth hormone from the anterior pituitary gland causes dwarfism or giantism, respectively. The secretion of adequate amounts of ovarian hormones is of paramount importance for prepuberal females aspiring to become well-endowed movie sex symbols. Similarly, the secretion of androgens transforms boys to young men and their fantasies to realities.

Nervous System Function

The activities of the autonomic and central nervous systems, as well as behavioral patterns, are modified by hormones. A baby born without thyroid function, a cretin, may suffer from irreversible mental retardation if not given thyroid hormone during the first few postnatal months. The hypothyroid adult is generally observed to be physically and mentally sluggish, has a low rate of body metabolism, low blood pressure, and a poor appetite. His hyperthyroid counterpart exhibits diametrically opposite symptoms. Injection of sex hormones into newborn animals has been shown to markedly alter their adult sexual behavior and expression of emotions; their reaction to stress is also changed. Some investigators have suggested that hormones from the adrenal cortex may play a role in regulating and limiting the size of certain animal populations. As the consequence of such hormonal influences, animals including the muskrat, woodchuck, deer, and rabbit avoid the hazard of destroying their environment and causing their own extinction. Whether humans will respond to these population density–dependent social pressures remains to be seen.

Hormonal Mechanisms of Action

The precise sites and mechanisms by which hormones act are not fully understood at this time. In general, hormones affect cell membranes, enzyme functions and protein synthesis. Some of these effects are mediated by a "second messenger," cyclic AMP.

Transport Across Cell Membranes

Some hormones are capable of increasing or decreasing the transport of chemicals across cell membranes, thereby increasing or decreasing their intracellular concentration and, in the former case, providing sources of energy or starting materials for the synthesis of compounds that are essential for maintaining the function of the organism. The hormone insulin enhances the ability of the muscle and other selected tissues to actively take up glucose from the blood and more effectively utilize this sugar as a source of intracellular energy. On the other hand, cortisol is believed to inhibit the transport of glucose into cells and thereby is an antagonist to insulin.

Stimulation of Protein Synthesis and Enzymes

Steroid hormones released by the adrenal gland, ovaries, and testes are capable of increasing the synthesis of proteins within cells. The steroid hormone enters the cell and binds to a specific cytoplasmic receptor protein; both enter the nucleus of the cell where they activate specific chromosomal genes to form messenger RNA (mRNA) which enters the cytoplasm and promotes the formation of new protein molecules. These proteins are undoubtedly enzymes which catalyze specific functions of the cell.

Effects Mediated by Cyclic AMP

One of the most significant recent findings in endocrinology has been the discovery of the role of cyclic AMP as a mediator of hormonal action.[2] **Cyclic AMP** or cyclic adenosine-3', 5'-monophosphate is a nucleotide[3] found in virtually all animal cells. Many hormones are now thought to act indirectly through the mediator substance, cyclic AMP, which, in turn, is directly responsible for triggering the physiological responses associated with the hormone's actions (Figure 22–2). The specific responses elicited are dependent upon the particular hormone and the cell or target tissue. Let us examine the sequence of events.

---

[2] For pioneering this concept while at Vanderbilt University, Earl Sutherland (1915–1974) received the 1971 Nobel Prize.

[3] A nucleotide is a molecule consisting of a purine or pyrimidine base with sugar and phosphate units.

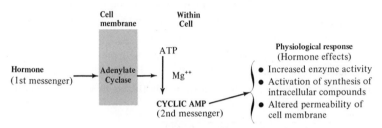

Cyclic AMP (cyclic adenosine-3', 5'-monophosphate)

FIGURE 22-2. The Role of Cyclic AMP as a Mediator of Hormonal Action. A hormone activates the enzyme adenylate cyclase located in the membrane of a target tissue. Adenylate cyclase promotes the formation of cyclic AMP, which produces the physiological response associated with the hormone's effects. Cyclic AMP is broken down to an inactive product 5'-AMP, a reaction catalyzed by the anzyme phosphodiesterase.

The hormone or "first messenger" interacts with adenylate cyclase, an enzyme found in the membrane of the target cell. Adenylate cyclase then catalyzes the immediate conversion of intracellular adenosine triphosphate (ATP) to cyclic AMP. Depending upon the hormone and tissue, cyclic AMP, the "second messenger," mediates such physiological responses as an increase in enzyme activity, an enhancement in the synthesis of important compounds within the cell, or an alteration in the permeability of the cell membrane to water, electrolytes, or other compounds required by the cell.

Regulation of Endocrine Activity

The endocrine glands are not functionally autonomous structures that capriciously release hormones. Just as the three branches of our federal government are subject to checks and balances, so are the endocrine glands. The activity of these glands is regulated by influences arising in the central nervous system, the actual blood levels of hormones and other biochemicals, and the activity of other endocrine glands.

The **anterior pituitary or adenohypophysis** has been classically viewed as the master gland responsible for controlling the activities of most of the individual endocrine glands. However, in recent years it has been ascertained that the anterior pituitary is the target of excitatory and inhibitory stimuli arising in the central nervous system, in particular from the **hypothalamus.** This supreme command post of the endocrine system directs the activity of the anterior pituitary by neurosecretory mediator substances called **releasing factors.** The hypothalamus receives field reports from the external environment and within the body; for example, it receives neuronal messages from other parts of the central nervous system that are activated by stress, visual stimuli, smell, and other sensory inputs. In addition, blood-carried signals of changes in hormone, nutrient, and electrolyte concentrations make the hypothalamus aware of alterations taking place within the internal environment of the body. All these inputs enable the hypothalamus to maintain a constant and optimal internal environment termed *homeostasis* that is essential for the survival of the organism.

Homeostatic mechanisms are biological examples of *negative feedback control* systems, which seek to minimize the differences between the actual condition of the system and the optimal functional level. The design of the

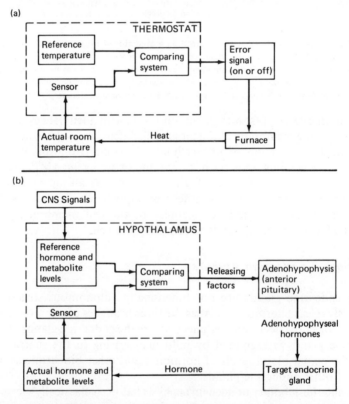

FIGURE 22-3. Negative Feedback Systems. (a) Furnace under thermostatic control. (b) Endocrine gland under hypothalamic control. Both systems consist of (1) a sensor to measure the actual existing conditions; (2) a comparing system to detect the error signal, that is, the difference between the ideal reference conditions (for example, hormonal levels) and the actual conditions; and (3) an effector mechanism that must be available to reduce this error signal to a minimal level.

household thermostat is based upon a similar principle [Figure 22–3 (a)]. An analogous negative feedback system exists to control endocrine function and hormonal secretions [Figure 22–3 (b)]. The hypothalamus, acting as does the thermostat, is the master collecting and integrating unit, and it determines what optimum levels of hormones are most consistent with maintaining homeostasis within the body. After the actual blood levels of hormones, other biochemicals, or electrolytes are detected, this information is compared with the ideal reference levels. Should higher concentrations of hormones be required, releasing factors from the hypothalamus stimulate the secretion of adenohypophyseal tropic hormones from the anterior pituitary which activate their respective endocrine glands to secrete their hormones. The detection of excessive hormonal levels advises the hypothalamus to cease secreting releasing factors.

THE PITUITARY GLAND

The **pituitary gland** or **hypophysis** is a relatively small structure located at the base of the brain and is connected to the hypothalamus by the hypophyseal stalk (Figure 22–4). The human pituitary gland, which is about 1 cm (0.4 in) long and 1 to 1.5 cm in width, weighs only about 0.5 g (1/60 oz). Anatomically

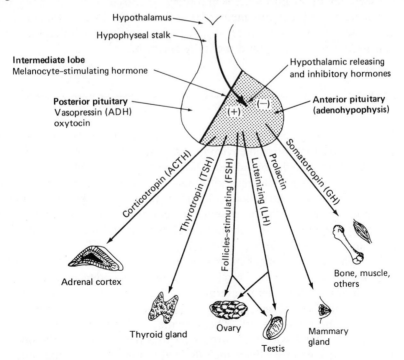

FIGURE 22-4. The Hypothalamus, Hypophyseal Hormones and the Target Endocrine Glands and Tissues of the Adenohypophyseal Hormones.

and functionally, the hypophysis is divided into two separate and independent portions: the adenohypophysis or anterior pituitary gland and the neurohypophysis or posterior pituitary gland. Separating these two parts is the intermediate lobe.

The **anterior pituitary** produces at least six hormones whose release is activated by specific releasing factors arising from the hypothalamus (Table 22-2). The adenohypophyseal hormones regulate the growth of body tissues, and some, the tropic hormones, regulate the release of hormones by endocrine glands located in the periphery. The **posterior pituitary** releases two hormones, antidiuretic hormone (vasopressin) and oxytocin. After the synthesis of these small protein molecules, they travel down nerve fibers terminating in the posterior pituitary, where chemical, physical, and emotional stimuli cause the release of these hormones into the blood and to their target organs.

As you might anticipate, aberrations in the function of the pituitary gland of an adult may cause profound changes in the activity of the endocrine glands, as well as changes in the homeostatic balance of the body. What are the physiological consequences of pituitary insufficiency, a state arising from disease or the surgical removal of the pituitary gland? The adrenal cortex atrophies, causing a decrease in the release of glucocorticoids, such as cortisol, with an ensuing reduction in the resistance to stress. The gonads also atrophy, and the secretion of sex hormones is markedly decreased, leading to a cessation of the female reproductive or menstrual cycle and the loss of secondary sex characteristics. As a consequence of a reduction in thyroid function, the individual becomes physically and mentally sluggish.

SUMMARY

The endocrine system, in conjunction with the nervous system, functions to maintain a constant internal environment, a state termed homeostasis. Hormones, the chemical mediators of the endocrine glands, generally exert their actions on specific target tissues, although a few hormones affect tissues throughout the body. The general biological functions of hormones include regulation of the rates of the biochemical reactions occurring within the body; control of the organism's growth and development; and modification of nervous system function, including behavior.

Although the precise mechanisms underlying the actions of hormones are not fully known at this time, there is a large body of evidence to suggest that many hormones act through the intermediary "second messenger" cyclic AMP. The hormone or "first messenger" activates adenylate cyclase, an enzyme present in the membrane of the cell. This enzyme catalyzes the formation of intracellular cyclic AMP which, in turn, is responsible for causing the observed physiological effects. Such effects include facilitation of the cellular uptake of essential endogenous compounds and enhancement of protein, enzyme, and

TABLE 22-2. THE PITUITARY HORMONES AND THEIR PHYSIOLOGICAL FUNCTIONS

Hormones	Physiological Functions
Anterior pituitary	
Somatotropin (STH) or growth hormone (GH)	Promotes the growth of all tissues throughout the body; influences protein, carbohydrate, and fat metabolism; used clinically to treat growth failure
Corticotropin or adrenocorticotropic hormone (ACTH)	Controls the synthesis and release of hormones from adrenal cortex; hormones affect metabolism of carbohydrates, proteins, and fats and mineral balance
Thyrotropin or thyroid-stimulating hormone (TSH)	Controls release of hormones from thyroid gland
Follicle-stimulating hormone (FSH)	Stimulates formation of ovarian follicles (eggs) in females and sperm formation (spermatogenesis) in males (Chapter 23)
Luteinizing hormone (LH) or interstitial- cell-stimulating hormone (ICSH)	Female: Stimulates ovarian follicles; ovulation; formation of corpus luteum Male: Stimulates interstitial cells of testes to secrete male hormones (androgens) (Chapter 23)
Prolactin or leuteotropin	Initiates production of milk after childbirth
Posterior pituitary	
Antidiuretic hormone (ADH) or vasopressin	Conserves body water via an action on the kidneys; used clinically to treat diabetes insipidus
Oxytocin	May facilitate contractions of uterus at childbirth; promotes flow of milk during nursing ("milk letdown")
Intermediate lobe	
Melanocyte-stimulating hormone (MSH) or intermedin	Coloration of skin—may be of greater importance in lower animals than in humans; effects on human behavior (?)

451

RNA synthesis. The specific hormone and target tissue upon which it acts determines the nature of the effect produced.

The release of hormones by a number of endocrine glands is controlled by the hypothalamus and the anterior pituitary gland. The hypothalamus releases specific releasing factors which activate the anterior pituitary; this latter structure secretes hormones that in turn cause certain peripheral endocrine glands to secrete their hormones.

The pituitary gland consists of two separate parts: the anterior and posterior pituitary, separated by the intermediate lobe. At least nine physiologically important hormones are released from this gland.

SUPPLEMENTARY READINGS

Berson, S. A., and R. S. Yalow, *Peptide Hormones.* New York: American Elsevier Publishing Co., 1973.

Fisher, L., ed., *Neuroendocrine Integration: Basic and Applied Aspects.* New York: Raven Press, 1975.

Sachs, B. A., ed., "The Brain and the Endocrine System," *Medical Clinics of North America* **62** (2):227–426 (1978).

Tepperman, J., *Metabolic and Endocrine Physiology.* 3rd ed. Chicago: Year Book Medical Publishers, 1973.

Thomas, J. A., and M. G. Mawhinney, *Synopsis of Endocrine Pharmacology.* Baltimore: University Park Press, 1973.

Ville, D. B., *Human Endocrinology: A Developmental Approach.* Philadelphia: Saunders, 1975.

Williams, R., ed. *Textbook of Endocrinology,* 5th ed. Philadelphia: Saunders, 1974.

Zimmermann, E., W. H. Gispen, B. H. Marks, and D. deWied, eds., "Drug Effects on Neuroendocrine Regulation," *Progress in Brain Research* **39**:1–502 (1973).

23

The Sex Hormones and Control of Fertility

The upsurge in the growth of human population constitutes the major problem for the immediate future of man.

—Philip Handler (1970)

The sex hormones are essential for the normal development, function, and maintenance of the reproductive organs and secondary sex characteristics. In addition, the pregnant female requires hormones for the successful maintenance of pregnancy. The sex hormones consist of the estrogens and progestins (progesterone) of the female and the androgens, the male hormones. In this chapter we shall discuss the physiological functions of these hormones and their use in the treatment of endocrine disorders and as oral contraceptives. Hormones are also employed to promote the growth of animals used as food and by athletes to enhance muscle development; these applications will also be examined. Let us first consider the female sex hormones.

FEMALE SEX HORMONES

The **ovary,** the female gonad, is both the site of the formation of the ovum or egg and the endocrine organ responsible for the release of hormones that control the activity of the female reproductive tract and determine secondary sex characteristics. Prior to the onset of puberty, the ovary is relatively inactive. At puberty, perhaps in response to activating influences arising in the central nervous system, ovarian function begins and is heralded by the start of the menstrual cycle. This cycle continues for three or four decades and then ceases at menopause.

The Menstrual Cycle

To permit us to gain an overview of the female reproductive system, and the mechanisms by which oral contraceptives exert their action, we shall first outline the sequence of events in the normal menstrual cycle (Figure 23–1).

Under the influence of releasing factors from the hypothalamus, *follicle-stimulating hormone (FSH)* is discharged from the anterior pituitary. This gonadotropic hormone travels in the blood to the ovary, where it stimulates the maturation of follicles from which an ovum will develop. FSH also activates the secretion of estrogen from the mature ovarian follicles.

By eight to ten days after the start of menstruation, and several days after the initiation of estrogen release, estrogen causes the uterine mucosa or endometrium to proliferate (increase in size). About day 10, high estrogen blood levels trigger two hypothalamically mediated effects on the anterior pituitary: Additional FSH release is suppressed, and there is a stimulation of *luteinizing hormone (LH)* secretion from the anterior pituitary. Estrogen blood concentrations peak by day 14.

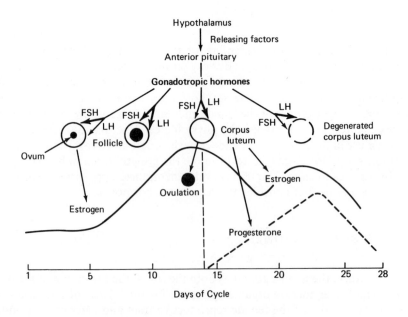

FIGURE 23–1. Sequence of Events in the Normal Menstrual Cycle. Day 1 is the first day of menstruation. See text for description.

LH travels via the blood to the ovary, where, on approximately day 14, it triggers the release of the ovum from the follicle. After ovulation has occurred, the ovum moves down the fallopian tube and into the uterus where it is available for fertilization by a sperm cell. The remaining follicle is now converted to the corpus luteum, a structure capable of secreting estrogen and progesterone. The woman's most fertile time is between days 14 and 18.

During the second half of the monthly cycle, progesterone activates changes in the uterine mucosa that provide a suitable environment for the implantation of a fertilized ovum. The cells of the uterus begin to stockpile fat and carbohydrate nutrient materials, and the local blood supply to the area is markedly enhanced; the thickness of the uterine mucosa is also greatly increased. Progesterone also reduces the normal contractions of the smooth muscles of the uterus (myometrium).

About days 23–25, blood levels of estrogen and progesterone reach a postovulation peak. If fertilization of the ovum has failed to occur, several events take place. High blood concentrations of progesterone initiate a negative feedback mechanism, via the hypothalamus, which suppresses the output of LH from the anterior pituitary. Reduced levels of LH cause a degeneration of the corpus luteum, which in turn ceases its secretion of estrogen and progesterone. In the absence of hormonal support of the uterine mucosa, there is a breakdown in its cells and menstruation begins. Falling estrogen levels serve as a stimulus to the anterior pituitary, via the hypothalamus, to start releasing FSH, thus initiating the next cycle.

If fertilization does occur, generally between days 14 and 18, the presence of a fertilized ovum in the uterine wall signals the corpus luteum to continue secreting estrogen and progesterone for the first three months of pregnancy. Estrogen continues to stimulate the enlargement of the uterine wall, whereas progesterone causes the glands to secrete necessary fluids. During the second month of pregnancy, the placenta assumes greater importance and begins secreting hormones. The high levels of estrogen and progesterone prevent the secretion of FSH, which precludes the development of additional ova by the ovarian follicles. This last point is of fundamental importance for an understanding of the mechanism of action of the oral contraceptives.

The Estrogens

Estradiol is the most important estrogen secreted by the ovaries. This steroid hormone is required for the development of the female reproductive organs (vagina, uterus, and fallopian tubes) at puberty and for secondary sex characteristics, including the development of the breasts, appropriate distribution of body fat around the breasts and hips, soft texture of the skin, growth and distribution of hair, and the nature of the feminine voice. The female hormones also permit the maintenance of these characteristics throughout the adult life.

During the monthly cycle, estrogen and progesterone stimulate the development of the uterine wall. When fertilization of the ovum fails to occur, the levels of these hormones precipitously drop, causing a shedding of cells and menstruation. Estrogens suppress FSH release from the anterior pituitary; this action will prove to be of importance when we discuss the mechanism of action of the oral contraceptives.

Natural and synthetic estrogen-like compounds are available for the treatment of hormone-deficient conditions. Unlike the natural estrogens, synthetic derivatives have been developed that possess considerable activity after oral administration (Table 23-1). A major therapeutic use of the estrogens is to relieve the distressing symptoms associated with *menopause,* "the change of life." With the onset of menopause, occurring between the ages of 45 and 55, there is a gradual cessation of the ability of the ovaries to secrete estradiol and other natural estrogenic hormones. The absence of estrogen causes the characteristic signs of menopause, which include "hot flashes," fatigue, anxiety, and irritability, and in some cases, psychotic aberrations termed involutional melancholia. Replacement therapy with estrogens generally provides relief from these highly distressing symptoms. However, it should be noted that the risk of endometrial cancer in postmenopausal women receiving estrogen therapy for extended periods is estimated to be 4.5 to 14 times greater than in nonusers. Hence, when estrogens are employed for the management of menopausal symptoms, the lowest effective dose should be prescribed for the shortest possible time. Moreover, women should be medically evaluated on a semiannual basis to determine whether a continued drug need exists.

Estrogens are also used to treat a large variety of menstrual disorders, to relieve engorgement of the breasts and suppress lactation after childbirth, and to provide improvement in patients with cancer of the prostate in males and cancer of the breast in postmenopausal women.

TABLE 23-1. REPRESENTATIVE FEMALE SEX HORMONES

Type	Generic Name	Selected Trade Names
ESTROGENS		
Natural and	Estrone	Theelin
semisynthetic	Estradiol	Duragen, Valergen
	Ethinyl estradiol	Estinyl, Feminone
	Estrogenic substances, conjugated	Premarin, Conestron, Genisis
Synthetic	Chlorotrianisene	Tace
	Diethylstilbestrol (stilbestrol)	
PROGESTINS		
Natural	Progesterone	Progelan
Synthetic	Dydrogesterone	Duphaston, Gynorest
	Hydroxyprogesterone	Delalutin
	Medroxyprogesterone	Provera
	Norethindrone	Norlutin

Estradiol	Ethinyl estradiol	Diethylstilbestrol
(Natural estrogen)	(Semisynthetic steroidal estrogen)	(Synthetic nonsteroidal estrogen)

Diethylstilbestrol (DES), a nonsteroidal estrogen-like compound effective after oral administration, has been widely used for three decades. Recent reports have appeared that have linked the maternal use of diethylstilbestrol during pregnancy with the occurrence of vaginal cancer in their female offspring many years later. Although there is, at present, only an *association* between diethylstilbestrol use and cancer, additional studies are currently being conducted to establish whether a cause-and-effect relationship exists. The use of diethylstilbestrol as a "morning-after" contraceptive is discussed below.

A former and controversial use of diethylstilbestrol was as a *growth promoting agent* in cattle. When this hormone was injected or added to cattle feed, it enhanced the growth of beef up to 25 percent above normal, and yet the animals ate the same amount of grain. The economic benefits to the cattle raiser were obvious; however, in recent years, critics have argued that since diethylstilbestrol is a known carcinogen, its use in beef should be prohibited. The arguments, to a large measure, revolve about the presence or absence of drug residues in animal carcasses, and what constitutes a minimally safe level that is not injurious to health. In 1973, the addition of diethylstilbestrol to cattle feed was prohibited.

Progestins

The most important natural progestin is **progesterone,** a hormone secreted by the corpus luteum and the placenta. This hormone induces changes in the uterine mucosa that provide a more favorable environment for the implantation of the fertilized ovum. During pregnancy, progesterone also induces mammary gland duct development and reduces the spontaneous activity of the uterine muscle. Pharmacological doses of progestins inhibit LH release from the anterior pituitary. This latter effect is important as will be observed when we discuss the use of progestins in oral contraceptive agents. Natural and synthetic progestins are clinically employed for the treatment of various menstrual disorders and as tests for pregnancy (Table 23–1).

CONTROL OF FERTILITY

Similarly excluded [is] every action which, either in anticipation of the conjugal act or in its accomplishment, or in the development of the natural consequences, proposes, whether as an end or as a means, to render procreation impossible.

—Pope Paul VI (1968)

It is unmistakably clear that unless something is done about the population explosion, we will be faced with an unprecedented catastrophe of overcrowding, famines, pestilence and war.

—Senator Gaylord Nelson (1970)

When each of us is confronted with the decision of planning the size of our family, many factors must be weighed. Most of us will undoubtedly consider financial resources: How many children can we afford to support? Medical considerations, such as the inherent dangers of pregnancy, in addition to psychological makeup (How many children can we emotionally tolerate?)—these are determining factors in planning a family. In some instances, additional children represent more hands to carry out work on the farm or in the family business. Strongly influencing these factors, either directly or indirectly, are religious beliefs and the desire to demonstrate one's virility or fertility, as manifested by a large family. Moreover, we cannot overlook widespread ignorance among many people about effective methods of precluding pregnancy.

For a moment, let us trace the trend in the growth of the world's population. From the birth of Christ, it took about 1650 years for the first doubling of the population, while only 200 years were required for the next doubling and only 80 years for the third. It is estimated that the present population of the world may increase twofold in 35 years and seven times in the next 100 years.[2] The age of the recluse may be rapidly concluding because of an inability to find an uninhabited region in which to escape from a rapidly enveloping horde of people encroaching upon one's privacy. Thus, we may view the need for population control on a microcosmic level, "I can't afford nor do I care to have more children"; or on a macrocosmic level,"In light of the rapidly diminishing natural resources on this planet, I shall limit my family size to two." Regardless of the level of concern, many people now believe, and even some insist, that the rate of population growth should be markedly reduced, perhaps with zero population growth the objective.[3]

[1] *Humanae Vitae (Of Human Life).*

[2] On March 14, 1980, the Environmental Fund's World Population Clock reached 4.5 billion; the Fund estimates that at the present rate of increase, the world's population should reach 5 billion in 1991.

[3] It should not be concluded from this discussion that overpopulation is a global problem necessitating a reduction in the growth rate of all nations. Each nation must evaluate this question according to its own population status and natural resources.

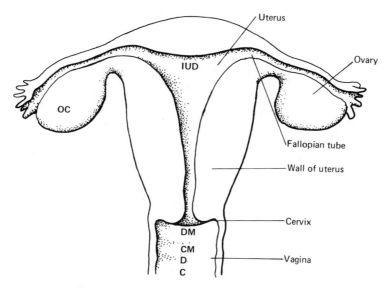

FIGURE 23-2. Sites of Action of Contraceptive Methods. Key to abbreviations: C= condom; CM = chemical methods; D = douche; DM = diaphragm; IUD = intrauterine device; OC = oral contraceptive.

While there are a wide variety of mechanical and chemical contraceptive methods available, with each possessing varying degrees of effectiveness, advantages, and disadvantages, the facts strongly indicate that the oral contraceptives are currently the most effective method for preventing pregnancy (Figure 23-2, Table 23-2).

Oral Contraceptives

All the oral contraceptive products currently available consist of estrogen and/or progestin ingredients. These oral contraceptives act by one or more of the following mechanisms: (1) preventing ovulation by blocking the release of FSH and LH from the anterior pituitary; (2) increasing the thickness of the cervical mucus, thereby creating an unfavorable environment for sperm penetration and subsequent conception; and (3) inducing other changes in the cervical mucosa that prove to be unfavorable for the implantation of the fertilized egg. Oral contraceptives are classified as combination products and the "minipills" (Table 23-3) and differ with respect to their ingredients, pharmacological actions, relative effectiveness, side effects, and schedule of administration.[4]

[4] *Sequential oral contraceptives* were formerly available for use. Preparations of this type (Norquen, Oracon, Ortho-Novum SQ) consisted of an estrogen (taken for 15–16 days monthly) and an estrogen-progestin-containing tablet (taken for the subsequent 5–6 days). The sequentials, clinically observed to be less effective than the combination products, were withdrawn from the American market in 1976 when their use was shown to be associated with a higher risk of thromboembolic (clotting) disorders and malignant tumors.

TABLE 23-2. CONTRACEPTIVE METHODS

Method (Synonym)	% Effectiveness† Theoretical/Actual use	What it is/How it works	Remarks
Oral contractive* ("the pill") Combination Minipill	99.66/90-96 98.5-99/90-95	Synthetic female hormones. Prevents development and/or release of egg.	Must be taken 20-21 days per month (combination) or daily (minipill). Only suitable for motivated user. Almost 100% effective. Use not related to sex act. Potentially dangerous adverse effects (see text). Most expensive.
Intrauterine device* (IUD)	97-99/95	Small plastic or copper object (coil, loop, "T") which is placed in uterus. May act by preventing implantation of fertilized egg in uterine wall.	Insertion generally simple and rapid. Progesterine-containing IUD (Progestasert) must be replaced annually. Highly effective. Useful for women unwilling or unable to take the pill. Spontaneous IUD expulsion by 10-15% of women in first year. Risk of pelvic inflammatory disease. Problems: cramping, irregular bleeding (spotting), heavy menstrual bleeding.
Diaphragm* with spermicide	97/83	Dome-shaped rubber cup inserted into vagina and covers cervix. Mechanical barrier to sperm penetration.	More effective when used with spermicidal jelly or cream. Must be correctly fitted by physician. Must be left in place six hours after intercourse.
Condom (rubber, prophylactic)	97/90	Rubber or skin (animal membrane) sheath worn on the penis. Prevents entrance of sperm into vagina.	Highly effective, harmless, simple to use, readily available. Most useful for occasional or unexpected intercourse. Only contraceptive method that protects against venereal disease. Use objectional to some.

Chemical methods	97/78	Vaginal foams, jellies, creams, suppositories, tablets containing spermicidal compounds. Kills sperm; may provide mechanical barrier to sperm passage.	Provides protection for about one hour. Some individuals experience irritation or burning sensation. Harmless to adults or baby if ineffective in preventing pregnancy. Suppositories and tablets are least effective and not recommended.
Douche	?/60	Flush vagina after intercourse with water (with or without spermicidal agent) immediately after intercourse to remove or destroy sperm.	Totally unreliable method of contraception. Sperm enter cervical canal within 90 seconds after ejaculation.
Rhythm*	87/79	Abstinence from sexual intercourse during time of month when female is fertile.	Highly effective when correctly practiced in women with regular menstrual cycles. Success requires abstinence for at least 8 days per cycle and usually longer. Fertile period can be determined by changes in body temperature. For most women, this method is not effective.

*Methods requiring consultation with physician.

†Theoretical effectiveness if method is used correctly and consistently. Actual use effectiveness based upon percentage of American women who became pregnant within one year after initiation of use of method. Data from K.A. Hatcher et al., *Contraceptive Technology 1978-1979*, 9th rev. ed. (New York: Irvington Publishers, 1978).

TABLE 23-3. REPRESENTATIVE ORAL CONTRACEPTIVES

Trade Names (Relative Dominance*)	Estrogen	Progestin
Combination products†		
Brevicon (I)	Ethinyl estradiol	Norethindrone
Demulen (I)	Ethinyl estradiol	Ethynodiol diacetate
Enovid 5 mg (E), Enovid-E (E)	Mestranol	Norethynodrel
Lo/Ovral (P), Ovral (P)	Ethinyl estradiol	Norgestrel
Loestrin 1/20 (P) and		
1.5/30 (P)	Ethinyl estradiol	Norethindrone acetate
Modicon (I)	Ethinyl estradiol	Norethindrone
Norinyl 1 + 50 (I), 1 + 80 (I)		
and 2 mg (E)	Mestranol	Norethindrone
Norlestrin 1/50 (I) and		
2.5/50 (P)	Ethinyl estradiol	Norethindrone acetate
Ortho-Novum 1/50 (I), 1/80 (I),		
2 mg (E), and 10 mg (P)	Mestranol	Norethindrone
Ovcon-35 (I)	Ethinyl estradiol	Norethindrone
Ovulen (E)	Mestranol	Ethynodiol diacetate
Minipill‡		
Micronor (P)	—	Norethindrone
Nor-Q.D. (P)	—	Norethindrone
Ovrette (P)	—	Norgestrel

*E = estrogen dominant; P = progestin dominant; I = intermediate estrogen-progestin balance. The varying amounts of each hormonal component are intended to fit each woman's unique requirement.

†Some of the combination products are taken on a daily basis for 20 to 21 days, starting on day 5 of menstrual cycle; others, taken for the entire 28-day cycle, contain 21 tablets with estrogen-progestin and 7 inert tablets.

‡The "minipills" contain only a progestin component and are taken on a daily basis throughout the year.

The *combination products,* consisting of tablets containing a synthetic estrogen and progestin, are taken from day 5 through day 24 of the cycle; withdrawal bleeding occurs 3 to 4 days after the last dose. Contraception is thought to occur by all of the above mechanisms. It is generally believed that the most important effects are an inhibition of the development of the ovarian follicles and the prevention of ovulation. How may we explain these effects? High blood levels of estrogen, supplied by "the pill," inhibit the release of FSH, the hormone essential for the maturation of the ovarian follicles. Moreover, elevated progestin concentrations inhibit the secretion of LH, which is responsible for triggering ovulation.

The "minipill," the most recent type of oral contraceptive agent available for use in the United States, contains only a progestin ingredient. Whereas the combination and sequential products are taken for about three weeks of every month, the "minipill" is used every day of the month throughout the year. It is believed that the estrogen component of the combination and sequential products is responsible for the increased incidence of the thromboembolic diseases (see below). The "minipill" attempts to reduce this problem by eliminating estrogen.

When all doses of the oral contraceptives are taken according to the prescribed schedule, both the combination and sequential products represent the most effective method of contraception, with the rate of pregnancy less than one per 100 women-years.[5] When doses are missed, the pregnancy rate is somewhat higher with the sequential products. With the "minipill," approximately three pregnancies might occur per 100 women-years. After estrogen-progestin therapy is terminated, over half the women regain their fertility within three cycles after taking the last dose and about 90 percent within one year.

Side Effects and Possible Hazards

Undesirable side effects are observed in 15 to 35 percent of all women employing oral contraceptives. The most common of these are symptoms observed during pregnancy and include nausea, vomiting, breast fullness, weight gain, headache, dizziness, fatigue, and depression. Breakthrough bleeding or failure to menstruate may also occur. The relative incidence of many of these adverse effects is dependent upon the amounts of estrogen or progestin taken (Table 23–4). Unpredictable bleeding is most commonly observed with the progestin-only products, which is a major disadvantage.

TABLE 23-4.   RELATIONSHIP OF SIDE EFFECTS TO RELATED HORMONAL DOMINANCE OF ORAL CONTRACEPTIVES

Hormone	Excess	Deficiency
Estrogen	Nausea Dizziness Fluid retention Breast swelling and tenderness Uterine and leg cramps Thromboembolic (clotting) disorders* Myocardial infarction (heart attack)*	Early and midcycle spotting Decreased menstrual flow Hot flashes
Progestin	Increased appetite and weight gain Tiredness and fatigue Depression Decreased sex drive Acne, hair loss Decreased days menstrual flow Hypertension*	Late breakthrough bleeding and spotting Heavy menstrual flow and spotting Delayed onset of menstrual bleeding

*Increased risk

[5] The rate of pregnancies during a given time period is a measure of the failure rate for that method. If we assume that ovulation occurs 13 times per year, for each woman there exist 13 opportunities for contraception to occur, or 1300 per 100 woman-years.

Although the oral contraceptives are among the newer classes of drugs, they are also among the most extensively used in the United States and in other parts of the world. The first experimental clinical studies were instituted in Puerto Rico in 1955, and they were approved for use in this country five years later. Hence, the clinical experience gained from the extended use of these drugs is rather limited, and many of the potential dangers associated with their chronic administration have not as yet been resolved.

Cardiovascular disorders. Of greatest concern is the relationship between the use of "the pill" and *thromboembolic diseases* such as thrombophlebitis, the presence of blood clots in the veins. The major hazard associated with thrombophlebitis is pulmonary embolism, a condition where a blood clot blocks the pulmonary artery, causing difficulty in breathing as well as circulatory failure; death may possibly occur. The results obtained from a number of studies indicate that the relative incidence of thromboembolic diseases is five to ten times higher in women taking oral contraceptives than in women of the same age who are not using these drugs. These blood clotting disorders are generally believed to be caused by the estrogen component. At this time there is no evidence that the use of combination products containing low levels of estrogen or the estrogen-free "minipills" are totally devoid of this risk.

Oral contraceptives cause *high blood pressure* in a significant number of women. The incidence of hypertension appears to be correlated with the duration of time the woman has taken the oral contraceptive and the level of progestin contained in the product. Pill-induced hypertension is generally mild to moderate in severity, with blood pressure usually returning to normal levels within one to three months after the discontinuation of drug administration.

The risk of *myocardial infarction* (heart attack) is increased by oral contraceptives. This risk is augmented in women over 40 years of age as well as in those having other risk factors including hypertension, cigarette smoking, diabetes mellitus, elevated cholesterol and triglyceride levels, and obesity. The incidence of heart attack with one risk factor has been reported to be increased fourfold above those with no risk factors and 10 and 78 times higher in women with two and three or more risk factors, respectively.

Other potential dangers. Considerable controversy currently rages in the literature concerning whether or not oral contraceptives increase the risk of cancer of the breast and reproductive tract (cervical and endometrial carcinomas). Prolonged use of estrogens for the control of postmenopausal symptoms has been shown to increase the risk of endometrial cancer. Other clinical reports document increases in the incidence of benign liver tumors (potentially resulting in fatal internal bleeding) and gallbladder diseases among oral contraceptive users.

Certain women are advised not to take oral contraceptives, and they include those with histories of thromboembolic disorders, cancers of the breast and genital tract, migraine headaches, and liver, heart or kidney diseases. If the possibility of pregnancy exists, these drugs should not be used because of possible progestin-induced masculinization of the fetus.

Alternative Methods of Fertility Control

Early in the nineteenth century, Thomas Malthus proposed that the world's population was capable of geometrically expanding, thus rapidly exhausting both natural and manufactured resources. Fortunately, his fears have not been realized. In addition to the oral contraceptives, a variety of alternative approaches that produce successful interference with pregnancy are in usage (Table 23–2).

"The Shot"

"The shot," used by approximately one million women in 64 countries outside the United States in 1978, consists of the progestin medroxyprogesterone acetate (Depo-Provera) or norethindrone ethanate. A single injection at 90-day intervals is about as effective in preventing pregnancy as combination oral contraceptive products and eliminates the necessity for taking the pill on a daily basis. Because of its carcinogenic hazard and potential risk of causing permanent infertility, the Food and Drug Administration rejected approval of this drug as a contraceptive agent in the United States.

Intrauterine Devices

While the antifertility effects of foreign bodies placed in the uterus have been long recognized, in only recent years have **intrauterine devices** (IUDs) achieved widespread popularity in the United States.

IUDs come in various sizes and shapes (loops, coils, "7" and "T"), and often consist of a polyethylene strip containing a copper wire and sometimes progesterone. The antifertility effects of IUDs do not result from a single action; they appear to act by preventing implantation of the fertilized egg and the subsequent development of the embryo. The actual use effectiveness of IUDs closely approximates their theoretical effectiveness (Table 23–2) since there are very few errors the user can make once the device has been properly inserted.

Worldwide 15 million women use IUDs. The Lippes Loop, introduced in 1964 and the most popular of any developed thus far, can be left in place indefinitely. The copper-containing IUDs (Cu-7 and Cu-T) are more effective in preventing pregnancy and should be replaced at three-year intervals. Progestasert, introduced in 1976, must be replaced annually because of progesterone depletion from the stem of the "T".

Unlike oral contraceptives, IUDs do not interfere with the normal hormonal balance of the body nor do they produce systemic adverse side effects resulting from this imbalance. Complications associated with the use of IUDs include painful menstrual periods, heavier menstrual flow (both effects most pronounced during the first three months after insertion), and pelvic inflammatory disease; the last is associated with severe infection and potentially causes complete tubal obstruction which may result in ectopic (outside the uterus) pregnancy and infertility.

Postcoital Contraception

Unprotected intercourse during midcycle is not an uncommon occurrence and carries with it a 2 to 30 percent risk of pregnancy. Following such intercourse many women seek postcoital contraception. Such "morning-after" contraceptives are not only useful when intercourse occurs infrequently but are also employed in the cases of rape or incest. These products, most practical if self-administered by the patient after occasional intercourse, would overcome the expense, inconvenience, and adverse side effects and potential hazards associated with the daily administration of oral contraceptives.

Diethylstilbestrol. A synthetic compound, possessing estrogenic activity, diethylstilbestrol has been approved for use in emergency situations requiring the termination of pregnancy when, for example, there is a high risk of teratogenic or other adverse effects to the fetus, or when the mother's physical or mental well-being is jeopardized as the result of pregnancy. When taken within 72 hours after sexual intercourse, this drug has been found to be highly effective in preventing pregnancy. However, because of the potential dangers associated with the use of diethylstilbestrol (see above), it should not be employed as a contraceptive agent on a routine or frequent basis.

IUD. Morning-after IUD insertion effectively prevents pregnancy probably by a mechanism involving prevention of implantation of the fertilized egg. This contraceptive approach is not employed in rape or in women who have had intercourse with multiple partners and in whom the risk of exposure to venereal disease is high.

Male Fertility Control

Practical attempts to chemically modify male fertility have not been successful. Although some compounds have been found to markedly, yet temporarily, inhibit the production of sperm, they have also impaired sexual desires or had other undesirable side effects. Let us assume for a moment that a safe, totally effective and nonpermanent antisperm compound were developed. Would men widely use it, or would the loss of the ability to procreate be equated to a loss of masculinity? In this regard, in recent years, vasectomies have become widespread and, in some circles, even fashionable.

Fertility Drugs

One of the approaches taken to control fertility was to develop an estrogen antagonist. *Clomiphene (Clomid)* possesses such properties, but, more significantly, it has been shown to stimulate ovulation in many women with various disorders that had previously rendered them infertile. The precise mechanism responsible for promoting ovulation has not been conclusively proved. Normally, high blood levels of estrogens exert an inhibitory influence on the hypothalamus which in turn suppresses the release of gonadotropic hormones by the anterior pituitary. This is an example of a negative feedback system. Clomiphene is an estrogen antagonist and may act by blocking the inhibitory effects of estrogens on the hypothalamus, thus promoting the release of gonadotropins and stimulating ovulation. About 80 percent of the women given this drug respond by ovulating, with about half becoming pregnant. In addition to such adverse effects as hot flashes, the incidence of *multiple births* is about 8 percent, which is higher than normal.

MALE SEX HORMONES

The male sex hormones or **androgens** are responsible for the normal development and maintenance of the male secondary sex characteristics, sex organs and related structures, and for the synthesis of sperm. **Testosterone,** the primary androgen, has a steroid nucleus and a chemical structure similar to that of progesterone.

Testosterone
(Male hormone)

Progesterone
(Female hormone)

Among the major effects produced by androgens are those concerned with protein *anabolism,* the buildup of proteins of body cells. Testosterone promotes the retention of nitrogen by the body, which is needed for the synthesis of proteins. Androgens account for the male's larger muscle mass.

TABLE 23-5. REPRESENTATIVE MALE SEX HORMONES

Type	Generic Name	Selected Trade Names
Androgen replacement therapy	Testosterone	Delatestryl, Oreton
	Methyltestosterone	Metandren, Oreton Methyl
Anabolic steroids *	Ethylestrenol	Maxibolin
	Fluoxymesterone	Halotestin, Ora-Testryl
	Nandrolone	Durabolin
	Oxymetholone	Adroyd, Anadrol
	Stanozolol	Winstrol

*Whereas testosterone and methyltestosterone have approximately equivalent androgenic (male hormonal) and anabolic (retention of nitrogen) effects, the anabolic steroids possess two to three times more of the latter activity.

Research efforts have been directed toward developing synthetic compounds that possess minimal virilizing effects, while retaining their anabolic activity. These drugs, termed **anabolic steroids** (Table 23–5), are used to reverse nitrogen loss after surgery, debilitating diseases, or malnutrition.

Anabolic steroids are also used by some body-builders aspiring to be Mr. Universe, weight lifters, football players, and other athletes seeking to increase their muscle mass and weight. Although few critical studies have been conducted, it is the general consensus among authorities in sports medicine that the anabolic steroids produce no increase in strength or physical performance and are harmful when improperly used. The apparent increase in muscle mass has been attributed to fluid retention and not functional gold medal–winning muscle.

Among the potential dangers associated with the use of anabolic steroids are testicular shrinkage, loss of sex drive, edema, and liver and bone damage. If administered prior to the attainment of full height, the anabolic steroids cause a premature hardening (calcification) of the ends of long bones, thereby preventing further elongation of bones. These drugs also produce masculinizing effects in women, such as deepening of the voice, growth of facial and body hair, and a regression of the breasts. Anabolic steroids will probably remain a behind-the-scenes part of some athletes' medicine chests until definitive studies unequivocally prove them to be ineffective and actually harmful when employed without medical supervision.

SUMMARY

Adequate secretions of the sex hormones are required for the development, function, and maintenance of the reproductive organs and secondary sex characteristics. The female sex organs synthesize the estrogen estradiol and the progestin progesterone. Estrogens are used clinically to replace hormone deficiencies, such as during menopause, and these drugs and the progestins are also used for the treatment of menstrual disorders. The estrogens and progestins are most commonly used as oral contraceptives and act by altering the normal reproductive cycle in the female.

The menstrual cycle is initiated by the release of FSH from the anterior pituitary, which stimulates the ovarian follicles and the developing ovum. The ovary secretes estrogen, a hormone that stimulates the uterine mucosa to increase in size. High blood levels of estrogen inhibit further release of FSH, and also promote the output of LH from the anterior pituitary. LH triggers the release of the egg from the follicle (ovulation) and converts the follicle to the corpus luteum. The corpus luteum secretes progesterone and estrogen, the former causing structural and functional changes in the uterine mucosa conducive to receiving and nourishing an implanted fertilized egg. If fertilization does not occur, progesterone blood levels inhibit additional LH release, resulting in degeneration of the corpus luteum and cessation of hormonal output, with shedding of the uterine mucosa and menstruation.

Oral contraceptives act by inhibiting the release of FSH and LH from the anterior pituitary, thus preventing the development and release of the egg. They also create an unfavorable environment for implantation of the fertilized egg.

A great variety of adverse effects are associated with the use of oral contraceptives, some of which include nausea, breast fullness, edema, headache, and breakthrough bleeding. Liver diseases, such as jaundice, and thromboembolic disorders are more serious problems linked with the use of these drugs. Only time will determine what long-term adverse effects are associated with the chronic use of these drugs. Other contraceptive methods are compared in Table 23–2.

The androgens, or male sex hormones, have virilizing and anabolic effects. Testosterone is used to replace deficient testicular androgen secretion and to treat breast cancer in females, while the anabolic steroids are employed to build up patients after debilitating disorders. At best, the use of anabolic steroids by athletes is ineffectual in building up functional muscle mass; if improperly employed, they may be dangerous, and in some cases irreversible, adverse changes can occur.

SUPPLEMENTARY READINGS

Bingel, A. S., and P. S. Benoit, "Oral Contraceptives: Therapeutic versus Adverse Reactions, with an Outlook for the Future," *Journal of Pharmaceutical Sciences* **62**:179–200, 349–62 (1973).

Brotherton, J., *Sex Hormone Pharmacology*. New York: Academic Press, 1976.

Chan, L., and B. O'Malley, "Mechanism of Action of Sex Steroid Hormones," *New England Journal of Medicine* **294**: 1322–28, 1372–81, 1430–37 (1976).

Ewing, L. L., and B. Robaire, "Endogenous Antisperm Agents: Prospects for Male Contraception," *Annual Review of Pharmacology and Toxicology* **18**: 167–87 (1978).

Garattini, S., and H. W. Berendes, eds., *Pharmacology of Steroid Contraceptive Drugs.* New York: Raven Press, 1977.

Hafez, E. S. E., and T. N. Evans, eds., *Human Reproduction: Conception and Contraception.* New York: Harper & Row, 1973.

Hatcher, R. A., et al., *Contraceptive Technology 1978–1979.* 9th rev. ed. New York: Irvington Publishers, 1978.

Jackson, H., *Antifertility Compounds in the Male and Female.* Springfield, Ill.: Charles C Thomas, 1966.

Kellie, A. E., "Pharmacology of the Estrogens," *Annual Review of Pharmacology* **11**: 97–112 (1971).

Martini, L., and M. Motta, eds., *Androgens and Antiandrogens.* New York: Raven Press, 1977.

Rahwan, R. G., "Pharmacological Approaches to Birth Control: Contraceptives, Interceptives, Abortifacients," *U.S. Pharmacist* **2** (9): 30-42; (10): 56-72 (1977).

24

Insulin and Oral Antidiabetic Agents

In the course of our experiments we have administered over seventy-five doses of extract from degenerated pancreatic tissue to ten different diabetic animals [dogs]. Since the extract has always produced a reduction of the sugar of the blood and of the sugar excreted in the urine, we feel justified in stating that this extract contains the internal secretion of the pancreas.

—Frederick G. Banting and Charles H. Best (1922)

Diabetes is probably the most common endocrine abnormality, with estimates suggesting there are about 8 million diabetics in the United States today. A little over a half-century ago, the prognosis for a child with this disorder was almost certain death prior to maturity. Since that time, insulin, although not producing cures, has permitted the diabetic to enjoy a full and productive life.

In this chapter we shall consider the hormone insulin and its use in controlling diabetes mellitus, a disease that results from inadequate functional blood levels of insulin. In addition, oral antidiabetic agents, first introduced in the mid-1950s and now widely used by many diabetics, will be discussed. The role of glucagon in diabetes mellitus and the treatment of this disorder with somatostatin will be discussed in the last section of this chapter.

INSULIN

History

In 1889 von Mering and Minkowski demonstrated that when the pancreas of a dog was surgically removed, within several days the animal exhibited symptoms that were identical to those observed in human diabetes. In particular, these scientists noted high concentrations of sugar in the urine. Unfortunately, they were primarily interested in the digestive functions of the pancreas and failed to pursue these significant findings.

The trail was picked up in the summer of 1921 at the University of Toronto by Frederick Banting, a young Canadian surgeon and his assistant, Charles Best, a graduate student in physiology. Banting theorized that previous attempts to isolate the hormone of the pancreas were unsuccessful because pancreatic enzymes, normally participating in the digestion of proteins in the diet, were destroying insulin, a protein, during the extraction process. When a ligature was tied to close the pancreatic ducts, the exocrine cells of the pancreas responsible for manufacturing these digestive enzymes would degenerate, while the endocrine cells of the pancreas that synthesized insulin would not be affected. Two months later, Banting and Best succeeded in obtaining this selectively degenerated pancreas, extracts of which when injected into a severely diabetic dog reduced the highly elevated blood sugar concentration to almost normal levels within one hour. Similar results were obtained in nine other dogs, one of whom was kept alive for 70 days by daily injections of the extract. Shortly thereafter, similarly beneficial effects of pancreatic extracts containing insulin were demonstrated in human diabetic patients.

Banting as well as John MacLeod, in whose laboratory Banting and Best conducted their experiments, won the 1923 Nobel Prize. In passing, it should be noted that Professor MacLeod provided the young workers with no stipend or technical assistance for their summer work, only the use of his laboratory and ten dogs; moreover, MacLeod was gone during this summer. Banting split his share of the prize money with Best.

Insulin was extracted in pure crystalline form in 1926, its chemical structure was established by Sanger[1] in 1954, and this hormone was first synthesized in the laboratory by Katsoyannis in 1966.

Chemistry and Source

Insulin is a protein having a molecular weight of about 6000 and consists of two chains of amino acids joined by two disulfide (—S—S—) bridges. The precise sequence of these 51 amino acids has been determined, and we now know that subtle differences in the order of these amino acids exist among different animal species. Since insulin is a protein, it cannot be administered by mouth. The enzymes of our digestive system would act on this hormone as they would on any other protein in our diets and would break the protein molecule down into small units, and thereby inactivate insulin, rendering it devoid of hormonal activity.

The **pancreas** is both an exocrine and endocrine gland. Ducts convey pancreatic juice containing enzymes for the digestion of foods from the pancreas to the intestines; this is the exocrine function of the gland. The endocrine activities

---

[1] In 1958, Frederick Sanger, a British biochemist, received the Nobel Prize in Chemistry.

of the pancreas are carried out by a small group of cells, the islets of Langerhans, that comprise only about 1.5 percent of the total weight of the pancreas. The islets contain several types of cells: the alpha cells which secrete glucagon and the beta cells, which manufacture, store, and release insulin.

Glucagon promotes the breakdown of liver glycogen (glycogenolysis), causing the release of glucose and a rise in blood sugar levels. This action is opposite to that of insulin. Recent evidence suggests that a relative or absolute excess of glucagon (hyperglucagonemia) may be involved in the development of diabetes. We shall consider the experimental use of the hormone *somatostatin* to suppress glucagon release in the last section of this chapter.

Metabolic Actions of Insulin

Diabetes mellitus is a highly complex disease. This is not surprising when we realize that insulin has a profound effect on the regulation of carbohydrate, fat, and protein metabolism in many parts of the body.

Carbohydrates

If we were to inject a normal or diabetic subject with insulin, the most prominent effect observed would be a rapid reduction in the levels of glucose in the blood. This effect results from an insulin-induced enhancement of the ability of this sugar to cross cell membranes and enter the cell. Once inside the cell, glucose is utilized as a raw material for the generation of energy required to carry out normal cellular activities. Not all glucose circulating in the blood is immediately utilized to provide energy, and large amounts are stored in the liver and muscle as glycogen. When the energy requirements of the body are increased, such as during exercise or emergencies, glycogen is broken down, thereby making glucose available. Insulin promotes the conversion of glucose to glycogen (glycogenesis), and in the absence of this hormone, normal storage of glycogen is impaired.

Fats and Proteins

In addition to being stored as glycogen, excess glucose is held in reserve in adipose tissue in the form of triglycerides.[2] Insulin is required for the synthesis of triglycerides; this hormone also inhibits the enzyme lipase which promotes the breakdown of triglycerides to free fatty acids. We shall soon observe that the aberration of fat metabolism in uncontrolled diabetes is the principle cause of death in this disease.

In the absence of insulin, protein synthesis is depressed and protein breakdown to amino acids is accelerated; failure to grow normally is one of the symptoms of diabetes in children. Insulin enhances the cellular uptake of amino acids and promotes the synthesis of proteins from amino acid building blocks.

[2] Triglycerides are esters consisting of glycerol and two or three different fatty acids.

Control of Insulin Release

The rate of insulin release is primarily dependent upon the concentration of blood glucose. A rise in blood glucose activates the secretion of insulin; when blood glucose levels are low or normal, insulin is released at a low rate. Subnormal blood sugar concentrations stimulate the release of epinephrine from the adrenal medulla and glucagon from the liver. Both these hormones are capable of activating the enzyme phosphorylase which breaks down liver glycogen into glucose, a process termed glycogenolysis. These hormones are thought to act by increasing levels of adenylate cyclase, an enzyme which, in turn, promotes the formation of cyclic AMP, the second messenger (Chapter 22); cyclic AMP may directly activate phosphorylase. Tolbutamide (Orinase) and related sulfonylurea compounds used for the oral treatment of diabetes act by enhancing the release of insulin from the pancreas (see below).

DIABETES MELLITUS

Having considered the normal physiological functions of insulin, let us now examine the consequences of inadequate insulin secretion or function that are manifested clinically in **diabetes mellitus.** The name of this hormonal disorder gives us some clues regarding two of its symptoms. Diabetes means "a running through" and mellitus denotes "sweet," or more precisely, "honeyed." Thus, diabetes mellitus is a disease in which there is an excessive output of urine (polyuria) and the urine contains sugar (glycosuria). In addition to polyuria and glycosuria, the untreated diabetic has high blood sugar levels (hyperglycemia), excessive thirst and hunger, marked weakness, and loss of weight. Impairment of normal fat metabolism causes acidosis or an excess of body acids. We shall briefly consider the basis for these symptoms.

Normally, the body frugally manages its sugar content. Some is immediately utilized to provide energy, while the remainder is stored as glycogen or fat, with very little excreted in the urine. Diabetics are incapable of adequately utilizing glucose or storing it, and, therefore, high concentrations are present in the blood (hyperglycemia). When blood sugar levels become sufficiently elevated, about 180 mg/100 ml, the excess is excreted in the urine and glycosuria results. Sugar acts as a diuretic agent, and accompanying its excretion is the loss of large volumes of water (polyuria). With the loss of body water in the urine, there is dehydration of the tissues, causing diabetics to be excessively thirsty. Notwithstanding the high concentrations of glucose in their blood, diabetics are unable to trap this great potential source of energy within their cells; hunger, weakness, and loss of weight result. Such individuals are virtually "starving in the midst of plenty." You will recall that an insulin deficiency has detrimental effects on protein metabolism, namely, increased breakdown of protein, impaired protein synthesis from amino acids, and enhanced conversion of proteins to glucose. These effects all contribute to loss of weight.

The initial problems of diabetes result from an impairment of carbohydrate metabolism, but it is the aberration in fat metabolism that is often responsible for the death of the patient. Normally, 30 to 40 percent of the ingested glucose is stored as fat in the form of triglycerides. In diabetes, we find that less than 5 percent is stored as fat, and very high blood levels of free fatty acids are present. These fatty acids are converted to ketone bodies, such as acetoacetic acid, acetone, and β-hydroxybutyric acid. The presence of high concentrations of acetoacetic acid and β-hydroxybutyric acid causes changes in the acid-base balance of the body (acidosis) and leads to a loss of body electrolytes and water resulting in impaired respiration, drowsiness, unconsciousness, or *diabetic coma,*[3] and, if not treated, death.

High cholesterol levels are usually observed in diabetes, favoring the development of atherosclerosis. Impaired circulation to the extremities and diabetic gangrene are among the chronic effects of this disorder.

Types of Diabetes

In our discussion thus far, you might be led (or misled) into concluding that diabetes is simply the result of the inability of the pancreas to produce adequate amounts of insulin. This view is only partially correct. If we were to analyze the pancreas for insulin content, we would observe that some diabetics have little or no insulin, while others have normal pancreatic concentrations of insulin. These two types are classified as juvenile and maturity-onset diabetes, respectively.

Juvenile diabetes (insulin-deficient diabetes, acute-onset diabetes, insulin-dependent diabetes) may occur at any age, although it usually makes its appearance prior to maturity. Seen in about 10 percent of all diabetics, this type is more severe and is often complicated by acidosis. Both the insulin content and the number of beta cells of the islets of Langerhans are virtually absent. **Maturity-onset diabetes (non-insulin-dependent diabetes),** which develops later in life, most often during middle age, is mild and acidosis is rare. The insulin content and beta cells are generally normal. It has been argued by some investigators that antagonists are present in the plasma which interfere with the actions of insulin.

Heredity is now viewed to be a major factor in diabetes which results from a defect in one or more genes controlling carbohydrate metabolism. The disease is fortunately a recessive characteristic which is present in about one-fifth of the population. We might predict that about 4 percent of us will develop diabetes, to at least some degree, during the course of our lifetimes. Maturity-onset diabetes is more commonly observed in older persons who are obese than in nonobese individuals.

---

[3] Persons found on the street in diabetic coma are sometimes mistaken for intoxicated individuals; however, rather than having the smell of alcohol on their breath, the diabetic often, but not always, has the odor of acetone.

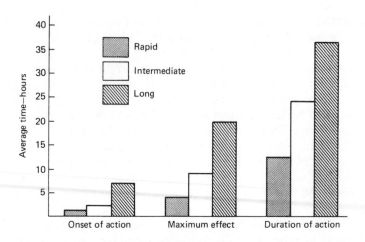

FIGURE 24–1. The Times of Onset, Duration of Action, and Maximum Effect of Insulin Preparations. The effect measured is the depression of blood glucose concentrations; the times depicted on this figure vary among the different insulin preparations within each group. *Rapid-acting insulins:* Crystalline zinc (regular) insulin; Semilente. *Intermediate-acting insulins:* Globin zinc; Lente; NPH; Isophane. *Long-acting insulins:* Protamine zinc (PZI); Ultralente.

Therapeutic Uses of Insulin

Insulin is commercially obtained from beef and pork pancreas. The various insulin preparations differ with respect to their onset, time of peak activity, and duration of action (Figure 24–1). The principal use of insulin is for the symptomatic treatment of diabetes, when the disease cannot be controlled by modifications in diet alone. Prior to the introduction of insulin, and even currently in mild cases, a carefully controlled diet represents an essential element of successful treatment.

Unlike with most other drugs, we do not speak of average doses of insulin. Based upon the amount of insulin endogenously released by the pancreas, as well as diet, level of exercise, and other concurrently existing illnesses or stresses, each diabetic must determine the dose that best fulfills his or her unique requirements. Inadequate amounts of insulin will not fully control the disease symptoms, while an overdose will produce weakness, nervousness, anxiety, seizures, coma, and even death resulting from a profound reduction in blood sugar (*hypoglycemia*).

The diabetic injects insulin under the skin, subcutaneously, usually into the loose tissues of the arms or thighs. Insulin does not cure diabetes but rather serves as a replacement for the inadequate amounts released by the pancreas. As long as proper amounts of insulin are administered, the patient no longer suffers the risk of diabetic coma and death, the major acute problems in the preinsulin era. Nevertheless, diabetes is the fifth leading cause of death in the United States. While insulin does control the symptoms of diabetes, the underlying complications associated with this disorder continue, and these include degenerative changes in the arteries, kidneys (diabetic nephropathy), and retina (diabetic retinopathy). Reduced arterial blood flow to the extremities causes cold hands and feet, slow healing of wounds, infections, ulceration, and gangrene. The diabetic has a greater risk of atherosclerosis and coronary artery disease than the nondiabetic. Among the most striking effects of diabetes is diabetic retinopathy which can cause significant impairment of vision; diabetes is the second leading cause of blindness in the United States.

ORAL ANTIDIABETIC AGENTS

While insulin has dramatically altered the prognosis for the diabetic patient, for many decades attempts were made to develop **hypoglycemic agents**—drugs that reduce blood sugar—which would be effective after oral administration.

During clinical trials conducted in 1942 with an antibacterial sulfonamide intended for the treatment of typhoid fever, it was observed that patients experienced hypoglycemia. In 1955, carbutamide was introduced in Europe as the first oral hypoglycemic agent. Shortly thereafter, tolbutamide was marketed in the United States, but unlike carbutamide it possessed no antibacterial activity. **Tolbutamide** and chemically related hypoglycemic agents are collectively referred to as the **sulfonylureas** (Figure 24–2).

About one-half century ago, several guanidine derivatives were shown to produce hypoglycemia in animals, but toxicity precluded their use in humans. Interest in these compounds was renewed when the sulfonylureas were shown to be clinically effective as oral hypoglycemic agents. **Phenformin**, a **biguanide**, is the only member of this drug class used in this country. As we shall soon observe, its mechanism of action differs from that of the sulfonylureas. Let us first discuss the sulfonylureas.

Sulfonylureas

Several oral hypoglycemic sulfonylurea agents are currently used in the United States, including tolbutamide (Orinase), acetohexamide (Dymelor), chlorpropamide (Diabinese), and tolazamide (Tolinase); these drugs differ primarily with respect to their duration of action.

The sulfonylureas act by stimulating the release of insulin from the beta cells of the islets of Langerhans. In the absence of the pancreas, or in cases of juvenile diabetes where the pancreas is grossly deficient in its ability to secrete insulin, the sulfonylureas are ineffective. We find that these drugs are of greatest value in the treatment of mild maturity-onset diabetes, where the pancreas continues to be rich in its insulin supply.

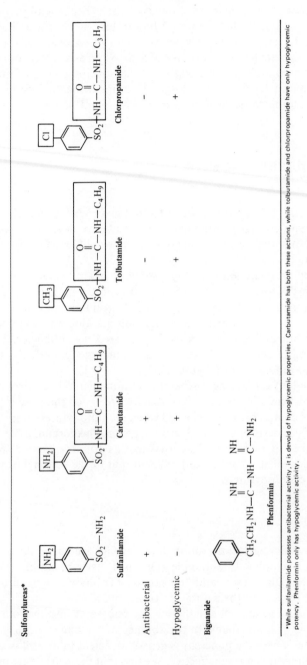

FIGURE 24-2. Representative Oral Hypoglycemic Agents.

*While sulfanilamide possesses antibacterial activity, it is devoid of hypoglycemic properties. Carbutamide has both these actions, while tolbutamide and chlorpropamide have only hypoglycemic potency. Phenformin only has hypoglycemic activity.

Biguanides: Phenformin

The mechanism underlying the hypoglycemic effects of phenformin (DBI) in diabetic patients is not clear. This drug does not activate the release of insulin from the pancreas, nor does it induce hypoglycemia in nondiabetic subjects. It appears that phenformin may act by accelerating the intracellular oxidation of glucose, a process which is depressed in the absence of insulin. Phenformin is used alone for the treatment of maturity-onset diabetes and in combination with insulin in juvenile diabetes. While clinically effective, phenformin was withdrawn from the general American market in 1977 because of its close association with the potentially fatal metabolic disorder lactic acidosis. This drug may be obtained directly from the manufacturer for use in selected patients. Neither biguanide nor sulfonylurea agents are recommended for the treatment of diabetes during pregnancy.

Oral Hypoglycemic Drug Interactions

A large number of pharmacologically unrelated drugs have been shown to interfere with the therapeutic effectiveness of the oral hypoglycemic agents and the control of stable blood sugar levels. Several examples of these drug-drug interactions include diuretics which themselves increase blood sugar; aspirin and other salicylates which can lower blood sugar concentrations, thus enhancing the effects of hypoglycemic agents; and, the antibacterial sulfonamides and monoamine oxidase inhibitor antidepressants which potentiate the effects of hypoglycemic agents.

Adrenergic agents promote glycogen breakdown, and thereby antagonize the effect of oral hypoglycemic agents or insulin by increasing blood sugar levels. Many of these drugs, including ephedrine, phenylephrine, and phenylpropanolamine, are found in nonprescription cold and allergy remedies. Amphetamine and related compounds used as appetite suppressants have mild hyperglycemic effects. Alcohol has been clinically shown to greatly enhance the hypoglycemic effects of insulin in diabetic patients.

It is far beyond the scope of this text to discuss these drug-drug interactions in detail. The author merely intends to point out the potential dangers to diabetic patients and encourage such individuals to consult with a physician or pharmacist prior to taking any other medications with their prescribed hypoglycemic agents.

UGDP Controversy

In 1970 a report appeared,[4] initiated in 1961, and designed to evaluate the effectiveness of antidiabetic therapy in preventing or reducing the incidence of vascular disease in diabetic patients. Eight hundred non-insulin-requiring

[4] University Group Diabetes Program, "A Study of the Effects of Hypoglycemic Agents on Vascular Complications in Patients with Adult-Onset Diabetes," *Diabetes* **19** (Supplement 2): 747–830 (1970).

patients at twelve different university based clinics (University Group Diabetes Program or *UGDP*) were compared for periods of up to eight years. The patients in this study received one of the following treatments: dietary modification and placebo, insulin, tolbutamide, or phenformin. Most unexpectedly, it was observed that the incidence of cardiovascular mortality was *highest* in those patients receiving tolbutamide and phenformin.

Many investigators have interpreted the results of this study to indicate that tolbutamide and dietary modifications may be less effective than diet alone or than diet and insulin in reducing cardiovascular mortality. The American Diabetic Association has advised that an attempt be made to control maturity-onset diabetes (in the absence of ketosis) with diet. If control cannot be achieved with diet, they suggest that insulin rather than oral hypoglycemic agents be used because insulin is more effective and probably safer.

The results of the UGDP report have generated considerable and, oftentimes, heated arguments both supporting and refuting these conclusions. Whether or not the conclusions of the UGDP report are valid, it is generally accepted that *proper diet* and *weight reduction* are of critical importance in the successful management of maturity-onset diabetes.

Future Treatment Approaches

For over one-half century, the management of insulin-dependent diabetes has remained essentially unchanged, namely, dietary restrictions and the need for intermittent subcutaneous injections of insulin. This approach does not completely restore glucose homeostasis to normal and, as a consequence, the diabetic is never normoglycemic throughout the entire course of a day. It has been suggested that this failure may be responsible for or contribute to the chronic complications that inevitably accompany even "well-controlled" diabetes.

At present, there is an intensive effort underway to develop alternative or supplementary methods that will more effectively control the diabetic hyperglycemia. New approaches include pancreatic transplantation, islet cell transplantation, artificial beta cell devices, and somatostatin. Unfortunately, all remain in the experimental stage at this time, and none have been sufficiently perfected to be used on a routine clinical basis.

Pancreatic transplantation. Among the earliest experimental approaches explored to lower elevated blood sugar levels was whole pancreas transplantation to serve as a source of insulin. This approach has not proven to be successful for a variety of reasons including tissue rejection (a problem encountered when any organ is being transplanted), vascular thrombosis (clot formation within the blood vessels), inflammation of the pancreas, and digestion of the host (recipient's) tissue by exocrine pancreatic enzymes. While acute and chronic tissue rejection remains the major obstacle, the most promising techniques involve the transplantation of pancreatic segments adapted to permit the drainage of the exocrine pancreas.

Islet cell transplantation. In an attempt to circumvent the inherent problems associated with transplantation of the whole or a partial pancreas, interest has been directed toward transplanting only the islet cells. While this has been successful in controlling experimentally induced diabetes in animals, to date this approach has not proved to be clinically fruitful in humans because the available isolation techniques do not yield a sufficiently large amount of islet cells available for transplantation.

Artificial beta cell. Considerable interest has been focused upon the development of an "artificial beta cell" device that would be sufficiently compact to permit its implantation into the body of a diabetic. Such a device would ideally constantly monitor the glucose concentration of the blood (or another suitable fluid) and control a self-contained unit to deliver insulin as needed to maintain normoglycemia. While existing devices fail to provide perfect control of blood glucose levels and are too cumbersome to permit the complete implantation of a closed-loop system, the positive results obtained in early studies are encouraging.

Somatostatin. It has been classically believed that an insulin deficiency is responsible for diabetes mellitus. This concept originated with the 1921 experiments of Banting and Best who demonstrated that the experimental diabetes resulting from the removal of the pancreas could be managed by the administration of insulin-containing pancreatic extracts. It is now clear that almost all types of clinical and experimental diabetes are also associated with a relative or absolute increase in blood glucagon levels or *hyperglucagonemia.*[5] **Glucagon** is a potent glycogenolytic, gluconeogenic, and lipolytic and ketogenic hormone whose actions are opposed by insulin and intensified by a deficiency of insulin. It now appears that the metabolic abnormalities associated with diabetes, namely hyperglycemia and hyperketonemia (ketoacidosis), are not the exclusive consequence of an insulin deficiency but result from both an insulin deficiency *and* a glucagon excess. Hence, if hyperglucagonemia plays a major contributory role in these metabolic abnormalities, and if dietary restrictions and the administration of insulin are insufficient to adequately normalize blood glucose levels, it would seem reasonable to attempt to control elevated blood glucagon levels.

During the course of studies designed to isolate from the hypothalamus a substance thought to stimulate the secretion of growth hormone (somatotropin), in 1973 Roger Guillemin[6] and his co-workers at the Salk Institute in

---

[5] R. H. Unger, "Diabetes and the Alpha Cell" (Banting Memorial Lecture), *Diabetes* **25**: 136–51 (1976).

[6] Guillemin was the co-recipient of the 1978 Nobel Prize for his studies on the chemistry and biology of hypothalamic peptides (Chapter 22).

LaJolla, California were surprised to discover that this substance inhibited somatotropin release; it was determined to be a 14-amino acid polypeptide and called **somatostatin.** Among the many actions that administration of this compound has on both endocrine and nonendocrine tissues is its ability to reduce plasma levels of both insulin and glucagon, causing a fall in blood glucose levels in both normal and diabetic human subjects. Infusion of somatostatin has been shown to significantly lower the insulin requirements of insulin-dependent diabetics and more effectively control blood glucose levels than insulin alone, as well as prevent hyperketonemia and alleviate other signs and symptoms of diabetes. Somatostatin is not suitable for routine clinical use because it must be given intravenously, is enzymatically inactivated within minutes, and lacks specificity of action. Attempts are now being made to develop synthetic somatostatin derivatives with greater specificity of action that have a longer duration of action.

SUMMARY

Diabetes mellitus is a disorder arising from a deficiency in insulin secretion and excess glucagon secretion from the pancreas or from an interference with the biological actions of the former hormone. Insulin lowers blood glucose levels by enhancing the tissue uptake of this sugar and promoting the storage of excessive glucose as carbohydrates (glycogen) or fats (triglycerides). The amount of insulin released from the beta cells of the pancreas is controlled by the concentration of glucose in the blood, as well as by a number of more complex factors that have not been discussed in this chapter.

The symptoms of diabetes include high blood sugar, excessive urinary output, excretion of sugar in the urine, hunger, weakness, and loss of weight. Impaired utilization of carbohydrates leads to disturbances in fat metabolism which, if not properly controlled, results in acid buildup in the body with a loss of alkaline reserves (acidosis), diabetic coma, and death. Complications of controlled diabetes, which may slowly appear over several decades, include degenerative changes in the arteries of the extremities and in the capillaries of the retina. Hereditary factors appear to be important in the development of diabetes. In juvenile diabetes, the pancreas contains little or no insulin, while patients with maturity-onset diabetes have almost normal pancreatic levels of insulin.

Insulin is destroyed by enzymes in the gastrointestinal tract and must, therefore, be administered by injection. The insulin preparations commercially available differ with respect to their time course of action. Hormonal replacement must be continued throughout life.

The sulfonylurea oral hypoglycemic agents (tolbutamide) are used for the treatment of stable maturity-onset diabetes and act by stimulating the release of insulin from the beta cells of the pancreas. These compounds are probably less effective than insulin and may increase the risk of cardiovascular mortality.

The acute problems associated with uncontrolled diabetes can now be successfully managed, yet one of the major challenges of biomedical research is to better understand the basis for the degenerative changes that continue even when this disorder is well controlled. Among the experimental approaches being investigated to control the hyperglycemia associated with diabetes include pancreatic and islet cell transplantation, the development of artificial beta cell devices, and the preparation of synthetic derivatives of the hypothalamic hormone somatostatin, a polypeptide that lowers blood glucose levels by inhibiting the secretion of glucagon.

SUPPLEMENTARY READINGS

Cuatrecasas, P., ed., "Symposium: Insulin—Its Synthesis, Release, Interaction with Receptors, and Mechanism of Action," *Federation Proceedings* **34**: 1537–69 (1975).

Fajans, S. S., ed., *Diabetes Mellitus,* Fogarty International Center Series of Preventive Medicine, Vol. 4. Washington, D.C.: Department of Health, Education and Welfare, 1976.

Foa, P. P., J. S. Bajaj, and N. L. Foa, eds., *Glucagon and Its Role in Physiology and Clinical Medicine.* Berlin: Springer-Verlag, 1978.

Karam, J. H., S. B. Martin, and P. H. Forsham, "Antidiabetic Drugs After the University Group Diabetes Program (UGDP)," *Annual Review of Pharmacology* **15**: 351–66 (1975).

Knowles, H. C., Jr., ed., "Fiftieth Anniversary Insulin Symposium," *Diabetes* **21** (Supplement 2): 385–714 (1972).

Larner, J., "Insulin and Oral Hypoglycemic Drugs; Glucagon," in *Goodman and Gilman's The Pharmacological Basis of Therapeutics.* Edited by A. G. Gilman, L. S. Goodman, and A. Gilman, 6th ed., Chap. 64, pp. 1497–1523. New York: Macmillan, 1980.

Podolsky, S., ed., "Symposium on Diabetes Mellitus," *Medical Clinics of North America* **62** (4): 625–869 (1978).

Raskin, P., "Treatment of Diabetes Mellitus: The Future," *Diabetes* **28**: 780-96 (1979).

Shen, S.-W., and R. Bressler, "Clinical Pharmacology of Oral Antidiabetic Agents," *New England Journal of Medicine* **296**: 787–93 (1977).

Steiner, D. F., and N. Freinkel, eds., "Endocrine Pancreas," in *Handbook of Physiology, Vol. 1: Endocrinology,* Sec. 7. Washington, D.C.: American Physiological Society, 1972.

Williams, R. H., and D. Porte, Jr., "The Pancreas," in *Textbook of Endocrinology.* Edited by R. H. Williams, 5th ed., pp. 502–626. Philadelphia: Saunders, 1974.

Drugs Affecting the Gastrointestinal and Respiratory Systems

25

Drug Treatment of Acid-Related Gastrointestinal Disorders

The longer I live, the more I am convinced . . . that half the unhappiness in the world proceeds from little stoppages, from a duct choked up, from a vext duodenum, or an agitated pylorus.

—Sidney Smith (1771–1845)

INDIGESTION, n. A disease which the patient and his friends frequently mistake for deep religious conviction and for the salvation of mankind.[1]

—Ambrose Bierce (1842–1914?)

Many of the most common disorders afflicting us are those affecting the gastrointestinal tract. Digestive disorders account for 16 percent of all absences from work, as well as countless hours of discomfort, agony, or even virtual disability while at work or school or while attempting to escape from the pressures of these activities.

In this chapter, we shall consider drugs used to treat acid-related gastrointestinal (GI) disorders, in particular peptic ulcer disease, while in the next chapter the management of constipation and diarrhea will be discussed. The reader will undoubtedly recognize many of these drugs having seen their virtues extolled ad nauseam in untold numbers of TV advertisement dramatizations designed to subliminally but instantaneously affect the function of your GI tract in a manner necessitating the immediate purchase of one or more of these wonder drugs.

[1] *The Devil's Dictionary.*

ACID-RELATED DISORDERS

In excess of $140 million are spent annually by the American public in search of relief of "sour stomach," "heartburn," "acid indigestion," "upset stomach," and other descriptive synonyms denoting indigestion or GI discomfort. To provide "instant relief" to these tens of millions of "upset stomachs," pharmaceutical manufacturers have made available 8000 gels, suspensions, tablets, powders, and gums.

After considering the physiology of gastric secretion and the nature of peptic ulcer disease, we shall consider the pharmacology of antacids, anticholinergic agents, and H_2-receptor antagonists.

Physiology and Pathophysiology of Gastric Secretion

The upper segment of the GI tract consists of the esophagus, stomach, and small intestine, the latter subdivided into the duodenum, jejunum, and ileum. Glands in the mucosal lining of the stomach secrete *gastric juice* which consists of a mixture of hydrochloric acid, pepsinogen, and gastrin. The acidic (low pH) environment of the stomach favors the conversion of pepsinogen to *pepsin,* an enzyme that participates in the breakdown and digestion of proteins. Why doesn't the gastric juice digest the inner walls of the GI tract as it would any other piece of meat? The mucosal membrane lining the esophagus, stomach, and duodenum is coated with a thick layer of mucus which is normally resistant to the digestive effects of the gastric juice.

Under certain conditions, the gastric juice produces irritation and erosion of the mucosal lining causing discomfort. When stomach acid bubbles up into the lower end of the esophagus, a warm or burning sensation is experienced, and this is commonly referred to as "heartburn." Chronic inflammation of the lining of the stomach, termed gastritis, and the sourness, bloated feeling, and belching associated with it (which the nonmedical sufferer calls "dyspepsia" or "indigestion") are usually managed by neutralizing the gastric acid with an antacid.

Peptic Ulcer Disease

The most severe of the acid-related disorders is **peptic ulcer,** an acute or chronic condition afflicting 10 to 15 percent of the general population. In this disorder, sharply circumscribed areas of the esophagus, stomach, or duodenum are digested and become eroded by the gastric juice; this lesion is termed an *ulcer.* In milder cases, this erosion is limited to the uppermost mucosal layer. In more severe and potentially fatal cases, the ulcer may extend down into deeper layers, breaking through large blood vessels (resulting in extensive internal bleeding) and even perforating the walls of the stomach or duodenum (resulting in peritonitis).

While gastric acid and pepsin must always be present for ulcer formation to occur, the etiology of peptic ulcer disease is not clearly understood. It remains a mystery why and how the normal resistance of the mucosa to acid and pepsin digestion is lost. A number of factors appear to play a role in the development of stomach (gastric) and/or duodenal ulcers: (1) a higher incidence in males than in females suggesting the involvement of hormonal factors; (2) prolonged excessive gastric secretion (gastric hyperacidity) may be present; (3) rapid gastric emptying time resulting in larger than normal amounts of unbuffered acid spilling into the duodenum; (4) emotional factors, such as stress, anger, and hostility; and (5) genetic factors, as suggested by a higher incidence of duodenal ulcers in patients with positive family history of this disorder or blood type O.

A number of *drugs* have been identified as being potentially **ulcerogenic.** Drugs are rarely the sole cause of peptic ulcer disease but more often aggravate or precipitate a pre-existing ulcer. Among such drugs are aspirin, anti-inflammatory drugs such as phenylbutazone (Butazolidin) and indomethacin (Indocin), the antihypertensive agent reserpine (Serpasil), and many anticancer agents including methotrexate. Alcohol, caffeine, and nicotine (tobacco smoking) should be avoided by patients with peptic ulcer disease because these agents stimulate the secretion of gastric acid.

Common complaints voiced by patients with chronic gastric ulcers include "heartburn," nausea, and substernal pain. This pain, located in the pit of the stomach, occurs about one hour after meals and is usually relieved by eating or taking antacids. Pain during the night or early morning is more commonly experienced by patients with duodenal ulcers, a condition ten times more common than gastric ulcers. The pain associated with duodenal ulcers is variously described as gnawing, burning, cramp-like, or as a "heartburn"; some patients, however, may be symptom-free.

As noted above, there are potentially severe complications associated with untreated peptic ulcer disease. Moreover, a number of more serious disorders, such as gastrointestinal cancers, cause ulcer-like pain. Hence, extended periods of self-medication with proprietary antacids, which may mask the symptoms of more severe gastrointestinal disorders, can be dangerous and should be strongly discouraged. If the temporary use of antacids fails to provide sustained relief from gastrointestinal pain, the patient should consult a physician.

DRUG TREATMENT OF ACID-RELATED DISORDERS

The primary objective in the treatment of peptic ulcer disease is to relieve the pain and promote the healing of the ulcer. *Pain* results from gastric acid activating nerve endings in the area of the ulcer leading to spasms of the sur-

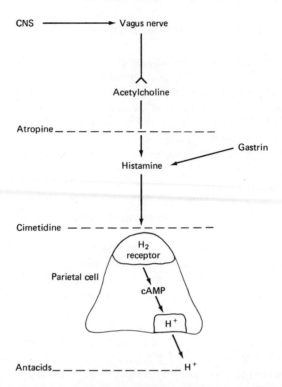

FIGURE 25-1. Diagrammatic Representation of Acid Secretion and Mechanisms of Antiulcer Drugs. Acetylcholine or gastrin can stimulate the release of histamine which activates the H_2-receptor resulting in acid (H^+) secretion; cyclic adenosine monophosphate (cAMP) is involved in acid secretion. Antiulcer drugs may act by: (1) inhibiting the action of acetylcholine at the cholinergic receptor responsible for histamine release (atropine); (2) antagonizing the action of histamine at its H_2-receptor (cimetidine): (3) inhibiting acid release by a mechanism that involves blocking cAMP synthesis; and (4) neutralizing the acid released into the stomach (antacids).

rounding smooth muscle. The *ulcer* results from the digestive action of the proteolytic enzyme pepsin on the GI mucosa; pepsin's proteolytic activity is maximum in a highly acidic environment between pH 1 and 2. Relief of pain and ulcer healing may be fostered by neutralizing the gastric acid or by reducing its secretion.

Acetylcholine, histamine, gastrin (a GI hormone), and the prostaglandins appear to be involved in the release of gastric acid; modifying the activity of one or more of these endogenous compounds in the GI tract represents a potentially fruitful approach to ulcer therapy. The secretory activity of the gastric mucosa is influenced in part by input transmitted from the central nervous system via the vagus (cholinergic) nerve. Vagal stimulation (induced by the sight, smell, taste, or even the thought of food) increases the release of acetylcholine from the postganglionic nerve endings (Figure 25-1). Experimental evidence suggests that acetylcholine or gastrin is able to promote the release of histamine from cells in the gastric mucosa. Histamine, in turn, activates H_2-receptors[2] of parietal cells causing the release of gastric acid. Some prostaglandin derivatives (PGE_2; Chapter 14) appear to play a role in the physiological control of gastric acid secretion.

Examination of Figure 25-1 suggests four of the potential mechanisms by which antiulcer drugs might act:

1. The actions of acetylcholine can be antagonized at the cholinergic (muscarinic) receptor responsible for activating the release of histamine. Atropine and many synthetic anticholinergic agents act by this mechanism.
2. The action of histamine at its H_2-receptor on parietal cells can be blocked with specific H_2-receptor antagonists such as cimetidine.
3. Synthetic prostaglandin derivatives, such as dimethyl-prostaglandin E_2, have been shown to inhibit the release of gastric acid and pepsin by a direct effect on secretory cells by a mechanism that appears to involve inhibition of cyclic adenosine monophosphate (cAMP) synthesis.
4. Antacids can be used to neutralize gastric acid after its release from parietal cells.

Drugs such as carbenoxolone (Biogastrone), isolated from licorice, are thought to promote ulcer healing by increasing the secretion of mucus, which protects the mucosal lining against the corrosive effects of the gastric juices. No drug has been developed as yet that is capable of specifically inhibiting gastrin, an extremely potent stimulant of gastric acid secretion.

Antacids

Antacids, traditionally the mainstay of peptic ulcer therapy, are very widely used to treat indigestion and to relieve the pain and promote the healing of GI ulcers. These drugs are not necessarily capable of preventing the recurrence of ulcers.

The beneficial effects of antacids are attributed to two primary mechanisms: neutralization of gastric acid and reduction in the proteolytic activity of pepsin. Elevation of the pH of the gastric contents to more than pH 4-5 results in the virtually complete inactivation of the enzyme pepsin and, at this pH, the damaging effects of gastric acid to the mucosa are minimal.

To provide maximum benefit, the antacid must remain in the stomach for a sufficiently long period of time to neutralize the acid present. When administered to fasting individuals, however, most antacids are effective for only 20 to 30 minutes before being emptied into the duodenum; this period of time is too short to effect a significant reduction in stomach acidity. Maximum secre-

---

[2] Two types of histamine receptor sites exist (Chapter 27). H_1-receptor activation increases the contraction of intestinal and bronchial smooth muscle; these effects are readily antagonized by classical antihistamines (H_1-receptor antagonists). H_2-receptor activation causes enhanced secretion of acid by the stomach, increased heart rate, and inhibition of contractions of the rat uterus; these effects are not modified by H_1-receptor antagonists.

tion of gastric acid occurs about one hour after meals, and this is the most rational time for the administration of antacids.

Selection of Antacids: General Considerations

Antacids can be purchased without a prescription, and consumers are entreated to rely upon the kindly advice provided by Mother Tums or Speedy in their selection of products to deal with the GI problems the morning after attending a party hosted by Bob and Babs Bacchus. The reassuring tone imparted by these TV ads suggests that there is nothing fundamentally wrong with gorging oneself with food (limited only by the elastic stretch provided in your trousers or skirt) or alcoholic beverages (until the last case of wine is drained) when "relief is only a swallow away."

Contrary to the impression one gains from these TV ads, the stomach is not merely an acid-containing beaker, nor is the most effective antacid the one that neutralizes acid in the shortest period of time or with the smallest dose. No antacid is ideal for all patients, nor best for all acid-related disorders, nor free of causing adverse side effects. The product you select for the rapid relief of distress arising from occasional gluttony ("sour stomach," "gas pains") is not necessarily the same product you should choose for the chronic treatment of peptic ulcer disease; the latter choice would require careful consideration if you had a preexisting kidney disease or were attempting to maintain a salt (sodium)-restricted diet.

Antacids have been traditionally classified as being systemic (absorbable) or nonsystemic (nonabsorbable). The former enter the blood after oral administration and, if taken in sufficiently high doses, may modify the electrolyte balance or alter the pH of the extracellular fluid resulting in systemic (metabolic) alkalosis. Nonabsorbable antacids act exclusively in the gastrointestinal tract, and their adverse effects are generally limited to changes in bowel function, that is, diarrhea or constipation. It is now recognized that some antacids, previously believed to be nonabsorbable, have the potential for causing systemic toxicity (see below).

Liquid antacid preparations are generally more effective than tablets containing the same ingredient(s) because they have a greater surface area available for interaction with and neutralization of gastric acid. Thorough chewing of tablets before swallowing them increases their effectiveness. In addition to considering the relative capacity of an antacid to neutralize an acid,[3] other factors to be taken into consideration when selecting an antacid include its onset and duration of action, palatability, cost, side effects, the patient's medical history, and any other drugs the patient may be taking.

---

[3] The *neutralizing capacity* of antacids can be calculated and compared by determining the volume (ml) of antacid required to neutralize an equivalent amount of acid in vitro (in a test tube); the smaller the volume of antacid required, the higher the drug's neutralizing capacity. For comparison of commercial antacids see J. S. Fordtran, S. G. Morawski, and C. T. Richardson, "In Vivo and In Vitro Evaluation of Liquid Antacids," *New England Journal of Medicine* **288**: 923–28 (1973).

Antacids can potentially **interact** with other drugs the patient is taking. The best documented and most clinically relevant of these involves an interaction with the *tetracycline antibiotics*. Antacids containing calcium, magnesium, or aluminum form a nonabsorbable chelate with members of this antibiotic class causing a substantial decrease in blood levels and a potential reduction in their anti-infective effects. Other interactions may result from the ability of the antacid to alter the pH of the stomach and urine and thereby modify the extent to which coadministered drugs are absorbed and excreted in the urine, respectively. Although the clinical significance of these latter interactions has not been established, it is wise not to take orally administered drugs within one to two hours after taking an antacid.

Specific Antacids

In this section, we shall examine the general properties of some of the most common ingredients in nonprescription antacid products, namely, sodium bicarbonate, calcium carbonate, aluminum- and magnesium-containing compounds, and aluminum-magnesium combinations. The names of selected commercial antacids and their distinguishing properties are summarized in Table 25-1.

Sodium bicarbonate. Baking soda has been used in households for generations as an inexpensive, effective, rapid-acting remedy for the treatment of "sour stomach." Sodium bicarbonate reacts with hydrochloric acid to liberate carbon dioxide:

$$NaHCO_3 + HCl \longrightarrow NaCl + H_2O + CO_2 \uparrow$$

Unfortunately, sodium bicarbonate overneutralizes the gastric acid and elevates the pH of the stomach contents above the optimal 4–5; this results in a rapid increase in acid secretion or "acid rebound" and a short duration of pain relief.

Regular use of this systemic antacid leads to the absorption of significant amounts of drug to potentially cause metabolic alkalosis and sodium loading, the latter a major problem for the patient being maintained on a sodium-restricted diet. Chronic administration of sodium bicarbonate with milk (intended to soothe ulcer pain) leads to an increase in calcium absorption and may result in the *milk-alkali syndrome*. This condition is characterized by greater than normal levels of calcium in the blood (hypercalcemia), impairment of kidney function, and systemic alkalosis which may cause nausea, vomiting, headache, and mental confusion. Hence, while sodium bicarbonate or a very popular effervescent product containing this antacid (Alka-Seltzer) is useful for occasional relief from overeating or indigestion, it should not be used on a chronic basis.

Calcium carbonate. Calcium carbonate, a chalky tasting compound, is a potent and effective antacid with a rapid onset and long duration of action.

TABLE 25-1. COMPARATIVE PROPERTIES OF SELECTED ANTACIDS

Generic Name (Synonym)	Selected Trade Names	Remarks
Sodium bicarbonate (baking soda)	Alka-Seltzer	Widely used, rapid-acting, potent, effective. Disadvantages: acid rebound, risk of systemic alkalosis, sodium overloading. Not recommended for regular use.
Calcium carbonate (precipitated chalk)	Dicarbosil Titralac Tums	Rapid, prolonged, effective acid neutralization. Disadvantages: acid rebound, milk-alkali syndrome, tendency to constipate, chalky taste.
Aluminum Compounds		
Aluminum hydroxide gel	Amphojel Alu-Cap Basaljel Robalate Rolaids	Aluminum compounds: relatively low neutralizing capacity; constipation common; some systemic absorption.
Aluminum carbonate		
Dihydroxyaluminum aminoacetate		
Dihydroxyaluminum sodium carbonate		
Magnesium Compounds		
Magnesium carbonate (carbonate of magnesia)		Magnesium salts: have tendency to cause diarrhea; slightly absorbable and should not be used by patients with impairment of kidney function.
Magnesium hydroxide (milk of magnesia)		
Magnesium oxide		
Magnesium trisilicate		
Aluminum/Magnesium Combinations	Aludrox A.M.T. Creamalin DiGel Gelusil Kolantyl Gel Maalox Malcogel Mylanta Trisogel Win Gel	More palatable products with greater neutralizing capacity than aluminum hydroxide. Aluminum-induced constipation and magnesium-induced diarrhea balanced. Most contain high salt content (except magaldrate).
Magaldrate	Riopan	

$$CaCO_3 + 2HCl \longrightarrow CaCl_2\downarrow + H_2O + CO_2\uparrow$$

Although only a limited amount of calcium is absorbed when the drug is used frequently, chronic administration may cause hypercalcemia and the milk-alkali syndrome.

Aluminum-containing antacids.   Aluminum-containing antacids possess relatively low acid-neutralizing capacity but do not cause acid rebound or systemic alkalosis.

$$Al(OH)_3 + 3HCl \longrightarrow AlCl_3 + 3H_2O$$

Their most common side effect is constipation which may lead to intestinal obstruction in elderly patients or those individuals with decreased bowel motility.

Aluminum hydroxide binds to and decreases the intestinal absorption of phosphates contained in the diet; it is used on a regular basis for the management of hyperphosphatemia (elevated blood phosphate levels) in chronic kidney dialysis patients. The results of recent clinical studies[4] reject the time-honored belief that insoluble aluminum salts are not absorbed and are non-toxic. Patients who have taken aluminum salts for several years develop a progressive neurological disorder termed *dialysis encephalopathy* or dialysis dementia that is associated with a high mortality rate; such patients have been found to have much higher than normal levels of aluminum in the gray matter of their brains.

Magnesium-containing antacids.   Magnesium salts have a higher acid neutralizing capacity than aluminum hydroxide gel and do not produce systemic alkalosis. Diarrhea is the most common side effect associated with their use.

$$Mg(OH)_2 + 2HCl \longrightarrow MgCl_2 + 2H_2O$$

Magnesium accumulates in the bodies of patients with impaired kidney function which can result in low blood pressure, depressed reflexes, respiratory depression, and coma. Hence, magnesium salts should not be used by patients with disorders of the kidney interfering with its function.

Aluminum-magnesium combinations.   A very large number of commercially available antacids contain a mixture of aluminum and magnesium salts (Table 25–1). Such preparations are more pleasant tasting and provide greater acid neutralizing capacity than aluminum hydroxide. The rationale underlying this combination is to balance the constipation and diarrhea normally caused by each of the ingredients.

[4] A. C. Alfrey, "Dialysis Encephalopathy Syndrome," *Annual Review of Medicine* **29**: 93–8 (1978).

Anticholinergic Agents

Surgical vagotomy (cutting the vagal nerve fibers to the acid-secreting cells of the stomach) effectively suppresses gastric acid secretion, but is a rather radical procedure not without risk. Anticholinergic agents produce a chemical vagotomy by preventing the action of acetylcholine at cholinergic receptors involved in the secretion of acid and pepsin.

More specifically, atropine and related anticholinergic (antimuscarinic) agents reduce gastric acid secretion, decrease smooth muscle motility, and delay gastric emptying time. Since an ulcer does not form in the absence of acid, and part of the pain associated with this disorder is caused by smooth muscle contractions, anticholinergic agents should, at least in theory, be ideally suited for the management of peptic ulcer disease. In practice, however, this has not been the case. While these drugs are believed by many physicians to be of benefit when used in conjunction with modifications in diet and antacid administration, their ability to prevent ulcer recurrences over extended periods of time has not been well established.

The high doses of atropine-like drugs required to substantially reduce gastric acid secretion are almost always accompanied by such adverse effects as dry mouth, blurred vision, increase in heart rate, and difficulty in urination (Chapter 8). The ability of these drugs to slow gastric emptying time prolongs the time available for antacids to neutralize gastric acid. However, this advantageous effect may be offset by the fact that the continued presence of food in the stomach provides a stimulus for the prolonged secretion of acid. These drugs are contraindicated for those with gastric ulcers because the delay in emptying time prolongs the duration of contact between the gastric contents and the ulcer. Atropine antagonizes acetylcholine-induced motility by blocking muscarinic sites on smooth muscle, and this is the basis for its antispasmodic effects.

Choice of Drugs

The naturally occurring belladonna alkaloids atropine and scopolamine are highly effective in reducing the motility and secretory activity of the GI tract. However, these drugs readily cross the blood-brain barrier and may produce adverse behavioral effects, such as restlessness, tremors, delirium, and hallucinations.

Synthetic quaternary ammonium compounds have been developed (Table 25–2) that possess anticholinergic activity. Although less reliably absorbed after oral administration, these drugs cause minimal central side effects.

Other chemical derivatives primarily possess antispasmodic activity with little anticholinergic properties (Table 25–2). These drugs are used to relieve a wide variety of GI conditions characterized by spasms and excessive motility of the small intestine and colon. They are also employed in conjunction

TABLE 25-2. ANTIMUSCARINIC ANTISPASMODIC AGENTS

Generic Name	Selected Trade Name
Belladonna alkaloids	
Atropine sulfate	–
Belladonna tincture	–
Scopolamine (hyoscine) hydrobromide	–
Belladonna alkaloids and phenobarbital	Bellergal, Donnatal
Belladonna alkaloids, quaternary ammonium derivatives	
Methscopolamine bromide	Pamine
Synthetic quaternary ammonium compounds	
Anisotropine methylbromide	Valpin
Diphemanil methylsulfate	Prantal
Glycopyrrolate	Robinul
Hexocyclium methylsulfate	Tral
Isopropamide iodide	Darbid
Mepenzolate bromide	Cantil
Methantheline bromide	Banthine
Oxyphenonium bromide	Antrenyl
Propantheline bromide	Pro-Banthine
Tridihexethyl chloride	Pathilon
Synthetic antispasmodic agents*	
Dicyclomine hydrochloride	Bentyl, Dyspaz
Methixene hydrochloride	Trest
Oxyphencyclimine hydrochloride	Daricon

*Antispasmodic activity with little or no antimuscarinic activity and little effect on gastric acid secretion.

with other drugs for the management of mild diarrhea and nonobstructive cramping.

H_2-Receptor Antagonists

> *The discovery of new specific antagonists to endogenous active compounds is usually of great importance in Pharmacology. Such antagonists provide powerful tools for mapping out the localization of receptors and may become useful therapeutic agents. The discovery of H_2-receptor antagonists . . . is thus an important development.*[5]

—Andres Goth (1976)

After an eight-year search involving the synthesis and biological evaluation of more than 700 compounds, J. W. Black and his British co-workers[6] reported their discovery of the first specific H_2-receptor antagonist. This compound,

[5] *Federation Proceedings* **35**: 1923 (1976).

[6] J. W. Black, W. A. M. Duncan, C. J. Durant, C. R. Ganellin, and E. M. Parsons, "Definition and Antagonism of Histamine H_2-Receptors," *Nature* **236**: 385–90 (1972).

burimamide, was found to block gastric acid secretion stimulated by pentagastrin and by feeding but not by vagal stimulation or the administration of the cholinergic receptor agonist carbachol.

Burimamide, ineffective when taken by mouth and a relatively weak antagonist, was succeeded in clinical trials by the orally active metiamide; trials were discontinued when metiamide was found to cause agranulocytosis, a potentially lethal blood disorder.

In 1977, **cimetidine** (Tagamet) became the first clinically available H_2-antagonist and is currently very widely used for the treatment of acid-pepsin-related disorders of the GI tract. These conditions include, but are not limited to, ulcers of the stomach, duodenum, and esophagus. It should be noted that while cimetidine has proved to be highly effective in promoting the healing of these ulcers after three to six weeks of drug administration, there is a high rate of ulcer recurrence after the discontinuation of therapy.

Cimetidine is considered by many biomedical investigators to be one of the most significant new drugs to be developed in the 1970s, a compound that has revolutionized the management of acid-related GI disorders. Unlike the anticholinergic agents, which may now be rendered obsolescent, cimetidine is a relatively safe drug with a low incidence of side effects. It appears highly likely that many "me, too" cimetidine-like drugs will be marketed in the near future.

SUMMARY

Acid-related GI disorders such as indigestion may result from occasional overindulgence in food and/or drink; ulcers are caused by acid-pepsin erosion of the GI mucosa. While the presence of gastric acid (hydrochloric acid) and pepsin appear to be prerequisites for ulcer formation, the reasons for the loss of the natural resistance of the GI mucosa to their erosive properties are not well understood.

Most commercially available antacids are relatively safe and effective drugs when used as directed for the relief of occasional indigestion. When the GI upset persists and the antacid fails to provide sustained relief, the patient should consult a physician to determine the cause of the discomfort. The selection of the most appropriate antacid for the long-term management of peptic ulcer disease must take into consideration the inherent properties of the drug (acid-neutralizing capacity, onset and duration of action, taste), cost, and medical history of the patient.

Anticholinergic (antimuscarinic) agents have been used for generations for the management of peptic ulcer disease despite their high incidence of troublesome side effects and questionable clinical effectiveness. These drugs inhibit acid secretion (chemical vagotomy) and reduce the motility and spasms of GI smooth muscle. In recent years, highly selective antagonists of histamine-stimulated gastric acid secretion (an H_2-receptor mediated effect) have been developed; cimetidine appears to be safer and more effective than anticholinergic agents in its ability to inhibit acid secretion, relieve pain, and promote ulcer healing, and has inaugurated a new era in the treatment of acid-related GI disorders.

Advances in our understanding of the role of the prostaglandins in GI function suggests that drug-induced inhibition of their synthesis (such as by aspirin and indomethacin) may be responsible for the ulcerogenic effects of these drugs. Conversely, synthetic prostaglandin derivatives are being actively evaluated for their ability to inhibit acid secretion via a cAMP-mediated mechanism; the clinical availability of such drugs in the future for the treatment of GI disorders appears highly likely.

Other approaches being investigated for the management of peptic ulcer disease include the search for antagonists of gastrin, an extremely potent physiological stimulant of gastric acid secretion, and drugs that will enhance the secretion of mucus, the natural armor that protects our GI mucosal membrane against a lifelong onslaught by gastric juices.

SUPPLEMENTARY READINGS

Bass, P., "Gastric Antisecretory and Antiulcer Agents," *Advances in Drug Research* **8**: 205–328 (1974).

Burland, W. L., and M. A. Simkins, eds., "Cimetidine," *Proceedings of the Second International Symposium on Histamine H_2-Receptor Antagonists*. Amsterdam: Excerpta Medica, 1977.

Garnett, W. R., "Antacid Products," *Handbook of Nonprescription Drugs*. 6th ed. APhA Staff Project. Washington, D.C.: American Pharmaceutical Association, 1979.

Hirschowitz, B. I., "H-2 Histamine Receptors," *Annual Review of Pharmacology and Toxicology* **19**: 203–44 (1979).

Sleisenger, M. H., and J. S. Fordtran, eds., *Gastrointestinal Disease: Pathophysiology, Diagnosis, Management*. 2nd ed. Philadelphia: Saunders, 1978.

26

Laxatives
and Antidiarrheal Agents

I hav finally kum to the konklusion, that a good reliable sett ov bowels iz wurth more tu a man, than enny quantity ov brains.[1]

—Henry Wheeler Shaw [Josh Billings] (1818–1885)

The vast army of hypochondriacs, who are never happy unless their stools conform to an ideal which they have invented for themselves, can only be cured by making themselves realize that feces have no standard size, shape, consistency, or colour.

—Sir Arthur Hurst (1935)

Disorders of bowel function, either real or imagined, are very common medical problems. In this chapter, we shall briefly discuss the physiology of defecation and then consider constipation and diarrhea and the drugs that are used (and often misused) to manage these conditions.

PHYSIOLOGY OF DEFECATION

The alimentary tract is essentially a long, hollow tube surrounded by layers of smooth (involuntary) muscle. Coordination between adjacent layers of circular and longitudinal smooth muscle types controls the movement of the intestinal contents. When circular muscle activity (intestinal *tone*) is increased, the intestinal lumen becomes occluded, and there is a resistance to flow of the intestinal contents; opiates produce constipation by this action. Conversely, when the activity of the circular muscle is decreased and more flaccid, the intestinal lumen opens more widely presenting little or no resistance to the flow of the intestinal contents; castor oil induces diarrhea by this mechanism (Figure 26–1).

Normal *intestinal motility* and peristalsis are maintained by the smooth muscles and the intrinsic nerves. Activation of cholinergic nerves stimulates intestinal motility, while blockade of cholinergic activity with atropine and related antimuscarinic agents reduces intestinal motility. Stimulation of the stretch receptors or sensory receptors of the intestinal mucosa by increasing the bulk of the intestinal contents can also promote the propulsive peristaltic activity of the intestines.

After reaching the colon (large intestine), undigested and unabsorbed food residues, termed *chyme,* move slowly and are mixed in a manner that facilitates the absorption of water and electrolytes from the intestinal lumen and results in the solidification of the stool. Subsequent movement of the stool into the rectum triggers the *defecation reflex* which can be consciously facilitated or inhibited by higher centers in the brain. If this reflex is inhibited, the rectum slowly relaxes and the defecation stimulus slowly dissipates.

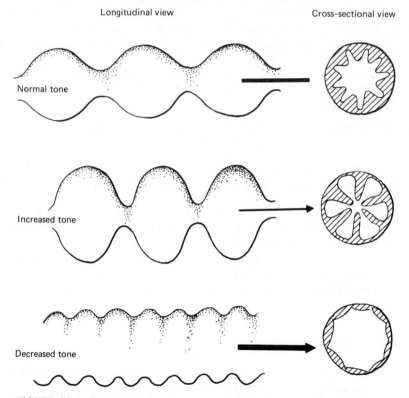

Longitudinal view   Cross–sectional view

Normal tone

Increased tone

Decreased tone

FIGURE 26–1. Relationship between Circular Muscle Tone and Movement of Intestinal Contents. *Top:* normal muscle tone. *Middle:* increased muscle tone, impaired movement of contents, possible resulting in constipation; may be induced by opiates (morphine). *Bottom:* decreased muscle tone, increased movement of contents, possibly resulting in diarrhea; may be castor oil–induced. (Modified from T.S. Gaginella, "Management of Gastrointestinal Disorders. Part 2: Use and Abuse of Laxatives," *Journal of Continuing Education in Pharmacy* 2 [2]: 20 [1978].)

CONSTIPATION AND LAXATIVES

An interest in, preoccupation with, or an obsession about bowel function is a health concern that strongly links us with the past. The Ebers papyrus (1550 B.C.) recommends chewing the seeds of the ricinus plant for constipation; castor oil, extracted from these seeds, may have been among the first effective drugs known. The Greek historian Herodotus (485?–425? B.C.) wrote that the Egyptians attempted to maintain internal cleanliness by evacuating the intestinal tract for three consecutive days each month. The terms "cathartic" and "purge" are derived from Greek and Latin words, respectively, meaning "to cleanse."

Into the nineteenth century, purging, along with bleeding and self-induced vomiting, were among the most common forms of treatment prescribed by physicians for a variety of medical disorders. This practice did not go unnoticed by earlier writers and served as a focal point of literary satire directed at the medical profession. As the curtain to Moliere's *le Malade imaginaire* (1673) rises, we find the hypochondriac Argan perusing his latest physician's bill:

> Item, on the twenty-fourth, a small injection preparatory, insinuative and emmollient, to lubricate, loosen, and stimulate the gentleman's lower intestine: thirty sous.

In *Gulliver's Travels*, written by Jonathan Swift 50 years later, the hero describes the habits of his countrymen to the Houyhnhnms:

> They take in at the orifice above a medicine equally annoying and disgustful to the bowels, which relaxing the belly drives down all before it; and this they call a purge.

Constipation may be loosely defined as an infrequent or difficult passage of feces; more precisely, it is a decrease in the frequency of bowel movements, accompanied by a prolonged and difficult passage of stool followed by a sensation of incomplete evacuation. Contrary to the impression one might gain from TV advertisements, the normal frequency of bowel movements may vary from several times daily to once or twice weekly. Hence, one individual's regularity is another's constipation.

Causes of Constipation

There are many diverse causes of constipation, some of which include: (1) *psychological factors*: failure to respond to the defecation stimulus or to acquire the habit of regular defecation; emotional stresses; (2) *nutritional factors:* a diet containing insufficient bulk or containing foods that harden the stools; severe dieting, starvation, dehydration; (3) *diseases*: hypothyroidism, tumors obstructing the intestinal tract, hemorrhoids, fissures, paraplegia; (4) *drugs:* aluminum-containing antacids, anticholinergic agents, phenothiazine antipsychotic agents, tricyclic antidepressants, iron-containing salts, opiates, and laxatives when used at frequent intervals (see below); (5) *miscellaneous factors:* pregnancy, after childbirth, decreased physical activity, old age.

Laxatives

Drugs used to induce defecation are perhaps the most ancient type of internal medication and were, for a long time, the only drugs so administered. Until relatively recently, it was commonplace to classify these drugs on the basis of their intensity of action. The terms *laxative* or *aperient* were used to refer to "mild" drugs that produced a formed stool in the absence of griping or intestinal cramps, while the terms *cathartic* or *purgative* were used to denote "harsh" drugs that produced watery feces usually accompanied by abdominal cramping. This distinction, now happily falling into disfavor, is fundamentally unsound because the differences in the intensity of the effect produced are largely dose-related. In contemporary writings, the terms *laxative* and *cathartic* are commonly used interchangeably to refer to all drugs used to induce defecation.[1]

Laxatives are commonly classified in the modern literature on the basis of their presumed mechanism of action. The reader should be forewarned, however, that this classification is by no means absolute because the mechanisms by which these drugs act are not completely understood in all cases, and some drugs produce their effects by more than one action. With these limitations in mind, we shall classify laxatives into the following categories: stimulants, saline laxatives, bulk-forming agents, emollients (lubricants), and fecal softeners (wetting agents). Representative examples of nonprescription drugs from each of these categories are listed in Table 26–1.

Stimulant Laxatives

Drugs in the stimulant category increase the propulsive peristaltic activity of the intestinal tract by one or more of the following mechanisms: stimulation of the stretch receptors or sensory nerves of the intestinal mucosa or direct stimulation of intestinal smooth muscle, inhibition of water and electrolyte reabsorption from the intestinal lumen, or enhancement of secretion of water into the intestinal lumen. Both of the latter actions result in an increase in the pressure within the lumen of the intestine (intraluminal pressure), thereby stimulating peristalsis. The primary site of action of castor oil is the small intestine, while most of the other stimulant laxatives act in the colon.

---

[1] In a typical textbook of pharmacology and therapeutics written at the turn of the century, it was not uncommon to find the recommended "purgatives" (numbering 40–50) placed into five or six "useful" clinical categories. While laxatives are now employed to relieve constipation and to evacuate the bowel prior to surgery or diagnosis, the 12th edition of *Cushny's Pharmacology and Therapeutics* (1940) speaks favorably of their virtues in the early phases of the treatment of malaria and syphilis; in acute fevers "perhaps through the congestion of the bowel withdrawing the blood from the rest of the body . . ."; for congestion of the brain; and to remove excess fluids from the body in cases of dropsy (edema).

TABLE 26-1. REPRESENTATIVE NONPRESCRIPTION LAXATIVES

Classification	Generic Name	Selected Trade Names (Common Name)
Stimulant laxatives	Castor oil	
	Glycerin suppositories	
	Bisacodyl	Dulcolax
	Phenolphthalein	Alophen
	(yellow)	Ex-Lax
		Feen-A-Mint
		Phenolax
Anthraquinone	Aloe	Carter's Little Pills*
derivatives	Aloe & cascara	Nature's Remedy
	sagrada	
	Cascara sagrada	
	fluid extract	
	Casanthranol	Peristim Forte
	Senna	Fletcher's Castoria
		Gentlax*
		Senokot
		X-Prep
	Sennosides A & B	Glysennid
		Nytilax
	Danthron	Dorbane
		Modane
	Danthron & dioctyl	Doctate-P
	sodium sulfosuccinate	Dorbantyl
		Doxan
		Magcyl
Saline laxatives	Magnesium carbonate	(Carbonate of magnesia)
	Magnesium citrate	(Citrate of magnesia; Citrate)
	solution	
	Magnesium sulfate	(Epsom salts)
	Milk of magnesia	(Magnesium hydroxide mixture; MOM; Cream of magnesia)
	Potassium sodium	(Rochelle salt)
	tartrate	
	Sodium phosphate	(Dibasic sodium phosphate)
	Sodium phosphate &	Fleet Phospho-Soda
	sodium biphosphate	Fleet Enema
	Sodium sulfate	(Glauber's salt)
Bulk-forming	Carboxymethylcellulose	
laxatives	Psyllium muciloid	Effersyllium
		Konsyl
		Metamucil
		Mucilose
	Psyllium & mineral	Petro-Syllium
	oil	
Emollient laxatives	Mineral oil	Kondremul*
(Lubricants)		Nujol
		(Liquid petrolatum)
	Glycerin suppositories	

*Contains other ingredients with laxative properties.

TABLE 26-1. CONTINUED

Fecal softeners (wetting agents)	Dioctyl calcium sulfosuccinate	Surfac
	Dioctyl sodium sulfosuccinate (DSS)	Colace
		Colocytyl
		Comfolax
		Dosinate
		Doxidan
		Doxinate
		Modane Soft
	DSS & casanthranol	Casa-Laud
		Comfolax Plus
		Disanthrol

Stimulant laxatives are most useful for the treatment of acute constipation that fails to respond to milder drugs. It is for this reason that this class of laxatives is most widely misused (see below). They are also used to clear the gastrointestinal tract prior to diagnostic examinations.

The intensity of action of these drugs is dose-related and varies from a mild laxative effect to one causing severe griping and catharsis and resulting in excessive loss of electrolytes (in particular, potassium) and fluids. Castor oil should not be used during pregnancy because of the risk of inducing an abortion.

Phenolphthalein, used in chemical laboratories as an indicator when titrating acids with bases, is a common ingredient in proprietary laxative products (Ex-Lax, Feen-A-Mint). This compound colors alkaline urine pink and may cause a persistent pink-to-purple skin rash in hypersensitive individuals. Since *anthraquinone derivatives* (Table 26–1) are excreted into the milk of nursing mothers at levels that may cause a laxative effect in the infant, it is generally recommended that these drugs be avoided by such mothers.

Saline Laxatives

Saline laxatives consist of nonabsorbable or poorly absorbable cations (magnesium, potassium, sodium) and anions (citrate, phosphate, sulfate, tartrate). A hypertonic solution[2] of these salts causes the osmotic retention of a significant volume of water in the intestinal lumen. The resulting increase in intraluminal pressure mechanically stimulates stretch receptors which increases peristalsis. In addition, the magnesium ion may activate the release of the stomach hormone cholecystokinin (CCK), and this hormone stimulates intestinal motility and inhibits fluid absorption from the intestine. Both actions are thought to contribute to the observed laxative effects.

Saline laxatives are used to empty the bowel prior to surgery and diagnostic procedures involving the gastrointestinal tract; to speed up the elimination of orally ingested poisons remaining unabsorbed in the gastroin-

---

[2] A hypertonic solution has an osmotic pressure greater than an isotonic solution such as plasma.

testinal tract; and to remove worms after the administration of anthelmintic agents.

The relative palatability of saline laxatives differs rather considerably, and this represents one consideration in the selection of medication. Magnesium citrate solution and milk of magnesia[3] have relatively pleasant tastes; on the other hand, while sodium sulfate enjoys a time-honored reputation for effectiveness, it is rarely used because of its very bitter taste.

Bulk-Forming Laxatives

After the ingestion of these nondigestible polysaccharide and cellulose derivatives, they absorb and retain large volumes of water in the intestinal tract.[4] By increasing the bulk of the intestinal contents, they increase intraluminal pressure and stimulate peristalsis which facilitates movement of the stool. Whereas stimulant and saline laxatives generally act within 2 to 8 hours, 12 to 24 hours are generally required with bulk-forming agents, with a complete effect sometimes being delayed for up to three days.

This group of laxatives is relatively safe, least subject to misuse, and represents a good first choice to employ for the treatment of constipation. These drugs are commonly used by women after childbirth and by elderly individuals.

Emollient Laxatives (Lubricants)

Mineral oil is the most commonly used emollient laxative. It has been suggested that it acts by softening the fecal matter by retarding the absorption of water from the intestinal lumen. Mineral oil may also act by coating the mucosal lining and fecal material, thus facilitating the "smooth passage" of the stool down the bowel. The drug is commonly used in patients whose medical conditions would be worsened by straining during defecation, for example, after abdominal surgery, hernia, heart attack, or hemorrhoids.

Chronic administration of mineral oil may interfere with the absorption of food and fat-soluble vitamins (A, D, E, K), potentially resulting in a nutritional deficiency. This laxative should not be used during pregnancy because it can reduce the availability of vitamin K to the fetus which may result in clotting disorders.

Fecal Softeners (Wetting Agents)

The dioctyl sulfosuccinates (Table 26–1) soften the stool by lowering the surface tension, thus permitting the stool to be penetrated by intestinal fluids. In addition, these drugs are thought to produce their laxative effects by inhibiting

---

[3] In lower doses, milk of magnesia is used as an antacid.

[4] Bulk-forming drugs, such as carboxymethylcellulose or methylcellulose are commonly included as one of several ingredients in nonprescription *appetite suppressants* (Anorexin, Appedrine, Diet-Trim, Odrinex, Slim Line, Spantrol). These drugs are reported to produce a sense of fullness in the stomach by the same sponge-like mechanism described above; their clinical effectiveness has not been established (see Chapter 15).

fluid and electrolyte absorption by the intestine. These drugs are employed clinically for the same conditions as the emollient laxatives.

Dioctyl sulfosuccinates (DSS) are often combined in proprietary preparations with other laxatives, a potentially dangerous practice having questionable therapeutic justification. The surfactant properties of DSS tend to enhance the systemic absorption of other drugs, which may result in an exaggerated laxative effect and greater toxicity.

Laxative Misuse

The excessive and, at times, compulsive use of laxatives by large segments of the population (most often the elderly) arises primarily from erroneous concepts about the normal physiology and pathophysiology of the digestive and excretory systems. Many individuals employ laxatives to expurgate the body of toxic substances they believe will be absorbed into the blood in the absence of a daily bowel movement. While some people think that weakness and headaches result from constipation, others use laxatives for the treatment of the common cold, anger, or depression.

While the *occasional* use of laxatives for the treatment of constipation is not associated with major risk, their regular use can cause fluid and electrolyte depletion and vitamin deficiency and often results in the development of a habit that is extremely difficult to break. Consider the following all-too-commonly played scenario: After taking a laxative, the bowel is completely evacuated of all food residues, and two to three days may be required for the accumulation of sufficient contents in the colon for a bowel movement to occur. Many individuals fail to appreciate that this delay is normal and to be anticipated. In the absence of a natural bowel movement, an additional dose of "Bowel-Purge" or "Clear-Colon" may be taken or a stronger drug employed (commonly a stimulant laxative) thereby perpetuating this vicious cycle. With the regular use of laxatives, normal defecation reflex mechanisms become blunted eventually resulting in the total reliance upon these drugs for defecation. Successful treatment involves changes in the diet to increase the intake of bulk-producing foods (such as unrefined bran), increased physical exercise, and professional assistance to establish regular bowel habits.

DIARRHEA AND ANTIDIARRHEAL AGENTS

Diarrhea is the frequent passage of semisolid or fluid stools. Acute episodes of diarrhea are generally self-limiting and require little, if any, drug therapy. In other cases, such as cholera or diarrhea in infants, immediate diagnosis and effective treatment are essential to avoid excessive electrolyte losses and dehydration.

Causes of Diarrhea

Acute diarrhea may arise from many factors including (1) *microbial causes:* infectious organisms, usually bacteria in adults and viruses in infants and young children; traveler's diarrhea resulting from exposure (generally via food and drink) to a markedly different population of microbes; (2) *toxic causes:* including botulism and other types of food poisoning; (3) *nutritional causes:* foods that are excessively spicy or fatty or that contain a high percentage of roughage; allergic responses to food; (4) *drug-induced causes:* antibiotic-induced diarrhea is relatively common and may result from the mildly irritating properties of these drugs or superinfections, caused by drug alteration in the normal intestinal flora (Chapter 28), or from drugs that alter the autonomic control of intestinal motility, such as cholinergic agents and certain drugs used for the treatment of high blood pressure (reserpine, guanethidine, methyldopa).

Chronic diarrhea often poses a great diagnostic challenge and may be a symptom of an emotional disorder, cancer of the rectum and colon (among the most common sites of cancer), one of several dozen diseases of the gastrointestinal tract, or a postoperative consequence arising from a surgical removal of certain segments of the bowel.

Antidiarrheal Agents

Diarrhea is a symptom of a disorder, and its control should not be interpreted as a cure for its underlying cause. Since more than 50 different disorders may be responsible for its occurrence, attention must be directed toward determining its cause and, if appropriate, instituting specific treatment such as administering an antimicrobial agent to control a bacterial infection.

Antidiarrheal agents should not be used for more than two days if a high fever is present or in children less than 3 years of age unless so directed by a physician. In this chapter, we shall consider three of the most commonly used classes of antidiarrheal agents, namely, the opiates, anticholinergic agents, and the adsorbents.

Opiates

For over 1000 years opium has been used for the treatment of diarrhea and dysentery, and its employment as an antidiarrheal agent long predated its use as an analgesic agent. The actions of morphine (the major active component in opium; Chapter 13) on the gastrointestinal tract are highly complex. Morphine reduces the rate at which chyme is transported through the small intestine and colon; this effect has been attributed to drug-induced inhibition of effective peristaltic movements and/or an increase in the circular smooth muscle tone of the intestines (Figure 26-1).

Paregoric (camphorated opium tincture) and other opium-containing preparations are generally considered to be safe and effective at the normally prescribed doses. The antidiarrheal doses are considerably lower than those required to produce analgesia. At these reduced doses, when used for the control of acute diarrhea, the abuse potential of the natural opiates is low. Moreover, these opiates are not sufficiently well-absorbed after oral administration to cause alterations in mood.

Diphenoxylate, a compound chemically related to meperidine (Demerol), is a highly effective antidiarrheal drug. The combination of diphenoxylate and atropine is marketed as Lomotil, with the antimuscarinic agent included to discourage diphenoxylate abuse. Lomotil has low abuse potential and is preferred for the management of chronic diarrhea. High doses of this product cause respiratory depression. *Loperamide* (Imodium) is a recently introduced drug with diphenoxylate-like properties. It is more potent, has a longer duration of action, and since it does not readily cross the blood-brain barrier, causes less central depression than diphenoxylate.

Anticholineric Agents

The use of anticholinergic agents (Table 25–2) for the treatment of diarrhea is based upon their ability to reduce the motility of the intestinal tract. The use of effective doses of these drugs, equivalent to 0.6 to 1.0 mg of atropine, is associated with a high incidence of side effects. Anticholinergic agents have a narrow margin of safety, especially in young children. Donnagel is a widely used nonprescription antidiarrheal product containing a mixture of belladonna alkaloids (Chapter 8) and the adsorbents kaolin and pectin (see below).

Adsorbents

Adsorbents are the most frequently used class of antidiarrheal agents contained in nonprescription products. The process of adsorption is not specific. These drugs not only adsorb toxins, bacteria, and other noxious materials that are responsible for causing diarrhea, but also nutrients, digestive enzymes, and a variety of orally administered drugs and vitamins.

Generally taken as liquid suspensions, a dose is commonly taken after each loose bowel movement until the diarrhea is controlled; hence, large doses must be taken over relatively short periods of time. It is generally believed that while these drugs are safe when taken at the usual doses, insufficient evidence is available to determine whether they are more effective than placebos in controlling diarrhea.

The most commonly used adsorbents are attapulgite, bismuth salts, kaolin, and pectin, and these are usually employed in combination with other antidiarrheal agents. *Attapulgite,* a hydrous magnesium aluminum silicate, is the primary antidiarrheal ingredient in Quintess and Rheaban. *Bismuth* salts such as the subnitrate and subsalicylate are employed in antidiarrheal preparations (Corrective Mixture, Pepto-Bismol) as adsorbents, astringents, and protectives. *Kaolin,* long used in the Orient for the management of diarrhea and dysentery, is a native hydrated aluminum silicate. *Pectin* is a purified carbohydrate extracted from the rind of citrus fruit or from apple pomace. Kaolin and pectin are used in combination in such nonprescription products as Kaopectate, Pargel, and Pektamalt, and with paregoric in Parepectolin.

SUMMARY

Constipation and diarrhea are very common medical disorders and, in some instances, prompt medical treatment may be required to control the latter.

Laxatives, commonly referred to as cathartics, are used to relieve constipation, to evacuate the bowel prior to surgery or diagnostic procedures, and with specific anthelmintic agents to rid the intestinal tract of worms. These drugs act by one or more of the following mechanisms: stimulant laxatives (castor oil, phenolphthalein) activate propulsive peristaltic movements by stimulating stretch receptors, sensory nerves, or the circular smooth muscle directly, or by increasing intraluminal pressure. Saline laxatives (magnesium citrate solution, milk of magnesia) and bulk-forming agents (psyllium) increase intraluminal pressure by causing the osmotic retention of water and by increasing the bulk of the intestinal contents, respectively. The emollient laxatives (mineral oil) soften the fecal material and facilitate its passage down the bowel, while fecal softeners (dioctyl sulfosuccinates) act as surfactants and permit the fecal material to be penetrated and softened by intestinal fluids.

Regular use of laxatives leads in time to dependency upon them for bowel function to occur. This laxative habit, not uncommon in the elderly, is difficult to break even with professional assistance.

The major classes of drugs used for the management of diarrhea are the opiates, the anticholinergic agents, and the adsorbents. Natural and synthetic opiates (paregoric, diphenoxylate), the most effective available antidiarrheal agents, reduce the intestinal transport of its contents. Anticholinergic agents, used either as a mixture of the natural belladonna alkaloids or as individual antimuscarinic agents, reduce intestinal motility; these drugs cause a relatively high incidence of side effects at clinically effective doses. The adsorbents are generally safe at their usual doses but, notwithstanding their very extensive usage, have not been clearly established to be effective antidiarrheal agents; these drugs are also capable of adsorbing nutrients, vitamins, and a number of other orally administered drugs.

SUPPLEMENTARY READINGS

Binder, H. J., "Pharmacology of Laxatives," *Annual Review of Pharmacology and Toxicology* **17**: 355–67 (1977).

Darlington, R. C., and C. E. Curry, Jr., "Laxative Products," in *Handbook of Nonprescription Drugs*. 6th ed., pp. 37–54. APhA Project Staff. Washington, D.C.: American Pharmaceutical Association, 1979.

Gaginella, T. S., "Management of Gastrointestinal Disease. Part 3: Diarrheal Disease and Antidiarrheal Therapy," *Journal of Continuing Education in Pharmacy* **2** (3): 41–51 (1978).

Gaginella, T. S., and P. Bass, "Laxatives: an Update on Mechanism of Action," *Life Sciences* **23:** 1001–10 (1978).

Long, R. L., "Antidiarrheal and Other Gastrointestinal Products," in *Handbook of Nonprescription Drugs.* 6th ed., pp. 25–36. APhA Project Staff. Washington, D.C.: American Pharmaceutical Association, 1979.

Pietrusko, R. G., "Use and Abuse of Laxatives," *American Journal of Hospital Pharmacy* **34:** 291–300 (1977).

27

Treatment of the Common Cold, Allergic Disorders, And Asthma

I am at this moment
Deaf in the ears,
Hoarse in the throat,
Red in the nose,
Green in the gills,
Damp in the eyes,
Twitchy in the joints,
And fractious in temper
From a most intolerable
And oppressive cold.

—Charles Dickens (1812–1870)

In this chapter, we shall consider the treatment of the all-too-common cold, allergic disorders, and bronchial asthma. The decision to place these three disorders together in a single chapter was based upon two primary considerations; namely, they primarily affect the respiratory system[1] and are managed, in some cases, by similar drugs.

Many of the drugs that we shall consider will be familiar to the reader. All of us have fallen victim to the common cold—on the average of two to three times per year—and have, at least on occasion, sought symptomatic relief from

---

[1] While allergic rhinitis (hay fever) affects the respiratory system, the symptoms of other allergic disorders can be manifested throughout the body.

its ravages by taking a nonprescription cold product; not infrequently this product has been recommended by our private medical advisor on the "tube." These products generally contain a nasal decongestant, one or more ingredients for cough, an antihistamine, and an analgesic agent. Many other individuals attribute their excellent health to their unfailing daily use of vitamin C.

THE COMMON COLD

The common cold, considered to be the most expensive single illness in the United States, is responsible for the loss of more time from work and school than the combined total of all other diseases; it annually accounts for almost one million person-years lost from work. The suffering American public spends about $500–700 million each year for the purchase of nonprescription cough, cold, and allergy preparations. Countless others in the United States and abroad attempt to manage the common cold by relying upon home remedies and the advice of friends.

> . . . I went on borrowing handkerchiefs and blowing them to atoms, as had been my custom in the early stages of my cold, until I came across a lady . . . [who] had from necessity acquired considerable skill in the treatment of simple "family complaints." I knew she must have had much experience, for she appeared to be a hundred and fifty years old.
>
> She mixed a decoction composed of molasses, aquafortis, turpentine, and various other drugs, and instructed me to take a wine-glass full of it every fifteen minutes. I never took but one dose; that was enough, it robbed me of all moral principle, and awoke every unworthy impulse of my nature. Under its malign influence my brain conceived miracles of meanness, but my hands were too feeble to execute them; . . . until I took that medicine I had never reveled in such supernatural depravity, and felt proud of it. At the end of two days I was ready to go doctoring again. I took a few more unfailing remedies, and finally drove my cold from my head to my lungs.[2]

The common cold is caused by *viruses;*[3] in excess of 120 different viral strains have been isolated that are capable of producing cold symptoms in humans. More than one-half of all adult colds are caused by different rhinovirus types.

Regardless of whether you call it a "cold," acute rhinitis, coryza, or catarrh, the most frequently encountered symptoms include nasal discharge

---

[2] Mark Twain, "Curing a Cold," in *The Complete Humorous Sketches and Tales of Mark Twain,* ed. C. Neider (Garden City, N.Y.: Doubleday, 1961), pp. 26–7.

[3] Influenza is also a viral disorder that is generally more severe than a common cold and causes greater susceptibility to secondary bacterial complications. The flu epidemic of 1918–1919 was responsible for more than 20 million deaths throughout the world, of which one-half million were in the United States.

and nasal congestion, cough, laryngitis, fever, aches, and pains. No remedies are capable of curing the common cold or shortening its duration. The available medications only provide temporary symptomatic relief while the uncomplicated routine cold runs its course over a one-to two-week period.

Nasal Decongestants

Nasal congestion and nasal discharge are the most often described symptoms associated with the common cold; these symptoms in combination with nasal irritation give rise to sneezing. *Sympathomimetic amines* (Chapter 6) are the primary class of nasal decongestants. These vasoconstrictor agents act by stimulating α-adrenergic receptors on the smooth muscles of the arterioles of the nasal mucosa causing a reduction in the blood flow in the engorged swollen nasal area. This vasoconstriction results in the shrinkage of the swollen nasal membranes which promotes drainage and creates an unobstructed air passage facilitating breathing and relieving the feelings of stuffiness. Examples of commonly used sympathomimetic vasoconstrictors are listed in Table 27-1. These drugs differ primarily with respect to their duration of action and route of administration.

TABLE 27-1. COMMONLY USED NASAL DECONGESTANTS

Generic Name	Selected Trade Names	Duration of (hours) Action
Topical preparations (drops, sprays, mists)		
Ephedrine	I-Sedrin	4
Naphazoline	Privine	6
Oxymetazoline	Afrin; Duration	8-12
Phenylephrine	Allerest;* Contact Nasal Mist; Coricidin;* Dristan; Sinex; Super Anahist	4
Xylometazoline	Otrivin; Sine-Off	8-10
Oral preparations (tablets, capsules, syrups)†		
Ephedrine		4
Phenylephrine	Neo-Synephrine	4
Phenylpropanolamine	Propadrine	4
Pseudoephedrine	Sudafed	4
Inhalers		
Levodesoxyephedrine	Vicks	Several
Propylhexedrine	Benzedrex; Vicks	Several

*Contains other active ingredients.

†Orally active sympathomimetic vasoconstrictors are commonly included in combination cold products containing antihistamines and analgesics.

Decongestants are either topically (locally) administered as sprays, drops, and inhalants or are orally ingested in the form of capsules, tablets, and liquids. *Topically* administered nasal decongestants provide immediate, but very temporary, symptomatic relief. The indiscriminate use of these products may result in an impairment of normal ciliary activity, damage to the nasal mucosa, and chronic nasal congestion, termed "rebound congestion." The response on the part of the patient is usually the administration of more drug, thus perpetuating this vicious cycle, and leading to habituation, a form of drug misuse.

Oral administration of sympathomimetic nasal decongestants provides a more effective means of reaching the nerves, via the bloodstream, regardless of the amount of mucus present. This route of administration does not disrupt the mucosal environment, is longer acting, and reduces the incidence of "rebound congestion." Unfortunately, oral administration usually produces more widespread undesirable sympathomimetic effects.

The use of these products, both topically and orally, are not without hazards. Undesirable side effects have been observed, including nervousness, insomnia, palpitations of the heart, elevation of blood pressure, and sweating. Central nervous system depression, coma, and a marked reduction in body temperature may occur in infants and children.

Cough Remedies

The **cough** is a protective reflex that acts to clear the respiratory tract of foreign bodies that might otherwise block this passageway and obstruct free breathing. The *cough reflex* may be initiated by mechanical (fish bones) or chemical (sulfur dioxide fumes, chlorine gas) activation of nerve endings located in the trachea, bronchi, or bronchioles. Such activation triggers an impulse along sensory nerves which ultimately stimulates the cough center, located in the medulla. A message from the medulla sets into motion a sequence of events in the respiratory tract that occur when we cough.

A cough may be viewed as being useful or useless depending upon the stimulus initiating it. A *productive cough* serves the very important function of removing accumulated fluids from the respiratory tract, fluids which may contain entrapped dust particles and bacteria. Certainly, the expulsion of foreign particulate matter from the respiratory tract is highly useful. In general, no attempt is made to suppress a productive cough, and in some instances it is highly desirable to facilitate expectoration. A *nonproductive cough*, by contrast, is not only useless and troublesome but may also be painful and fatiguing. These coughs often cause irritation of the mucosal linings of the larynx, pharynx, and trachea and perpetuate the cough reflex cycle.

Cough remedies contain drugs that suppress the cough and often have other ingredients that increase the production of respiratory tract fluids; we refer to these drugs as antitussives (from Latin *tussis*, "cough") and expectorants, respectively.

Antitussive Agents

Antitussive agents, drugs that inhibit or suppress the act of coughing, may depress the cough center located in the medulla or may block the peripheral sensory receptors of the nerves responsible for transmitting the tussal (cough) impulses to the cough center. The most commonly used antitussive agents are those that act centrally, including codeine and dextromethorphan. Benzonatate possesses both central and peripheral antitussive activity, but the latter is thought to be of greater importance.

Codeine.   For over a century, the narcotics (Chapter 13) have been recognized as the most effective drugs available to suppress cough. The naturally occurring opium alkaloid codeine, a common ingredient in nonprescription cough mixtures, is particularly useful for the relief of a painful cough because of its antitussive and analgesic actions. When compared with morphine, its advantages include less respiratory and behavioral depression, a lower incidence of nausea and constipation, and a relatively low abuse potential. The narcotic agents suppress the cough reflex by depressing the cough center in the medulla, thereby elevating the central threshold to sensory impulses arising from noxious stimuli in the respiratory tract.

Dextromethorphan.   Unlike levorphanol (Levo-Dromoran), a narcotic analgesic agent, dextromethorphan, its methylated dextro-isomer, possesses no analgesic activity, has low potential for abuse, and is not a respiratory depressant. Dextromethorphan is among the most extensively used nonnarcotic antitussive compounds employed in proprietary products (Romilar hydrobromide), either alone or in combination with expectorants (see below). This compound approaches the effectiveness of codeine in its ability to suppress cough, is less prone to abuse (although abuse of this compound has been reported), and causes fewer adverse side effects.

Benzonatate.   Benzonatate (Tessalon) is chemically related to the local anesthetic tetracaine and is thought to act, in part, by blocking the sensory (stretch) receptors located in the lungs.

Expectorants

Expectorants are used for the treatment of useless or nonproductive coughs resulting from irritation of the respiratory tract or are used to liquify and thereby facilitate the removal of mucus. Some drugs stimulate the secretion of respiratory tract fluids, while others reduce their viscosity (thickness). The widespread use of expectorants in almost all nonprescription cough products is primarily based upon time-honored tradition and subjective clinical impressions rather than the results obtained in carefully controlled clinical studies. In short, there is little evidence that these drugs are effective. Among the most widely used expectorants are guaifenesin, ammonium chloride, ipecac syrup, and terpin hydrate.

High fluid intake and the inhalation of moist air facilitate respiratory tract fluid mucus production and represent an important component in the treatment of the common cold. Mucus production can be enhanced by increasing fluid intake to six to eight glassfuls daily and by employing a cool mist or hot steam vaporizer.

Antihistamines

Although antihistamines are included in virtually all cold products, there is no evidence that they prevent or reduce the duration of the common cold. They are included to decrease the secretion of mucus and relieve the running nose. Proof of their effectiveness at the doses contained in cold remedies has not been well established. The pharmacology and therapeutic uses of antihistamines will be considered in detail below.

Analgesic-Antipyretics

Aspirin and acetaminophen (Datril, Tylenol) are extensively used to relieve the aches and pains commonly associated with the common cold. Moreover, these drugs are highly effective in reducing fever (Chapter 14). In adults, 325–650 mg (1–2 tablets) of aspirin or acetaminophen, taken every four to six hours, represent effective doses. For children, aspirin in doses of 65 mg (1 grain) per year of age, up to 650 mg for a 10-year-old, may be taken at four-to-six-hour intervals. The following doses of acetaminophen are often recommended by physicians: under 1 year, 60 mg; 1–2 years, 60–120 mg; 2–6 years, 120 mg; 6–12 years, 250 mg. These doses may be repeated at four-to-six-hour intervals.

Ascorbic Acid (Vitamin C)

In his 1970 book, *Vitamin C and the Common Cold,*[4] the Nobel Prize winning chemist Linus Pauling advocated the daily use of 1–5 g of ascorbic acid to prevent the cold and up to 15 g to treat it.[5] Although numerous studies have been conducted to test this hypothesis, at this time, on the basis of the results obtained, it is not clear whether this drug prevents or reduces the severity or duration of the cold. The most common side effect associated with large doses of vitamin C is diarrhea, and there exists the risk of kidney stone formation.

[4] San Francisco, W. H. Freeman.
[5] The recommended daily dietary allowance of vitamin C in adults is 60 mg.

ALLERGIC DISORDERS

Some men also have strange antipathies in their natures against that sort of food which others love and live upon. I have read of one that could not endure to eat either bread or flesh; of another that fell into a swooning fit at the smell of a rose. . . . There are some who, if a cat accidentally come into the room, though they neither see it, nor are told of it, will presently be in a sweat, and ready to die away.

—Increase Mather (1639–1723)

We are all generally familiar with the term *allergy*. This is not surprising because approximately one out of every five persons suffers some adverse reaction when they encounter certain pollens, foods, plants, or drugs.[6]

The term **allergy** refers to a condition of unusual or exaggerated susceptibility to a specific substance, which in equivalent concentrations is harmless to most other individuals of the same species. Employing this general definition of allergy, we might include excessive stimulation and nervousness after drinking a cup of coffee. However, this extreme reaction or *hypersensitivity* to coffee is not an allergy. Let us be more explicit and redefine an allergy as an *exaggerated susceptibility to a substance which may be attributable to some underlying antigen-antibody reaction.*

This provoking substance or *allergen* we are referring to may come from a myriad of diverse sources. The most important class of allergens is the *inhalants*, which cause allergic symptoms in the respiratory tract. *Food* allergies are also relatively common. Manifestations of the allergic response may appear on the skin and mucous membranes, in the blood, in the respiratory tract, or in the form of fever. Let us now briefly discuss the underlying basis responsible for allergies.

Mechanisms Underlying Allergic Reactions

Allergies, regardless of etiology, arise as the result of an **antigen-antibody reaction.** An **antigen** is a large molecule, usually a protein, that is capable of stimulating the formation of specific **antibodies** (immunoglobulin E or IgE). Most drug molecules are too small to be antigenic, and they must first combine with a body protein to form a drug-protein complex that is antigenic. A drug or any other simple chemical that combines with a protein to form an antigen is termed a *hapten* and the protein is called a *carrier*. When the antigen is in-

[6] Adverse drug actions caused by drug allergies are discussed in Chapter 31.

518

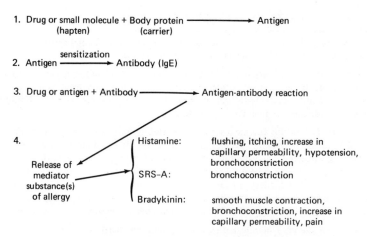

1. Drug or small molecule + Body protein ⟶ Antigen
   (hapten)   (carrier)

2. Antigen ⟶ sensitization ⟶ Antibody (IgE)

3. Drug or antigen + Antibody ⟶ Antigen-antibody reaction

4. Release of mediator substance(s) of allergy

   Histamine: flushing, itching, increase in capillary permeability, hypotension, bronchoconstriction

   SRS-A: bronchoconstriction

   Bradykinin: smooth muscle contraction, bronchoconstriction, increase in capillary permeability, pain

FIGURE 27–1. Mechanisms of Allergic Reactions.

troduced into the body for the first time, antibodies are formed and the body becomes sensitized to the antigen. This protein antibody may circulate in the plasma or it may be fixed in tissues. Upon reexposure to that specific antigen, an antigen-antibody reaction occurs, resulting in the release of mediator substances which are responsible for the allergic symptoms (Figure 27–1).

It was previously believed that histamine was the only mediator responsible for allergic disorders. If this were the case, specific antagonists of histamine, namely, the *antihistamines,* should be uniformly successful in treating all allergic diseases. Whereas clinical experience has shown antihistamines to be quite effective in managing some allergies such as early hay fever, antihistamines provide little or no relief from asthma. In humans, slow-reacting substance of anaphylaxis (SRS-A) is considered to be an important mediator. Most of our subsequent discussions regarding allergies and their treatment will focus upon histamine (see below), since more is known about this endogenous compound, and specific drugs are currently available that are capable of antagonizing its effects.

Allergic reactions are often categorized as being either immediate or delayed. *Immediate* reactions are generally observed after the antigenic substance has been rapidly absorbed; for example, after injection (foreign serums or a bee sting), ingestion (foods or drugs), or inhalation (pollens). By contrast, contactant allergens, or those injected into the skin are more slowly absorbed and cause a *delayed reaction.* In an immediate reaction such as anaphylactic shock, within minutes after reexposure to the antigen the patient complains of anxiety and headache, which are followed by circulatory and respiratory failure and shock. Unless prompt medical treatment is rendered, death often results. Delayed reactions generally manifest themselves by symptoms on the skin. Table 27–2 provides a glossary of common allergic disorders.

TABLE 27-2. GLOSSARY OF ALLERGIC DISORDERS

Allergic rhinitis: A condition characterized by seasonal or perennial sneezing, runny nose, nasal congestion, with itching and congestion of the eyes.

Hay fever: A seasonal variety of allergic rhinitis that results from hypersensitivity to pollens, grass, or ragweed. *Perennial allergic rhinitis,* unlike hay fever, is not seasonal, but occurs continuously, with oscillations in the severity of the symptoms. Common causes include dust, animal dander, and foods.

Bronchial asthma: In this allergic disorder, the smooth muscles of the bronchioles constrict and the mucous membranes become swollen. These obstructions to the airway impair breathing; wheezing is a characteristic symptom of asthma. Half the patients suffer from extrinsic asthma, where there exists hypersensitivity to such external allergens as pollens and animal danders. In the other patients, with intrinsic asthma, infections of the respiratory tract serve as precipitants for asthmatic attacks. Slow-reacting substance (SRS) and bradykinin, as well as histamine, have been suggested as mediators of asthma.

Gastrointestinal allergy: Manifested by nausea, vomiting, diarrhea, and abdominal pains, and induced by specific food allergens and drugs administered by mouth or by injection.

Urticaria (hives): Smooth, somewhat elevated patches of reddened skin; itching is usually present. Allergies to food or drugs, especially penicillin, are the most common causes. *Angioneurotic edema (giant urticaria)* is similar to urticaria, but the areas of edema are larger and involve the skin and subcutaneous tissues. Increased capillary permeability leads to tissue edema in the mucosa of the respiratory tract, which may impair breathing.

Serum sickness: An allergic reaction, which may occur immediately after or up to one to two weeks after the administration of a foreign serum. It is characterized by an urticarial rash, fever, pains in the joints, and swelling of the lymph nodes. Whereas mild cases may be of two or three days in duration, this condition may prove fatal in highly susceptible individuals.

Anaphylactic shock: A severe and often fatal reaction occurring in a previously sensitized person commencing within minutes after the administration of a foreign serum or certain drugs.

Histamine

Since 1910, histamine has been known to be present in both plants and animals. This compound is present in most mammalian tissues and body fluids, has profound effects on many tissues of the body, and participates in the human allergic response. Over the years, many alluring hypotheses have been presented that have attempted to ascribe a normal physiological function to histamine, yet to date, histamine's definite raison d'etre remains obscure.

A large percentage of the total body histamine is present in the granules of *mast cells,* where this compound is bound to heparin. While comfortably reposing in these granules, histamine is not subject to inactivation by enzymes nor is it physiologically active. We shall soon observe the biological consequences of histamine release by drugs, chemicals, physical factors, and antigen-antibody reactions.

$$HC = C-CH_2CH_2NH_2$$

$$HN \quad N$$

$$C$$

$$H$$

Histamine

Pharmacological Effects

Let us first examine the gross pharmacological effects that result after the injection of a moderate dose of histamine under the skin. Because histamine is rapidly inactivated by intestinal bacteria, it exerts little effect after oral administration.

We first observe itching or pain and swelling at the site of injection. A headache and flushing of the face and upper part of the body ensue, and blood pressure precipitously falls. With small doses of histamine, blood pressure rapidly returns to normal, whereas high doses cause the pressure to remain at low levels. In an attempt to combat circulatory failure, the heart rate is accelerated. Difficulty in breathing is experienced, which may be especially pronounced or even life-threatening for the asthmatic. In addition to bronchoconstriction, the smooth muscles of the stomach contract and there is a marked increase in gastric acid secretion. The highly susceptible individual may die as a result of impaired circulation and shock. Analysis of these effects reveal effects on the cardiovascular system and smooth muscles and exocrine glands. Let us now briefly look at these effects and examine the underlying mechanisms responsible for their occurrence.

Histamine produces its biological effects as the result of interactions with *histamine receptors.* These receptors have been subdivided into two types: H_1 and H_2.[7] Contraction of nonvascular smooth muscles is mediated by activation of H_1-receptors, while histamine-mediated enhanced gastric acid secretion involves interactions with H_2-receptors; relaxation of vascular smooth muscle and increased capillary vasodilation appear to be mediated by both H_1- and H_2-receptor types. The actions of histamine on nonvascular smooth muscle and exocrine glands (gastric acid secretion) can be antagonized by specific blockers of each of these receptor types (that is, H_1- and H_2-antagonists, respectively), while a combination of both receptor antagonists is required to block the actions of histamine on capillaries.

The effects of histamine on the *cardiovascular system* are relatively complex and vary greatly among the species studied. Most of the major cardiovascular effects of histamine in humans can be attributed, directly or indirectly, to vasodilation of the smallest blood vessels, namely, the capillaries and venules. As

[7] The concept of multiple receptor types activated by a common chemical will be recalled from Chapter 5; epinephrine (and to a lesser extent, norepinephrine) activate α-, β_1-, and β_2-adrenergic receptors, while acetylcholine activates both muscarinic and nicotinic receptor types.

a direct consequence of this widening of these vessels, the permeability of the capillary membranes is increased, permitting the movement of plasma proteins and fluids into the extracellular spaces. This fluid accumulation results in edema. Moreover, when sufficient amounts of plasma have escaped from vessels, there is a reduction in the circulating volume of blood, a decrease in blood pressure, and eventually shock. The reduction in blood pressure reflexly activates a compensatory stimulation in heart rate in an attempt to restore the circulation of an adequate amount of blood around the body. Profound vasodilation also produces flushing of the face and upper trunk.

In humans, especially those suffering from respiratory diseases, constriction of the bronchioles—hence, impaired breathing—is an important adverse effect associated with exposure to histamine.

Histamine has been shown to be a very potent stimulant of gastric acid (hydrochloric acid) and pepsin secretion from the cells of the gastric mucosa and may act as the "final common mediator" responsible for the normal physiological release of gastric acid by the parietal cells of the stomach (Chapter 25).

Histamine Release

With the realization that histamine is at least in part responsible for allergic reactions, considerable effort has been directed toward learning more about the factors and mechanisms responsible for the release of histamine from mast cells, either with, or in the absence of, gross destruction of these cells.

Curare-like componds (d-tubocurarine), morphine, and stilbamidine are drugs capable of releasing histamine. In some instances histamine liberation can have fatal consequences, which result from anaphylactic reactions, while in other cases, less extreme side effects result. Shortly after stilbamidine was administered to West African natives suffering from kala-azar (Black fever), the patients began to vigorously scratch themselves and complained of "ants." The itching experienced was the consequence of histamine liberation from the skin. The plasma substitutes, dextran and polyvinylpyrrolidone (PVP), are also histamine releasers as are some iodine-containing contrast media used for diagnosis of gallbladder disease.

Insect venoms often contain histamine and/or histamine-releasing substances, as well as compounds that are toxic to red blood cells and nerves. Susceptible individuals may experience profuse sweating, a drop in blood pressure, circulatory failure, and bronchoconstriction, which may result in respiratory failure. Individuals with heart disease and asthma are most susceptible to fatally succumbing after insect stings. These effects are the result of an antigen-antibody reaction (see below). Although most of us consider bees, hornets, and wasps to be merely unwelcome guests at a summer picnic, stings from insects of the *Hymenoptera* order resulted in 229 fatalities from 1949–1959; in a very high percentage of these cases, death occurred in less than one hour.

Possible Physiological and Pathological Roles

Histamine has long suffered an identity crisis. This highly potent compound is widely distributed throughout the body; hence, we might assume that its presence is indicative of some important physiological function. Although the precise nature of this function remains obscure, its role in some human allergic disorders is generally accepted. Far more speculative is histamine's importance in tissue growth and repair, maintenance of pregnancy, regulation of microcirculation, and as a neurotransmitter in the nervous system.

Antihistamines (H₁-Antagonists)

> *Perhaps no better definition could be given of an antihistaminic subtance than to state that it is a counter-poison having no specific activity of its own on the normal animal, its properties appearing only when it can manifest a detoxifying power against the action of histamine.*

> —Daniel Bovet (1950)

Although we now recognize that several natural substances in the body act as mediators of the allergic response, let us restrict our attention to the best studied of these, namely, histamine. How can we, in theory at least, prevent or antagonize the action of histamine, and, thereby, prevent the allergic reaction from occurring? We might prevent the synthesis of histamine by inhibiting the essential enzyme histidine decarboxylase, or attempt to increase the rate at which the enzymes of the body inactivate histamine, or chemically "neutralize" histamine in a manner not unlike the way a base neutralizes an acid. Perhaps you might suggest that we deplete mast cells of histamine, or, conversely, develop a drug that will prevent the release of histamine from mast cells. Some of these approaches have been investigated and have proved unsuccessful, whereas others are in various stages of fruition. At present, two different modes are employed for the treatment of allergic disorders.[8] These involve the use of physiological antagonists of histamine, such as adrenergic agents, and the use of pharmacological antagonists of the antihistamine class (Chapter 3).

Physiological antagonists exert a biological action that is diametrically opposed to that produced by histamine. Whereas histamine causes bronchoconstriction, the *adrenergic agents* epinephrine and isoproterenol relax the bronchial smooth muscles and actively produce bronchodilation, thus restoring open airways essential for free breathing. These physiological antagonists do not directly interact with histamine, nor do they modify the activity of the histamine receptor site. *Pharmacological antagonists* compete with histamine

---

[8] **Cromolyn** is a unique drug introduced in 1973 for the treatment of chronic bronchial asthma. It has no bronchodilator, antihistaminic, or anti-inflammatory activity. This drug prevents antigen-induced release of histamine and slow-reacting substance (SRS) from mast cells (see below).

for a common receptor site. Unlike the physiological antagonists, antihistamines do not exert a positive action themselves, but rather restore normal function without improving upon it. Anaphylactic shock or an acute asthmatic attack are acute life-threatening conditions that undoubtedly result from the release of one or more mediator substances in addition to histamine. Adrenergic agents rather than antihistamines are used for the treatment of these medical emergencies. The former drugs have a more rapid onset of action and, because they are physiological antagonists, they are able to produce bronchodilation, regardless of the specific mediator of bronchoconstriction.

History

Prior to 1937, the physiological antagonists, epinephrine, for example, were the only class of drugs available for reversing histamine's actions. In that year, Bovet and Staub, working at the Pasteur Institute in Paris, begin their search for specific histamine antagonists. Bovet noted that acetylcholine, epinephrine, and histamine were all naturally occurring compounds that had a common chemical group, that is:

$$-\overset{|}{\underset{|}{C}}-\overset{|}{\underset{|}{C}}-N\overset{\diagup}{\diagdown}$$

Moreover, if compounds could antagonize acetylcholine and epinephrine, why could a histamine antagonist not be developed? The first antihistamine (H_1-antagonist) was *929F*, a compound capable of protecting guinea pigs against five lethal doses of histamine. Unfortunately, its high toxicity precluded its use in man. Antergan was the first successful antihistamine suitable for clinical application. This drug, introduced in France in 1942, was about twenty times more active than 929F and was less toxic. The financial success of diphenhydramine (Benadryl) and tripelennamine (Pyribenzamine) in 1945–1946 in the United States led to the introduction of approximately 30 other antihistamines which are currently available.

Prior to 1972, only histamine antagonists that were capable of blocking the actions of histamine at its H_1-receptor sites were developed. Histamine-mediated increase in gastric acid secretion was conspicuously refractory to blockade by the classical histamine antagonists. In 1977, the first specific H_2-antagonist was approved for clinical use in the United States. This drug, cimetidine (Tagamet), represents a totally new concept in the treatment of peptic ulcer disease and is discussed in Chapter 25.

Prior to the development of H_2-antagonists, the term *antihistamine* was understood to be synonymous with a H_1-antagonist. Although somewhat imprecise, we shall give way to tradition and retain this designation. By contrast, cimetidine and related drugs will be referred to as H_2-antagonists.

Antihistaminic (Anti-H$_1$) Actions

Antihistamines are able to antagonize the actions of histamine by a mechanism that is directly analogous to atropine's antagonism of acetylcholine. Namely, antihistamines act by occupying the histamine receptor sites, thereby precluding histamine from interacting at these sites (Chapters 2 and 8). Notwithstanding their strong affinity for the histamine receptor site, antihistamines have minimal activity of their own. We have previously noted that these agents do not chemically inactivate histamine nor do they impair the release of this mediator substance.

The antihistamines are able to antagonize histamine-mediated vasodilation (which results in hypotension) and increased capillary permeability. Whereas antihistamines are highly effective in blocking histamine-induced bronchoconstriction, they offer a fraction of this protection (1/10,000) against antigen-mediated bronchoconstriction. What accounts for this very marked difference? Undoubtedly, the true answer will explain why antihistamines are not useful in the treatment of asthma. It has been argued that after an antigen-antibody reaction, massive amounts of histamine are released in the immediate area of the histamine receptor site. Antihistamines may not be able to reach sufficiently high concentrations at these sites to effectively antagonize histamine. A more widely held hypothesis suggests that histamine is not the only mediator substance released as a consequence of an antigen-antibody reaction. Antihistamines are not capable of blocking the effects of such mediators as slow-reacting substance of anaphylaxis and bradykinin, and so, at best, are only partially effective in reversing bronchoconstriction.

Other Actions of Interest

All antihistamines competitively inhibit histamine at its receptor site. This constitutes the primary action of this class of drugs. In addition, antihistamines have a myriad of other actions, most of which cannot be readily explained on the basis of histamine antagonism. Some of these include effects on the central nervous system, suppression of motion sickness, anticholinergic activity, and anti-Parkinson and local anesthetic actions.

Central nervous system. Antihistamines in both therapeutic and toxic doses have pronounced effects on the central nervous system. In this regard infants and very young children are particularly sensitive. In young children, toxic doses of these drugs produce signs of stimulation—excitement, hallucinations, muscle tremors, and convulsions. While some older children and adults may become restless, nervous, and unable to sleep, more frequently central nervous system depression is observed. In normal doses, almost all antihistamines induce some degree of drowsiness, while high doses may produce coma. Tolerance develops to this drowsiness after several days of repeated doses.

Other antihistaminic actions resulting from effects of these drugs on the central nervous system include prevention of motion sickness and an anti-Parkinson effect. Neither of these actions is universally possessed by all antihistaminic agents. Whereas we cannot correlate these effects with the histamine antagonizing properties of these drugs, conversely, we cannot summarily exclude the possibility of a histamine interaction. Many of these centrally acting antihistamines also possess atropine-like properties which may be responsible for these effects. Indeed, dryness of the mouth is a common side effect associated with antihistamines. Hence antagonism of cholinergic receptors in the brain must be considered as a possible mechanism responsible for their beneficial effects in motion sickness and Parkinson's disease.

Therapeutic Uses of Antihistamines

There are, at present, over 30 antihistamines available, yet none of these drugs is completely effective therapeutically while also being totally devoid of undesirable side effects. It has been said of antihistamines that, "perhaps in no other class of therapeutic agents does the physician enjoy a wider choice of preparations; but in no other group of drugs does a discerning choice offer less reward." The differences among antihistamines are summarized in Table 27-3. Inspection of the label of your favorite nonprescription cold capsule or sleep aid will probably reveal one of these antihistamines or a chemically related compound.

Antihistamines are among the more extensively used class of drugs. If you do not suffer from an allergic disorder, perhaps this past winter has left you with a cough or a cold. Possibly, the anticipation of your summer cruise to Europe this summer aboard a tramp steamer has caused you some sleepless nights. Do you suffer from motion sickness? When any of these problems arise, an antihistamine may be the class of drugs to which you turn. In some instances, these drugs provide symptomatic relief, in other cases, their placebo effect may be beneficial. Unfortunately, antihistamines never cure the underlying disease.

Allergies.   The most effective method of dealing with allergic disorders is to remove the patient from the noxious allergen or the allergen from the patient. If the allergic symptoms can be traced to eating lobster Newburg or to wearing a sable fur coat, one can, if absolutely imperative, resort to dining on tuna fish and donning a cloth coat. What realistic course of action is open to the handsomely remunerated Hoosier steel worker, residing in Gary, when he discovers that the cause of his allergy is some airborn particles continuously belching from the chimneys of his plant? Although his respiratory difficulties may dramatically disappear in the clear air over Arizona, so might his income. Finally, for some individuals, the allergen cannot be uncovered; or conversely, the allergen may be so common that it cannot be successfully eluded.

Because of wide differences in etiology, sweeping generalizations cannot be made concerning the effectiveness of antihistamines in treating allergic disorders. Moreover, the effectiveness of the same drugs for the same condition,

TABLE 27-3. DIFFERENCES AMONG CLASSES OF ANTIHISTAMINES

Class of Antihistamine	Generic Name	Selected Trade Names	Properties of the Class	Remarks
Ethanolamines	Diphenhydramine Dimenhydrinate Carbinoxamine Doxylamine	Benadryl Dramamine Clistin Decapryn	High incidence of drowsiness; atropine-like effects; gastrointestinal upset less frequent	Dimenhydrinate: motion sickness. Doxylamine: used in some nonprescription sleep aid products.
Ethylenediamines	Tripelennamine Pyrilamine Methapyrilene	PBZ Neo-Antergan	Lower incidence of drowsiness; gastrointestinal upset frequent	Pyrilamine: the most specific antihistamine; 40,000 times more active against histamine than acetylcholine; most commonly used antihistamine in nonprescription sleep aids (Compoz, Nytol, Sleep-Eze, Sominex, Sure-Sleep). Methapyrilene: formerly used sleep aids; withdrawn after shown to produce tumors in animals.
Alkylamines	Chlorpheniramine Brompheniramine	Chlor-Trimeton Teldrin Dimetane Disomer	Most potent class of histamine antagonists; low incidence of drowsiness	
Piperazine	Cyclizine Meclizine	Marezine Bonine	Lower incidence of drowsiness; used primarily for motion sickness	High doses of cyclizine have been shown to produce fetal abnormalities in animals. Relevancy of these findings to humans has not been established, but contraindicated during pregnancy.
Phenothiazines	Promethazine	Phenergan		Promethazine: motion sickness; marked sedation. Methdilazine and trimeprazine: relieve itching; mild-to-moderate sedation.
Miscellaneous	Methdilazine Trimeprazine Cyproheptadine Diphenylpyraline	Tacaryl Temaril Periactin Diaphen Hispril		Cyproheptadine: histamine and serotonin antagonist; antipruritic; moderate sedation.

528   *Sec. 6   Drugs Affecting the Gastrointestinal and Respiratory Systems*

such as hay fever, varies at different times of the year. Antihistamines are highly effective (80%) early in the season for the symptomatic treatment of *hay fever.* These agents relieve sneezing, runny nose, and itching of the eyes, nose, and throat. Later in the season, as the pollen (allergen) count rises, the favorable drug effects proportionately decrease. Similarily, in *perennial allergic rhinitis,* antihistamines may help only 50 percent of the patients. Antihistamines are of great value in relieving the itching associated with urticaria or *hives;* swelling and redness respond less favorably.

In acute life-threatening allergic disorders such as *angioneurotic edema* or *anaphylactic shock,* physiological antagonists (epinephrine and isoproterenol, for example) are employed to actively reverse the respiratory distress arising from bronchoconstriction. In such conditions, it is imperative to provide prompt and positive bronchodilation. Although antihistamines may be of some value in mild cases of *asthma,* they are ineffective in arresting an acute attack. As we have previously observed, it is quite likely that mediators other than histamine may be responsible for the observed bronchoconstriction.

Common cold.   In 1949, the North Atlantic Treaty Organization treaty was signed and the New York Yankees won their first of five consecutive world championships. Yet, by far, the most significant news of that year was the startling announcement that the *common cold could be prevented and cured.* The *Reader's Digest*[9] called it "the best health news of the year."

The public response to the ensuing multidimensional promotion was wildly enthusiastic, as were the manufacturers of antihistamines who were capitalizing on a $100,000,000 business. As might be anticipated, some individuals with vested scientific or financial interests were content with putting aside several gross shortcomings in the design and analysis of their studies. For example, colds were not carefully differentiated from allergic disorders; patients supplied their own subjective reports after medication, without objective professional examinations; and, in addition, double-blind studies were not utilized, leading to natural, and perhaps unavoidable physician bias. When carefully controlled studies were finally conducted, antihistamines were found to be no more effective than placebos in preventing, curing, or reducing the duration of the common cold. These investigations revealed that 25 to 50 percent of the subjects treated with placebos reported effective results. At present, medical experts believe that, at best, antihistamines provide only *symptomatic relief* of the runny nose associated with the common cold; this effect has been attributed to the atropine-like actions of these drugs. Virtually all preparations now marketed for cold symptoms contain an antihistamine.

Motion sickness.   Motion sickness is a complex phenomenon that is strongly influenced by the fullness of the stomach, visual and olfactory stimuli, and the effects experienced by traveling companions. The continuous and rhythmic movement of a ship is generally acknowledged to be without equal in

---

[9] P. deKruif, "Is This at Last, Goodbye to the Common Cold?" *Reader's Digest,* December 1949, pp. 16–18.

evoking motion sickness. Prevention of its occurrence is far easier than producing a cure as this English sailor's proverb suggests: "The only cure for seasickness is to sit on the shady side of an old brick church in the country."

The belladonna alkaloids (Chapter 8), notably scopolamine, have been used to treat seasickness since 1869. However, little scientific enthusiasm was shown in evaluating the most effective therapy for the prevention of vomiting until the ominous black clouds of war hung over England 70 years later. The incentive for such research was elementary: "When a landing has to be made in the face of resistance, it is easy to see that seasickness might on occasion become a handicap." Extensive studies conducted during World War II have clearly established the effectiveness of *scopolamine* for the prevention and relief of motion sickness arising from trips of short duration, that is, of about six hours. *Antihistamines* were found to be beneficial after it was astutely observed that a woman's usual car sickness was unexpectedly absent after she took dimenhydrinate (Dramamine) for her allergy. Not all antihistamines are capable of preventing nausea and vomiting; diphenhydramine (Benadryl), promethazine (Phenergan), cyclizine (Marezine), meclizine (Bonine), and dimenhydrinate (Dramamine) are most useful, and the last three drugs are available without a prescription. In general, the antihistamines are recommended for trips of greater than six hours because they cause fewer side effects than scopolamine. Although drowsiness may not prove to be a serious liability for a passenger embarking upon a trans-Atlantic cruise, it may be a real problem for the ship's captain.

Morning sickness.   Unlike scopolamine, antihistamines have been shown to be useful in preventing nausea and vomiting arising from causes other than motion. The most common of these is *morning sickness of pregnancy.* There is a lack of unanimity among physicians regarding the desirability of women taking any drugs during pregnancy. To further complicate these arguments, cyclizine has been shown to produce fetal abnormalities in several rodent species.

Sedation.   The Americans of the early 1970s were indeed fortunate that so many nonprescription products were available to provide them with "safe and restful sleep" or to relieve their "nervous tension," without exposing them to "harmful, habit-forming barbiturates." It was an age of specialization. This fact was well appreciated by the manufacturer of proprietary drugs who marketed products for simultaneous relief of nervous tension and for the promotion of sleep (Compoz, Sominex, Sleep-Eze), for the relief of pain and tension and for the aid of sleep (Cope, Excedrin P.M.), and, finally, products for the alleviation of cold symptoms and for the facilitation of sleep (NyQuil). Advertisements for many of these products suggested that this nonbarbiturate was new and had been conclusively shown to rapidly induce sleep. *Pyrilamine,*[10] an antihistamine, has been marketed for 30 years, and in the concentrations

---

[10] Prior to 1979, **methapyrilene** was the antihistamine used in these products but was voluntarily withdrawn by manufacturers and replaced by pyrilamine or doxylamine after methapyrilene was shown to cause tumors in animals.

contained in the above-mentioned products, it is questionably effective. At these dose levels, it usually produces drowsiness at best, and tolerance develops with repeated administration. Notwithstanding the relatively mild effects these drugs have on the central nervous system, the reader should still avoid taking antihistamine-containing products with alcoholic beverages before driving a motor vehicle. Alcohol-potentiated antihistamine drowsiness is suspected as being the cause of many traffic accidents.

Toxicology of Antihistamines

Although undesirable side effects occur with even normal doses of anti-histamines, severe adverse effects rarely occur. When we consider the very extensive uses of this class of drugs by the public, the number of fatalities resulting from over-dosage or idiosyncrasy are extremely low indeed. The undesirable effects associated with antihistamines affect three major areas: the central nervous system, the gastro-intestinal tract, and the autonomic nervous system.

The most common problem associated with the use of antihistamines is depression of the central nervous system, an effect that may vary in intensity from slight drowsiness to an inability to concentrate, to dizziness with muscle weakness, to deep sleep. These effects are dependent upon the specific antihistamine employed, its dosage, and the susceptibility of the patient. In in-fants and children, antihistamines can act as stimulants and may cause hyper-activity, confusion, muscle twitching, and convulsions. Most of the reported deaths resulting from antihistamines have occurred in children, thus reinforcing the importance of keeping such medicines out of their reach. Adults should avoid taking antihistamines with alcohol, barbiturates, and other depressant agents. Unfortunately, no specific antidotes have been developed to combat acute antihistamine poisoning.

Side effects include loss of appetite, nausea, vomiting, diarrhea, and gastric upset. These unpleasantries may be minimized by taking antihistamines with meals. Since many antihistamines also possess anticholinergic activity, it is not surprising that we see many atropine-like effects, namely, dryness of the mouth and blurred vision.

BRONCHIAL ASTHMA

Bronchial asthma, a chronic disease characterized by respiratory distress resulting from obstruction of airflow, affects 1 to 2 percent of the population. An asthmatic attack, lasting in duration from a few minutes to several hours, usually begins with tightness in the chest, followed by coughing, wheezing, and difficulty in breathing; exhalation of air is more difficult than inhalation. These symptoms result from excessive secretion of bronchial fluids, bronchial mucosal edema, and constriction of the bronchial smooth muscle.

Asthma is generally classified as being either extrinsic or intrinsic. *Extrinsic (atopic, allergic) asthma* has an allergic basis, generally appears early in life in children and young adults, occurs in patients with a family history of allergy, and exhibits seasonal variation in symptoms; elevated circulating serum levels of IgE are present. By contrast, *intrinsic asthma* occurs later in life (after 35 years of age), in patients with no family history of allergy, elevated IgE levels, or aspirin intolerance.

In patients with extrinsic (allergic) asthma, the interaction of an allergen (antigen) with the IgE antibody bound to the membrane of a sensitized mast cell reduces intracellular levels of cyclic adenosine 3', 5'-monophosphate (cyclic AMP) and results in the release of chemical mediators such as histamine and slow-reacting substance of anaphylaxis (SRS-A). These chemicals cause contraction of bronchial smooth muscle which is clinically manifested as bronchospasms. By contrast, drug-induced increased intracellular levels of cyclic AMP prevent the release of these chemical mediators from sensitized mast cells (Figure 27-2).

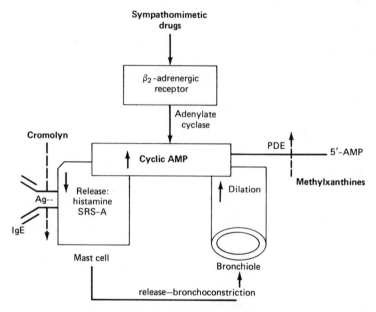

FIGURE 27-2. Pharmacological Basis for Antiasthmatic Agents. In patients with extrinsic asthma, the antigen-IgE antibody interaction results in release of histamine and SRS-A from sensitized mast cells. These mediators cause contraction of smooth muscle and bronchoconstriction. Increased levels of cyclic adenosine 3', 5'-monophosphate (cyclic AMP) inhibit mediator release from mast cells and cause smooth muscle relaxation and bronchodilation. Sympathomimetic drugs (ephedrine, isoproterenol, terbutaline), via activation of the β_2-adrenergic receptor, enhance the synthesis of cyclic AMP in mast cells and bronchioles. Methylxanthines (theophylline, aminophylline) increase cyclic AMP levels by inhibiting phosphodiesterase (PDE), the enzyme responsible for its inactivation. The antiasthmatic effects of corticosteroids (beclomethasone, hydrocortisone) result from multiple actions and may involve enhancement of the sensitivity of the β_2-receptor to endogenous catecholamines. Cromolyn stabilizes the mast cell membrane preventing the release of chemical mediators after antigen-IgE interactions. Intrinsic asthma may involve inadequate β-adrenergic activation and/or excessive cholinergic activity causing bronchoconstriction.

Bronchial smooth muscle tone, which determines the diameter of the bronchioles and their resistance to airflow, is controlled by a balance between opposing sympathetic (adrenergic) and parasympathetic (cholinergic) influences. Activation of β-adrenergic receptors in the bronchioles (in particular, the β_2-receptors) causes bronchodilation, while stimulation of cholinergic receptors causes bronchoconstriction (Figure 27–2). It has been suggested that intrinsic asthma and asthmatic bronchoconstriction may result from excessive cholinergic activity or inadequate β-adrenergic activation.

Drug Treatment of Asthma

Drugs used for the treatment of bronchial asthma include the bronchodilator sympathomimetics and methylxanthines (the actions of both classes of these drugs involve cyclic AMP), corticosteroids, and cromolyn (Table 27–4). The bronchodilators are the mainstay of asthma therapy and are employed to both prevent and terminate acute attacks.

TABLE 27-4. REPRESENTATIVE ANTIASTHMATIC AGENTS

Generic Name (Synonym)	Selected Trade Names	Distinguishing Properties
Sympathomimetic bronchodilators		
Ephedrine	—	Orally used to prevent asthmatic attacks.
Pseudoephedrine	Novafed Sudafed	Activates α-, β_1-, and β_2-adrenergic receptors.
Epinephrine (adrenaline)	Adrenalin Medihaler-Epi Primatene Mist	Administered by subcutaneous injection and by inhalation to arrest acute attack; rapid onset, short duration of action. Some adverse effects on heart.
Isoproterenol	Isuprel Medihaler-Iso Norisodrine	Potent β-adrenergic stimulant and bronchodilator used for relieving acute asthmatic attacks.
Metaproterenol	Alupent Metaprel	Similar to isoproterenol but greater β_2 specificity (lower incidence of adverse effects on heart) and longer duration of action.
Terbutaline	Brethine Bricanyl	β_2-specific causing minimal adverse effects on the cardiovascular system.
Albuterol (salbutamol)	—	β_2-specific available in Canada and Europe.
Isoetharine + phenylephrine	Bronkosol Bronkometer	
Methylxanthine bronchodilators		
Theophylline	Aerolate Bronkodyl Elixophyllin	Administered orally and rectally for management of mild-to-moderate asthma. Plasma drug levels monitored

TABLE 27-4. CONTINUED

Generic Name (Synonym)	Selected Trade Names	Distinguishing Properties
	Marax* Quadrinal* Quibron* Tedral* Theon Theophyl	to increase therapeutic response and decrease toxicity.
Aminophylline (theophylline ethylenediamine)	—	Administered orally and rectally; IV injection used to relieve acute attacks.
Dyphylline	Dilot Lufyllin Neophylline	Reported to be more consistently absorbed and less irritating after oral administration than theophylline and
Oxtriphylline (choline theophylline)	Choledyl Brondecon*	aminophylline.
Adrenocorticosteroids		
Beclomethasone dipropionate	Vanceril	Administered by inhalation for chronic management of asthma; causes few adverse systemic effects.
Dexamethasone	Decadron	Inhalation; some systemic toxicity.
Hydrocortisone	Solu-Cortef	Administered by IV to arrest severe
Methylprednisolone	Solu-Medrol	acute asthmatic attacks.
Prednisolone	Hydeltrasol	
Miscellaneous		
Cromolyn (disodium cromoglycate)	Intal	Inhalation of dry contents of capsule to prevent attacks.

*Mixtures containing methylxanthine.

Sympathomimetics

Activation of β_2-adrenergic receptors by sympathomimetics increases the synthesis of cyclic AMP which causes relaxation of bronchial smooth muscle and bronchodilation. Ephedrine (Chapter 6) is the oldest of the commonly used sympathomimetic antiasthmatic agents.

Ephedrine. Ephedrine is widely used for the treatment of mild-to-moderate cases of bronchial asthma, as well as to relieve nasal congestion. Although ephedrine is 100 times less potent than epinephrine (adrenaline) as a bronchodilator, its effectiveness after oral administration and prolonged duration of action (four hours) make it a valuable drug for the prevention of asthmatic attacks. However, its relatively slow onset of action (about 60 minutes) precludes its usefulness in arresting acute attacks.

Epinephrine. Epinephrine has a rapid onset of action (several minutes) and a duration of action of two to three hours after injection or inhalation making it a highly useful drug for the management of an acute moderate-to-severe asthmatic attack. In addition to its β_2-mediated bronchodilatory activity, epinephrine-induced α-adrenergic receptor activation causes vasoconstriction of the bronchial mucosal blood vessels causing a reduction in congestion and edema.

Selective β-adrenergic agents. Isoproterenol (Isuprel) is the most potent β-adrenergic stimulant and is a powerful bronchodilator agent. This drug is highly effective after inhalation for the treatment of acute asthmatic attacks. Since isoproterenol and epinephrine activate both β_1- and β_2-adrenergic receptors, the primary adverse effects are β_1-mediated and involve the heart (arrhythmias and anginal pain).

In recent years, more selective β_2-adrenergic stimulants have been developed for the treatment of asthma. These drugs, including metaproterenol (Alupent, Metaprel) and terbutaline (Brethine, Bricanyl), are reported to produce fewer undesirable effects on the heart.

Methylxanthines

Methylxanthines are the other major class of bronchodilators employed for the treatment of bronchial asthma. Drugs in this group produce their beneficial therapeutic effects via actions that result in increased levels of cyclic AMP by a mechanism that differs from the sympathomimetics. Cyclic AMP is inactivated by the enzyme phosphodiesterase, and this enzyme is inhibited by *theophylline* and related methylxanthines (Figure 27–2). Since these drugs have fewer pronounced effects on the heart than epinephrine and isoproterenol, they are often preferred for use in patients with heart disease.

Corticosteroids

For patients who fail to respond to standard antiasthmatic medications, it may be necessary to initiate corticosteroid (glucocorticoid, adrenocorticoid, steroid) medication. These drugs often provide dramatic and sometimes life-saving effects. Their potential therapeutic usefulness is limited by the wide range of potentially severe adverse effects associated with their chronic administration. The mechanism by which the corticosteroids produce their antiasthmatic effects is not well understood but thought to involve multiple actions on blood vessels, bronchial smooth muscle, and IgE formation.

Corticosteroids can be administered orally or by inhalation for the chronic management of asthma and by intravenous injection to arrest acute life-threatening attacks. *Beclomethasone dipropionate* (Vanceril), a highly effective new steroid, is administered by inhalation. It is not systemically absorbed after inhalation and, therefore, causes few of the adverse side effects generally associated with other corticosteroids. This drug is used for the chronic treatment of asthma.

Cromolyn (Disodium Cromoglycate)

Cromolyn sodium (Intal) possesses a unique mode of action. This compound is not a bronchodilator nor does it possess anti-inflammatory (corticosteroid-like) or antimediator (antihistamine-like) activities. The antiasthmatic properties of this drug have been attributed to its ability to stabilize the membrane of the sensitized mast cell and thereby *prevent the release of chemical mediators* (including histamine and slow-reacting substance of anaphylaxis) normally associated with an antigen-antibody (IgE) interaction. This drug, administered by inhalation of the dry contents of a capsule via a special device, is most useful for preventing attacks in young patients with extrinsic asthma. Cromolyn is also employed successfully in adult patients with intrinsic asthma and in exercise-induced bronchospasm.

SUMMARY

The common cold, allergic disorders, and bronchial asthma are three extremely common disorders causing impairment of respiratory function.

The common cold, the most frequently encountered and most expensive illness affecting Western society, is caused by viruses. A very large number of nonprescription remedies have been extensively and aggressively promoted for relief from the symptoms of the common cold. These products contain most of the following constituents: a sympathomimetic nasal decongestant (phenylephrine); an antitussive agent (codeine, dextromethorphan) to inhibit the nonproductive cough; a questionably effective expectorant (guaifenesin) to facilitate the removal of mucus from the respiratory tract; an antihistamine (chlorpheniramine, pyrilamine) to reduce mucus secretion and stop the runny nose; and an analgesic-antipyretic (aspirin, acetaminophen) for the relief of aches and pains and the reduction of fever. The rational basis for such a wide conglomeration of ingredients in a single product has very often not been clinically or scientifically substantiated. With the addition of each component, the incidence of adverse side effects may be expected to increase. Regulation of the often misleading advertising of these products would undoubtedly provide a great asset in protecting the public's health and wallet.

An allergy is an extreme sensitivity to a substance resulting from an antigen-antibody reaction. This reaction causes the release of a mediator substance such as histamine that is directly responsible for the allergic response. Most of the total body histamine is found in mast cells and, as such, is physiologically inactive. After its release from mast cells by drugs, chemicals, or physical stimuli, histamine exerts profound effects on the cardiovascular system, smooth muscles, and exocrine glands. Histamine-induced capillary vasodilation causes a drop in blood pressure, flushing of the face, and headache.

Bronchial smooth muscle constricts, which impairs breathing, and the secretion of gastric acid from the stomach is markedly enhanced.

The drug manufacturer and other benefactors of human health have shown a keen interest in developing newer and better antihistamines (H_1-antagonists) in an attempt to treat the allergies from which 20 percent of us suffer. False hopes were raised, as were stock market prices, with the later disproved hypothesis that antihistamines could prevent and cure the common cold. These compounds provide relief for cold symptoms, nothing more. Some antihistamines prevent motion sickness, morning sickness of pregnancy, and itching. Nonprescription sleep aids are among the most common uses of antihistamines. Whereas some of the above effects can be attributed to competitive antagonism of histamine at its tissue receptor sites, the mechanisms underlying other effects are far more obscure. H_2-antagonists are used for the treatment of peptic ulcer disease (Chapter 25).

Bronchial asthma, characterized by wheezing, coughing, and difficulty in breathing, may or may not have an allergic basis. Reduced levels of cyclic AMP promote the release of histamine, SRS-A and other mediators of bronchoconstriction. Sympathomimetic amines activate the β_2-adrenergic receptor increasing cyclic AMP levels in the mast cells and bronchioles; some of these drugs are used to prevent asthmatic attacks (ephedrine), while others arrest an acute attack (epinephrine, isoproterenol). New drugs (terbutaline) are specific β_2-adrenergic agonists. Methylxanthines (theophylline, aminophylline) produce bronchodilation by inhibiting the enzymatic inactivation of cAMP. Cromolyn prevents the release of chemical mediators from sensitized mast cells, while the effects of corticosteroids (beclomethasone) are less well understood and have been attributed to multiple mechanisms. In recent years, the fundamental biochemical etiology of allergic disorders and asthma have become better understood. This knowledge will permit the rational development of more specific and effective drugs with reduced adverse effects.

SUPPLEMENTARY READINGS

Austen, K. F., and L. M. Lichtenstein, eds., *Asthma: Physiology, Immunopharmacology, and Treatment.* New York: Academic Press, 1973.

Bach, M. K., *Immediate Sensitivity: Modern Concepts and Developments.* New York: Marcel Dekker, 1978.

Beaven, M. A., *Histamine: Its Role in Physiological and Pathological Processes.* Basel: S. Karger, 1978.

Brand, J. J., and W. L. M. Perry, "Drugs Used in Motion Sickness," *Pharmacological Reviews* **18**: 895–924 (1966).

Cormier, J. F., and B. G. Bryant, "Cold and Allergy Products," in *Handbook of Nonprescription Products.* 6th ed., pp. 73–114. Washington, D.C.: American Pharmaceutical Association, 1979.

Kahlson, G., and E. Rosengren, *Biogenesis and Physiology of Histamine.* London: Edward Arnold Ltd., 1971.

Kaliner, M., and K. F. Austen, "Immunologic Release of Chemical Mediators From Human Tissue," *Annual Review of Pharmacology* **15**: 177–89 (1975).

Paton, W. D. M., "Histamine Release by Compounds of Simple Chemical Structure," *Pharmacological Reviews* **9**: 269–328 (1957).

Rocha e Silva, M., ed., *Histamine: Its Chemistry, Metabolism and Physiological and Pharmacological Actions. Handbook of Experimental Pharmacology.* Vol. 18, Part 1. Berlin: Springer-Verlag, 1966.

Rocha e Silva, M., ed. *Histamine II and Anti-Histaminics: Chemistry, Metabolism and Physiological and Pharmacological Actions.* Vol 18, Part 2. Berlin: Springer-Verlag, 1978.

Schacter, M., ed., "Histamine and Antihistamines," in *International Encyclopedia of Pharmacology and Therapeutics.* Vol. 1, Sec. 74. Oxford: Pergamon Press, 1973.

Weiss, E. B., and M. S. Segal, eds., *Bronchial Asthma—Mechanisms and Therapeutics.* Boston: Little, Brown, 1976.

Wilson, A. F., and J. J. McPhillips, "Pharmacological Control of Asthma," *Annual Review of Pharmacology and Toxicology* **18**: 541–61 (1978).

Ziment, I., *Respiratory Pharmacology and Therapeutics.* Philadelphia: Saunders, 1978.

section seven

Chemotherapeutic Agents

28

Introduction to Chemotherapy

In order to pursue chemotherapy successfully we must look for substances which possess a high affinity and high lethal potency in relationship to the parasites, but have a low toxicity in relation to the body, so that it becomes possible to kill the parasites without damaging the body to any great extent. We want to hit the parasites as selectively as possible.

—Paul Ehrlich (1909)

During the Middle Ages, the infamous Black Death or bubonic plague ravaged the Western World, and it is reported that this bacterial disease killed 25 million persons, one-quarter of the entire European population. While 19 million men died in battle in the nineteenth century, there were almost twice as many victims of tuberculosis. In 1900, 23 percent of all deaths in the United States were caused by influenza, pneumonia, and tuberculosis, with 2.3 percent of the population succumbing from diphtheria. At the turn of the century, a diagnosis of such communicable diseases as cholera, meningitis, scarlet fever, various streptococcal and staphylococcal infections, typhus, and typhoid fever were all virtual death warrants for the unfortunate patients, as were syphilis and gonorrhea. What do we observe at present? Today only viral pneumonia remains on mortality lists of the ten principal causes of death in this country. The remainder of the previously mentioned infectious diseases have ceased to be major health problems in the United States or are amenable to treatment.

Many factors have contributed to the reduction in deaths from infectious diseases and to the increase in our life spans; they include advances in preventive medicine, more sensitive tests to permit early diagnosis of disease, improved training and acumen of physicians, more effective public health laws, and better living conditions. However, the most significant single factor, perhaps, has been the development of effective chemotherapeutic agents.

Chemotherapy is a general term referring to the *use of a drug to kill or weaken invading cells or organisms without unduly harming the patient.* Such invading organisms may be bacteria, protozoa, worms, and viruses or tumors. Hence, if we wish to be more precise in designating a chemotherapeutic agent, we may speak of antibacterial, antiprotozoan, anthelmintic, antiviral, or antitumor drugs. **Antibiotics** are *chemotherapeutic agents produced or derived from microorganisms which kill or inhibit the growth of other microorganisms or tumor cells.* We shall also consider antibiotics to be drugs that are synthetic or semisynthetic derivatives of compounds naturally produced by living cells.

All clinically useful chemotherapeutic agents are more toxic to the organism than to the patient and may be used internally to treat systemic infections. *Antiseptics* or *disinfectants* are chemicals capable of destroying microorganisms on inanimate objects or on the surface of the skin or mucous membranes, but are generally far too toxic to be taken internally. Iodine tincture, phenol, Merthiolate, Mercurochrome, gentian violet, Zephiran, and hexachlorophene are representative examples of local anti-infective agents; these drugs will not be considered in our subsequent discussions.

In this chapter we shall introduce some basic concepts about microorganisms and disease and then discuss general principles concerning the therapeutic and nontherapeutic uses of chemotherapeutic agents. Chapters 29 and 30 will deal with specific antimicrobial and anticancer agents, respectively. The study of microbiology and chemotherapy is very extensive, yet despite the fascinating nature of these subjects, the author has, with great reluctance, been obliged to reduce this discussion to but a few short pages. Let us begin by considering the nature of the relationship between the host and the invading organism.

HOST-PARASITE RELATIONSHIPS AND DISEASE

Humans and their fellow animals are under a constant state of siege from a very large number of microorganisms and worms. When these invaders entrench themselves as guests on or in another living organism or **host** and use the host to provide nutrients and a suitable environment for their growth and reproduction, yet contribute nothing of benefit to the host in return, they are referred to as **parasites.** This state is not unlike the invasion of our home by an uninvited idle in-law. Just as this in-law does not necessarily harm us by his or her presence, it should not be inferred that the parasite necessarily dangerously harms the host organism. In a successful host-parasite relationship, the host's life or health is not seriously jeopardized. By contrast, a state of mutualism or *mutualistic symbiosis* is said to exist when each partner benefits from the other's presence.

Classification of Microorganisms

The cardinal principle underlying chemotherapy is **selective toxicity**; that is, the *chemotherapeutic agent must be more toxic to the parasite than to its host.* Selective toxicity can only be realized if there are fundamental differences between the host and the parasite or else the drug will be equally toxic to both. In this chapter we shall outline the different types of microorganisms that produce disease in humans and consider the differences between the cells of higher organisms and microbes. These differences serve as the focal point of attack of chemotherapeutic agents.

Prior to the nineteenth century, all living organisms were classified as plants or animals. With the realization that microorganisms also inhabit the earth and, at times, aggressively demonstrate their presence, this simple plant-animal classification of life was reevaluated. Any child can readily distinguish the differences between a blade of grass and a dog, fish, or butterfly; however, not even a competent biologist can unequivocally classify all fungi, blue-green algae, bacteria, and protozoa into either the plant or animal kingdoms. Many of these organisms possess characteristics that are common to both kingdoms. To resolve this dilemma, a third kingdom of living organisms was established, **protista,** and was subdivided into higher and lower protists (Table 28–1) on the basis of two different cell types.

The higher protists, including plants, animals, protozoa, fungi, and most algae, possess a highly differentiated **eucaryotic cell.** The less differentiated **procaryotic cell** is the unit of structure in bacteria and blue-green algae. While chemically both cell types consist of similar proteins, carbohydrates, fats, and nucleic acids and both employ similar metabolic machinery, the selective toxicity of many antibiotics is predicated upon several fundamental differences between procaryotic and eucaryotic cells, for example, the presence of a cell wall in bacteria and differences in the size of ribosomes (the site of protein synthesis) between these cell types.

HISTORY OF CHEMOTHERAPY

Prior to this century, few effective chemotherapeutic agents were available. These included an extract prepared from cinchona bark, the natural source of quinine, which was successfully employed since the early seventeenth century for the treatment of malaria; ipecacuanha root, from which the alkaloid emetine is obtained, was observed to be useful for the management of amebic dysentery; and mercury, which for 400 years was the principal drug used for the treatment of syphilis, notwithstanding the high incidence of toxicity to the patient.

TABLE 28-1. CLASSIFICATION OF MICROORGANISMS

Organism	Characteristics	Representative Organism – Disease
I. HIGHER PROTISTS (Eucaryotic cell type)		
A. Algae (except blue-green)	Chlorophyll-containing	—
B. Protozoa	Unicellular Nonphotosynthetic Mobile	*Entamoeba*–amebic dysentery *Plasmodium*–malaria *Trypanosoma*–African sleeping sickness
C. Fungi	Nonphotosynthetic Higher forms grow as a mass of branching interlacing filaments (hyphae) Myocoses (fungal infections) cause tissue damage not by toxins but by allergic reactions	*Actinomyces*–actinomycosis *Candida (Monilia)*–moniliasis *Coccidioides*–San Joaquin Valley fever *Histoplasma*–histoplasmosis *Microsporum*–ringworm of scalp *Trichophyton*–athlete's foot
D. Slime Molds	Resemble fungi	
II. LOWER PROTISTS (Procaryotic cell type)		
A. Bacteria*	Unicellular–3 cell types: cocci (round), bacilli (rods), spirilla (spiral) Thick, rigid cell walls Nonphotosynthetic Mobile	Greatest single cause of disease! **Gram-positive:** *Bacillus*–anthrax *Clostridium*–botulism, gas gangrene, tetanus *Corynebacterium*–diphtheria *Pneumonococcus*–pneumonia, meningitis *Staphylococcus*–pimples, boils, abscesses, and other pus-forming infections *Streptococcus*–scarlet fever, pneumonia, peritonitis, rheumatic fever, meningitis, "strep throat" **Gram-negative:** *Hemophilus*–influenza, whooping cough (pertussis) *Neisseria*–gonorrhea, meningitis

II. LOWER PROTISTS (cont.)

A. Bacteria* (cont.)

Gram-negative: (cont.)

Pasteurella—plague

Proteus and Pseudomonas—urinary tract infections

Salmonella—typhoid fever

Shigella—bacillary dysentery

Vibrio—cholera

Miscellaneous bacteria

Mycobacterium—tuberculosis, leprosy

Treponema—syphilis

B. Rickettsiae

Intermediate in size between bacterium and virus

Small cocci or rods

Grow only on living cells

Rocky Mountain spotted fever

Typhus fever

Q fever

III. VIRUSES

Most primitive and minute form of life

Consist of DNA or RNA wrapped in protein cover

Can only exist and multiply in living cells which supply nutrients and energy

Adenovirus—respiratory diseases

Arbovirus—yellow fever

Herpes virus—cold sore, fever blister, warts

Myxovirus—influenza

Paramyxovirus—measles, mumps

Picornavirus—polio

Poxvirus—small pox

Rhabdovirus—rabies

Tumor viruses—animals, humans(?)

*Bacteria, one type of microorganism, are categorized as being gram-positive or gram-negative. These designations refer to the ability or inability of certain microbes to be stained by a method devised in 1884 by the Danish physician Christian Gram. In addition to the importance of this stain for the identification of microbes, we find that each bacterial group responds somewhat similarly to antibiotics. That is, some antibiotics are useful for the treatment of gram-positive diseases, while other antibiotics are more effective against gram-negative diseases. Broad-spectrum antibiotics are capable of treating diseases caused by both gram-positive and gram-negative bacteria, as well as by some chlamydia and rickettsiae.

Paul Ehrlich (1854–1915), the father of chemotherapy, devoted the first twenty years of his scientific career to studying the selective staining of cells and tissues by dye substances. He noted that while some tissues possessed an affinity for the dye and were colored, other tissues remained uncolored. Moreover, other dyes stained microorganisms, but not animal tissues. Ehrlich theorized that drugs could be developed that would be selectively toxic to a parasite and yet be harmless to the host. Seeking such a "magic bullet," Ehrlich experimented with organic arsenical compounds in an attempt to discover a cure for syphilis. The 606th compound in the series, arsphenamine (Salvarsan), was clinically introduced in 1910, and when injected over a period of a few months, cured syphilis.

Before 1935, it was generally believed that only infections caused by protozoa were sensitive to the effects of chemotherapeutic agents. A new era of chemotherapy began in 1935 with the clinical introduction of the red azo ($-N=N-$) dye *Prontosil,*[1] the first compound in a long line of **sulfonamides,** drugs effective for the treatment of a broad spectrum of bacterial infections. When added to a tube containing certain bacteria, Prontosil is inactive, but it does possess antibacterial activity after it is administered to bacterially infected animals and humans. Workers at the Pasteur Institute demonstrated that animals convert the inactive Prontosil to **sulfanilamide,** an active antibacterial agent. With the realization that the simple sulfanilamide molecule was responsible for the observed biological activity, organic chemists set to work synthesizing analogs of this compound. Over the years, 5000 such sulfonamides have been prepared, and over a score of these have proved to be clinically useful. Suitable chemical modification of these compounds has given rise to drugs useful for diseases other than infections, for example, diuretic agents such as chlorothiazide (Diuril; Chapter 21) and oral antidiabetic agents including tolbutamide (Orinase; Chapter 24).

Prontosil
(Inactive)

Sulfanilamide
(Active)

Triaminobenzene
(Inactive)

---

[1] Gerhard Domagk (1895–1964), Director of the Pathological Laboratory of the I.G. Farbenindustrie in Germany, was responsible for the development of Prontosil and was the first to demonstrate its clinical effectiveness as an antibacterial agent. One of the first successfully treated patients was Domagk's own daughter who was experiencing streptococcal septicemia ("blood poisoning"), a previously inevitably fatal disease. Domagk received the Nobel Prize in Medicine in 1939.

The ability of one microorganism to inhibit the growth of another microbial species was recognized in 1877 by Pasteur and Joubert. Over the next half-century, there were some clinical attempts to combat bacterial infections with micoorganisms or their products, but these efforts were generally unproductive.

The need for effective antibacterial agents was obvious to **Alexander Fleming** (1881–1955) who, while serving as a military surgeon during the Great War of 1914–1918, stood by helplessly while soldiers died from wound infections. During the course of his studies on staphylococcal bacteria at St. Mary's Hospital in London in 1928, Fleming noted that his culture plate was contaminated by a large colony of the airborne fungus *Penicillium*. Many bacteriologists before Fleming had experienced the same problem but, undoubtedly, discarded their contaminated plates in disgust. We are told that chance only favors the prepared mind, and so it was in this laboratory. With respect to this culture plate contamination, Fleming wrote:

> This itself did not call for comment but what was very surprising was that the staphylococcal colonies in the neighbourhood of the mould, which had been well developed, were observed now to be showing signs of dissolution—this was an extraordinary and unexpected appearance and seemed to demand investigation.[2]

Fleming isolated the mold, demonstrated that it possessed antibacterial activity against some, but not all, microbes, and noted that **penicillin,** the name he gave to the metabolic product obtained from the fungus, was nontoxic to animals even after very large doses. Lacking both training in chemistry and support from his colleagues, he was unable to isolate pure penicillin from the mold, thus precluding clinical studies. An account of these observations appeared in 1929 in the *British Journal of Experimental Pathology* and collected dust for the next decade.

With England's entry into World War II in 1939, interest in Fleming's penicillin was revitalized. At Oxford, Howard Florey, a pathologist, and Ernst Chain, an accomplished chemist, confirmed Fleming's earlier observations and also partially purified penicillin.[3] Subsequent clinical trials demonstrated the effectiveness of this antibiotic in treating human infections. With an appreciation of penicillin's therapeutic potential to meet military needs, mass production was undertaken in the United States on a cash basis by three pharmaceutical companies and the Department of Agriculture. While only two ounces were produced in January 1943, by the end of the war, the monthly output was in excess of 1000 pounds. In 1943, 600 mg of penicillin G cost $200; by 1954 the cost of the same quantity was a mere 2 cents!

Whereas the source of Fleming's penicillin was an airborne mold, René Dubos began his search for antibiotics in the ground. Animals are continually

---

[2] A. Fleming, ed., *Penicillin, Its Practical Applications* (Philadelphia: Blakiston, 1946), pp. 2–3.

[3] Fleming, Florey, and Chain shared the 1945 Nobel Prize in Medicine.

dying of infectious diseases, they discharge bacteria into the earth, and yet these disease-causing bacteria are absent from the earth. Dubos theorized that microorganisms living in the soil were capable of killing bacteria. In 1939 he isolated tyrothricin from the soil bacterium *Bacillus brevis* and found this compound to be destructive to pneumococcus, a microbe that causes pneumonia. Although tyrothricin proved too toxic for systemic use in animals, Dubos's efforts served as an impetus for the search for other soil microbes that produce antibiotics. Table 28–2 lists some major antibiotics and their spectrum of antimicrobial activity.

MECHANISMS OF ACTION OF CHEMOTHERAPEUTIC AGENTS

Some chemotherapeutic agents are able to kill bacteria, while others only suppress their growth and reproduction; these drugs are classified as **bactericidal** or **bacteriostatic** agents, respectively (Table 28–2). Such effects are often concentration-dependent; that is, at low doses, a bactericidal antibiotic may exert a bacteriostatic effect. While bacteriostatic agents are able to inhibit the growth of bacteria, the *host defense mechanisms,* including white blood cells and antibodies, must be operative to eradicate the disease-causing microbe. In the absence of such mechanisms, bacteriostatic drugs merely retard the spread of infection, and the patient often relapses after discontinuation of medication. Bactericidal drugs also require the cooperation of host defense mechanisms to be most effective. These drugs are only active against rapidly growing bacteria, while bacteriostatic drugs are effective in combating both growing and inactive microbes.

If one antibiotic is good, is the combined use of two different drugs twice as beneficial? The answer to this clinically relevant question depends upon the antibiotics in question. An additive antibacterial effect often results when two bactericidal or two bacteriostatic drugs are combined. By contrast, the combined effects of a bactericidal and bacteriostatic drug may be antagonistic to one another. Why should this occur? Bactericidal drugs kill multiplying bacteria most efficiently, and if growth is suppressed by a bacteriostatic agent, the growth requirement is eliminated. For example, it was clinically demonstrated that the combination of chlortetracycline (bacteriostatic) and penicillin (bactericidal) cured fewer patients with pneumococcal meningitis than did the same dose of penicillin when used alone.

Let us now discuss the mechanisms by which antimicrobial agents are more toxic to the parasite and less toxic to the host. These drugs act by one or more of the following five mechanisms: competitive antagonism, inhibition of cell wall synthesis, impairment of cell membrane function, inhibition of protein synthesis, and inhibition of nucleic acid synthesis (Table 28–2).

TABLE 28-2. ANTIBIOTICS, THEIR SPECTRUM OF ANTIMICROBIAL ACTIVITY AND MECHANISM OF ACTION

Antibiotic (Selected Trade Names)	Primary Spectrum of Activity	Mechanism of Action*	Bactericidal (Bc) or Bacteriostatic (Bs)
Penicillins (PCN) (Table 29-2)	Gram +	CW	Bc
Cephalosporins (Keflin, Loridine)	Gram +, some Gram –	CW	Bc
Erythromycin (Ilosone, Ilotycin, Erythrocin)	Gram +	PS	Bs
Vancomycin (Vancocin)	Resistant *Staphylococcus*	CW (CM)	Bc
Tetracyclines (Table 29-3)	Gram +, Gram –, rickettsiae	PS	Bs
Chloramphenicol (Chloromycetin)	Gram +, Gram –, rickettsiae. Use: severe Gram –, typhoid fever	PS	Bs
Streptomycin	Antituberculosis, PCN-resistant *Staphylococcus*, severe Gram –	PS	Bc
Rifampin (Rifadin)	Antituberculosis	NA	Bc
Gentamicin and Aminoglycosides (Table 29-4)	Gram –	PS	Bc
Bacitracin	Gram + (local use)	CW (CM)	Bc
Polymyxin B (Aerosporin)	Gram –	CM	Bc
Amphotericin B (Fungizone)	Antifungal	CM	Fs
Griseofulvin (Fulvicin, Grifulvin)	Antifungal	NA	Fs

*Key to abbreviations: CW = inhibition of cell wall synthesis; PS = inhibition of protein synthesis; CM = inhibition of cell membrane function; NA = inhibition of nucleic acid synthesis; Fs = fungistatic.

Competitive Antagonism

Some antibacterial agents act by interfering with the utilization of nutritional substances that are essential for microbial growth. For many microorganisms, para-aminobenzoic acid (**PABA**) is an essential dietary requirement for the synthesis of the vitamin *folic acid,* a building block in the manufacture of purines and eventually nucleic acids. Whereas few bacteria are capable of absorbing preformed folic acid from their environment, mammals are able to utilize dietary folic acid directly. It is now generally believed that the antibacterial *sulfonamides,* which closely resemble PABA chemically, interfere with the microbial synthesis of folic acid from PABA. The latter acid and the sulfonamide antimetabolites both compete for the same enzyme that catalyzes the incorporation of PABA into folic acid. Animals and microbes that require preformed sources of folic acid, and who, therefore, do not require PABA, are not susceptible to the growth-inhibiting effects of the sulfonamides.

Inhibition of Cell Wall Synthesis

One of the fundamental differences between the procaryotic cells of bacteria and the eucaryotic cells of mammals is the presence of a rigid cell wall in the former. In addition to providing the microbe with a definite shape, the cell wall enables the microbe to maintain much higher internal pressure than is present in the external environment. The cell wall consists of carbohydrate (polysaccharide) chains that are cross-linked with amino acids; some of the individual sugar and amino acid components are not present in mammals. *Penicillin* blocks cell wall synthesis of daughter cells of multiplying bacteria by preventing the cross-linking of amino acids on the polysaccharide chains. Some other antibiotics also act by inhibiting cell wall synthesis, although not necessarily by the same mechanism as does penicillin.

Inhibition of Cell Membrane Function

The cell membranes of microbial and animal cells act as barriers for the selective transfer of compounds between the external environment and the cell. Damage to the membrane results in a loss of essential intracellular constituents and the uncontrolled admission of other compounds into the cell resulting in its death. *Polymyxin B* forms a complex with the phospholipid constituent of the cell membrane of gram-negative bacteria causing a nonselective increase in membrane permeability. *Amphotericin B* also impairs cell membrane function, but unlike polymyxin B, acts only on the membranes of fungi and other eucaryotes.

Inhibition of Protein Synthesis

Many of the most clinically useful antibiotic agents act by inhibiting protein synthesis via several different complex mechanisms. *Chloramphenicol* and *erythromycin* are thought to attach to one of the two subunits of the ribosome and block the formation of peptide bonds between amino acids; chloramphenicol may also prevent the attachment of messenger RNA to the ribosome. *Tetracyclines* are believed to inhibit protein synthesis by blocking the binding of the amino acid-transfer RNA complex to ribosomes. *Streptomycin* binds to the ribosome in such a manner that incorrect amino acids are laid down, thus resulting in the formation of a nonfunctional protein.

Inhibition of Nucleic Acid Synthesis

Cell replication requires the continuous synthesis and normal function of DNA, and once DNA is destroyed, the cell is incapable of replacing it. Antibiotics and other drugs that combine with and alter the function of nucleic acids, DNA in particular, are toxic to both bacteria and humans. Although the use of such compounds is not practical for the treatment of microbial infections, some have been found to be useful as anticancer and antiviral agents.

DRUG RESISTANCE

When penicillin G was first introduced into therapeutics about four decades ago, almost all infections caused by *Staphylococcus aureus* responded favorably to this drug. Resistant strains of this microbe soon appeared, and today about 90 percent of hospital staph infections are resistant to penicillin G. In 1943, most strains of *Neisseria gonorrheae,* the bacterium causing gonorrhea, were inhibited in the culture tube by 0.01 units/ml of penicillin G, with virtually no strain able to survive 0.06 units/ml. Twenty-five years later, 14 percent of the strains tested required more than 0.5 units/ml to inhibit growth of this microbe.

Resistance to an antibacterial agent is said to exist when a strain of microorganisms is less sensitive or totally insensitive to drugs that ordinarily inhibit their growth or cause their death. The acquisition of resistance should not be confused with natural resistance, which is observed when an antibiotic is administered to a given population of susceptible bacteria, with the resulting death of some individual microbes more readily than others. The development of drug-resistant bacterial strains is of obvious importance when attempting to treat infectious diseases.

A variety of different mechanisms has been shown to be responsible for the emergence of bacterial resistance to antimicrobial agents. (1) Microbes can become resistant to certain antibiotics by producing enzymes that are capable of inactivating these drugs by chemically altering critical portions of the molecule required for antimicrobial activity. Staphylococci resistance to penicillin G has been attributed to the ability of certain strains of these bacteria to form *penicillinase,* an enzyme capable of hydrolyzing and cleaving the β-lactam ring of penicillin. Synthetic penicillin derivatives have been developed that are not susceptible to penicillinase inactivation. (2) Resistance may result from an alteration in normal pathways of bacterial metabolism to overcome or circumvent the ability of the antibacterial drug to inhibit their growth. Some sulfonamide-resistant bacteria have acquired the ability to directly utilize preformed folic acid and do not, therefore, require PABA from the environment. (3) Changes may occur in the structure of the microbe that restricts the entry of the antimicrobial agent into the interior of the microbial cell. Resistance to chloramphenicol, tetracyclines, aminoglycosides, and polymyxins have been associated with alterations in microbial cell wall permeability. (4) The microbial strain may become resistant because of an alteration of the target structure normally attacked by the antibiotic or in the ability of the drug to bind to such target structures. L-forms of bacteria become resistant to penicillin and other antibacterial agents that act by interfering with cell wall synthesis by adapting to and surviving without a cell wall. Certain gram-negative rods possess plasmid-bound antimicrobial resistance factors (*R factors*) which, by an enzymatic action, attach certain organic groups to an antibiotic and block the biologically active parts of the drug molecule. Because these R factors can be transferred from one species of gram-negative bacteria to another, they represent a major potential threat in the treatment of infections caused by such organisms, particularly in a hospital setting where patients are exposed to multiple microbes.

THERAPEUTIC USES AND MISUSES
OF ANTIMICROBIAL AGENTS

Let us now discuss some of the factors that must be considered when antibiotic agents are employed for the treatment of a bacterial disease. When used rationally, these drugs are capable of producing dramatic and even miraculous effects. By contrast, the improper use of antibiotics has resulted in deaths from antibiotic-induced allergy and toxicity and has been responsible for both the development of infections far more severe than those originally present and the appearance of resistant strains of microorganisms.

The first step in the proper use of antibiotics is the determination of an accurate *diagnosis* of the disease, based upon the clinical symptoms present, as well as a laboratory identification of the microbe responsible for the disorder. Knowledge of the natural disease process permits the physician to decide whether other additional therapeutic measures should be instituted, as well as to evaluate the patient's response to the antibiotic. While some diseases have only one microbial cause, other diseases, such as pneumonia and wound and urinary tract infections, may be caused by several different microbes. If the patient's illness is not the result of a microbial infection, or if the infection is caused by organisms that are not responsive to antibiotics, for example viruses, antibiotics should not be prescribed. Moreover, a bacteriological diagnosis will predict whether the particular microbial strain is susceptible or resistant to certain antibiotics.

The **misuse** of antibiotics by patients is undoubtedly widespread. Antibiotics left over from a previous illness are often used by the patient or a member of the family to treat a disease with apparently similar symptoms. Drug-induced toxicity or allergy or delay in receiving proper medical attention are only a few of the dangers associated with this kind of self-medication. Assuming that an accurate diagnosis has been made by the physician and that the most effective drug has been chosen for use, it is then necessary to employ an adequate dosage of this chemotherapeutic agent for an optimal period of time. An inadequate dose, or the proper dose not administered for a sufficiently long period of time, may lead to the development of drug-resistant bacterial strains and a clinical relapse. Hence, it is very unwise to stop antibiotic therapy as soon as you "feel better."

As we have observed with all other classes of drugs, antibiotics are capable of producing adverse effects. While some of these toxic effects are highly specific for a given drug, hypersensitivity and superinfection are common problems associated with the use of many antibacterial agents.

Hypersensitivity reactions are particularly common in patients with allergic disorders or who are allergic to other drugs; these effects have been attributed to antigen-antibody reactions (Chapter 27). Such adverse drug responses vary in type and severity from a mild skin rash to a fatal anaphylactic reaction. Unless it is absolutely imperative to use the offending antibiotic and no alternative drug exists, that drug should not be readministered after such a reaction has been observed. Moreover, the patient should avoid the use of drugs related to the one causing the allergic response, such as all penicillin derivatives.

Superinfection (or suprainfection) is the development of a new infection, either bacterial or fungal in origin, during antibacterial treatment of the primary infection. While the incidence of superinfection is low with narrow-spectrum antibiotics such as penicillin, it is a common occurrence with tetracycline and other broad-spectrum antibiotics. Suppression of the growth of normal nonpathogenic inhabitants of the gastrointestinal, genitourinary, and respiratory tracts disrupts the natural microbial balance, with other bacteria and fungi now able to freely proliferate. Often disease-producing microbes appear that are highly resistant to existing antimicrobial agents.

NONMEDICAL USES OF ANTIMICROBIAL AGENTS

Contrary to popular belief, antimicrobial agents are also extensively employed for nonmedical purposes. Approximately 30 to 40 percent of the total production of antibiotics in the United States is used to *promote animal growth* and to *prevent diseases in both animals and plants.* Antibiotics also have limited applications in some countries for the preservation of foods. About one-half of the field crops are spoiled by microbes before reaching the ultimate consumer.

The most important nonmedical application of antibiotics is their uses as feed additives to stimulate the growth rate of such livestock as poultry, swine, dairy calves, beef cattle, and sheep. Animals treated with antibiotics have a lower incidence of illness and death and attain a marketable weight in a shorter period of time with only a modest increase in food consumption. Although antibiotics have been used as growth promoters for over 30 years, the precise mechanism underlying this effect has not been fully elucidated. The reduction in disease-causing organisms from the host permits it to realize its maximal potential for growth. Experimental studies suggest that antibiotics also reduce the thickness of the intestinal wall and thereby enhance the absorption of nutrients. Although, at present, there is no evidence that the antibiotic residues found in animal tissues constitute a present danger to human health, we cannot overlook this possibility. Potential hazards include toxicity, hypersensitivity reactions, superinfections, and the development of resistant strains of microorganisms. Thus, new antibiotics must be developed for exclusive use in animals.

Antibiotics, such as streptomycin and griseofulvin, are also used to control various plant diseases. In the United States streptomycin is used to control bacterial diseases of the apple, pear, tomato, bean, and tobacco, while in India this same drug controls infections of cotton, rice, and citrus fruits. Economic and public health considerations have limited the use of these drugs in plant diseases.

SUMMARY

Advances in the prevention and treatment of infectious diseases have been highly instrumental in increasing the average American life span almost fifteen years since the beginning of the twentieth century. In this regard, the development of effective chemotherapeutic agents represents one of the most tangible contributions of pharmacology to society.

Chemotherapeutic agents are drugs that are selectively toxic to the parasite (bacterium, fungus, virus, worm) and yet cause minimum harm to the host or patient. Some of these drugs kill the parasite while others inhibit parasitic growth. These effects are accomplished by competitive antagonism of the synthesis of essential compounds by the parasite (sulfonamides); inhibition of cell wall synthesis (penicillin); impairment of normal cell membrane function (polymyxin B is an antibacterial agent, while amphotericin B is effective against fungi); inhibition of protein synthesis (chloramphenicol), and nucleic acid synthesis (mitomycin C). Few safe and effective chemotherapeutic agents are currently available for the treatment of systemic infections caused by viruses and fungi.

The emergence of drug-resistant strains of disease-causing bacteria has proved to be a major problem in the successful treatment of infectious diseases. By a variety of biochemical and physiological mechanisms, resistant microbes acquire the capacity to withstand the normally toxic effects of chemotherapeutic agents, a very dynamic example of evolution in action. This clinical problem has provided a major incentive for the development of new drugs to which the parasites are susceptible. Judicious prescribing of antibiotics by physicians and more careful adherence to dosage regimens by patients are essential factors in delaying the development of bacterial resistance.

Nonmedical applications of antibiotics include their use to prevent plant and animal diseases and to promote the growth of livestock. These applications have contributed to increasing the available food supply.

SUPPLEMENTARY READINGS

Albert, A., *Selective Toxicity,* 6th ed. New York: John Wiley, 1979.

Conn, H. F., ed., "Efficacy of Antimicrobial and Antifungal Agents," *Medical Clinics of North America* **54:** 1075–1354 (1970).

Garrod, L. P., H. P. Lambert, and F. O'Grady, *Antibiotic and Chemotherapy.* 4th ed. Baltimore: Williams & Wilkins, 1973.

Kagan, B. M., ed., *Antimicrobial Therapy.* 2nd ed. Philadelphia: Saunders, 1974.

Klastersky, J., ed., *Clinical Use of Combinations of Antibiotics.* New York: John Wiley, 1975.

Lerner, P. I., M. C. McHenry, and E. Olinsky, eds., "Symposium on Infectious Diseases," *Medical Clinics of North America* **58:** 463–708 (1974).

Lowbury, E. J. L., and G. A. J. Ayliffe, *Drug Resistance in Antimicrobial Therapy.* Springfield, Ill.: Charles C Thomas, 1974.

Mandell, G. L., R. G. Douglas, Jr., and J. E. Bennett, eds., *Principles and Practices of Infectious Diseases.* New York: John Wiley, 1979.

Pratt, W. B., *Chemotherapy of Infection.* New York: Oxford University Press, 1977.

Sande, M. A., and G. L. Mandell, "Chemotherapy of Microbial Diseases," in *Goodman and Gilman's The Pharmacological Basis of Therapeutics.* Edited by A. G. Gilman, L. S. Goodman, and A. Gilman, 6th ed., Sec. 12, Chap. 48–54, pp. 1080–1248. New York: Macmillan, 1980.

Sanders, W. E., Jr., and C. C. Sanders, "Toxicity of Antibacterial Agents: Mechanism of Action on Mammalian Cells," *Annual Review of Pharmacology and Toxicology* **19:** 53–83 (1979).

29

Sulfonamides and Antibiotics

One of the greatest achievements of all time by man has been the discovery, practical manufacture, and use of antibiotics.[1]

—Philip Handler (1970)

This chapter on chemotherapeutic agents could not have been written five decades ago. At that time sulfonamides or "sulfa" drugs were first being tested for antibacterial activity in animals and few people were cognizant of Fleming's experiments with penicillin. Four decades ago, only the sulfonamides were widely employed in therapeutics, with pencillin's availability limited to military use. The newer semisynthetic pencillins had not yet been developed and other antibiotics still remained nature's secret. Indeed, it has only been within our generation that antibiotics have become available to the practicing physician. Antibiotics are among the most widely prescribed class of drugs and account for one out of every five prescriptions in the United States.

We shall discuss in this chapter the pharmacology of the sulfonamides and some of the more important of the many antibiotic agents currently employed in therapeutics. The sulfonamides are totally synthetic compounds, not derived from living cells, and therefore, precisely speaking, they cannot be classified as antibiotics. Among the antibiotics we shall consider are the penicillins, streptomycin and the aminoglycosides, the tetracyclines, chloramphenicol, erythromycin, polymyxin B, and one antifungal antibiotic, griseofulvin.

SULFONAMIDES

With the realization that Prontosil's antibacterial activity resided in the simple sulfanilamide molecule (Chapter 28), many thousands of derivatives were synthesized after 1935 in an attempt to optimize the pharmacological and

[1] *Biology and the Future of Man.*

R = H, Sulfanilamide

therapeutic properties of this compound. Most of these derivatives contain various chemical substitutions of the R-group. The earliest sulfonamides had limited solubility in acidic urine and had a tendency to precipitate and block the kidney tubules. Today, all sulfonamides in common use are sufficiently soluble in urine to preclude this danger. By contrast, in some therapeutic situations, it is advantageous to reduce the solubility of the sulfonamide in order that it not be absorbed from the intestines nor enter the blood. Addition of appropriate chemical substituents to the free amino ($-NH_2$) group gives rise to insoluble sulfonamides whose antibacterial activity is limited to the gastrointestinal tract (Table 29–1).

TABLE 29-1. COMMONLY USED SULFONAMIDES

Generic Name (Selected Trade Names)	Remarks
Short-acting systemic sulfonamides Sulfadiazine Sulfamerazine Sulfamethazine Sulfisoxazole (Gantrisin)	Majority of widely used agents; rapid onset and short (4-hour) duration of action; used for systemic infections. The first three are combined in a mixture (trisulfapyrimidines) containing 1/3 the full dose of each.
Long-acting systemic sulfonamides Sulfamethoxypyridazine (Midicel) Sulfamethoxazole (Gantanol)	Long duration of action; long-term prophylactic or suppressive therapy; greater potential danger of toxicity
Insoluble sulfonamides Sulfasalazine (Azulfidine) Phthalylsulfathiazole (Sulfathalidine)	Poor absorption from intestinal tract; used to suppress intestinal bacteria
Topical sulfonamides Mafenide (Sulfamylon) Sulfadiazine silver (Silvadene)	Treatment of burn infections

Therapeutic Uses

The sulfonamides compete with para-aminobenzoic acid (PABA) for incorporation into folic acid (Figure 29–1). As a consequence, these drugs are able to inhibit the growth and reproduction of microbes that are unable to utilize preformed dietary folic acid. Although sulfonamides are active against many gram-positive bacteria and some gram-negative microorganisms, newer, more effective, and safer antibiotics have limited the contemporary therapeutic applications of these drugs. At present, these drugs are most commonly used to treat urinary tract infections where they continue to enjoy widespread pop-

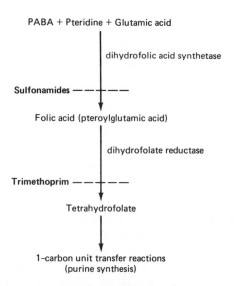

PABA + Pteridine + Glutamic acid

dihydrofolic acid synthetase

Sulfonamides — — ┼ — —

Folic acid (pteroylglutamic acid)

dihydrofolate reductase

Trimethoprim — — ┼ — —

Tetrahydrofolate

1-carbon unit transfer reactions
(purine synthesis)

FIGURE 29-1. Folic Acid Synthesis and Utilization in Microorganisms and Inhibition by Sulfonamides and Trimethoprim. The sulfonamides and trimethoprim inhibit the enzymes dihydrofolic acid synthetase (required for utilization of PABA into folic acid synthesis) and dihydrofolate reductase, respectively. Tetrahydrofolate is not formed and cannot serve as a cofactor in biochemical reactions required for microbial survival.

ularity because of their established effectiveness and relatively low toxicity and cost. The insoluble sulfonamides are sometimes employed to reduce the bacterial population of the intestines prior to abdominal surgery.

The systemic sulfonamides are potentially dangerous and can cause allergic disorders, as well as adverse effects involving the urinary tract and blood. They are capable of displacing bilirubin from plasma proteins, and this can lead to a potentially fatal degeneration of nerve cells in the brain (kernicterus) in newborn babies; these drugs are, therefore, contraindicated during pregnancy and in nursing mothers.

Sulfonamide-Trimethoprim Combination

Sulfonamides competitively inhibit the enzyme dihydrofolic acid synthetase and thereby prevent the bacterial synthesis of folic acid from PABA (Figure 29-1). For folic acid to become biochemically active in 1-carbon unit transfer reactions (for example, purine synthesis and subsequent nucleic acid manufacture), it must be converted to tetrahydrofolate via a reduction reaction catalyzed by dihydrofolate reductase. Trimethoprim inhibits this reaction (Figure 29-1). The combination of trimethoprim (a nonsulfonamide) and sulfamethoxazole (Bactrim, Septra) act by inhibiting consecutive steps in the bacterial synthesis and utilization of folic acid. The combination increases the antimicrobial spectrum (beyond that of the individual components) and markedly decreases the development of resistant bacterial strains.

Some clinicians consider this combination to be the treatment of choice for acute and chronic urinary tract infections, and useful in the treatment of typhoid fever, uncomplicated gonorrhea, cholera, and malaria.

Sulfones and Leprosy

> *The leper in whom the plague is . . . shall cry, Unclean, unclean.*
> —Leviticus 13:45

From biblical days, leprosy has been regarded as among the most dreaded disorders afflicting mankind. It was formerly believed that leprosy was a highly contagious disease and, therefore, all noninfected individuals took great lengths to avoid contact with the ostracized leper. We now know that this disease is only mildly contagious and that nurses and doctors working at leper colonies are rarely infected. At present, most cases of leprosy are confined to hot, moist climates such as Central Africa and the west coast of India.

The most effective drugs available for the treatment of leprosy are the **sulfones,** which are chemical derivatives of the sulfonamides. Sulfones, such as DDS, must be administered for many years to alleviate the skin lesions and other clinical manifestations of this disease.

$$H_2N-\langle\bigcirc\rangle-SO_2-\langle\bigcirc\rangle-NH_2$$

Diaminodiphenylsulfone
(DDS, dapsone)

PENICILLINS

The pencillins were the first antibiotics discovered and remain today the second most widely used class of drugs for the treatment of bacterial infections. Penicillins include the natural products of the mold *Penicillium* or are semisynthetic derivatives of these products. The most important natural penicillin is benzylpenicillin, which is more commonly designated **penicillin G.**

Although penicillin G is the most potent of all penicillin derivatives, it suffers from several major disadvantages. It is subject to breakdown by gastric acid in the stomach and is poorly and irregularly absorbed after oral administration. In addition, many disease-producing staphylococci are able to produce penicillinase (β-lactamase), an enzyme capable of inactivating penicillin G; penicillinase-producing bacteria are resistant to this antibiotic. Finally, penicillin G possesses a rather limited spectrum of antibacterial activity, being primarily effective against only gram-positive bacteria. In 1957, *6-aminopenicillanic* acid, the basic penicillin nucleus, was isolated. By the addition of suitable chemical starting materials to the penicillin fermentation vats, semisynthetic penicillin derivatives have been prepared that have overcome most of the inherent limitations of penicillin G. Many of these newer compounds are stable in gastric acid, resist attack by penicillinase, and are active against both gram-positive and gram-negative bacteria (Table 29-2).

Antimicrobial Activity

All penicillin derivatives product their bactericidal effects by inhibition of cell wall synthesis of daughter cells of multiplying bacteria, more specifically, by preventing the cross-linking of peptides on the mucosaccharide chains. Blockade of cell wall formation leads to an increase in the flow of water into the cell resulting in the bursting of the bacterial cell.

With the exception of ampicillin and carbenicillin, most penicillins have a narrow spectrum of antibacterial activity. That is, penicillins are far more effective in killing susceptible gram-positive bacteria (staphylococci, streptococci) than they are in their activity against gram-negative microbes. Notable exceptions are the gram-negative bacteria responsible for gonorrhea and the spirochete that causes syphilis. In the absence of natural or acquired bacterial resistance and host allergy, penicillin G remains among the most useful antibacterial agents known.

Toxicity and Adverse Effects

For all practical purposes, when administered to a patient with normal kidney function, penicillin is a nontoxic compound. One patient was given 144 g (1/3 lb) of penicillin intravenously on a daily basis for six weeks without producing toxicity. By contrast, penicillin causes irritation, tremors, and seizures when injected into the central nervous system. Patients who are given high doses of penicillin and who are unable to excrete this drug normally as a consequence of impaired kidney function may show the same symptoms as central nervous system penicillin toxicity. Other less severe signs of the irritating properties of this antibiotic are manifested by pain and inflammation at the site of an intramuscular injection and nausea and diarrhea after its oral administration.

The major adverse effects associated with penicillin use are **allergic** reactions to this drug. It has been estimated that between 5 and 10 percent of all American adults are hypersensitive to penicillin, and this probably represents the most common drug allergy. In addition to its presence in drugs, traces of penicillin are sometimes found in cosmetics and foods, especially milk. The severity of the allergic reaction may range from a slight rash to anaphylactic shock and death. Unfortunately, at present, diagnostic skin tests for penicillin hypersensitivity have not proved to be reliable and may themselves be dangerous. Patients allergic to one pencillin are generally allergic to all other penicillin derivatives.

TABLE 29-2. COMMON PENICILLIN DERIVATIVES

6-Aminopenicillanic Acid

(Site of penicillinase attack)

R	Generic Name (Selected Trade Names)	Antibacterial Spectrum	Distinguishing Characteristics	
			Acid Stability	Penicillinase Resistant
	Penicillin G, benzylpenicillin	Highly active Gm + Weakly active Gm − (narrow spectrum)	No	No
	Penicillin V, phenoxymethyl penicillin (Compocillin-V K, Pen-Vee K, V-Cillin K)	Same as penicillin G	Yes	No
	Methicillin (Staphcillin)	Less active than penicillin G but same spectrum	No	Yes

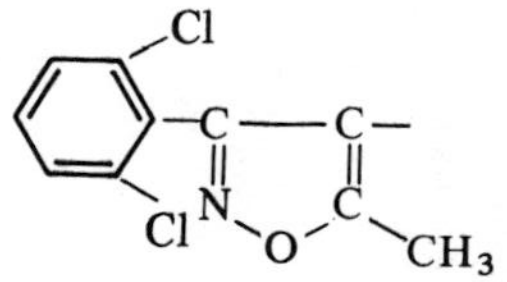	Dicloxacillin (Dycill, Dynapen, Pathocil, Veracillin)	Same as methicillin	Yes	Yes
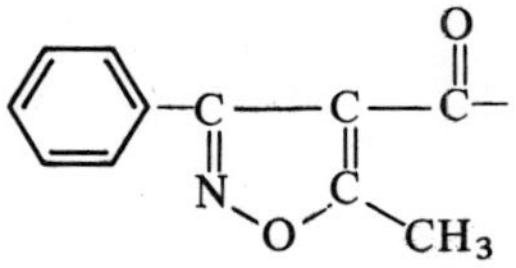	Oxacillin (Prostaphlin, Resistopen)	Same as methicillin	Yes	Yes
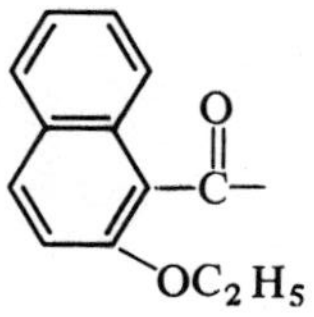	Nafcillin (Unipen)	Same as methicillin	No	Yes
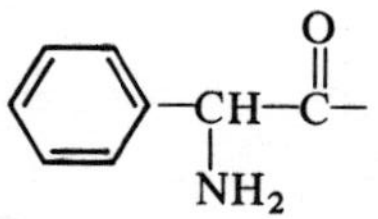	Ampicillin (Amcill, Omnipen, Penbritin, Polycillin)	Active against Gm + and Gm – (broad spectrum)	Yes	No
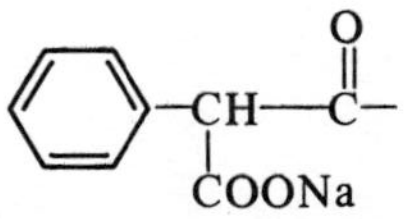	Carbenicillin (Geopen, Pyopen)	Same as ampicillin but greater activity vs Gm –	Yes	No

Therapeutic Uses

Notwithstanding the development of many new antibiotics, penicillins remain among the most widely used antibacterial agents for the treatment of gram-positive and selected gram-negative infections. Their major virtues are high potency, a bactericidal action, and low toxicity, while disadvantages include possible allergic reactions and the development of drug-resistant strains of bacteria. Many of the newer semisynthetic penicillins are not broken down by penicillinase and are therefore useful for the treatment of infections caused by resistant staphylococcal strains. Unfortunately, these newer derivatives are less potent than penicillin G. However, ampicillin[2] and carbenicillin have been shown to be of value against many urinary tract infections caused by gram-negative pathogens.

CEPHALOSPORINS

The *Cephalosporium* fungus was first isolated in 1948 off the coast of Sardinia in the sea near a sewer outlet. The cephalosporin antibiotics resemble the penicillins with respect to their chemistry and mechanism of action (that is, they exert their bactericidal effects by inhibiting cell wall synthesis).

The antimicrobial spectrum of the cephalosporins is broader than penicillin G and more closely resembles ampicillin. They are less active than the pencillins against gram-positive bacteria but are generally penicillinase-resistant. These antibiotics are effective in the treatment of infections caused by some gram-negative bacteria. In general, the cephalosporins represent useful alternatives for the management of a variety of infectious disorders that are nonresponsive to the penicillins.

Orally active cephalosporin derivatives include cephalexin (Keflex), cephaloglycin (Kafocin), cephradine (Anspor, Velosef), and Cefaclor (Ceclor). The following derivatives are not well absorbed after oral administration and must be administered by intramuscular and/or intravenous injection: cephalothin (Keflin), cephaloridine (Loridine), cefazolin (Ancef, Kefzol), cephapirin (Cefadyl), and cefamandole (Mandol).

TETRACYCLINES

Of all the antibiotic agents in common usage, the tetracyclines have the broadest spectrum of antimicrobial activity. Drugs in this class are the most widely used group of antibiotics for the treatment of a great number of diseases caused by gram-positive and many gram-negative bacteria, rickettsiae, some

[2] The second and third most frequently prescribed drug in the United States in 1978 and 1979, respectively.

TABLE 29-3. TETRACYCLINES

Tetracycline

Generic Name	Selected Trade Names	Remarks
Chlortetracycline	Aureomycin	First of class to be isolated (1948)
Oxytetracycline	Terramycin	Second member isolated (1950)
Tetracycline	Achromycin, Panmycin, Tetracyn, and others	Most widely used of the tetracyclines since its introduction in 1953
Demeclocycline	Declomycin	Allergic photosensitivity reactions more common than with other members of class
Methacycline	Rondomycin	
Rolitetracycline	Syntetrin	Very water-soluble, used for injections
Doxycycline	Vibramycin	Excreted very slowly, thus only one dose required daily in many patients
Minocycline	Minocin, Vectrin	Excreted very slowly, long duration of action; active against some strains normally resistant to tetracycline

protozoa, and chlamydia. They are not active against yeasts, fungi, or true viruses.

The original tetracyclines were isolated from different strains of *Streptomyces,* from 1948 to 1953, with the most recent derivatives prepared by chemically modifying the naturally occurring tetracyclines (Table 29–3). Although some minor differences exist among these compounds, since they all have the same general antimicrobial, pharmacological, and therapeutic properties, they will be collectively discussed under the general designation tetracycline.

Absorption, Distribution and Excretion

All tetracyclines are incompletely absorbed from the gastrointestinal tract and are distributed throughout the body after oral administration. In an attempt to reduce the gastric upset often associated with the oral use of these drugs, it was formerly recommended that the tetracyclines be taken with milk.

Subsequent studies showed that calcium present in milk and milk products interferes with the absorption of tetracyclines and reduces their concentration in the blood by forming an insoluble calcium complex with these drugs. This is an example of a drug-food interaction. To prevent this problem these antibiotics should be taken approximately one hour prior to meals.

Tetracyclines are stored in the bones and teeth. Administration of these drugs has been shown to cause brown discoloration of the teeth, an effect most prominent when tetracyclines are taken between the ages of two months and two years, when permanent teeth are calcified. The intensity of discoloration is dependent upon the total dose of antibiotic administered to the child. Similarly, administration of tetracyclines to pregnant patients, especially during mid-pregnancy, has been shown to produce discoloration of their offspring's teeth.

Some tetracyclines are more slowly excreted in the urine than others, thus accounting for the selective differences in duration of action (Table 29–3).

Therapeutic Uses

The tetracyclines have gained widespread popularity as antimicrobial agents because of their effectiveness after oral administration, relatively low toxicity, and broad spectrum of antimicrobial activity. Among the many infectious diseases for which they have proved useful are streptococcal and staphylococcal disorders, acne, pneumonia, gonorrhea, syphilis, urinary tract infections, Rocky Mountain spotted fever, typhus, lymphogranuloma venereum (a venereal disease), and trachoma (a disease of the eyes that is prevalent in the Middle East and Far East). Tetracyclines are believed to inhibit bacterial protein synthesis by blocking the binding of the amino acid–transfer RNA complex with the ribosome.

The broad spectrum of tetracycline's antimicrobial action has led to its indiscriminate use for the treatment of minor disorders, resulting in the development of bacterial resistance even in microbes that were once highly susceptible to this drug's actions. Fortunately, the emergence of these resistant strains has been relatively gradual.

Adverse Effects

Although the tetracyclines are considerably more toxic than penicillin, they produce few frequently encountered adverse effects. The most common of these include nausea, vomiting, and diarrhea, which may be caused by local irritation of the gastrointestinal tract or by superinfection resulting from an alteration of the normal microbial population of the intestines. Superinfection by resistant staphylococci represents a potentially life-threatening situation.

Tetracyclines may also cause discoloration of the teeth and liver damage. Demeclocycline has been shown to cause phototoxicity in some patients, where severe burns develop when susceptible patients are exposed to sunlight.

CHLORAMPHENICOL

Chloramphenicol (Chloromycetin) is a broad-spectrum antibiotic that possesses antimicrobial activity resembling that of the tetracyclines. Although this drug was originally isolated from a soil microbe, *Streptomyces venezuelae,* at present it is the only commonly used antibiotic that is totally prepared synthetically.

Chloramphenicol inhibits the growth and reproduction of both gram-positive and gram-negative bacteria as well as rickettsiae. It inhibits protein synthesis by attaching to the bacterial ribosome and interferes with the formation of peptide bonds between amino acids.

The routine use of chloramphenicol has been sharply limited because of its tendency to cause *aplastic anemia,* an irreversible and often fatal blood disorder characterized by a marked reduction in all blood cells. Aplastic anemia, which results from a drug-induced effect on bone marrow, is not seen in all patients and is thought by some investigators to be a genetically determined idiosyncrasy to this antibiotic.

In older children and adults, chloramphenicol is readily inactivated by a glucuronic acid conjugation reaction. Newborn infants lack glucuronyl transferase, the enzyme needed to catalyze this biochemical reaction, and, as a consequence, chloramphenicol levels become markedly elevated. The resulting "gray syndrome" in infants is manifested by vomiting, a drop in body temperature, an ashen gray color, circulatory failure, shock, and, in some instances, death. The effects may be obviated by reducing the dosage of chloramphenicol administered to the newborn.

Chloramphenicol   Chloramphenicol glucuronide

The potential danger of bone marrow toxicity with resulting aplastic anemia has markedly reduced the therapeutic applications of chloramphenicol to all but the most serious infectious diseases for which other, less dangerous antibiotics are ineffective. Chloramphenicol's accepted therapeutic uses include salmonella infections (including typhoid fever), Rocky Mountain spotted fever and other severe rickettsial infections, and meningitis caused by *Hemophilus influenzae.*

STREPTOMYCIN AND RELATED AMINOGLYCOSIDES

The aminoglycosides are a group of antibiotics sharing common chemical, antimicrobial, pharmacological, and toxicological characteristics. The oldest and most intensively studied member of this class is streptomycin; other aminoglycosides are compared in Table 29–4.

TABLE 29-4. AMINOGLYCOSIDES

Streptomycin

Generic Name	Selected Trade Names	Remarks
Streptomycin		Treatment of tuberculosis and gram-negative infections; rapid development of bacterial resistance; administered only intramuscularly; potential impairment of kidney function and ototoxicity with all aminoglycosides.
Neomycin	Mycifradin	High systemic toxicity; primarily used topically for local infections.
Gentamicin	Garamycin	Widely used aminoglycoside for treatment of gram-negative infections (especially *Pseudomonas*) of urinary tract, eye, skin; effective against some gram-positive bacteria (staphylococci); administered intramuscularly and topically.
Kanamycin	Kantrex	Not absorbed orally, used for intestinal infections; useful for gram-negative septicemia ("blood poisoning") after injection.
Tobramycin	Nebcin	New drugs similar to gentamicin.
Amikacin	Amikin	
Paromomycin	Humatin	Primarily used for treatment of acute and chronic amebiasis (amebic dysentery); more effective drugs are available.

Streptomycin

Streptomycin was isolated from *Streptomyces griseus*[3] by Selman Waksman in 1944. This antibiotic was first isolated from the gizzard of a chicken and later from soil samples. Although this drug is effective against many gram-negative microorganisms, it is primarily used for the treatment of tuberculosis. Streptomycin binds to the bacterial ribosomes and is thought to inhibit protein synthesis by causing a misreading of the messenger RNA information.

This drug suffers from three limitations: poor absorption, development of bacterial resistance, and toxicity. Streptomycin is very poorly absorbed after oral administration and must therefore be administered by injection. Bacterial resistance develops very rapidly, within a few days to several weeks, after the initiation of drug therapy. The development of *Mycobacterium* (microbe causing tuberculosis) resistance can be delayed by coadministering other antitubercular drugs with streptomycin. Moreover, under appropriate conditions, it has been demonstrated that certain microbes become dependent upon streptomycin and require this drug for their normal growth and multiplication.

After the administration of streptomycin in normal therapeutic doses for the treatment of tuberculosis for about one month, almost all patients experience difficulty in maintaining their sense of balance and develop impairment of normal hearing. These effects have been attributed to a direct toxic effect on the eighth cranial nerve. Patients suffer from vertigo or dizziness and are only able to retain their balance standing or sitting when their eyes are open. Hearing losses first affect high-pitched sounds and may in time progress to total deafness. Kidney toxicity and hypersensitivity reactions are also caused by this drug.

Streptomycin was the first drug shown to be effective for the treatment of tuberculosis, and, notwithstanding some significant disadvantages, it remains one of the most important chemotherapeutic agents available for the management of this disease; it is rarely used for the treatment of gram-negative infections.

Newer Aminoglycosides

The aminoglycoside derivatives developed after streptomycin (Table 29–4) are active against aerobic gram-negative rods, particularly sensitive strains of *Enterobacter (Aerobacter), Proteus, Pseudomonas,* and *Serratia.* Although some gram-positive bacteria such as staphylococci are inhibited by the aminoglycosides, far safer antibiotics are available for clinical use.

[3] In addition to producing streptomycin, the genus *Streptomyces,* a mold-like fungus, is also the source of such antibiotics as chloramphenicol, tetracycline, erythromycin, neomycin, and cycloheximide.

These antibiotics are very extensively employed (by parenteral administration) to treat bacteremia ("blood poisoning") and infections of the respiratory system, soft tissues (including burn infections), bone, and urinary tract caused by gram-negative rods that are resistant to less toxic antibiotics. These drugs, like streptomycin, may potentially cause ototoxicity and kidney impairment.

OTHER ANTIMICROBIAL AGENTS

Erythromycin

First isolated in 1952 from *Streptomyces erythreus,* erythromycin possesses antimicrobial activity similar to penicillin against such gram-positive bacteria as streptococci, staphylococci, and pneumonococci, as well as corynebacteria, microbes responsible for causing diphtheria. Erythromycin is highly effective against *Legionella pneumophila,* the bacterium responsible for Legionnaires' disease. This antibiotic has a low order of host toxicity and is often used to treat patients who are allergic to penicillin. Bacterial strains, especially staphylococci, appear to develop marked resistance to this antibiotic, thus limiting its usefulness.

Erythromycin and its salts are available for oral administration or injection and are marketed under a variety of trade names including E-Mycin, Erythrocin, Ilosone, Ilotycin, Pediamycin, and Robimycin.

Polymyxin B

Polymyxin B (Aerosporin) is a polypeptide antibiotic produced by the soil microbe *Bacillus polymyxa.* This drug possesses its greatest antimicrobial activity against gram-negative bacteria and is used to treat infections of the urinary tract, skin, and ears. Polymyxin attaches to the cell membrane of bacteria, disrupting its function and causing the loss of essential intracellular materials. Application of this antibiotic to the surface of the skin is relatively safe, whereas nerve and severe kidney damage are hazards associated with its systemic administration.

Griseofulvin

Human *fungal* (mycotic) infections may be of deep skin layers, bones, and internal organs, or they may be limited to the outer skin layer (epidermis), hair, and nails. The latter, so-called superficial mycotic infections, include such familiar diseases as ringworm of the body, scalp, feet, and nails. Unfortunately, successful treatment and cure is often complicated by a high rate of reinfection and the limited distribution of topical antifungal agents to the sites of infestation.

Griseofulvin (Fulvicin, Grifulvin, Grisactin) is an antifungal antibiotic that is isolated from a *Penicillium* mold. This drug is not effective when administered directly on the skin, nor is it useful for the treatment of deep mycotic infections or those caused by bacteria. It is administered orally for the treatment of various ringworm infections. Griseofulvin binds to the keratin cells that will eventually differentiate into skin, hair, and nails and makes these cells resistant to fungal infection, presumably by inhibiting nucleic acid synthesis by the fungus. In time, griseofulvin-containing keratin replaces fungal-infected keratin, a process that may require several weeks for treatment of ringworm of the skin or many months for infections of the nails.

CHALLENGES FOR THE FUTURE

Although antibiotic chemotherapy has radically altered the prognosis for patients suffering from many infectious diseases of bacterial and rickettsial etiology, many major problems still remain for the future. Two such problems, unique to our study of chemotherapy, include the increasing emergence of resistant strains of bacteria as well as the discovery of new antibiotics that will be useful for the treatment of other diseases that are presently refractory to these drugs. Although many effective antibiotics are available for the treatment of gram-positive bacteria, most antibiotics that are active gram-negative microbes are quite toxic to the host.

Drug resistance is the consequence of genetic changes occurring within the microbe and may occur even in the absence of exposure to chemotherapeutic agents.

Antibiotics eliminate susceptible strains and provide a more favorable environment for the growth and reproduction of resistant mutants. Thus, to successfully deal with the problem, humans must always be several steps ahead of the microbes and have at their disposal reserve agents to which resistance has not yet developed. Such antibiotics must be employed judiciously and reserved only for life-threatening infections.

The development of safe and effective anticancer and antiviral agents remains one of the greatest challenges for the future. In recent years, progress has been made in the chemotherapy of cancer, although, as we shall observe in the following chapter, the failures far outnumber the triumphs. Most drugs now used for the treatment of **viral infections** are capable of *preventing disease,* for example, immunization against polio, smallpox, measles (rubeola), German measles (rubella), mumps, and rabies, or providing symptomatic relief once the viral disease is present. Synthetic or antibiotic antiviral agents are needed that will *cure* viral infections once they are present. A major obstacle exists which has limited success thus far. Viruses are only capable of living and reproducing within living cells and, unfortunately, existing drugs that are able to inhibit the reproduction of viruses also significantly interfere with the normal cellular function of the host. The relative absence of selective toxicity makes the therapeutic use of such agents hazardous to the host. There also exists a need for better antibiotics or synthetic chemotherapeutic agents that will be more effective for the treatment of naturally resistant gram-negative bacteria and fungi that are responsible for causing deep infections.

Approximately one-third of the world's population is infested with parasitic worms or helminths. While roundworm and pinworm are most common in North America, *schistosomiasis* (caused by blood flukes) is a chronic, serious infection afflicting 200 million inhabitants of Asia, Africa, the Caribbean, and South America. Worldwide there are almost an equal number of cases of *malaria,* with 2 million people dying annually as the result of this protean infestation. The need for more effective, less toxic, inexpensive, and readily administered chemotherapeutic agents to prevent, treat, and cure these parasitic disorders is all too apparent.

SUMMARY

In this chapter we have surveyed the general properties of frequently employed antibiotics and sulfonamides. While some of these drugs are effective primarily against gram-positive (penicillin, erythromycin) or gram-negative bacteria (streptomycin, polymyxin B), other antibiotics including the tetracyclines and chloramphenicol are active against both gram-positive and many gram-negative bacteria, rickettsiae, and chlamydia. Griseofulvin lacks antibacterial potency but is useful for the treatment of superficial fungal infections such as ringworm.

Chemotherapeutic agents represent one of the few classes of drugs that are capable of *curing* a disease, while in most other instances we have previously considered, drugs only alleviate the symptoms of disease. Although all the chemotherapeutic agents discussed are selectively toxic to the parasite, the use of such agents is not without hazard; potential dangers include allergies (penicillin, sulfonamides), superinfection (tetracyclines), drug-induced blood disorders (sulfonamides, chloramphenicol), impairment of hearing and normal balance (streptomycin), and kidney damage (streptomycin, polymyxin B). All drug therapy involves an evaluation of the relative benefits anticipated with the potential risks. In many instances, the potential benefit of antibiotic therapy is the rescue of a patient from an otherwise fatal outcome.

SUPPLEMENTARY READINGS

Note: For general references, see Supplementary Readings at the end of Chapter 28.

Arnold, H. C., and P. Fasal, *Leprosy: Diagnosis and Management.* 2nd ed. Springfield, Ill.: Charles C Thomas, 1973.

Barza, M., and R. T. Schiefe, "Antimicrobial Spectrum, Pharmacology and Therapeutic Use of Antibiotics, Part 1: Tetracyclines," *American Journal of Hospital Pharmacy* **34:** 49–57 (1977).

Bauer, D. J., *The Specific Treatment of Virus Diseases.* Baltimore: University Park Press, 1977.

Flynn, E. H., ed., *Cephalosporins and Penicillins: Chemistry and Biology.* New York: Academic Press, 1972.

Graham, R. C., Jr. "Antibiotics for Treatment of Infections Caused by Gram-Positive Cocci," *Medical Clinics of North America* **58:** 505–17 (1974).

Hoeprich, P. D., "Chemotherapy of Systemic Fungal Diseases," *Annual Review of Pharmacology* **18:** 205–31 (1978).

Lorian, V., "The Mode of Action of Antibiotics on Gram-Negative Bacilli," *Archives of Internal Medicine* **128:** 623–32 (1971).

Marois, M., ed., *Development of Chemotherapeutic Agents for Parasitic Diseases.* Amsterdam: North-Holland Publishing Co., 1975.

Most, H., "Treatment of Common Parasitic Infections of Man Encountered in the United States," *New England Journal of Medicine* **287:** 495–98, 698–702 (1972).

Pinsker, K. L., and S. K. Koerner, "Chemotherapy of Tuberculosis," *American Journal of Hospital Pharmacy* **33:** 275–83 (1976).

Rollo, I. M., "Chemotherapy of Parasitic Diseases," in *Goodman and Gilman's The Pharmacological Basis of Therapeutics.* Edited by A. G. Gilman, L. S. Goodman, and A. Gilman, 6th ed., Sec. 11, Chaps. 44-47, pp. 1013–79. New York: Macmillan, 1980.

Thompson, P. E., and L. M. Werbel, *Antimalarial Agents: Chemistry and Pharmacology.* New York: Academic Press, 1972.

Thrupp, L. D., "Newer Cephalosporins and Expanded-Spectrum Penicillins," *Annual Review of Pharmacology* **14:** 435–67 (1974).

Tilles, J. G., "Antiviral Agents," *Annual Review of Pharmacology* **14:** 469–89 (1974).

Woodward, T. E., and C. L. Wisseman, Jr., *Chloromycetin (Chloramphenicol).* New York: Medical Encyclopedia, Inc., 1958.

30

Cancer Chemotherapy

While there are several chronic diseases more destructive to life than cancer none is more feared.

—Charles H. Mayo (1926)

Cancer cells are the anarchists of the body, for they know no law, pay no regard for the commonwealth, serve no useful function, and cause disharmony and death in their surrounds.[1]

—William Boyd (1971)

Cancer does not discriminate against the sexes, races, national origin, or age groups. Moreover, humans have no monopoly on tumors, for these growths are seen in plants, in almost all species of vetebrates, and in many invertebrates including worms, mollusks, lobsters, bees, ants, and *Drosophila,* the fruit fly. Second only to cardiovascular disease, cancer is a major cause of death in the United States, claiming in excess of 350,000 victims annually. Each year almost twice this number of people receive a diagnosis of cancer, with the eight most common types accounting for seven out of every ten cases. The anatomical site and annual incidence of these cancers in this country are as follows: colon and rectum, 100,000; lung, 91,000; female breast, 88,000; prostate gland, 56,000; uterus, 46,000; bladder and kidney, 43,000; lymphatic structures, 29,000; white blood cells, 21,000.

In this chapter we shall consider general concepts concerning cancer—a general term used to refer to dozens of different diseases possessing common characteristics—and then discuss the present status of cancer chemotherapy.

[1] *An Introduction to the Study of Disease.*

CANCER

In many disease states, we observe *hyperplasia,* an increase in the number of cells found in a tissue or organ. When iodine is deficient or absent from the diet, the thyroid gland increases in size—a hyperplastic state referred to as a goiter. Liver cell hyperplasia occurs when chemicals, injury, or disease destroys part of the liver. In both these situations, the reproductive propensity of the cells are under the *control* of the body. Moreover, these newly formed cells do not infringe upon the territorial boundaries of contiguous cells, they maintain their normal morphological characteristics and physiological function, and they generally pose no threat to the health and well-being of the host organism.

Tumors

A tumor or **neoplasm** is a mass of new cells, the growth of which is not under the control of the organism and which serves no useful function for the host. Such neoplasms are classified as being either *benign* or *malignant.* Whereas benign neoplasms, such as warts or moles, remain at the site of their origin, **malignant neoplasms** spread or *metastasize* to parts of the body which may be distant from their origin. The term *benign* does not denote whether the neoplasm has deleterious effects on the host; such benign tumors may prove harmful because of their size and anatomical location and may endanger the host by compressing surrounding tissues or organs.

All tumors, both benign and malignant, are characterized by uncontrolled growth. Malignant tumors, collectively termed **cancer,** are morphologically abnormal, invasive, and are capable of setting up secondary growths in other parts of the body (Table 30-1).

Uncontrolled Growth

When normal cells are placed on the surface of a culture tube, they actively move until they make contact with other cells. This cell-to-cell contact causes cessation in locomotion, a decline in the rate of cell division and replication (mitosis), and a substantial reduction in the rate at which substances are synthesized by the cell. This phenomenon, termed *contact inhibition,* limits the excessive proliferation of cells. Malignant cells do not exhibit the property of contact inhibition and therefore they attain a much higher population density than normal cells. A better understanding of the factors responsible for the absence of this essential control mechanism in tumors will undoubtedly provide an important clue for the design of anticancer agents.

TABLE 30-1. A COMPARISON OF THE CHARACTERISTICS OF BENIGN AND MALIGNANT TUMORS

	Benign Tumor	Malignant Tumor
Nomenclature (suffix)	–oma (e.g., adenoma)	–carcinoma: epithelial tumor (e.g., adenocarcinoma) –sarcoma: nonepithelial tumor (e.g., lymphosarcoma)
Gross characteristics of tumor	Circumscribed, may have surrounding capsule	Invasive
Increase in size	By compression of surrounding tissue	By invasion
Metastatic growth	Absent	Present
Deviation among similar cells	Uniform size and shape	Variation in size, shape, and arrangement
Mitosis (cell division)	Few	Frequent; may be atypical
Invasion of surrounding tissues	Absent	Present

Morphology

Malignant neoplasms lose the distinguishing morphological characteristics of their cells of origin and revert to a more primitive and undifferentiated cell type; we term this *dedifferentiation.* Normal cells are arranged in an orderly, systematic manner, while malignant tumor cells are irregularly arranged. The cells of a malignant neoplasm differ in size and shape from normal cells, as well as from each other. These microscopic differences are of crucial importance to pathologists when examining a tissue, because, based upon these considerations, they will inform the surgeon whether the patient has a benign or malignant neoplasm.

Invasiveness

This term describes the capacity of malignant tumors to encroach upon the territorial boundaries of neighboring cells. While benign tumors compress normal cells, malignant neoplasms actively invade and penetrate between these cells, usurping their nutrients and vascular supply and utilizing these resources to support their often rapid rate of growth and cell division. This voracious appetite leads to the ultimate destruction and death of normal cells.

Metastases

Malignant cells may set up secondary growths or **metastases** in parts of the body that are far removed from their sites of origin. This spread is not an expansion of the primary growth, and there is no physical continuity between these

TABLE 30-2. GLOSSARY OF DIFFERENT TYPES OF CANCER

Burkitt's lymphoma: A malignant tumor of the bones of the face afflicting African children.

Cancer: A malignant tumor; a collective term used to refer to dozens of diseases that are characterized by uncontrolled growth, invasiveness and metastatic growth.

Choriocarcinoma: A malignant tumor derived from cells of fetal origin.

Hodgkin's disease: A chronic disease characterized by progressive enlargement of the lymph nodes of the neck and other sites and often the spleen and liver. It is generally classified as a lymphoma.

Leukemia: A neoplastic disorder characterized by a marked increase in the number of white blood cells (leukocytes); e.g., lymphocytic leukemia is an increase in lymphocytes; myelocytic leukemia is an increase in granulocytes (neutrophils). Whereas in chronic leukemias the survival time is about three to four years after clinical onset, in the absence of effective treatment, acute leukemias may result in death within a few weeks to six months.

Lymphoma: A tumor derived from lymphocytes which may be present in any of the lymphatic structures and includes lymphosarcomas and Hodgkin's disease.

Lymphosarcoma: A tumor arising from the lymph nodes or lymphatic tissues, especially of the gastrointestinal tract. Enlargement and spread to surrounding tissues and lymphatics occurs.

Multiple myeloma: A malignant tumor of the bone and bone marrow.

Neuroblastoma: A malignant tumor of the nervous system (most commonly the adrenal gland) that is primarily observed in young children.

Wilms' tumor: A neoplasm of the kidneys affecting children.

sites. The cancer cell travels via blood from its original locus. The prognosis for a cancer patient with extensive metastases is generally poor.

Although there are rare instances of spontaneous tumor regressions in the absence of treatment, surgery, radiation (including x-ray), or chemotherapy, death is usually the inevitable result of cancer that is not diagnosed and treated during the early stages. General symptoms include fever, pain, weakness, and extreme weight loss. Malignant tumors may grow at rates that are much faster than normal and nourish themselves at the expense of the normal cells of the body. A glossary briefly defining the different types of cancers appears in Table 30-2.

Possible Causes of Cancer

> *Even to the astute observer of biological processes, cancer is a bewildering illness that defies simple categorization. It is a multifactorial disease, and depending on the nature of the population and the environment, the initiation of the disease process may involve interactions between two or more of the following: carcinogenic chemicals present in cigarette smoke, industrial pollutants, and the diet; radiation; oncogenic viruses; chronic mechanical or thermal trauma; parasitic infection; genetic predisposition; and the aging process.[2]*

—William B. Pratt and Raymond W. Ruddon (1979)

[2] *The Anticancer Drugs.*

At the outset we should state that the exact cause of cancer is unknown. Furthermore, it is unlikely that there is only one cause responsible for the extensive group of diseases we collectively term cancer. While a large number of chemical, biological, physical, and environmental factors have been associated with the development of malignant tumors in humans and animals, the specific mechanism(s) responsible for the aberrations in the control of normal growth and replication are not well understood at present, although much progress has been made in recent years.

Chemicals

In 1775, Percival Pott observed that cancer of the scrotum was an occupational hazard associated with the then popular chimney sweep vocation—a fact undoubtedly expurgated from the movie *Mary Poppins.* Pott hypothesized that the coal tars found in soot contain an active carcinogen; one such compound, now known to be a carcinogen, is 3, 4-benzpyrene, one of the "tars" found in tobacco smoke. Cancer and other health hazards associated with tobacco smoking are considered in Chapter 32.

3, 4-Benzpyrene

The widespread use of flame retardants in infants' and children's sleepwear began in 1973. To meet the then newly established federal regulations, most manufacturers selected polyester into which the flame retardant *Tris* could be readily dissolved by a heat treatment. This chemical, tris (2, 3-dibromopropyl) phosphate, was effective, inexpensive, and apparently safe. Four years later, the manufacture and sale of Tris-treated sleeping garments was abruptly banned after laboratory studies showed that this chemical caused kidney cancer in animals and could be absorbed across their skin. To date there is no evidence that Tris causes cancer in humans. Whether or not the hundreds of thousands of children who wore Tris-treated sleepwear have sustained changes that will increase their risk of kidney cancer is still a question.

By contrast, it is now well established that occupational exposure to *asbestos* fibers increases the risk of lung cancer six to ten times after a latent period of 20 to 40 years. Asbestos miners, millers, and insulation, construction, shipyard, and textile workers are at highest risk. Inhalation of asbestos fibers and cigarette smoking contribute synergistically to the development of lung cancer in humans. Additional aspects of chemical carcinogenesis are discussed in Chapter 31.

Viruses

While viruses have been conclusively shown to be a cause of cancer in many animal species, similar evidence has not been unequivocally demonstrated in humans. However, many investigators believe that human leukemia and other tumors may be of viral origin. In 1935, Bittner described a form of breast cancer in young nursing mice that resulted from a transfer of a virus in the mother's milk. Removal of the offspring immediately after birth prevented tumor development in this strain of mice which normally shows a high incidence of breast tumors. Evidence suggests that viral DNA enters the host cell's chromosomes and displaces a normal gene, which results in marked aberrations in cellular metabolism, growth, and replication.

Radiation

Less than a decade after Roentgen's discovery of the x-ray in 1895, radiation was shown to cause cancer. Among the earliest victims were radiologists and x-ray technicians, who, unaware of the potential dangers, overexposed themselves to ionizing radiation and developed skin cancer. In 1920, bone cancer was observed to be an occupational hazard among painters of luminous radium clock and watch dials. They would use their lips to make a fine tip on their brushes, and in the process ingest the carcinogenic radioactive compound. Japanese survivors of the Hiroshima and Nagasaki atomic bomb blasts have shown an increase in the incidence of leukemia, with a direct relationship observed between the proximity of the victim to the hypocenter of the blast and the frequency of this cancer of the white blood cells. Fishermen, farmers, sailors, and other individuals exposed to direct sunlight for long periods of time have a higher than normal incidence of skin cancer.

Hormones

While it has not been clearly ascertained whether hormones are able to initiate cancer in humans, there is no doubt that some cancers are *hormone-dependent*. Cancer of the prostate gland in males can be treated by castration, thereby eliminating the major source of male testosterone, or by the administration of estrogen, the female sex hormone (Chapter 23). Conversely, in premenopausal women, removal of the ovaries or administration of testosterone has proved to be of value in the treatment of breast cancer.

CANCER CHEMOTHERAPY

Chemotherapy of microbial diseases has been far more successful than drug treatment of cancers. A brief review of the fundamental differences between microbes and malignant tumors will permit a better appreciation of the reasons for this differential success (Table 30–3).

TABLE 30-3. COMPARISON OF MICROBIAL DISEASES AND CANCER AND THEIR CHEMOTHERAPIES

Dimension	Microbial Disease	Cancer
Characteristics of disease		
Specific causes of disorder established	Yes	No
Invading cell	Foreign	Host's own cells
Anatomical/biochemical differences from host	Major	Minor or none
Cell population	Homogeneous	Heterogeneous
Diagnosis of presence of disease	Usually early	Usually late
Characteristics of chemotherapy		
Effectiveness of chemotherapy	Authentic cures	Increased incidence of five-year survival, few cures
Drug toxicity	Selective toxicity to parasite	Nonselective toxicity to normal and cancer cells
Margin of drug safety	Wide	Narrow
Acquired cell resistance during chemotherapy	Relatively rare	Common
Duration of treatment	Brief	Prolonged
Accessibility of drug at intended site of action ("pharmacological hideouts")	Generally good	Often limited
Host defense mechanisms (immunocompetence)	Strong	Weak and further decreased by disease and chemotherapy

Microbial cells have metabolic and nutritional requirements and cellular structures that are markedly different from their mammalian hosts (Chapter 28). Malignant neoplasms, by contrast, are derived from the cells of the host, and, consequently, in most respects bear great similarity to normal host cells. Hence, while the selective toxicity of antimicrobial agents is high, this is not the case for most cancer chemotherapeutic agents. Therapeutically effective doses of these drugs are toxic to both neoplasms and normal cells, with rapidly proliferating host cells particularly susceptible; these include the epithelial cells of the gastrointestinal tract and of the hematopoietic or blood cell-forming system. Commonly encountered adverse effects associated with the administration of anticancer drugs include ulceration and bleeding of the gastrointestinal tract, severe diarrhea, nausea and vomiting, hair loss, and a marked reduction in circulating blood cells. With the decrease in white blood cells (leukopenia) is a resulting suppression of the patient's immune response and enhanced vulnerability to microbial infections.

We have previously observed that host defense mechanisms are a very important factor for the successful eradication of microbial infections. It is not clear how effective and to what extent host immune systems participate in limiting the growth of tumors. At the time of a diagnosis of acute leukemia, one trillion (10^{12}) cancer cells are generally present and widely distributed throughout the body of the host. If an antileukemic agent were able to kill 99.9 percent of the cells present, patients would show symptomatic improvement although they would still harbor one billion (10^9) cancer cells capable of actively reproducing. A contemporary philosophy of cancer chemotherapy argues that attempts should be directed toward killing *all* cancer cells rather than attempting to achieve merely symptomatic patient improvement. The high host toxicity of these drugs usually serves as a limiting factor in realizing this goal.

Cell Cycle and Cancer Chemotherapy

Successful cancer chemotherapy often requires the use of multiple drugs that act at different phases of the cell cycle. The *cell cycle* is divided into four primary phases—G_1, S, G_2, and M (Figure 30-1). G_1, the first growth phase, occurs prior to DNA synthesis and after mitosis, and is associated with the synthesis of enzymes, structural proteins, and cellular organelles. S is the phase of DNA synthesis. The second growth phase, G_2, is a period of specialized protein and RNA synthesis as well as the manufacture of the mitotic spindle apparatus prior to the M phase of mitosis.

In normal adult tissues and most tumors, cells are in different phases of the cell cycle at a given time. After cell division has occurred, some cells enter a resting phase (G_0) of varying duration and do not reproduce. This noncycling phase serves as a reservoir from which resting cells can be drawn to supply cells for division in response to cell losses. Most anticancer drugs act by interfering with the replication of cycling cells with only a limited number of drugs

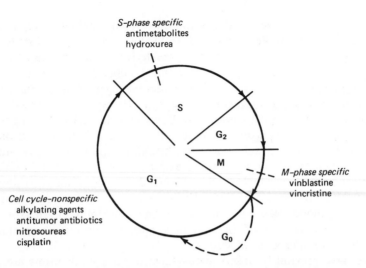

FIGURE 30-1. The Cell Cycle and Cancer Chemotherapeutic Agents. The cycling phases: G_1 is a growth phase between mitosis and DNA synthesis in which enzymes, other proteins, and structural organelles are synthesized; **S** is the phase of DNA synthesis; G_2 is a phase of protein and RNA synthesis and the manufacture of the mitotic spindle apparatus required in the mitotic phase **M**. G_0 is a resting or noncycling phase in which the cells are not involved in activities associated with cell division. Cytotoxic anticancer agents may inhibit cell replication at a specific phase in the cycle or may act at any phase in the cycle or on resting cells: examples of cell cycle–specific and cell cycle–nonspecific agents, respectively, appear in the figure.

affecting noncycling cells at concentrations that are nontoxic to normal growing cells. Cells can leave the cycle and enter G_0, thereby escaping from the otherwise lethal effects of many chemotherapeutic agents, and re-enter the cycle when drug levels fall below harmful concentrations or after the discontinuation of drug administration. A major problem in cancer chemotherapy is the eradication of drug-resistant resting or noncycling tumor cells.

The time-honored view that cancer cells proliferate at extremely rapid rates has been disproven, and available evidence now shows that there are few significant differences between normal and cancer tissues in their rates of cell division. Since both normal and neoplastic cells must carry out similar biochemical pathways for survival, it is not surprising that cytotoxic anticancer agents kill both types of cells, and that those tissues with the shortest generation times (hematopoietic, gastrointestinal, epithelial) are most susceptible.

Some cytotoxic agents are only capable of inhibiting cell replication during one phase of the cell cycle and are, therefore, referred to as **cell cycle–specific** (CCS) agents; for example, methotrexate and cytarabine (cytosine arabinoside) act in the S phase to inhibit DNA synthesis, while vinblastine and vincristine interfere with the M phase of mitosis (Figure 30–1). Other anticancer drugs are cytotoxic to both cycling and noncycling cells, although cycling cells are more vulnerable. Since these drugs are cytotoxic at any phase of the cycle, they are designated **cell cycle–nonspecific** (CCNS) agents. CCNS agents, which usually produce cell death by complexing with DNA, include the alkylating agents and the antitumor antibiotics. CCS agents have been found to be more effective clinically for the treatment of blood cancers (leukemias) and other tumors with a rapid rate of proliferation. CCNS agents, which act on cells regardless of their rate of proliferation, are often used for the treatment of solid tumors.

The strategy for developing optimal therapeutic regimens requires an understanding of the time course of the cell cycle of the specific tumor and the site(s) of action and toxicity of the individual chemotherapeutic agents. It is now recognized, for example, that CCS agents often produce greater beneficial effects after the administration of CCNS agents. Why? A rather large proportion of tumor cells may be in the resting G_0 phase at a given time. It has been suggested that CCNS drugs promote the "recruitment" of resting cells into actively cycling cells thereby enhancing their sensitivity to the toxic effects of CCS agents.

Let us now consider the following classes of cancer chemotherapeutic drugs: alkylating agents, antimetabolites, antibiotics, steroid hormones, and miscellaneous agents.

Alkylating Agents

When the Kaiser's soldiers employed sulfur mustard against the Allied forces in 1917, immediate interest was focused upon the blistering effects of this gas on the respiratory tract, skin, and eyes. It was subsequently noted that mustard gas caused a depression of the blood-forming and lymphoid tissues of the body. The *nitrogen mustards* were later developed as potential chemical warfare agents, and although never employed in combat during World War II, they were observed to be effective for the treatment of cancers of lymphoid tissue (Hodgkin's disease), white blood cells (leukemia), and neoplasms of the ovaries, testes, and breasts. While these drugs cause temporary remissions, they do not cure the cancer. Table 30–4 lists several of the more commonly employed alkylating agents.

Alkylating agents are *cytotoxic,* that is, they are general cell poisons that adversely affect both malignant tumors and rapidly growing normal cells. These drugs are cell cycle–nonspecific. In the water of the body, they are converted to highly reactive, positively charged (cationic) intermediate compounds that are able to chemically interact with negatively charged (anionic) groups in cells in a nonspecific manner. As a consequence of this chemical interaction, alkylating agents interfere with the activity of enzymes and other compounds responsible for the regulation of essential cellular functions. Among the most important of these interactions are those involving alkylation of the guanine molecule of chromosomal DNA. This attachment produces cross-linking of DNA strands which interferes with normal cellular mitosis and replication. These effects bear great similarity to those seen after ionizing radiation (x-ray), and hence alkylating drugs are frequently termed radiomimetic agents.

TABLE 30-4. ALKYLATING AGENTS AS ANTICANCER AGENTS

Generic Name	Selected Trade Names	Principal Therapeutic Uses
Busulfan	Myleran	Chronic myelogenous leukemia
Carmustine (BCNU)	BiCNU	Hodgkin's disease Brain tumors
Chlorambucil	Leukeran	Chronic lymphocytic leukemia Hodgkin's disease Lymphosarcoma
Cyclophosphamide	Cytoxan	Same as chlorambucil
Lomustine (CCNU)	CeeNU	Same as carmustine
Mechlorethamine (nitrogen mustard)	Mustargen	Same as chlorambucil
Melphalan	Alkeran	Multiple myeloma
Streptozocin (streptozotocin)	Zanosar	Pancreatic islet cell carcinoma (insulinoma)

The *nitrosourea* compounds (carmustine, lomustine) are alkylating agents whose most significant property is their ability to cross the blood-brain barrier. These drugs are particularly useful for the treatment of tumors that have invaded the brain.

Antimetabolites

The antimetabolites employed as anticancer agents chemically resemble endogenous compounds used as building blocks for the synthesis of the nucleic acids, DNA and RNA. These drugs inhibit nucleic acid synthesis (acting at the S-phase of the cell cycle) by attaching to an enzyme and thereby preventing it from catalyzing a necessary biochemical reaction, or by entering a synthetic pathway and being incorporated into the formation of a fraudulent end product that cannot be utilized by the cell for growth and reproduction (Chapter 28).

Antimetabolites may be antagonists of the normal metabolism of folic acid, purines, or pyrimidines, all of which ultimately play a role in the biosynthesis of nucleic acids (Figure 30-2). Table 30-5 summarizes the more commonly employed antimetabolite cancer chemotherapeutic agents.

Folic Acid Antagonists

Folic acid is a vitamin required for the synthesis of purines and pyrimidines which in turn are incorporated into nucleotides and nucleic acids (Figure 30-2). Antagonists such as *methotrexate* bind to and inhibit dihydrofolate reductase, the enzyme responsible for the conversion of dietary folic acid to tetrahydrofolate, a coenzyme involved in nucleic acid synthesis. Rapidly proliferating cells are particularly susceptible to the action of this drug; interference with mitosis results. Methotrexate, employed alone or in combination with other drugs, has produced remission in the symptoms of acute leukemia up to several years. This compound has also produced apparent cures (that is, no

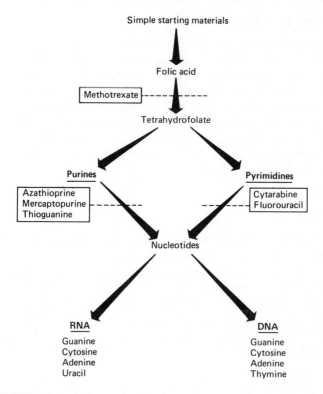

FIGURE 30–2. Antimetabolite Interference with Nucleic Acid Synthesis.

TABLE 30-5. ANTIMETABOLITES AS ANTICANCER AGENTS

Generic Name	Selected Trade Names	Principal Therapeutic Uses
Folic acid antagonist		
Methotrexate		Acute leukemia (children)
		Choriocarcinoma
Purine antagonists		
Mercaptopurine (6-MP)	Purinethol	Acute leukemia (children)
Thioguanine	6-TG	Acute leukemia (children)
Pyrimidine antagonists		
Cytarabine (cytosine arabinoside)	Cytosar, Ara-C	Acute leukemia
Fluorouracil	5-FU	Advanced cancers of rectum,
Floxuridine	FUDR	colon, breasts, and ovaries

reappearance of malignancy after five years) of choriocarcinoma, a relatively rare (one in 40,000 pregnancies) but highly lethal tumor arising from cells of fetal origin.

Purine and Pyrimidine Antagonists

Mercaptopurine, a chemical analog of the purine adenine introduced in 1949, is primarily used to treat acute leukemia in children. Remissions in this disease and prolongation of life have been reported. Azathioprine, structurally related to mercaptopurine, is chiefly used as an immunosuppressive agent to prevent the rejection of transplanted organs. This immunosuppressive effect has been attributed to azathioprine-induced depression of lymphatic tissues. Fluorouracil and cytarabine are pyrimidine antagonists that interfere with DNA synthesis. A highly toxic drug, flourouracil is used for the treatment of advanced cases of certain cancers.

Antibiotics

A number of antibiotics are currently employed for the treatment of cancers. Most of these drugs bind to and inactivate DNA, acting at the S-phase of the cell cycle, and produce inhibition of RNA synthesis. With the exception of bleomycin, all other antitumor antibiotics (Table 30–6) cause bone marrow depression. *Doxorubicin* (Adriamycin) has been found to possess a relatively broad spectrum of antineoplastic activity. Unfortunately, the potential usefulness of this antibiotic is limited by its propensity to produce severe and often irreversible adverse effects to the heart (cardiotoxicity) and bone marrow depression.

TABLE 30-6. ANTIBIOTICS AS ANTICANCER AGENTS

Generic Name	Selected Trade Names	Principal Therapeutic Uses
Bleomycin	Blenoxane	Squamous cell carcinoma of head, neck, penis, cervix Lymphomas Testicular carcinoma
Dactinomycin (actinomycin D)	Cosmegen	Wilms' tumor Choriocarcinoma Carcinoma of the testes
Daunorubicin (daunomycin)		Acute leukemia
Doxorubicin	Adriamycin	Acute lymphoblastic and myeloblastic leukemia Wilms' tumor Neuroblastoma Soft tissue and bone sarcoma Breast, bladder, bronchogenic, metastatic thyroid cancers
Mithramycin	Mithracin	Testicular carcinoma
Mitomycin	Mutamycin	Widespread stomach and pancreatic carcinomas

Steroid Hormones

Sex hormones, both male and female, and the glucocorticoid cortico-steroids have proved useful for the treatment of certain types of neoplastic conditions (Table 30–7). In contrast to other drugs used for cancer which act nonselectively on rapidly multiplying cells, the steroid hormones possess a relatively high degree of *selective toxicity,* with each hormone acting on specific tissues. The rationale underlying the use of this drug class is predicated upon the fact that cancers arising from tissues that are responsive to the effects of hormones retain the hormonal responsiveness of their tissues of origin. Depending upon the properties of the tissue of origin, changes in the hormone concentration present may cause the cancer to increase or decrease in size.

All human *breast cancers*[3] are thought to be responsive to hormones at some time, but later many become nonresponsive to hormonal stimulation; approximately one-third of all female patients with breast cancer have tumors that are hormone responsive or dependent. Circulating estrogen binds to a cellular *estrogen receptor protein* and stimulates DNA synthesis in hormone-dependent tumors. The presence of estrogen receptor proteins in tumor biopsies can now be readily determined by laboratory tests. If a premenopausal woman is found

[3] Approximately 35,000 women in the United States die each year as the result of breast cancer. This is the leading cause of death in women 40–44 years of age.

TABLE 30-7. STEROID HORMONES AS ANTICANCER AGENTS

Drug Class	Principal Therapeutic Uses
Female hormones (estrogens)	Prostatic cancer, males
Diethylstilbestrol	Breast cancer, in postmenopausal
Ethinyl estradiol (Estinyl)	females and males
Antiestrogen	
Tamoxifen (Nolvadex)	Breast cancer, postmenopausal
	females
Male hormones (androgens)	Breast cancer, females
Testosterone	
Anabolic androgens (little or no	Breast cancer, females
hormonal activity)	
Dromostanolone (Drolban)	
Testolactone (Teslac)	
Glucocorticoids	Acute leukemia
Cortisol (Cortef)	Lymphomas
Dexamethasone (Decadron)	Chronic lymphocytic leukemia
Prednisone (Deltasone)	

to have the receptor protein, surgical removal of the ovaries is indicated to remove the primary source of circulating estrogen; testosterone administration is frequently initiated. The antitumor effects of testosterone are independent of its androgenic activities (Chapter 23). *Testolactone* (Teslac) is a potent antitumor compound chemically related to testosterone that is relatively free of the natural hormone's masculinizing properties.

While estrogen administration prior to menopause promotes tumor growth, after menopause estrogen and such synthetic derivatives as diethylstilbestrol have proved useful in breast cancer. *Antiestrogenic agents* such as *tamoxifen* (Nolvadex) are now being used for the treatment of breast cancer in postmenopausal women having tumors with significant numbers of estrogen receptors. This new drug is believed to act by competing with circulating estrogen for receptor sites on the breast tumor thereby interfering with hormone-stimulated DNA synthesis and cell replication.

Cancer of the prostate has been successfully managed by the removal of the testes, the source of testosterone, and by treatment with diethylstilbestrol. Prolonged use of estrogens produces feminization of males, while testosterone causes masculinization of female patients.

Glucocorticoids, steroid hormones related to cortisol, cause a shrinkage of lymphatic tissues. These hormones have been useful for the treatment of acute leukemia and lymphomas, as well as advanced cases of breast cancer.

Miscellaneous Drugs

The last group of cancer chemotherapeutic agents we shall consider are classified as miscellaneous drugs because they lack a common mechanism of ac-

TABLE 30-8. REPRESENTATIVE MISCELLANEOUS ANTICANCER COMPOUNDS

Drug	Source	Class	Principal Therapeutic Uses
L-Asparaginase (Elspar)	*Escherichia coli* (bacterium)	Enzyme	Acute lymphoblastic leukemia
Cisplatin (cis-platinum, Platinol)	Synthetic	Simple organic molecule	Cancers of ovaries, testicles, bladder
Hydroxyurea (Hydrea)	Synthetic compound	Simple organic molecule	Chronic granulocytic leukemia
Interferon	Human blood; potentially recombinant DNA	Protein	Experimental, possible broad spectrum of cancers
Laetrile (Amygdalin; vitamin B-17)	Apricot pits	Sugar	None proven to be effective
Mitotane (o, p '-DDD; Lysodren)	Synthetic compound	Insecticide-like	Cancer of adrenal cortex
Procarbazine (Matulane)	Synthetic compound	Simple organic molecule	Hodgkin's disease
Sodium Phosphate P32 (Phosphotope)	Synthetic	Radioisotope	Polycythemia vera Chronic myelocytic leukemia
Vinblastine (Velban)	*Vinca rosea* (periwinkle plant)	Alkaloid	Hodgkin's disease Choriocarcinoma
Vincristine (Oncovin)	*Vinca rosea*	Alkaloid	Acute leukemia Lymphosarcoma Neuroblastoma Wilms' disease

tion and source from which they are obtained and have different therapeutic indications (Table 30–8).

L-Asparaginase

Derived from the bacterium *Escherichia coli,* the enzyme L-asparaginase represents an exciting therapeutic and theoretical advance in cancer chemotherapy. The use of this enzyme was predicated upon a known metabolic difference between malignant neoplasms and normal cells. Certain tumor cells require dietary sources of the amino acid L-asparagine for growth. L-asparaginase destroys exogenous L-asparagine and thereby inhibits the growth of these malignant cells. Since normal cells are able to synthesize their own L-asparagine, they are not adversely affected by the presence of L-asparaginase. This observation provides hope that other fundamentally different nutritional requirements exist between malignant and normal cells, with such differences serving as the focal point for the attack of cancer chemotherapeutic agents possessing selective toxicity (Chapter 28). L-asparaginase is used for the treatment of acute lymphoblastic leukemia. The rapid resistance that develops to this drug has been attributed to the ability of the tumor cell to synthesize L-asparagine.

Laetrile

Laetrile, also referred to as amygdalin and vitamin B_{17}, is a substance derived from pulverized apricot pits that has been widely promoted for the prevention, treatment, and cure of cancer. Although rigorous scientific and clinical proof establishing the anticancer activity of this drug is lacking, and its reputation is almost exclusively predicated upon patient and physician testimonials, intensive lobbying efforts by nonmedical groups have led to its legalization in approximately twelve states.[4] In 1980, the Food and Drug Administration (FDA) granted approval for laetrile to be evaluated in controlled clinical trials.

Amygdalin is believed to be metabolized to hydrogen cyanide and thiocyanate by the following (highly simplified) pathway:

$$\text{2-Glucose}-O-\underset{\underset{\text{Ph}}{|}}{\overset{\overset{H}{|}}{C}}-C\equiv N \quad \xrightarrow{\ \beta\text{-glucuronidase}\ } \quad 2\ \text{Glucose} \quad + \quad HO-\underset{\underset{\text{Ph}}{|}}{\overset{\overset{H}{|}}{C}}\diagup C\equiv N$$

Amygdalin   Mandelonitrile

$$\xrightarrow[\text{lyase}]{\text{Hydroxynitrile}} \quad O=\underset{\underset{\text{Ph}}{|}}{\overset{\overset{H}{|}}{C}} \quad + \quad CN^{-} \quad \xrightarrow{\ \text{Rhodanese}\ } \quad SCN^{-}$$

Benzaldehyde cyanide   Thiocyanate

---

[4] The author has elected to devote a perhaps excessively disproportionate amount of space to laetrile because, irrespective of the validity of the claims made for its safety and effectiveness, this drug has aroused considerable public interest; moreover, many of the arguments raised for and against its legalization seem worthy of careful scrutiny and philosophical consideration.

The constituents of prolaetrile lobbying groups and their fundamental arguments differ widely: Many individuals are undoubtedly terminal cancer victims or their relatives who view laetrile to be their last hope for survival and who ask for the freedom of choice in medication selection; others perceive antilaetrile laws as still another example of big government interference with the constitutional rights of the individual as guaranteed by the Fourteenth Amendment; a few are quacks, hucksters, and profiteers, extravagant and irresponsible in their claims, who are capitalizing upon the fears of actual and potential cancer victims; still other proponents argue that the "medical establishment" simply opposes laetrile because it represents "the greatest single threat to [medicine's] $20 billion a year cancer industry."

The FDA has and continues to oppose laetrile legalization because, contrary to the claims of its proponents: It is not completely nontoxic; it has not been proven to be effective in preventing or treating cancer; and there is no basis for the claim that it is a vitamin that plays an essential role in

E. T. Krebs, Jr., a leading scientific proponent of laetrile, has hypothesized that cancer cells contain high levels of β-glucuronidase, and that this enzyme actively participates in the metabolism of laetrile to cyanide, an extremely toxic substance that inhibits the respiration of cancer cells causing their death. By contrast, normal cells contain relatively modest amounts of β-glucuronidase and rather high amounts of rhodanese thus promoting the rapid breakdown of the poisonous cyanide to the relatively nontoxic thiocyanate. Krebs's "cyanide theory" remains to be proven.

Pro-laetrile advocates have staunchly maintained that the drug is harmless—"even less toxic than sugar." This myth was disproven in 1977 when an 11-month-old infant died of cyanide poisoning after ingesting not more than five tablets (500 mg per tablet) of laetrile. Other deaths (particularly in debilitated patients) ascribed to cancer may, in some cases, actually result from or be hastened by the cyanide liberated from laetrile. Chronic cyanide poisoning has been well-documented in geographic areas where ingestion of cyanogenic foods is common.

Interferon

While the medical establishment has been highly critical in their assessment of the potential therapeutic merits of laetrile, the guarded optimism expressed about interferon has, by contrast, been directly transmitted to the public by nationally recognized cancer specialists on television talk shows and in cover stories in *Saturday Review* and *Time.*

The discovery of interferon dates back to 1957 when investigators were attempting to determine why patients suffering from one viral infection were rarely ever the victim of a different viral infection at the same time. They knew that when a virus invades a cell, the cell machinery begins producing identical copies of the virus rather than engaging in the normal synthesis of proteins required for the health and survival of that cell. After the cell becomes filled to capacity with newly synthesized viruses, the cell bursts and discharges the viruses which are potentially free to attack other healthy cells thereby spreading the infection. These scientists determined that when the virus invades the first cell, it also triggers the cellular production of **interferon,** a compound which leaves the cell and activates surrounding uninfected cells to produce antiviral proteins.[5] These proteins prevent viral replication in uninfected cells or, if

---

human nutrition. Moreover, the FDA maintains that permitting the patient to employ laetrile may delay early diagnosis of cancer and the inception of use of medically and scientifically recognized chemotherapeutic agents. This last argument appears less compelling for the desperate terminal patient who is no longer deriving therapeutic benefit from approved anticancer medications while suffering from drug-induced adverse effects.

Arguments for laetrile appear in B. W. Halstead, *Amygdalin (Laetrile) Therapy,* Los Altos, Calif: Choice Publications, 1977; antilaetrile arguments are voiced in "Laetrile: The Making of a Myth," *FDA Consumer* **10** (December-January): 5–9 (1977).

[5] Some scientists have likened interferon to Paul Revere warning neighbors of an impending attack and invasion.

replication does occur, they prevent the newly synthesized viruses from leaving the cell, thus checking the spread of the infection.

Preliminary clinical trials reveal that administered interferon might be effective for the prevention and/or treatment of various *viral infections* including the common cold, chicken pox, and a highly contagious conjuctivitis commonly referred to as "pink eye." While interest in the potential antiviral properties of interferon persists, and this compound may represent a highly significant breakthrough in *antiviral chemotherapy,* public and scientific interest has been captured by its possible use as an anticancer agent.

Although no human cancer virus has been identified to date, some tumors appear to be linked to viruses. For this reason, interferon was tested as an anticancer drug. Highly encouraging preliminary responses were obtained in the treatment of a wide range of carcinomas including breast cancer, lymphoma, multiple myeloma, and osteogenic sarcoma, a rare but deadly bone cancer.

Extensive clinical trials are currently being hampered by the limited availability and high cost of interferon. In 1980, the world supply was sufficient to treat only several hundred patients at a daily cost of $150 and up to $30,000 for an entire course of anticancer therapy. Unlike insulin and thyroid hormone, which are obtained for human use from animal sources, the protein interferon is *species-specific;* that is, it is only active in the species of animal that produces it. In 1979 virtually all interferon for clinical use was obtained from human blood, with the efficiency for isolation relatively low; 45,000 liters (90,000 pints) of blood were processed to obtain 400 mg.

Among the many different approaches being evaluated for the economical mass production of interferon are those employing the *recombinant DNA technique.* In this promising approach, the gene containing the code for human interferon is chemically spliced into the DNA of a common laboratory bacterium *Escherichia coli* which then begins to manufacture this protein. Each individual bacterium is capable of producing only a minute amount of interferon. Under favorable growth conditions, the bacterium will begin to actively proliferate carbon copies of itself, each containing an interferon gene, and resulting in a cumulative output of interferon that is potentially enormous.

The mechanism underlying the anticancer properties of interferon are not well understood but it has been shown to be effective against tumors caused by chemicals and radiation rather than viruses. Interferon inhibits the growth of both healthy and abnormal cells by slowing their rate of cell division. Unlike most available cytotoxic agents, interferon does not directly kill cancer cells but inhibits their ability to proliferate. Moreover, it differs from existing drugs in its ability to act on resting cells rather than those that are rapidly dividing (Figure 30-1).

The enthusiasm generated for interferon to date is predicated upon the hope that this natural compound, unlike most existing anticancer agents, will be *relatively nontoxic* and prove to be active against a *broad spectrum of cancers.* Moreover, there is reason to believe that it might be potentially useful in *preventing* the development of cancer in high-risk individuals.

CANCER CHEMOTHERAPY IN PERSPECTIVE

In the two previous chapters we have spoken about the *cure* of microbial infections. In this chapter infrequent references are made to curing cancer, but rather to reducing the symptoms and prolonging life. Surgery and radiation therapy are able to cure about one-third of all cancer patients, and perhaps as many as 50 percent if they are diagnosed at the earliest stages; these treatments are capable of eradicating localized tumors but are not useful once the cancer has metastasized to distant parts of the body. Unfortunately, cancer chemotherapeutic agents have not adequately filled the void. With the exception of the sex hormones, virtually all the compounds we have discussed are potentially toxic to the host, and while these drugs may temporarily extend the patient's life and cause a remission in the symptoms, their administration is generally associated with a high incidence of very adverse effects.

In general, anticancer drugs have been found to be most useful for the treatment of malignancies with a high proportion of replicating cells, in particular, the leukemias and lymphomas. The most common cancers are "solid" tumors (colon, rectum, lung, breast) that have a low proportion of dividing cells; unfortunately, these cancers are generally less responsive to treatment employing only drugs.

No significant advances have been made in the five-year survival rates for the most common solid tumors since the 1940s, with reductions in the mortality rates resulting primarily from a decrease in the incidence of that tumor type. Drug cures of choriocarcinoma, Wilms' tumor, and Burkitt's lymphoma give us cause for optimism, as do the two-fold increase in the five-year survival rate for Hodgkin's disease and chronic lymphocytic leukemia. With a better understanding of the differences between the biochemistry and physiology of normal and malignant cells, effective drugs with selective toxicity against the tumor can be designed.

SUMMARY

Cancer is the second leading cause of death in the United States, claiming over 350,000 victims per year. Tumors or neoplasms are new cells that are primarily characterized by uncontrolled growth. In contrast to benign tumors, malignant tumors (collectively termed cancer) actively invade the territorial boundaries of surrounding cells and are able to propagate in regions of the body far removed from their primary site of origin; this is termed metastasis. Since "cancer" is a general term referring to dozens of diseases sharing common characteristics, it appears highly unlikely that a single cure for cancer can be discovered.

Many chemicals, coal tars for example, radiation, and sex hormones have been implicated in the initiation and/or promotion of tumor growths in humans and animals. Viruses have been shown to cause cancer in plants and many species of lower animals, and it is highly likely that they play some role in human cancer as well.

In contrast to antimicrobial agents, anticancer drugs produce few authentic cures, cause relatively nonselective toxicity to both normal and malignant cells (except for hormones), have a narrow margin of safety; acquired resistance to the anticancer agent is common, the duration of therapy is prolonged, and the host defense mechanisms are generally weak.

Cytotoxic anticancer agents may inhibit cell replication at a specific phase in the cell cycle (cell cycle–specific agents such as the antimetabolites) or they may act at any phase in the cycle or on resting (noncycling) cells (cell cycle–nonspecific agents such as the alkylating agents and antitumor antibiotics).

Anticancer drugs include the following major classes: (1) alkylating agents (nitrogen mustards), general cell poisons that cause a cross-linking of DNA and thereby inhibit cellular multiplication; (2) antimetabolites which prevent nucleic acid synthesis by interfering with the metabolic function of folic acid, purines, and pyrimidines; (3) antibiotics, such as dactinomycin, which interfere with the normal activity of DNA; (4) steroid hormones, the most specific and least toxic class of anticancer agents, including the glucocortical steroids and the male and female sex hormones; and (5) L-asparaginase, interferon, and other miscellaneous drugs; the clinical effectiveness of laetrile remains controversial.

Thus far, successful chemotherapy of cancer has been limited, with authentic cures observed in only rare tumor types. In other cancers, such as leukemias and lymphomas, remission of symptoms and a lengthening of life is obtained. Safer, more effective drugs will be developed only after a better understanding of the fundamental biochemical differences between normal and neoplastic cells is acquired.

SUPPLEMENTARY READINGS

Bertino, J. R., and W. M. Hryniuk, "Disorders of Cell Growth," in *Clinical Pharmacology.* Edited by K. L. Melmon and H. F. Morrelli, 2nd ed., Chap. 15, pp. 802–41. New York: Macmillan, 1978.

Busch, H., and M. Lane, chairmen, "Symposium: Cancer Chemotherapy," *Federation Proceedings* **38:** 94–114 (1979).

Calabresi, P., and R. E. Parks, Jr., "Alkylating Agents, Antimetabolites, Hormones, and Other Antiproliferative Agents," in *Goodman and Gilman's The Pharmacological Basis of Therapeutics.* Edited by A. G. Gilman, L. S. Goodman, and A. Gilman, 6th ed., Sec. 13, pp. 1249–1313. New York: Macmillan, 1980.

Cline, M. J., and C. M. Haskell, *Cancer Chemotherapy.* 2nd ed. Philadelphia: Saunders, 1975.

DeVita, V. T., and P. S. Schein, "The Use of Drugs in Combination for the Treatment of Cancer," *New England Journal of Medicine* **288:** 998–1006 (1973).

Hickey, R. C., ed., *Pharmacological Basis of Cancer Chemotherapy.* Baltimore: Williams & Wilkins, 1975.

Holland, J. F., and E. Frei, III, eds., *Cancer Medicine.* Philadelphia: Lea & Febiger, 1973.

McGuire, W., P. Carbone, and E. Vollmer, eds., *Estrogen Receptors in Human Breast Cancer.* New York: Raven Press, 1975.

Oberfield, R. A., ed., "Symposium on Malignant Disease," *Medical Clinics of North America* **59** (2): 237–504 (1975).

Pratt, W. B., and R. W. Ruddon, *The Anticancer Drugs.* New York: Oxford University Press, 1979.

Sartorelli, A. C., and D. J. Johns, eds., *Antineoplastic and Immunosuppressive Agents.* Berlin: Springer-Verlag, 1975.

Stoll, B. A., ed., *Endocrine Therapy in Malignant Disease.* Philadelphia: Saunders, 1972.

Zimmerman, A. M., G. M. Padilla, and I. L. Cameron, eds., *Drugs and the Cell Cycle.* New York: Academic Press, 1973.

section eight ————————

Toxicology

31

Introduction
To Toxicology

All things are poisons, for there is nothing without poisonous qualities. It is only the dose which makes a thing a poison.

—Paracelsus (1493–1541)

She had never forgotten that, if you drink too much from a bottle marked "poison," it is almost certain to disagree with you, sooner or later.[1]

—Lewis Carroll (1865)

Only within the last ten millennia have humans evolved from food-gatherers to food-producers. During this earlier food-gathering period, our nomadic ancestors were obliged to satisfy their nutritive needs by empirically sampling a wide variety of unknown flora and fauna and, in so doing, became the first students of toxicology. The poorer students—those who failed to emulate the culinary examples of their feathered and four-legged neighbors or neglected to heed the wise counsel of their elders—became the unwitting earliest victims in this emerging science. Our most astute forebears employed some of these same newly discovered poisons for hunting, at the tips of spears and arrows for use in combat against other members of the species, as instruments in pursuit of the ancient profession of poisoner, and, in lower doses, as medicines to treat diseases. Industrialization, a phenomenon of more recent times, and associated with the intentional and unintentional production of many hundreds of thousands of new chemicals, has extended the number of potential victims from a poor soul sipping from a chalice of poisoned wine or standing at the distance of an archer's bow to the inhabitants of our entire planet.

Toxicology is the *study of the adverse actions of chemicals on biologic systems.* The commonly used terms *toxic* and *poison* are somewhat more

[1] From *Alice's Adventures in Wonderland.*

TABLE 31-1. CLASSIFICATION OF RELATIVE TOXICITY OF TOXIC SUBSTANCES

Term Denoting Relative Degree of Toxicity	Probable Oral Lethal Dose for 70 kg (150 lb) Person	
Super toxic	< 5 mg/kg	A taste; < 7 drops
Extremely toxic	5–50 mg/kg	7 drops–1 teaspoonful
Very toxic	50–500 mg/kg	1 teaspoonful–1 oz
Moderately toxic	0.5–5 g/kg	1 oz–1 pint
Slightly toxic	5–15 g/kg	1 pint–1 quart
Practically nontoxic	> 15 g	> 1 quart (2.2 lb)

Source: Adapted from R. E. Gosselin, H. C. Hodge, R. P. Smith, and M. N. Gleason, *Clinical Toxicology of Commercial Products,* 4th ed. (Baltimore: Williams & Wilkins, 1976), inside cover.

difficult to define in a simple and unambiguous manner. In the context of our discussion, *toxic* is considered to be synonymous with *harmful* or *adverse*. While certain chemicals are nonselective in their ability to exert adverse effects on all living matter, other chemicals are selectively toxic to certain species and, within a given species, may exert adverse actions on only specific cells.

Assuming that we have identified the living organism and the specific site of the adverse action, mere reference to the chemical as being "toxic" is still not informative unless we know the amount (dose or concentration) required to produce toxicity. Knowledge of dose permits us to assess the *relative toxicity* of different chemicals (Table 31–1). The semanticist will raise similar questions regarding use of the term *poison,* which is generally defined as any chemical that is capable of producing a harmful effect in biologic systems. *No chemical is completely safe if administered in sufficiently large doses or for an excessively prolonged period of time.* Hence, a meaningful definition of a poison must take into account the circumstances and conditions under which exposure to the chemical has occurred.

The final section of this text consists of two chapters dealing with different subjects of toxicological interest. In this chapter, an overview of toxicology will be presented in which we shall examine the scope of toxicology, the nature of adverse effects produced by chemicals (including but not limited to considerations of mutagenicity, carcinogenicity, teratology, drug idiosyncrasy and allergy), and the treatment of acute poisoning. In the next chapter, we shall consider nicotine and tobacco smoking, the latter having been categorized as "the largest preventable cause of death in America."

SCOPE OF TOXICOLOGY

The ever-expanding boundaries of toxicology include, but are not limited to, three primary branches: environmental, economic, and forensic toxicology (Table 31–2).

TABLE 31-2. BRANCHES OF TOXICOLOGY

Environmental toxicology
  Air, water, food pollutants
  Soil residues
  Industrial chemicals
Economic toxicology
  Therapeutic agents—humans, animals
  Food additives
  Cosmetics
  Pesticides, insecticides
  Herbicides
Forensic toxicology
  Medical aspects—diagnosis, treatment
  Legal aspects—cause-and-effect relationships

Environmental Toxicology

During our day-to-day living, we are all exposed to a countless number of potentially dangerous chemicals. The most obvious of these are chemicals taken *voluntarily,* whether to treat a disease, to induce changes in our behavior, or, in the female, to prevent conception from occurring. In addition, as members of a technically advanced society, we are often *involuntarily* exposed to some of the over one-half million chemicals manufactured and used in this country. Such compounds are present in the air, water, and food and on the job. For the purposes of our discusssion in this chapter, we shall restrict our consideration of *environmental toxicology* to chemicals to which we are *involuntarily exposed.*

Most of these compounds are not injurious to health at the levels of normal exposure. By contrast, acute exposure to higher concentrations of the same chemicals, or the subjection to them at lower concentrations for protracted periods of time, may have toxicological consequences. Among such consequences are a wide array of illnesses which may ultimately culminate in death. Other potential dangers include the induction of malignant tumors, malformations of the fetus during pregnancy, and adverse genetic changes that may first appear during the lifetimes of our descendants (see below).

When an environmental pollutant has been clearly demonstrated to produce adverse effects at *high* concentrations, should society establish a "zero tolerance" for this pollutant, that is, totally ban its use? This question is being currently debated with considerable vigor by environmentalists and scientists with respect to the use of certain insecticides, food and gasoline additives, and industrial waste products.

The desire to obtain zero is causing consternation in the minds of many engineers and scientists. When people speak of zero they apparently mean different things. And even in the case of scientific analysis, zero has changed. A few years ago analytical methods might have indicated the absence of a particular chemical in a test sample. Today, with better analytical methods, the same sample would show the particular chemical present; we no longer have the zero we had a few years ago.[2]

The informed student must attempt to balance the benefits such chemicals confer on society with the real and potential risks associated with their use. We have repeatedly observed the same benefit-to-risk concept throughout this book with respect to the rational and safe use of drugs.

Since 1970, the United States *Environmental Protection Agency* (EPA) has been responsible for establishing and enforcing environmental standards to combat pollution. In an attempt to improve the quality of the air, standards have been set for the following major air pollutants: total suspended particulate matter, sulfur dioxide, hydrocarbons, carbon monoxide, ozone, and lead. Pollution of the air is not only aesthetically distasteful but also exposes vast segments of the population to a variety of potentially harmful chemicals, many of which are known or strongly suspected to cause both acute and chronic adverse effects on health; individuals with histories of respiratory and cardiovascular diseases are particularly at risk. We shall illustrate the hazards of environmental pollution with a consideration of the heavy metals lead and mercury.

Heavy Metals: Lead and Mercury

In former times, heavy metals were held in high esteem as therapeutic agents. The now yellowed pages of old and ancient medical texts devote great attention to the use of arsenic for the treatment of syphilis and to mercury as a disinfectant, astringent, laxative, and diuretic. At times, however, the cure was worse than the disease!

Some heavy metals continue to retain a role in modern therapeutics, although their grasp becomes progressively weaker with the continuous introduction of newer drugs that are both more effective and less toxic. Representative examples of such metals include organic arsenic-containing compounds for the treatment of certain protozoan infections such as sleeping sickness and amebic dysentery; bismuth salts are incorporated in antidiarrheal mixtures (Pepto-Bismol); and gold is sometimes used for the treatment of rheumatoid arthritis. Our interest in heavy metals is not predicated upon their limited therapeutic uses but rather upon their toxicological effects. In particular, we shall consider lead and mercury and their importance as environmental toxicants.

Lead poisoning.   Although lead ceased to be used in therapeutics several centuries ago, the nerve damage and death caused by lead poisoning remains a contemporary problem. Lead enters our body in food, water, and air, all of which are contaminated by leaded gasolines and industrial activity. The inclusion of tetraethyllead and chemically related antiknock additives to gasolines was formerly responsible for the annual deposition of 180,000 tons of lead into American air. Among the victims of such lead-contaminated air were animals

[2]Mitchell H. Bradley, "Zero—What Does It Mean?" *Science* **208**: 7 (1980).

residing in two New York City zoos. At the Staten Island Zoo, profound muscle weakness and the subsequent death of a leopard and several snakes were attributed to lead poisoning.

Leaded paints have been associated with lead poisoning in young children since the mid-1920s. Some children, most of whom are six years of age or younger, mouth, chew, or even eat paint chips or plaster. While the inclusion of lead salts to provide pigments to indoor paints has been condemned or even banned by all states, many old dwellings, primarily in urban slum areas, still have such flaking paint on their walls; lead-containing exterior paints continue to be widely used and remain a source of this metal for children with appetites for unnatural substances (pica). Ingestion of toys, crayons, telephone wires, and putty have also been implicated as causes of lead poisoning in children. More recently, the leaded glaze on pottery eating utensils has been recognized as a hazard.

There is no evidence to suggest that lead is an essential trace metal required in human metabolism, nor does the presence of this metal confer any benefit on the body. Under normal conditions, the amount of lead eliminated in exhaled air, urine, and the feces is equal to those quantities entering the body in the food, water, and air. Over 90 percent of the lead that does accumulate in the body is stored, without causing harm, in bones. At times of physiological stress, including severe injury, infection, or pregnancy, lead may be released from bones and enter the blood stream.

Exposure to massive amounts of lead, most commonly by inhalation of dusts and fumes, may result in acute lead poisoning; however, this is a relatively rare occurrence. *Chronic lead poisoning* does constitute a major problem and affects the blood, nervous system, and gastrointestinal tract. Symptoms of lead poisoning include anemia (a reduction in red blood cells), muscle weakness, *lead encephalopathy* (irritability, insomnia, and in advanced stages confusion, delirium, convulsions, and coma), and severe intestinal spasms, termed "lead colic."

In the absence of proper medical treatment, severe lead encephalopathy has a mortality rate of about 65 percent, with survivors often afflicted with brain damage, causing loss of muscle coordination and mental retardation. Ethylenediaminetetraacetic acid (EDTA), a chelating agent (Chapter 2 and below), is used for the treatment of lead poisoning. This compound removes lead from bones and forms a soluble EDTA-lead complex which is excreted from the body.

Some cases of chronic lead poisoning in children are *asymptomatic* or are characterized by mild and relatively nonspecific symptoms such as restlessness, short attention span, easy distractibility, crying, temper tantrums, and listlessness. Such a child may have behavioral problems in school and, on the basis of the first three symptoms, may be erroneously labeled by teachers as a hyperkinetic child (Chapter 15). While "normal" blood levels of lead are about 0.02 mg/100 ml, these children frequently have concentrations of lead in their blood two to three times as high, while not manifesting obvious signs of lead poisoning. The magnitude of this problem is illustrated by the results obtained in mass screening programs conducted in recent years in low socioeconomic urban neighborhoods of large cities. Among several hundred thousand children tested, 20 to 30 percent were found to have blood levels of lead in excess of 0.04 mg/100 ml.

Mercury poisoning. One of the less publicized results of Columbus's voyages to the New World was the introduction of syphilis into Europe during the 1490s. However, another school of thought vigorously contends that the Europeans were responsible for bringing syphilis to the New World. Mercury was found to be a useful chemotherapeutic agent and retained its preeminent position as the drug of choice for the treatment of syphilis until 1910 when Ehrlich's arsenical, Salvarsan, became clinically available. At present, mercury-containing compounds are used as antiseptics (Merthiolate, Mercurochrome) and in selected cases as diuretic agents (Chapter 21). In this section we shall consider the toxicological consequences of environmental pollution by mercury.

Mercury is principally obtained for commercial purposes from cinnabar ore, which is mercury sulfide. Vapors of mercury are naturally released into the air from the ore, with atmospheric contamination also resulting from the mining, refining, and smelting processes. Combustion of coal and petroleum products gives rise to mercury in amounts thought to approximate the natural runoff from lands into rivers and streams. The greatest commercial applications of mercury are in the production of chlorine and caustic soda, in the manufacture of electrical equipment, and in the paper and pulp industries. Mercury-containing wastes from these plants were, until recently, freely deposited in waterways. Some sources contend that, with the exception of coastal regions, human activities have only elevated the concentrations of mercury in the sea by 1 percent.

Toxicologically, mercury compounds may be categorized as being either inorganic or organic in nature. Inorganic refers to mercury present as the free metal, such as in a thermometer, or in the ionic state as a salt, for example, mercury chloride or nitrate. Inhalation of vapors of metallic mercury is primarily toxic to the central nervous system, while ingestion of inorganic mercury salts damages the kidneys.

$$Hg^0 \qquad HgCl_2 \qquad CH_3-Hg^+ \qquad CH_3-Hg-CH_3$$
Free Metal   Mercury Chloride   Methylmercury   Dimethylmercury

INORGANIC   ORGANIC

Organic compounds are those in which mercury is bound covalently to at least one other carbon atom. These include *methylmercury* and dimethylmercury, collectively referred to as alkylmercury. While some organic mercury compounds are stable, others break down in the body into inorganic mercury products. Conversely, many living organisms are able to convert inorganic mercury into methylmercury. Inorganic or phenylmercury compounds are rapidly removed from the body while methylmercury remains for longer periods of time. Methylmercury is concentrated in the biological food chains from diatoms (algae) to small fish to large marine animals including swordfish and tuna, where mercury contents may be 20 to 50 times in excess of present allowable limits in the United States.

Attention has been focused upon the dangers of ingesting methylmercury-contaminated fish and shellfish. Two separate outbreaks of methylmercury poisoning have been reported in Japan: one in Minimata Bay caused 121 cases of poisoning with 46 deaths, while the second, in Niigata in 1964–1965 claimed 72 individuals and 6 fatalities. In 1969, three members of a New Mexican family of nine were poisoned and suffered severe brain damage after eating a hog that was fed on grain containing methylmercury.

Symptoms of methylmercury poisoning, which do not often appear until weeks after ingestion of the contaminated food, include incoordination, marked deterioration of intellect, and loss of vision and hearing. Among the victims of the Minimata Bay disaster were 23 children (out of a total of 359) who were born of apparently healthy mothers. At birth, or shortly thereafter, these young children developed cerebral palsy-like symptoms (incoordination, spasticity, seizures and marked intellectual retardation) with death occurring in some cases. Poisoning of these infants is thought to have been caused by the passage of methylmercury across the placental barrier during pregnancy. Chelating agents are useful for the treatment of inorganic mercury poisoning, but have proved far less satisfactory in methylmercury toxicity.

Economic Toxicology

Economic toxicology concerns itself with the harmful effects of chemicals *intentionally* administered to living organisms to product a specified effect. Such chemicals include therapeutic agents employed in human and veterinary medical practice; food additives, cosmetics, and hair colorings; insecticides, pesticides, and herbicides, compounds employed by humans to specifically eliminate an undesirable species (at least from the perspective of *Homo sapiens*).

Many examples of the adverse effects of chemicals used as therapeutic agents appear throughout this book. As will be discussed below, some of these adverse effects are normal and to be anticipated when a given class of drugs is administered, while other adverse effects are unanticipated or abnormal. We shall consider food additives below; insecticides were previously discussed in Chapter 7.

Food Additives

The addition of spices, colors, and preservatives to foods dates back to ancient times. Then, as now, the skillful inclusion of flavoring and seasoning agents to foods often spells the difference between mere nourishment and a gourmet's delight. *Additives* are substances lacking in nutritive value that are primarily employed to modify the flavor of the foods, impart color, prevent spoilage, or improve texture.

Two fundamental questions have been asked with increasing frequency in recent years: Are these additives really essential? and, if so, Are these compounds devoid of potential danger to the consumer? In this country, the Food and Drug Administration has established a list of about 600 approved additives that are "generally recognized as being safe," commonly referred to as GRAS compounds.[3]

To test the safety of food additives, animals are fed very large amounts of the additive, quantities far in excess of those intended to be used in foods. Acute and chronic studies are designed to determine whether the additive adversely modifies growth rate, body function, and reproduction, as well as whether or not it induces tumors. The largest dose that results in no undesirable effects in animals is then reduced one hundredfold, and it is arbitrarily assumed that this amount, obtained from all dietary sources, can be safely consumed by a human on a daily basis for an entire lifetime.

The Delaney Amendment of the Food, Drug, and Cosmetic Act of 1958 sets a further important limitation; it prohibits the addition of any substance to foods, in *any* quantity, that has been shown to produce cancer in animals, regardless of the dosage employed to induce tumor growth. Critics of this amendment contend that because it is written in such unequivocal terms, no option is available for the exercise of good scientific judgment. In passing, it should be observed that there is little agreement among nations concerning the criteria of a safe food additive.

Over 2000 substances are used for more than 40 functions as food additives throughout the world. We shall briefly consider some relevant examples of additives that are or have been employed as flavors, colors, and preservatives, and we shall attempt to emphasize the problems associated with their use.

Flavors.   Approximately one-half of all food additives are flavors, and these are obtained from both natural and synthetic sources. Flavors are widely used in soft drinks, desserts, preserves, in medicines to mask bitter and other unpleasant tastes, and in simulated "meat" products that consist of vegetable ingredients. The controversy regarding the relative safety of the *artificial sweeteners* has spilled out of the laboratory and clinic and into the halls of the United States Congress.

> Thus, decisions concerning saccharin and other low-level exposures to other potentially hazardous substances can seldom be based on unequivocal scientific evidence. Those who make the decisions must reach beyond the available scientific base to what appears to be most prudent. Opinions on what is prudent are more numerous

[3] The annual per capita consumption of food additives in the United States is 3.5 lb.

than opinions on what is good science; it is this fact, not the quality of the scientific base, that explains much of the seemingly endless controversies over these issues.[4]

Saccharin is 500 times sweeter than sugar, yet contains no calories. Although many clinicians recommend its use as an adjunct in the treatment of diabetes, obesity, and tooth decay, the health benefits of this artificial sweetener have not been clearly established. Saccharin was introduced at the turn of the century but did not enjoy widespread popularity until the 1960s.[5] Storm clouds appeared in 1977 after the publication of a Canadian report demonstrating that large doses of saccharin (extrapolated to be in excess of the amount a human would receive drinking 800 containers of diet soda daily) caused bladder cancer in rats. Yielding to public pressure and extensive lobbying efforts by the diet food industry, the United States Congress blocked action by the Food and Drug Administration to enforce provisions of the Delaney amendment and remove saccharin from the market pending further assessment of the carcinogenic potential of this compound. Subsequent clinical studies have failed to support the conclusion that the use of saccharin is associated with an increase in the incidence of bladder cancer or other cancers in the general population. There are some indications, however, that persons who are both heavy cigarette smokers and heavy saccharin users may be at greater risk. Many responsible scientists and clinicians share the view that while saccharin may not pose an immediate threat to our health, the possibility that this compound is a weak carcinogen cannot be discounted. It would appear prudent to suggest that saccharin use by nondiabetic children and pregnant women and heavy use by other members of the general population should be strongly discouraged.

Colors. Our selection of foods at the market is often strongly influenced by an attractive color, and the color of certain foods also enhances our appreciation of their flavor. In addition to being safe, a suitable color must not deteriorate with prolonged storage or as a consequence of cooking. Notwithstanding the expansion of international commerce, no single dye is officially approved as being safe by all nations of the world. A number of dyes have been removed from the market over the years because of toxicity, or carcinogenic potential, among these butter yellow. Amaranth or *FDC Red No. 2* was formerly the most extensively used dye in the United States employed to color meats, fruits, salad dressings, jellies, soft drinks, lipsticks and other cosmetics, and liquid medications. The Food and Drug Administration banned its use in 1973 after receiving the results of animal studies suggesting that high levels of this dye may cause cancer and an increase in early fetal deaths.

[4] Robert Hoover, "Saccharin—Bitter Aftertaste," *New England Journal of Medicine* **302**: 573–74 (1980).

[5] Unlike saccharin, *cyclamate* has no bitter aftertaste and is stable in heat making it useful in cooking. It was withdrawn from the market in 1969 after being shown to produce bladder cancer in rats fed very high doses.

Preservatives. A large number of antimicrobial agents are used to prevent food spoilage by microorganisms. Mold growth in breads is retarded by sodium diacetate, monocalcium phosphate, and several propionate salts; sorbic acid and its salts prevent mold growth in cheese, syrups, and fruits; benzoic acid and sodium benzoate are preservatives in margarine, juices, and fruit juice concentrates; sulfur dioxide inhibits mold growth and deterioration in wines and fruit drinks; and, antioxidants prevent unsaturated fats and oils from becoming rancid. Although certain antibiotics are useful in preserving fish, meat, poultry, cheese, and bananas, their use as preservatives has been forbidden in the United States and many other countries because of the danger of human allergy and the emergence of resistant strains of microbes (Chapter 28).

Sodium nitrite is widely used as a preservative in meat, fish, and cheese and also in curing mixtures to fix the red color in frankfurters, sausages, and hams. The use of this compound as a food additive is currently being reviewed in many countries because of the possibility that, in the digestive tract, nitrites are converted to nitrosamines, potent carcinogenic and mutagenic agents.

$NaNO_2$

Sodium Nitrite   **Dimethylnitrosamine**

In conclusion, it would appear that safe food additives have had a very beneficial role by both increasing our food supply and enhancing the eye appeal and flavor of the foods that appear on our dinner plates. It is obviously incumbent upon manufacturers and the government to insure that such additives do not constitute a hazard to our health nor mislead us as to the quality of the foodstuffs purchased.

Forensic Toxicology

We shall never fully realize the historical scope of man's preoccupation with poison. Until a few centuries ago, fear of it was as common as today's dread of approaching baldness or the atomic bomb. . . . Elaborate precautions to escape being given a deadly potion were daily hygienic tasks. Petty jealousies, neighborhood quarrels, old hates, political intrigues, and family disagreements—all were too often reputedly solved by a deadly powder or draught.[6]

—Richard R. Mathison (1958)

"Always an awkward business, a poisoning case. Conflicting testimony of the experts—then doctors are usually so extremely cautious in what they say. Always a difficult case to take to the jury. No, if one must have murder . . . give me a straight-forward case. Something where there's no ambiguity about the cause of death."[7]

—Agatha Christie (1939)

[6]*The Eternal Search* (New York: Putnam's), p. 141.
[7]*Murder For Christmas* (New York: Dodd, Mead), p. 78.

Forensic toxicology deals with the *medical and legal aspects* of the adverse effects of chemicals on human subjects. The medical aspects are concerned with the diagnosis and treatment of poisoning, while the legal components attempt to determine whether a cause and effect relationship exists between exposure to the chemical and the adverse effects of that chemical. Accidental, homicidal, and suicidal exposure to chemicals all fall within the purview of forensic toxicology. In 1977, of the 43,316 cases of poisoning reported to involve individuals over 5 years of age, 41.5 percent were ascribed to successful or unsuccessful suicide attempts (see below).

ADVERSE EFFECTS CAUSED BY CHEMICALS AND DRUGS

The undesirable or adverse effects of chemicals and drugs can be subdivided into two general categories, namely, those that may be anticipated and those that are unanticipated.

Anticipated adverse effects resulting from the known pharmacological properties of the drug are normal and may be predicted prior to their occurrence. While anatomical, physiological, and/or biochemical differences between species and among members of the same species may account for individual differences in susceptibility to these adverse effects, all drugs are capable of producing *toxicity* in all members of a given species if sufficiently high doses are administered. The intensity of these adverse effects is generally directly proportional to the dose or concentration of the toxic chemical to which the victim is exposed. An inverse relationship commonly exists between the dose of the toxic chemical and the onset of the adverse reaction; that is, the higher the dose, the shorter the time required for the appearance of toxicity. As will be noted below, anticipated adverse effects may be nonselective or selective and may, in some instances, result in a mutagenic, carcinogenic, or teratogenic response.

Some adverse effects are *unanticipated* and could not be reasonably predicted based upon our knowledge of the drug nor upon the results of toxicity studies previously conducted in animals or human subjects. As will be noted below, *idiosyncratic reactions* are related to the genetic characteristics of the individual, while *drug allergies* arise as a consequence of antigen-antibody reactions.

Nonselective and Selective Toxicity

Nonselectively toxic chemicals produce their harmful effects at the site of initial exposure with the body, usually with the skin or respiratory tract. Examples of such chemicals include strong inorganic acids or bases that produce chemical burns on the surface of the skin; ammonia gas, which, when inhaled in high concentrations, can produce corrosive effects in the respiratory tract after its conversion to ammonium hydroxide; sulfur dioxide and nitrogen hydroxide, atmospheric pollutants in smog that cause lung damage after being converted to acids in the body.

Some chemicals produce nonselective systemic toxicity by interfering with functions that are essential for the viability of the cell. Compounds that impede the ability of the cell to carry out fundamental biochemical reactions, produce energy, utilize oxygen, or reproduce are referred to as *cytotoxic poisons;* examples of such chemicals include cyanide, the heavy metal arsenic, and many anticancer drugs.

In contrast to the contact or systemic nonselective chemicals, most of the therapeutic agents that were considered in the earlier pages of this text are relatively *selective* in their ability to cause toxic effects when administered at usual doses. These toxic effects primarily involve individual organs and can often be attributed to interactions with specific receptor types or to inhibition of enzymes. Examples of selectively toxic compounds include botulinum toxin causing muscle weakness and paralysis by inhibiting the release of acetylcholine from motor nerves; aminoglycoside antibiotics producing kidney toxicity and impairment of hearing and balance; and digitalis glycosides causing irregularities in the formation and conduction of electrical impulses in the heart.

Chemical Mutagenesis, Carcinogenesis, and Teratogenesis

Increasing emphasis has been directed in recent years toward assessing the mutagenic, carcinogenic, and teratogenic potential of drugs and environmental chemicals. The mechanisms underlying these potential hazards are complex and incompletely understood but are thought to result from toxic effects at the subcellular or molecular level.

Chemical Mutagenesis

Mutagenesis refers to a permanent alteration of the inherited genetic material (DNA of chromosomes) in the germ cell of the male (sperm) or female (ovum). Incorporation of a defective chromosome will produce a persisting change in the germ line of the species unless, of course, the alteration is incompatible with the survival of the individual.

Radiation and chemical agents have been demonstrated to produce mutations in living organisms. While many chemicals have been shown to cause mutations in animals and tissue cultures, no chemical has been demonstrated to be mutagenic in humans. In most cases, the chemically induced mutation is silent; that is, it is not expressed nor does it cause harm to the offspring. Among the chemicals found to be mutagenic under laboratory conditions are alkylating agents used for the treatment of cancer, sodium nitrite employed as a food preservative, caffeine, and certain fungicides.

Chemical Carcinogenesis

Eighty percent of all cancers have been postulated to be directly or indirectly caused by environmental chemicals present in the air, food, and water. As is true with other pharmacological and toxicological chemicals, the individual response to a chemical carcinogen varies with the species, strain, sex, and age of the animal and may be modified (intensified or antagonized) by other drugs and chemicals to which the individual is exposed.

By contrast, chemical carcinogens differ from other toxic agents in the following ways: (1) their action is generally irreversible; (2) although producing no apparent effect, single exposures to a chemical carcinogen act in an additive manner; and (3) synergistic effects with other carcinogenic and/or noncarcinogenic factors (such as diet) in the environment appear to be significant in human carcinogenesis.

Chemical carcinogenesis is thought to involve two separate processes, namely, initiation and promotion. *Initiation* entails the production of an irreversible cellular change; taken alone, this process is insufficient for the production of cancer. Tumor cells, unlike their normal cells of origin, lack the fundamental property of *contact inhibition,* that is, the capacity of a cell to cease dividing once it has come into contact with another cell. It has been suggested that during the initiation process the carcinogenic agent induces a permanent mutation in the chromosome of the cell causing a loss in a contact inhibitory protein; this concept is termed the *somatic mutation hypothesis. Promotion* is the process whereby a tumor develops in a tissue in which initiation has previously occurred. While some chemicals appear to have little or no carcinogenic activity themselves, they are capable of significantly enhancing or promoting the effects of carcinogens; such compounds are termed *cocarcinogens.* Table 31–3 lists representative common drugs and chemicals believed to possess strong carcinogenic potential.

As noted above, chemical carcinogens differ from most toxicological agents in the *temporal relationship* between the time of exposure and onset of the adverse effect. Drugs and other toxic chemicals exert their adverse effects very soon after administration, with the intensity of these effects progressively diminishing as the chemical is metabolized and eliminated from the body. By contrast, exposure to a chemical carcinogen may result in a chromosomal mutation, the visible and/or functional consequences of which may not be evident until after many multiplications of the initially mutated cell and its progeny. Hence, malignant cells may only make their appearance many months or even years after the initiation of the carcinogenesis process.

Under experimental conditions, increasing doses of the carcinogenic chemical increase the yield of the tumor and decrease the time required for its development. Moreover, in theory, exposure on only a single occasion to extremely small amounts of a carcinogenic chemical is capable of triggering the carcinogenesis process by inducing a single mutation in a single cell. For this

TABLE 31-3. SELECTED ESTABLISHED OR SUSPECTED HUMAN CARCINOGENIC DRUGS AND CHEMICALS

Drug/Class (Example)	Use/Source	Type of Cancer
Aflotoxin	Peanut contaminant	Liver
Alkylating agents (cyclophosphamide)	Anticancer drugs	Liver, urinary bladder
Aromatic amines (naphthylamine)	Dye industry	Urinary bladder
Arsenic	Industrial Medicines (Fowler's Solution)	Skin
Asbestos	Industrial	Lungs
Azo dyes ("butter yellow")	Food coloring	Liver, urinary bladder
Benzene	Industrial solvent and chemical	Leukemia
Carbon tetrachloride	Solvent	Liver
Diethylstilbestrol	Threatened abortion	Genital tract
Immunosuppressants (azathioprine)	Prevent rejection of tissue transplants	Leukemia
Nitrosamines (sodium nitrite)	Food preservative	Widespread throughout body
Phenacetin	Analgesic	Kidney (renal pelvis)
Polycyclic aromatic hydrocarbons (benzo(a)pyrene)	Tars—paving roads Tobacco & exhaust smoke	Skin Lungs
Polyvinyl chloride	Plastic industry	Liver
Safrole	Sassafras tea	Liver

reason, some individuals have argued that carcinogenic compounds should be *totally* removed from the environment.

Chemical Teratogenesis

Teratology literally denotes "the study of monsters"; the ancient Egyptians and Romans disposed of deformed infants (whom they perceived to be monsters) and their parents. A *chemical teratogen* is a chemical which, when administered to a pregnant female, induces structural and/or functional abnormalities in the fetus or newborn. The incidence of severe malformations in humans is about 3 percent; by one year of age, the incidence rises to 6–7 percent when some conditions, such as functional abnormalities, are first detected.[8]

The fetus is variably susceptible to the teratogenic effects of chemicals and physical factors during the three primary stages of gestation : (1) *Blastogenesis:* days 1 to 10 of pregnancy, when cells of the fertilized ovum repeatedly divide

[8] Not all teratogenic changes can be attributed to chemicals; physical teratogens include radiation (the most potent teratogen) and pressure. Furthermore, not all fetal abnormalities are teratogenic; some result from drug toxicity.

without differentiating. During this stage, chemicals can kill the blastula. (2) *Embryogenesis (organogenesis)*: days 10 to 60 of pregnancy, when cellular differentiation and organ development occur. This is the stage of greatest teratogenic sensitivity. Since organs and bodily structures are formed at different rates, exposure of the fetus to teratogens at different times during this stage cause dissimilar types of abnormalities. In humans, primary structural development of the nervous system occurs between days 15 and 25 of gestation; the heart, from days 20 to 40; the eyes, from days 24 to 40; and the arms and legs, from days 24 to 46. Thalidomide interference with limb development is primarily a hazard if this drug is administered during the second month of pregnancy, while rubella (German measles) induces malformations of the heart and eyes primarily between the fourth through the eighth weeks of gestation. (3) *Fetogenesis:* days 60 to parturition, when organs mature in size and function. Exposure to teratogens at this stage causes little structural damage but might be expected to interfere with function.

During the *postnatal period,* the central nervous system continues to functionally mature. Administration of an antithyroid drug during pregnancy or to a nursing mother can depress the thyroid function of the newborn, a condition which, if not diagnosed and treated at an early stage, can cause irreversible impairment of central nervous system function including mental retardation; this represents a classical example of *behavioral teratology.*

A number of generalizations can be made regarding chemical teratogenesis. The teratogenic risk associated with a drug cannot be safely predicted on the basis of its relative or absolute acute or chronic toxicity to children or adults. The judicious pregnant woman assumes that all drugs are potential teratogens and takes only those expressly prescribed by her physician that are *essential* for her health and well-being. While the incidence of malformations is proportional to the dose of some teratogens, an all-or-none response may be observed—that is, a single dose of certain drugs (such as thalidomide) taken at critical times during gestation is capable of producing pronounced malformations.

Table 31–4 summarizes chemicals known or strongly suspected to cause human teratogenesis. While this list is relatively short, a rather extensive number of chemicals (including many therapeutically useful drugs) have been shown to produce malformations in laboratory animals. Unfortunately, no single species of common laboratory animal is a perfect model for human teratogenesis. The ideal animal model must be capable of metabolizing all drugs and chemicals in a manner that is identical to that of humans and, as well, must have a placenta that is anatomically the same as the human female.

Unanticipated Drug Effects: Drug Idiosyncrasy and Allergy

As noted above, the *toxic* effects of drugs are associated with their therapeutic actions (and are, therefore, predictable) and are observed in all individuals exposed to a sufficiently large dose. By contrast, *idiosyncratic* and

TABLE 31-4. SELECTED ESTABLISHED AND SUSPECTED HUMAN CHEMICAL TERATOGENS

Drug/Class	Therapeutic Use(s)	Primary Types of Teratogenesis
Alcohol	Alcoholic beverages	Fetal alcohol syndrome (Chapter 12)
Androgens Anabolic steroids	Gynecological disorders and cancer in women; wasting diseases	Masculinization of external genitalia of female offspring

Anticancer agents
  Alkylating agents
  Antimetabolites
	Cancer chemotherapy	Widespread defects; very high incidence of teratogenesis

Anticoagulants (warfarin)	Retard blood clotting	Eye and nose defects
Anticonvulsants (phenytoin)	Epilepsy	Mental retardation, heart defects, cleft palate
Antithyroid agents Radioiodine	Diagnosis or therapy of thyroid disorders	Cretinism and mental retardation
Propylthiouracil	Treatment of hyper-thyroidism	
Estrogens (diethylstilbestrol)	Threatened abortion	Females: no menstrual cycle at puberty Males: defects in genital organs
Glucocorticoids (dexamethasone)	Anti-inflammatory disorders	Cleft palate
Meclizine	Motion sickness	Bone deformities
Oxygen	Premature infants	Blindness (at O_2 concentrations $> 40\%$)
Progestins	Component of oral contraceptives	Heart and limb defects
Tetracyclines	Antimicrobial chemotherapy	Yellow-brown discoloration of teeth
Thalidomide	Insomnia	Limb defects (phocomelia)
Vitamin D	Prevention or treatment vitamin deficiencies	Bone deformities

allergic responses to drugs are not caused by the typical pharmacological effects of drugs and occur only in a limited number of individuals rather than the entire population. The comparative characteristics of these three types of adverse drug reactions appear in Table 31–5. The incidence of these unpredictable adverse drug effects is comparatively low, and the relative number of drugs implicated in such reactions is small.

Drug Idiosyncrasy

A drug idiosyncrasy refers to a *genetically* determined abnormal response to a drug. This unusual response, observed at normal doses, may be manifested by a marked increase or decrease in the time course or intensity of drug action or may represent a totally novel drug response. A variety of mechanisms have been shown to underlie idiosyncratic drug reactions.

TABLE 31-5. COMPARISON OF ADVERSE DRUG REACTIONS RESULTING FROM TOXICITY, IDIOSYNCRASY, AND ALLERGY

	Toxicity	Idiosyncrasy	Allergy
In which individuals and with which drugs?	In all persons with sufficiently high concentrations of all drugs	In genetically susceptible persons and to a specific drug or class	Dependent upon the drug and the individual: mephenytoin: 90%, penicillin: 5-10%, caffeine: 0%
Influence of dose	Direct relationship	Extreme sensitivity to low dose, or great resistance to high dose, or unusual reaction to any dose	May occur at any dose
Is prior exposure to drug necessary?	No	No	Essential
Structure and specificity of drug	Adverse reaction determined by structure of drug; changes in chemical structure of the drug modify intensity of toxicity.	Adverse reaction determined by structure of drug; changes in chemical structure of the drug modify intensity and frequency of idiosyncrasy.	Adverse reaction results from antigen-antibody reaction after release of mediator substance. Chemically related drugs are capable of serving as antigens and provoking antigen-antibody reaction.
Basis underlying treatment of adverse drug reaction	Use antagonist of drug.	Use antagonist of drug.	Antagonize the effects of the mediator substance. Use of an antagonist to the antigenic drug after the occurrence of the antigen-antibody reaction would be ineffective.
Common drug examples	Heroin Barbiturates Alcohol Strychnine	Succinylcholine Isoniazid (INH) Primaquine Barbiturates	Penicillin Aspirin Sulfonamides

Abnormalities in drug-metabolizing enzymes. The very brief duration of action of the skeletal muscle relaxant succinylcholine has been attributed to its rapid inactivation by the plasma cholinesterase enzyme. In 1 of 3000 individuals, normal doses produce profound muscle relaxation and respiratory impairment of several hours in duration. This idiosyncratic reaction has been ascribed to a genetically determined trait resulting from the presence of an abnormal plasma cholinesterase possessing decreased activity.

The antitubercular drug isoniazid (INH) is inactivated after its biotransformation to an acetylated metabolite (Chapter 3). While some members of the population are "rapid inactivators" of this drug, others are classified as "slow inactivators." The latter group has been shown to have reduced quantities of this acetylation enzyme, and, when administered normal doses, is more susceptible than normal to drug-induced nerve toxicity. While approximately one-half of American whites and blacks are "slow inactivators," this genetically determined trait is seen in only 5 percent of Eskimos.

Abnormalities in enzymes unrelated to drug metabolism. The enzyme glucose-6-phosphate dehydrogenase participates in maintaining the integrity of the red blood cell membrane. In susceptible persons, administration of normal doses of the antimalarial drugs primaquine and quinine, as well as aspirin, phenacetin, and the sulfonamides, causes the breakdown (hemolysis) of a large number of erythrocytes resulting in hemolytic anemia; no similar response is observed in normal individuals even after receiving very large doses of these drugs. This male sex-linked trait is most common in blacks and Mediterraneans.

Other abnormalities. Other idiosyncratic reactions have been attributed to abnormalities in (1) *absorption*—inadequate absorption of vitamin B_{12} results in pernicious anemia; (2) *distribution*—Wilson's disease, the symptoms of which result from excessive distribution and deposition of free copper ions in the liver and brain; and (3) *sensory receptors*—decreased sensitivity of receptors mediating the senses of taste (for example, to detect phenylthiourea, an extremely bitter substance) and smell.

Drug Allergy

The term *allergy* refers to an exaggerated susceptibility to a substance resulting from an *antigen-antibody reaction;* the mechanism underlying allergic reactions has been previously described (Chapter 27). Prior exposure to the offending drug (antigenic agent) is essential for an allergic response to occur, with the nature and intensity of the response independent of the dose of the drug.

The incidence of allergic reactions to a given drug varies from none (caffeine) to virtually 100 percent (phenylethylhydantoin, an experimental antiepileptic agent). The incidence of allergic reactions to aspirin is 0.2 percent in the general population but may be as high as 20 percent in patients with a history of allergic disorders or bronchial asthma. The highest incidence of allergic reactions to a common drug is observed with penicillin (5–10 percent of the adult population).

The symptoms of a drug-induced allergic response may vary in severity from itching and hives to an anaphylactic-type reaction which may rapidly cause death resulting from circulatory collapse or respiratory failure.

ACUTE POISONING

> *Poisoning is now the most common medical emergency among young children: child deaths from poisoning exceed those from poliomyelitis, measles, scarlet fever, and diphtheria combined. Children, who learn by exploration, questioning, sampling, and trial and error, are constantly exposed to more than a quarter million products and to myriads of drugs now available and often present in the home.*[9]
>
> —Jay M. Arena (1979)

Each year several million persons are accidentally or intentionally poisoned in the United States, and for approximately 1 of every 200 of these, the outcome will be fatal. Official tabulations[10] contain only an estimated one-tenth of the actual number of poisonings. Of the 43,316 poisoning cases reported for 1977 involving individuals over 5 years of age (Table 31–6), 41.5 percent were suicide attempts, 7.3 percent involved drug or substance abuse, and 23 percent of the total required hospitalization.

Sixty-one percent of the poisoning cases reported in 1977 involved children under the age of 5 years. Examination of the trends in poisoning in this age group reveals an increase in reports involving poisonous plants (176 percent increase from 1972 to 1977, Table 31–7) and a very significant decrease in aspirin poisonings; aspirin was implicated in about 25 percent of all poisoning cases in 1966 and only 3.4 percent in 1977. Credit for this substantial turn-around may be attributed to improvements in the design and the extensive use of childproof containers, and to government and private health groups promoting public awareness of the potential dangers of storing drugs and other household chemicals within the reach of children. The time for self-approbation has not yet arrived! Since 72 percent of all reported poisoning cases in 1977 (across all age categories) were said to have resulted under accidental circumstances, considerable room remains for improving the public's often cavalier attitude about the relative safety of plants, drugs, and household chemicals.

---

[9] *Poisoning,* 4th ed. (Springfield, Ill.: Charles C Thomas), p. 3.

[10] Reports to the National Clearinghouse for Poison Control Centers are voluntarily submitted, and do not include patients advised or treated by private physicians or hospitals not associated with poison control centers. Of the total of 156,330 reports received in 1977, 94,949 involved patients under 5 years of age, and 43,316 involved patients 5-years-old and older; the ages were unspecified in 18,065 reports.

TABLE 31-6. FREQUENCY OF ACCIDENTAL INGESTION OF SUBSTANCES IN 1977

Type of Substance	Total Cases—All Ages		Under 5 Years of Age	
	Number	Percent	Number	Percent
Medicine*	73,317	46.9	36,859	38.8
Internal†	61,413	83.8	27,422	74.4
Aspirin	4,790	7.8	3,264	11.9
Other	56,623	92.2	24,158	88.1
External	11,904	16.2	9,437	25.6
Cleaning and polishing agents	17,990	11.5	14,050	14.8
Plants and plant substances	16,288	10.4	12,875	13.6
Cosmetics	11,594	7.4	10,375	10.9
Pesticides	9,099	5.8	5,316	5.6
Turpentine, paints, etc.	5,881	3.8	4,310	4.5
Petroleum products	4,648	3.0	2,948	3.1
Gases and vapors	1,895	1.2	107	0.1
Miscellaneous or unknown	15,613	10.0	8,105	8.5
Total of all categories	156,330	100.0	94,949	100.0

Source: Individual poison reports submitted to National Clearinghouse for Poison Control Centers by 340 centers in 42 states, the District of Columbia, Canal Zone, and military bases abroad. *Bulletin of National Clearinghouse for Poison Control Centers* 24 (4): 18-20 (April 1980).
*Totals include internal and external medicines.
†Totals include aspirin and other internal medicines.

Treatment of Acute Poisoning

The primary general rules in the first-aid treatment of acute poisoning are to *remove the patient from contact with the poison* and to *secure expert medical assistance at the earliest possible moment.* Supportive measures, such as artificial respiration, are often essential for the survival of the comatose patient. Poisoning most commonly results from local exposure to or ingestion of the toxic substance.

Local Exposure

Various chemicals, in particular acids and alkalis, are toxic to the skin, eyes, and mucous membranes. In most cases, injury results from direct irritation of the affected area, although some chemicals (chlorinated or organophosphate insecticides or those containing nicotine) can cause systemic toxicity after being absorbed through the skin.

Toxic materials spilled on the *skin* are best removed with large volumes of water, using soap if available. Vinegar (acetic acid) and baking soda (sodium bicarbonate) can be used to neutralize alkalis (lye) and acids, respectively. Exposure of the *eye* to caustic substances can cause chemical burns to the cornea and conjunctiva. The eye should be gently washed with very large volumes of water for at least five minutes, with the eyelids held open during this time; the patient should not be permitted to rub the eye. Expert medical assistance should be secured without delay.

Oral Ingestion

Oral ingestion of toxic chemicals may result in injury to the mucous membranes of the gastrointestinal tract or cause systemic toxicity after absorption. Treatment approaches include removal of the poison from the stomach by inducing emesis or employing gastric lavage; inactivation of the poison using local or systemic antidotes; or hastening the removal of the poison from the body.

Emptying the stomach. Induction of **emesis** (vomiting) is often the treatment of choice for the removal of poisons from the stomach. Compared to gastric lavage, emesis is more rapid, more efficient in emptying the stomach and duodenum, less traumatic to the patient, and more simple to perform. Neither emesis nor gastric lavage should be performed in patients experiencing seizures, or after the ingestion of strong acids or alkalis or petroleum distillates (gasoline, kerosene, cleaning fluids). Emesis should not be attempted in unconscious individuals.

Vomiting can be induced by mechanical stimulation or with drugs. **Syrup of ipecac** is a highly effective emetic agent which can be purchased at pharmacies at low cost and without a prescription. The syrup is about 90 percent effective in inducing emesis within 30 minutes. For children over one year of age, the usual

TABLE 31-7. COMMON POISONOUS PLANTS

Common Name [Synonyms] (Scientific Name)	Toxic Ingredients	Plant Part	Symptoms
Black elder *(Sambucus nigra)*	Sambuniarin (cyanide-producing glycoside)	Berries; leaves, shoots, bark	GI symptoms*
Castor bean *(Ricinus communis)*	Ricin	Seeds	Severe GI symptoms, convulsions, deaths reported
Dumb cane *(Dieffenbachia seguine)*	Calcium oxalate	All parts	Swollen tongue and loss of speech if ingested; itching and swelling of skin and mucous membranes
Holly *[Ilex]*		Berries	GI symptoms, stupor, stimulation
Jequirity bean [Rosary pea] *(Abrus precatorius)*	Abrin	Seeds	Severe GI symptoms, drowsiness, coma, circulatory collapse, kidney failure, fatalities reported
Jerusalem cherry *(Solanum pseudocapsicum)*	Alkaloids		Vomiting, local irritation, slowing of the heart
Jimson weed *(Datura stramonium)*	Stramonium, scopolamine, atropine	All parts	Fever, thirst, dry mouth, pupil dilation, skin flushed and dry, rapid heart rate, hallucinations

Plant	Toxin	Toxic parts	Symptoms*
Lantana (*Lantana camara*)	Lantanin	Unripened fruit	GI symptoms, muscle weakness, circulatory collapse, fatalities reported
Oleander (*Nerium oleander*)	Cardiac glycosides	Twigs (used as skewers); leaves; flowers	GI symptoms, cardiac irregularities, respiratory paralysis, fatalities reported
Philodendron (*Philodendron cordatum*)	?	Leaves	Skin rash; swelling of mouth and throat if ingested
Poinsettia (*Euphorbia pulcherrina*)	Milk white latex	All parts	Severe skin irritation; severe GI distress, if ingested
Poison hemlock (*Conium maculatum*)	Coniine	All parts	GI symptoms, muscle weakness, respiratory paralysis, convulsions
Pokeweed [Pokeroot] (*Phytolacca americana*)	Phytolaccatoxin (a saponin)	Roots, berries	Severe GI irritation, soreness of mouth and throat, lassitude, blurred vision, tremors
Wisteria (*Wisteria senensis*)	Wisterin	Pods, seeds	Severe GI symptoms, collapse
Yew (*Taxus*)	Taxine	Berry	Circulatory collapse, respiratory failure, convulsions, deaths reported

*Gastrointestinal symptoms include nausea, vomiting, diarrhea.

dose is one tablespoonful (15 ml, ½ oz) followed by a full of glass of water; this dose may be repeated in fifteen to twenty minutes if emesis has not occurred.

Apomorphine, a morphine derivative employed exclusively as an emetic agent, usually acts within three to five minutes after subcutaneous injection. The emesis induced by apomorphine is more complete than with ipecac syrup. Since this drug is only effective when injected, it cannot be recommended for routine inclusion in the household first-aid kit.

Gastric lavage is most useful in comatose, hysterical, or otherwise un-cooperative patients, and may be life-saving when employed within two to four hours after the ingestion of most poisons. Tap water is most commonly used as the lavaging fluid in adults, while normal saline solution (0.9% sodium chloride) is preferred in children. When the identity of the poison is known, specific lavage fluids may be used to inactivate or neutralize the poison (Table 31-8).

Inactivation of the poison.   Antidotes may antagonize poisons by virtue of their local or systemic actions (Table 31-8). *Local antidotes* act by either chemically neutralizing the poison remaining in the gastrointestinal tract or by physically combining with the poison and thereby preventing or retarding its absorption. **Activated charcoal** is a highly effective adsorbent that can be used to prevent the systemic absorption of a large number of poisons including most in-organic and organic toxic compounds; it is ineffective in the treatment of poisoning by cyanide, methanol, caustic alkalis, and mineral acids. This odorless, tasteless, fine black powder is generally administered as a freshly mixed slurry in water and is *never* swallowed dry.[11]

Systemic antidotes act systemically by specifically neutralizing the poison or by antagonizing its toxic effects. This antagonism may be pharmacological (competition for common receptor sites) or physiological (producing an effect that opposes that caused by the poison). Examples of specific antidotes appear in Table 31-8.

Hastening elimination of poison.   *Chelating agents,* such as EDTA and BAL, combine specifically or preferentially with certain toxic metals to form drug-metal complexes that are readily eliminated from the body.

Since relatively few specific and highly effective systemic antidotes are currently available, emergency treatment of acute poisoning frequently involves enhancing the rate at which the poison is excreted in the urine. Chemically, most drugs are weak acids or weak bases with only the nonionized forms of molecules capable of crossing the cell membranes of the kidney tubules and be-ing reabsorbed into the blood (Chapter 3). The degree to which acidic drugs such as aspirin and the barbiturates are ionized can be increased by alkalinizing the urine to pH 8 by administering sodium lactate or sodium bicarbonate.

---

[11] The time-honored "universal antidote" is totally undeserving of its laudatory reputation and should not be used. It consists of activated charcoal, tannic acid, and magnesium oxide. The last two ingredients are not only ineffective but may interfere with the beneficial properties of the activated charcoal.

Conversely, acidifying the urine with ammonium chloride or ascorbic acid enhances the urinary elimination of such basic drugs as the amphetamines and antihistamines.

Intravenous administration of large volumes of water, often containing an osmotic diuretic agent (mannitol, urea; Chapter 21), promotes water diuresis and facilitates elimination of the toxic agent; this is termed *forced diuresis*.

In the *dialysis* procedure, using an artificial kidney, toxic materials in the blood are allowed to diffuse across semipermeable membranes into a trapping solution (dialysate). Continuous replacement of the dialysate may be highly effective in removing the poison from the body.

SUMMARY

Toxicology is the study of the adverse effects of chemicals on biologic systems. No chemical is completely safe if administered in sufficiently large doses or for excessively protracted periods of time. Potential toxic chemicals include those to which we are involuntarily exposed, such as pollutants of our air, water, and food (environment toxicology); and those intentionally administered to produce a specified effect, either as medication, food additives, or pesticides (economic toxicology). Forensic toxicology includes the diagnosis and treatment of poisoning and any legal ramifications arising therefrom.

Many adverse toxic effects of chemicals can be predicted and often represent extensions of the normal pharmacological effects; adverse effects may range from the highly selective and specific to those that are relatively nonspecific. A number of environmental chemicals and therapeutic agents have been shown to be mutagenic (inducing permanent alterations in the DNA of germ cells), carcinogenic (malignant tumor-producing), and/or teratogenic (inducing structural and/or functional alterations in the fetus).

Idiosyncratic and allergic responses are atypical, unanticipated adverse drug effects observed in a limited number of subjects. Idiosyncratic reactions are genetically determined and differ from normal responses with respect to time course or intensity or may be totally novel and never observed in nonsusceptible persons. Allergic responses result from an antigen-antibody reaction; the symptoms are evoked by the release of histamine and other chemical mediators; the responses are independent of the dose and require more than one exposure to the chemical.

Acute poisoning is a major medical problem in children less than 5 years of age. In all poisoning cases, an attempt is made to remove the patient from contact with the toxic agent. After local exposure, this may be accomplished by washing the affected area with copious volumes of water. After oral ingestion, the toxic chemical can be removed by emptying the stomach by inducing vomiting (syrup of ipecac, apomorphine) or by gastric lavage; by preventing drug absorption (activated charcoal); by inactivating the poison, or by

TABLE 31-8. LOCAL AND SYSTEMIC ANTIDOTES AGAINT SELECTED POISONS

Poison (examples)	Antidote	Mechanism of Action
Locally acting antidotes against unabsorbed poisons		
Acids, corrosive*	Antacid or weak alkali	Neutralization of acid
Methanol		
Alkalis, caustic*	Weak acid (diluted vinegar)	Neutralization of alkali
Alkaloids	Potassium permanganate solution	Oxidation and inactivation
(nicotine, quinine, strychnine)		
Antidepressants, tricyclic	Activated charcoal (lavage)	Adsorption, retards absorption
Aspirin		
Propoxyphene (Darvon)		
Unknown poison		
Cyanide	Sodium thiosulfate	Precipitation, inactivation
Sodium hypochlorite (laundry bleach)		
Iodine	Starch or flour slurry in water	Inactivation
Iron	Sodium bicarbonate	Forms insoluble iron salt
	Deferoxamine	Forms iron chelate
Petroleum products* (gasoline, kerosene, cleaning fluids, paint thinner)	Mineral oil, followed by sodium bicarbonate lavage	Retards absorption
Systemically acting antidotes to heavy metal poisons		
Arsenic	Dimercaprol (BAL)	Chelation
Gold		
Mercury		

Poison	Antidote	Mechanism
Lead	Edetate calcium disodium (EDTA) (calcium disodium versenate)	Chelation
Copper Gold Lead Mercury	Penicillamine (Cuprimine)	Chelation
Iron	Deferoxamine (Desferal)	Chelation

Systemically acting antidotes for selected poisons

Poison	Antidote	Mechanism
Amphetamines	Chlorpromazine or haloperidol	Receptor blockade (behavioral effects)
	Propranolol	Receptor blockade (peripheral effects)
Anticholinergics Antidepressants, tricyclic	Physostigmine	Receptor blockade
Carbon monoxide	Oxygen inhalation	Hastens carboxyhemoglobin breakdown
Cyanide	Sodium nitrite and sodium thiosulfate	Cyanide inactivation
Methanol (wood alcohol)	Ethanol	Slows formation of toxic products
Narcotics Propoxyphene	Naloxone	Receptor antagonism
Strychnine	Diazepam	Controls convulsions

*Indicates emesis or initial use of gastric lavage not recommended.

antagonizing its effects; and/or by hastening its elimination by employing chelating agents, modifying the pH of the urine, or by dialysis.

In Chapter 1 we discussed the relevance of drugs to society, and emphasized that a general knowledge of drugs is essential for the well-informed citizen. When physicians, dentists, or veterinarians consider prescribing a drug for their patients, they must evaluate the benefit-to-risk ratio. The judicious consumer must also attempt to make a similar assessment, albeit armed with far fewer facts than the health professional. Successful solving of the problems of environmental toxicology involves many of the same basic principles discussed with respect to drugs. Moreover, the combined expertise and talents of medical, biological, environmental, chemical, physical, engineering, and social scientists will be required to find answers that best serve the needs of society.

SUPPLEMENTARY READINGS

Arena, J. M., *Poisoning: Toxicology, Symptoms, Treatment.* 4th ed. Springfield, Ill.: Charles C Thomas, 1979.

Doull, J., C. D. Klaassen, and M. O. Amdur, eds., *Casarett and Doull's Toxicology: The Basic Science of Poisons.* 2nd ed. New York: Macmillan, 1980.

Flamm, W. G., and M. A. Mehlman, *Mutagenesis.* New York: Halsted Press, 1978.

Gosselin, R. E., H. C. Hodge, R. P. Smith, and M. N. Gleason, *Clinical Toxicology of Commercial Products.* 4th ed. Baltimore: Williams & Wilkins, 1976.

Hardin, J. W., and A. M. Arena, *Human Poisoning From Native and Cultivated Plants.* 2nd ed. Durham, N.C.: Duke University Press, 1974.

Heinonem, O. P., D. Slone, and S. Shapiro, *Birth Defects and Drugs in Pregnancy.* Littleton, Mass.: Publishing Sciences Group, 1977.

Kaye, S., *Handbook of Emergency Toxicology.* 3rd ed. Springfield, Ill.: Charles C Thomas, 1977.

Loomis, T., *Essentials of Toxicology.* 3rd ed. Philadelphia: Lea & Febiger, 1978.

Martin, E. W., *Hazards of Medication.* 2nd ed. Philadelphia: Lippincott, 1978.

Sax, N. I., *Dangerous Properties of Industrial Materials.* 5th ed. New York: Van Nostrand Reinhold, 1979.

Schmahl, D., C. Thomas, and R. Auer, *Iatrogenic Carcinogenesis.* Berlin: Springer-Verlag, 1977.

Sunshine, I., *Handbook of Analytical Toxicology.* Cleveland, Ohio: Chemical Rubber Co., 1969.

Weiss, B., and V. G. Laties, eds., *Behavioral Toxicology.* New York: Plenum Press, 1975.

Wilson, J. G., and F. C. Fraser, eds., *Handbook of Teratology,* Vols. 1–4. New York: Plenum Press, 1977, 1978.

32

Nicotine and Tobacco Smoking

No research demonstrates that any ingredient as found in cigarette smoke causes cancer or cardiovascular, respiratory, or other illness in humans. No research has demonstrated any physiological process through which cigarette smoke results in illness.[1]

—The Tobacco Institute (1970)

[If] the government is to shift its health strategy toward preventive rather than curative medicine, it cannot ignore smoking. For smoking is the largest preventable cause of death in America. When demographers look at the death rates for diseases related to cigarette smoking, they identify 80,000 deaths each year from lung cancer, 22,000 deaths from other cancers, up to 225,000 deaths from cardiovascular disease, and more than 19,000 deaths from chronic pulmonary disease—every single one of them related to smoking. That is why smoking is Public Health Enemy Number One in America.[2]

—Joseph A. Califano, Jr. (1979)

Tobacco, a member of the nightshade family, is produced in all parts of the world. In recent years, production of the tobacco plant, *Nicotiana tabacum,* has increased, with a total of 11.7 billion pounds harvested throughout the world in 1975. Tobacco production is highest in Asian countries, followed by North America, Europe, and South America. The United States produced a total of 2.19 billion pounds in 1975, making this plant the fifth largest money crop in the nation. *Nicotiana tabacum,* a plant indigenous to the Americas, is used for the manufacture of cigarettes, cigars, pipe tobaccos, and, to a lesser extent, chewing tobaccos.

[1] "The Cigarette Controversy: Eight Questions and Answers" (Washington, D. C.; The Tobacco Institute, 1970).

[2] *Smoking and Health. A Report of the Surgeon General* (Washington, D. C.: U.S. Government Printing Office, 1979), p. ii.

After harvest, the green tobacco leaf is "cured" and aged, processes intended to improve the aroma and taste of products intended for smoking. These properties are further modified during the manufacture of cigarettes by blending and mechanically processing different tobaccos, by the addition of moisture-retaining and flavor-enhancing agents, and by wrapping the tobacco in cigarette paper with different burning qualities.

Of the more than 2000 compounds present in tobacco smoke, greatest attention has been focused upon *nicotine,* an alkaloid primarily responsible for both the organoleptic properties we generally associate with tobacco smoking as well as the proclivity for causing the smoking habit. After examining the pharmacology of nicotine, we shall consider some historical aspects of tobacco use, the nature of the smoking habit and the health hazards associated with it, and conclude by examining tobacco dependence and its treatment.

NICOTINE

Nicotine[3] is a volatile, colorless liquid, which, upon exposure to air, turns brown and emits an aroma characteristic of tobacco. The concentration of this alkaloid in the dried leaves of *Nicotiana tabacum* varies from about 2 to 8 percent.

Nicotine

Nicotine is a lipid-soluble (fat-soluble) compound that readily crosses cell membranes. It is readily absorbed across the intact skin and gastrointestinal tract (of toxicological significance), the oral cavity (chewing tobacco), and the lungs (smoking). After absorption into the blood, nicotine is metabolized rapidly, primarily by the liver; the plasma half-life of nicotine is about 40 minutes.

Pharmacology of Nicotine

The pharmacological actions of nicotine are complex, and this compound produces effects in many parts of the body. We shall primarily restrict our discussion to those aspects of nicotine pharmacology that are related to smoking.

---

[3]Nicotine was first isolated from the tobacco leaves in 1828 and named in honor of Jean Nicot, the French ambassador to Portugal, who was instrumental in introducing tobacco into France in 1559.

Mechanism Of Action

The actions of nicotine at the autonomic ganglion have been extensively studied. You will recall from Chapters 5 and 7 that the cholinergic receptors in autonomic ganglia are responsive to both acetylcholine (the endogenous neurotransmitter) and to nicotine. At low concentrations, nicotine interacts with the cholinergic receptor causing depolarization and acetylcholine-like stimulation. By contrast, higher nicotine doses produce initial stimulation followed by prolonged blockade of transmission. Nicotine has also been shown to stimulate the release of catecholamines from the adrenal medulla and norepinephrine from sympathetic (adrenergic) nerve endings.

Central Nervous System Effects

With the exception of caffeine (the pharmacologically active component of coffee, tea, and cola soft drinks), tobacco is undoubtedly among the most widely used substances intended to produce alterations in the mood. These effects are sufficiently reinforcing to motivate tens of millions to continue to smoke even after being fully convinced of the health hazards associated with this habit. Nicotine is the most likely component of tobacco responsible for the behavioral effects produced by smoking.

More than 90 percent of the nicotine inhaled after smoking is absorbed in the lungs and rapidly enters the blood. Nicotine reaches the brain almost twice as fast after inhalation as after an intravenous injection (7.5 sec versus 13.5 sec)!

Some individuals smoke because they seek stimulation or arousal, while others desire tranquilization with a reduction in feelings of anxiety and tension. Is tobacco a drug for all moods? Based upon our understanding of the actions of nicotine in the brain, we know that the speed and depth of inhalation of tobacco smoke are capable of producing these opposite behavioral effects. Shallow, infrequent puffs on a cigarette in a quiet room tend to be mentally activating, while rapid breathing, with deep inhalations, cause feelings of tranquilization.

At smoking doses, nicotine primarily *increases the level of arousal,* an effect resembling the normal arousal produced by a stimulating situation. This activation of the cerebal cortex is thought to be indirectly mediated via actions on the reticular activating system and hippocampus and may also involve nicotine-stimulated release of acetylcholine from the cortex.

Individuals very frequently smoke to relieve stress and achieve feelings of relaxation. While the pharmacological basis for this effect has not been clearly established, it has been suggested that smoking may reduce skeletal muscle tension. However, as we shall consider below, irritability is one of the primary symptoms associated with the cessation of the tobacco habit. The rapid dissipation of this irritability after smoking can be interpreted by the smoker as pleasurable tranquilization or, alternatively, through the skeptical eyes of the pharmacologist, as nicotine suppression of a nicotine withdrawal (abstinence) syndrome.

Peripheral Effects

Cardiovascular effects.   Regular tobacco smokers experience increases in heart rate (ranging from a few beats per minute to over 50), blood pressure, and basal metabolic rate (the rate at which energy is expended under resting or basal conditions), and vasoconstriction of the blood vessels of the skin causing a drop in skin temperature. The effects of smoking on heart rate and blood pressure, which may persist for up to one hour, have been attributed to nicotine-stimulated release of catecholamines from the adrenal medulla and norepinephrine release from sympathetic nerve endings in the heart.

Kidney.   Nicotine and tobacco smoking have an *antidiuretic effect,* with the nonsmoker more susceptible than smokers. You can demonstrate this effect with the following simple (and safe) experiment. Have two subjects drink about one quart of warm water and ask the nonsmoker to smoke one cigarette. After 60 minutes, diuresis or urine output should be considerably greater for the subject who has not smoked. These same effects occur in the experienced smoker who has had two or three cigarettes in succession.

Gastrointestinal effects and weight gain.   A common complaint of former smokers is their weight gain[4] after "kicking the habit." Is there any scientific basis for this observation, or can it be attributed to rationalizations by individuals who are incapable of curbing their voracious appetites? Nicotine has actions that might be responsible for a suppression of appetite. A single cigarette inhibits the hunger contractions of the stomach for 15 to 60 minutes. Although smoking exerts little effect on the normal blood sugar level, it elevates the fasting levels to normal for about one-half hour. You will recall that in Chapter 15 we discussed the stimulatory influence of blood sugar on the satiety center in the hypothalamus. Nicotine has been shown to numb the sensory nerves on the tongue responsible for taste. Benzocaine, a local anesthetic, is an alleged appetite suppressant that acts by a similar mechanism. The relative importance of these nicotine-induced effects in reducing appetite has not been fully assessed. Whereas many individuals respond to stress by smoking, still others find relief by eating. Perhaps the psychological considerations associated with smoking outweigh the pharmacological effects.

Acute Toxicity

Nicotine is among the most poisonous commonly encountered chemicals. Although it has no therapeutic uses, nicotine is the active ingredient in Black Leaf 40, an insecticide employed in the garden. Deaths have occurred within minutes after its absorption through the unbroken skin or after the accidental

---

[4] We are not referring to an increased wallet weight, which might approximate $500 annually for an individual who consumes two packs of cigarettes daily.

ingestion of this spray by children or gardeners. Administration of toxic amounts of nicotine produces nausea and vomiting, rapid breathing, behavioral disturbances, muscle weakness, convulsions, and respiratory failure. Death results from paralysis of the voluntary muscles responsible for breathing. The usual lethal dose of nicotine is between 5 and 60 mg, and yet, children have ingested tobacco products containing 20 to 30 mg of this alkaloid (about one pack of cigarettes)[5] and have survived. What accounts for their good fortune? The small amounts of nicotine initially absorbed into the blood stream cause vomiting, thus purging the young body of the remaining nicotine and tobacco. The small amount of nicotine still present in the body is then rapidly inactivated by normal biotransformation reactions.

Historical Background of Tobacco Use

> *For several centuries man has been possessed of a bizarre and apparently irresistible urge to inhale the smoke produced by burning the dried and shredded leaves of Nicotiana tabacum. Despite the evidence that life is shortened by about 12 min for every cigarette smoked, consumption continues unabated throughout the world.*
>
> —M. Lader (1978)

When Columbus arrived in the New World in 1492, he discovered a pleasure previously unknown to Europeans, but long enjoyed by the earliest Americans, namely, the smoking of tobacco leaves. While perhaps better remembered as the gentleman who provided his cape to carpet Queen Bess's feet from the mud, Sir Walter Raleigh—English explorer, soldier, historian, statesman, courier, and contemporary of Shakespeare—was also primarily responsible for promoting the introduction of tobacco in England in the 1570s and was instrumental in making smoking a fashionable habit at court and in polite company. Tobacco smoking soon became a habit enjoyed by all strata of Elizabethan society.[6] Tobacco was successfully cultivated in colonial Jamestown, Virginia, in 1611.

Smoking rapidly became the subject of controversy among Europeans. The pro-tobacco forces argued that this plant possessed virtually miraculous healing powers (*herba panacea*), and noted that it had been used by the Indians as a remedy for the relief of aches and pains in the abdomen and heart, for the treatment of snakebite, chills, convulsions, and skin diseases, and for the alleviation of feelings of fatigue, hunger, and thirst. One Nicholas Nomartes of Seville claimed that almost every disease of the gastrointestinal, respiratory, and urogenital tracts could be aided by a tobacco prescription. Among the cures he alleged to have obtained with tobacco syrups, tobacco enemas, or by

[5]In 1978, the sales-weighted average nicotine per cigarette was 1.1 mg down from 2.0 mg in 1959.

[6] "The Elizabethan age might be better named the beginning of the smoking era"—Sir James Barrie, author of *Peter Pan.*

inhalation of tobacco smoke were headaches, coughs, asthma, gout, stomach pains, constipation, kidney stones, flatulence, rheumatism, and toothaches.

The anti-tobacco forces in England were lead by King James I who stated that tobacco had "been taken in excess by a number of riotous and disorderly persons of mean and base condition who . . . spent most of their time in idle vanity, to the evil example and corruption of others." Moreover, he compared the black and smelly smoke of tobacco to vapors exhaled from hell. To protect the souls and bodies against "enslaving addiction," the Church and State enacted legislation proscribing its use; these laws, however, proved totally unsuccessful in curbing the ever-growing tobacco habit. Cardinal Richelieu in France and Charles I across the channel in England rapidly converted this moral defeat into a financial victory. They astutely recognized that whereas tobacco was sufficiently habit-forming to induce its faithful users to pay an onerous tax for its purchase, these same habit-forming properties were insufficiently potent to cause the moral and physical deterioration of their loyal subjects.[7]

Prior to the turn of the century in the United States, tobacco was most commonly smoked in pipes or as cigars, inhaled as snuff, and was chewed. The cigarette industry had its origin in the post–Civil War years with the opening of factories in North Carolina and Virginia. In 1870, an estimated 14 million cigarettes were manufactured, increasing to one billion in 1885, and achieving an annual average of 4.2 billion between the years of 1900–1909. The following decade, the average annual production increased almost six-fold to 24.3 billion[8] and has climbed over the years to 615 billion cigarettes in 1978—which were consumed by 54 million Americans. The rise in the per capita consumption of cigarettes and the corresponding decline in chewing tobacco from 1900 to 1975 is depicted in Figure 32–1.

Trends in Cigarette Smoking and Cigarette Products

The per capita consumption of cigarettes has decreased steadily in the United States since 1973. The estimated percentage of all adults who regularly smoked cigarettes in 1978 reached its lowest recorded point in over 30 years. From 1955 to 1978, the percentage of regularly smoking adult males declined from 53 to 38 percent. By contrast, the percentage of adult females who regularly smoked increased from 25 to 32 percent between 1955 and 1964; from 1965 to 1978 a decline was observed of no more than 3–4 percent. The decline in

---

[7] The practice of permitting citizens to handsomely pay their way to hell is still with us over three centuries later. Consider the taxes we are tendering when purchasing a tobacco product or an alcoholic beverage or are buying tickets to participate in a state-operated lottery or an off-track betting operation.

[8] The 1910–1920 decade marked the first time in American history when cigarette smoking surpassed tobacco chewing in popularity. Cigar consumption achieved its peak in 1920 when over 8 billion cigars were sold. By contrast, in 1976, 55-times as many cigarettes as cigars were consumed per capita in the United States.

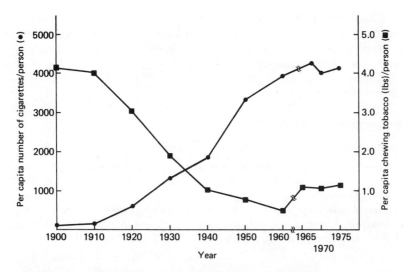

FIGURE 32-1. Consumption of Cigarettes and Chewing Tobacco in the United States, 1900-1975. Data from 1900-1960 represent the per capita consumption of tobacco products (for all males and females) 15 years of age and over, while the data from 1965-1975 represent the per capita consumption of cigarettes (for all males and females) and chewing tobacco (for males only) 18 years of age and over. (Data from *The Tobacco Situation* [U.S. Agricultural Marketing Service, 1977].)

the prevalence of adult male smoking occurred in all socioeconomic classes and age ranges, while the across-the-board smoking cessation among females was counterbalanced by the high rate at which smoking was initiated.

During the 1968 to 1974 period, there was little overall change in the percentage of teenage males who regularly smoked cigarettes (14.7 versus 15.8%). The percentage of *teenage female smokers,* by contrast, almost doubled from 8.4 to 15.3 percent and now exceeds the teenage male prevalence. Analysis of the available data suggests that the average age for the initiation of smoking among both males and females is declining.

The percent of market share of *filter-tip cigarettes* has increased from 0.6 in 1950, to 50.9 in 1960, to over 90 in 1978. By 1975, 85 percent of all regular cigarette smokers used filter-tip products. The average "tar"[9] and nicotine content of cigarettes has steadily declined since 1954 when reports linking cigarettes to lung cancer first appeared. From 1954 to 1977, the sales-weighted average "tar" content of a cigarette decreased from 36 mg to 17 mg, while from 1959 to 1978, the sales-weighted average nicotine content per cigarette dropped from 2.0 mg to 1.1 mg. From 1970 to 1978, the market share of cigarettes with "tars" less than or equal to 15 mg has increased from 3 to over 30 percent.

The available scientific evidence suggests that cigarettes with lower "tar" and nicotine are less hazardous to the health than are the high "tar" and nicotine cigarettes but that the health risks for smokers of these "safer" ciga-

[9] "Tar" refers to the particulate phase of cigarette smoke and excludes nicotine.

rettes still remain significantly greater than for nonsmokers. It should be noted that many individuals who shift to low "tar" and nicotine cigarettes may inhale more deeply, smoke the cigarette further down to the butt, or may simply increase their daily consumption of cigarettes to compensate for the lower concentration of nicotine.

THE SMOKING HABIT

> *Cigarette smoking is probably the most addictive and dependence-producing form of object-specific self-administered gratification known to man. . . Throughout history, no other single biologically unnecessary object has meant so much to so many people who, after so few initiating experiences, have needed to have it so often, so regularly, and for so many years, despite trying so hard to do without it; and for which there is no other adequate substitute.*[10]
>
> —Michael A. H. Russell (1976)

The smoking habit usually begins in the early or mid-teen years. The most important factors responsible for the *initiation* of smoking are the influence of friends and family. The best predictor of whether teenagers will initiate smoking is the smoking behavior of their friends; children with smoking parents or older siblings are also most likely to smoke.

Smoking is not a natural act—it must be learned and perfected with practice. Initial encounters with cigarettes are generally very unpleasant and often leave the smoker feeling sick and nauseated. In time, however, as these acute adverse feelings pass and smoking seems to satisfy the user's physiological and/or psychological needs, the habit becomes strengthened.

Six primary factors have been identified as being responsible for or influencing the *maintenance* of the smoking habit:

1. *Stimulation*—deriving a sense of increased energy or to relieve feelings of boredom.
2. *Sensorimotor manipulation*—getting satisfaction from handling or lighting the cigarette.
3. *Pleasurable relaxation*—rewarding oneself with a cigarette after the completion of a task, or to feel good, or to promote social interactions.
4. *Reduction of negative feelings*—as a tranquilizer to relieve or cope with feelings of anxiety, tension, anger, or restlessness.
5. *Addictive or craving*—to prevent or suppress the unpleasant feelings of withdrawal that are associated with physiological (physical) dependence upon cigarettes and nicotine.

[10] "Tobacco Smoking and Nicotine Dependence," in *Recent Advances in Alcohol and Drug Problems,* Vol. 3, ed. R. J. Gibbins, et al. (New York: John Wiley, 1976), p. 1.

6. *Habit*—smoking is tied to a specific situation (when having a cup of coffee, while conversing on the telephone, on a work break, after a meal, when reading, prior to bed).

Regardless of the precise reason(s) why individuals choose to continue to smoke, there is little doubt that for some it becomes an overwhelming compulsion that cannot be given up.[11] Tobacco dependence will be discussed in the last section of this chapter.

HEALTH CONSEQUENCES OF SMOKING

Today there can be no doubt that smoking is truly slow-motion suicide.
—Joseph A. Califano, Jr. (1979)

In a single year, the typical one-pack-a-day smoker takes 50,000 to 70,000 puffs of a cigarette whose smoke contains over 2000 known compounds. The presence of "tars," nicotine, and carbon monoxide in cigarette smoke have been implicated as causing or being associated with a variety of diseases. In this section, we shall summarize the health consequences of smoking as detailed in the 1979 comprehensive monograph, *Smoking and Health: A Report of the Surgeon General.* After presenting an overview of the influence of smoking on mortality and morbidity, we shall consider the relationship between smoking and cardiovascular diseases, cancer, respiratory diseases, gastrointestinal disorders, and pregnancy and infant health. Smoking-drug interactions and "second-hand smokers" will also be examined in this section.

Mortality and Morbidity

Mortality

The 1979 monograph *Smoking and Health* notes that, "Cigarette smoking is the single most important environmental factor contributing to premature mortality in the United States." While the mortality rates among smokers are particularly high for such diseases as lung cancer, chronic obstructive lung disease (emphysema, bronchitis), and cancer of the larnyx, coronary heart disease is the primary contributor to the excessive death rate among cigarette smokers.

The overall *mortality ratio*[12] for all male cigarette smokers, irrespective of the amount smoked, is 1.7 compared to nonsmokers. The mortality ratio has

---

[11] "I have made it a rule never to smoke more than one cigar at a time. . . . As an example to others, and not that I care for moderation myself, it has always been my rule never to smoke when asleep, and never to refrain when awake"—Mark Twain (1835–1910).

[12] Mortality ratio = death rate for a given classification of smokers divided by the death rate for a comparable group of nonsmoker volunteers.

been shown to increase: (1) as the number of cigarettes smoked increases—compared with the nonsmoker, the ratio for a two-pack-a-day male is 2.0; (2) the longer the individual has been a smoker; (3) the younger the age at which smoking was initiated; (4) the more smoke is inhaled; and (5) the higher the "tar" (T) and nicotine (N) content of the cigarette. For smokers of low T/N cigarettes (less than 17.6 mg T and 1.2 mg N), overall mortality rates are 50 percent greater than nonsmokers but 15 to 20 percent less than smokers of all cigarettes.

The life expectancy at a given age is significantly shortened by cigarette smoking; for example, a two-pack-a-day smoker between 30 and 35 years old has a life expectancy that is eight to nine years shorter than does a nonsmoker of the same age. The mortality ratios for male cigarette smokers who began smoking at ages 15–19 and 20–24 are 1.64 and 1.51, respectively. "Kicking the habit" appears to pay off. Former cigarette smokers experience declining mortality rates as their years of abstinence increase, and, after fifteen years, the mortality rates of former smokers are similar to those who have never smoked.

Pipe and cigar smokers show an overall mortality rate that is somewhat higher than the nonsmoker and, for the cigar smoker, is directly proportional to the number of cigars smoked daily. Smoking of cigars and pipes is associated with elevated mortality rates primarily resulting from cancers of the upper respiratory tract, including the oral cavity, the larnyx, and the esophagus.

Morbidity

A large body of evidence indicates that current cigarette smokers of both sexes experience more chronic illnesses than persons who have never smoked; among these conditions are chronic bronchitis and/or emphysema, peptic ulcer disease, and arteriosclerotic heart disease. A direct relationship has been generally observed between the amount smoked and the duration of smoking and the incidence and severity of these chronic conditions. This relationship has been the most dramatically demonstrated for respiratory disorders, where two-pack-a-day male and female smokers experience four and ten times the incidence of these illnesses, respectively, than nonsmokers. Moreover, compared with persons who have never smoked, current male and female smokers reported a 33 and 45 percent excess, respectively, in their work days lost.

Cardiovascular Diseases

Cigarette smoking has been closely linked with cardiovascular diseases, which, along with hypertension and high blood cholesterol, are important and significant risk factors for the development of coronary heart disease. More specifically, smoking increases the risk of fatal and nonfatal *myocardial infarction* (heart attack), the reoccurrence of a heart attack, and sudden cardiac death in adults. Among women of childbearing age, the risk of a nonfatal heart attack is doubled by the use of an estrogen-containing oral contraceptive, yet is increased by a factor of ten when oral contraceptive users also smoke.

The mechanisms responsible for the adverse influence of smoking on the cardiovascular system are varied and complex (Figure 32-2). Cigarette smoking indirectly affects the **heart** as the result of nicotine-enhanced catecholamine release from the adrenal medulla and norepinephrine release from sympathetic nerve endings causing a transient increase in heart rate and blood pressure for up to one hour. Catecholamines increase the adhesiveness of blood platelets promoting *clot formation*. The presence of a clot in the coronary arteries may mechanically obstruct the flow of blood thereby starving the heart muscle of essential nutrients and oxygen. Catecholamine release also increases the serum concentration of free fatty acids. These fats deposit in the walls of blood vessels, narrowing their lumen, and impairing blood flow through the coronary arteries. Cigarette smoke contains 1-5 percent *carbon monoxide* which preferentially combines with the hemoglobin in blood impairing its oxygen-carrying capacity. Thus, while smoking increases the demands placed on the heart muscle for oxygen, it produces changes that decrease the amount of oxygen available.

Smoking does not induce chronic high blood pressure (hypertension), nor has a conclusive association been demonstrated between smoking and angina pectoris or stroke. It should be noted, however, that smoking appears to lower the threshold for the onset of angina after exercise.

Cigarette smoking is a major risk factor for *atherosclerotic peripheral vascular disease* (PVD), and 90 percent of patients with PVD are cigarette smokers. This disorder primarily occurs as the result of occlusion of the arteries of the legs. As PVD progressively worsens, circulation to the legs may become inadequate to satisfy the increased need for oxygen and nutrients during exercise causing severe pain. Inadequate blood supply over long periods of time may potentially cause tissue wasting and gangrene.

Cancer

Cigarette smoke consists of a gaseous phase and a particulate phase. More than 2000 compounds have been identified which are retained by the filter; these compounds constitute the particulate phase and are commonly referred to by the collective term "tar." The gaseous phase, which constitutes more than 90 percent of the volume of the whole smoke, contains a much smaller number of compounds.

Compounds isolated from both the gaseous and particulate phases of tobacco smoke are involved in **tumor formation;** such compounds have been classified as carcinogens, tumor promoters, and cocarcinogens.[13] Among the most potent of these carcinogens is the polycyclic aromatic hydrocarbon *benzo(a)pyrene.*

---

[13] Chemicals that can induce the first steps of malignant transformation are known as *carcinogens* or *tumor initiators. Tumor promoters* are compounds which continue the process of tumor formation when applied to a tissue previously exposed to a chemical carcinogen. *Cocarcinogens* exert their effects when administered simultaneously with carcinogens but do not necessarily possess tumor-promoting properties themselves.

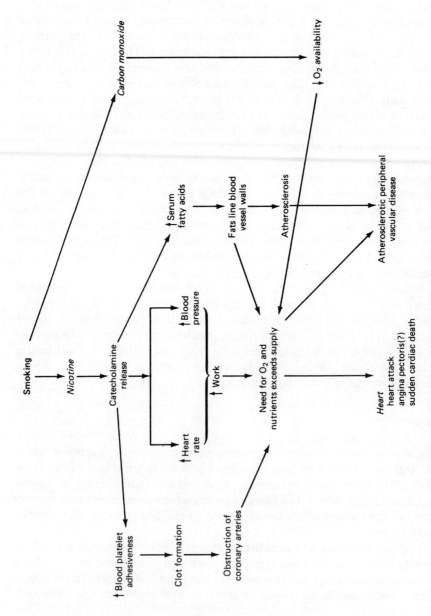

FIGURE 32–2. Influence of Smoking on Cardiovascular Disease.

The major cause of **lung cancer** in men and women is cigarette smoking, the risk of which is increased with increasing "doses" of smoking. Quantitative measures of smoking "doses" include the number of cigarettes smoked daily; the duration (years) of the smoking habit; the age at which smoking was initiated; the degree of inhalation; and the "tar" and nicotine content of the cigarettes smoked. In recent years, the mortality rates for lung cancer have been increasing more rapidly in females than in males and, if these present ominous trends continue in the coming decade, carcinoma of the lungs will become a leading cause of cancer death in women. Thus, the slogan, "You've come a long way, baby," may be subject to several interpretations.

Asbestos workers who smoke cigarettes carry eight times the risk of lung cancer than do smokers not exposed to asbestos. This has been estimated to be 92 times the risk of nonsmokers who do not work with asbestos.

Smoking is a significant factor in cancer of the oral cavity, larnyx, and esophagus, and there appears to be a synergistic effect between smoking and alcohol intake for these three cancer types. In both sexes, there is a significant association between cigarette smoking and cancer of the urinary bladder and, in males, between smoking and cancer of the kidney.

Respiratory Disease

Deaths resulting from *emphysema* and *bronchitis* are six times more prevalent in cigarette smokers than in nonsmokers. Emphysema, the most common chronic disease of the lungs, causes years of suffering for the patient. Emphysemic patients have marked difficulty in breathing, are short of breath (dyspneic), wheeze, and often have painful hacking coughs. This debilitating disease eventually prevents patients from working, causing them to be an emotional and financial liability to themselves, their families and society in general. Whereas coughing and expectoration are related to the number of cigarettes smoked, the incidence of these symptoms is only slightly greater than normal for cigar and pipe smokers. On the average, the physiological function of the lung is less efficient in cigarette smokers when compared with nonsmokers of the same age. The major problems involve a narrowing of the airways and impaired transfer of gases. When the young smoker stops smoking, respiratory function returns to normal. Advanced cases of respiratory disease show only modest improvement after cessation of smoking, although there may be significant relief from the hacking cough.

What is the underlying basis of these distressing respiratory symptoms? Irritating substances present in the tobacco smoke cause coughing and bronchoconstriction after the smoke is inhaled. These compounds increase the size of the mucus glands and the amount of secretions from these glands which causes expectoration; the normal movement of the cilia lining the walls of the bronchi is also impaired. These two effects lower the resistance of the cigarette smoker to bacterial infections of the bronchi.

Gastrointestinal Disorders

An increased frequency of *peptic ulcer disease* is observed among smokers, and smoking increases the mortality rate resulting from these ulcers of the stomach and duodenum. While smoking appears to have little or no effect on gastric (hydrochloric) acid secretion, it retards the healing of peptic ulcers. Nicotine inhibits the secretion of bicarbonate from the pancreas; the lack of this natural antacid reduces the body's capacity to neutralize gastric acid potentially favoring duodenal ulcer formation. Moreover, smoking increases the reflux of the duodenal contents (bile, pancreatic juice) into the stomach which might cause damage to the gastric mucosa (inner lining of the stomach) and which may contribute to the etiology of gastric ulcers.

Pregnancy and Infant Health

Babies born of smoking mothers are more likely to be aborted, to be stillborn (fetal death), or to die shortly after birth (neonatal death). This risk increases directly with increasing levels of maternal smoking.

Maternal smoking is a direct cause of a *reduction in birth weight.* Babies born of mothers who smoke during pregnancy weigh, on average, 200 g (7 oz) less than babies born of nonsmoking mothers; the more the mother smokes, the greater the reduction in birth weight. Since maternal smoking does not alter the average duration of pregnancy, the lower birth weight would appear to result from a retardation of fetal growth. Studies attempting to assess the effects of maternal smoking on long-term growth and development suggest that physical growth, mental development, and the behavioral (intellectual, emotional) characteristics of children may be impaired at least up to the age of 11 years.

The proportion of fetal deaths and live births that occur prior to term increase directly with the maternal level of smoking; it has been suggested that up to one-seventh of all preterm deliveries in the United States may be attributable to maternal smoking. Such smoking can be a direct cause of *fetal* or *neonatal death* in an otherwise normal infant. The immediate cause of most smoking-related fetal deaths is anoxia, and this oxygen deprivation often results from placental complications. In other cases, the presence of carbon monoxide in the maternal and fetal blood interferes with the availability of oxygen to satisfy the needs of the fetus. There is no support for the allegation that smoking increases the incidence of congenital malformations.

Nicotine is excreted in the *breast milk,* and its concentration in the milk is directly proportional to the number of cigarettes smoked by the nursing mother. There is insufficient evidence currently available to indicate whether maternal smoking modifies the adequacy of the milk supply.

Smoking-Drug Interactions

Tobacco smoke contains a number of compounds that are capable of modifying the activity of *liver microsomal drug-metabolizing enzymes* (Chapter 3). In light of the regular smoking habits practiced by one-third of the adult population of the United States, tobacco smoking might potentially represent a primary source of drug interactions. Polycyclic aromatic hydrocarbons (PAH), including benzo(a)pyrene, that are present in the "tar" (particulate) phase of cigarette smoke have been shown to act as inducers of selected drug-metabolizing enzymes. Moreover, it would be premature for us to exclude the possibility that PAH are acting by other mechanisms to hasten the pharmacological inactivation or removal of drugs.

In clinical studies, smokers have exhibited faster than normal rates of metabolism of phenacetin and pentazocine (analgesics), theophylline (bronchodilator used for the treatment of asthma and bronchitis), and imipramine (tricyclic antidepressant). The beneficial therapeutic effects or incidence of adverse effects associated with the administration of propoxyphene (analgesic), furosemide (diuretic), propranolol (cardiovascular agent), and diazepam (antianxiety agent) have been shown to be reduced in smokers versus nonsmokers by mechanisms that do not appear to involve an increase in the rates of metabolism of these drugs. Interpretation of the relationship between smoking and drug effects is complicated by the fact that cigarette smokers tend to consume more coffee and alcohol than nonsmokers as well as take more drugs for the relief of pain, insomnia, anxiety, and gastrointestinal disorders.

"Second-Hand Smokers"

The antismoking campaigns of the early 1900s attempted to protect the smoker against self-inflicted physical and mental decay, while those initiated in the 1970s sought to protect the innocent bystander against the hazards of "second-hand" smoke.

As the use of cigarettes increased after 1910, so did the intensity of the activities of antismoking leagues seeking to protect susceptible women and children[14] against the evils and dangers associated with the inhalation of the smoke of the tobacco leaf. Emulating the model of the antisaloon leagues and

---

[14] The nefarious effects of cigarettes on the young people of America were well known to cigar-smoking Thomas Edison and described to Henry Ford in a letter written in 1914. In contrast to cigar smoke, the smoke liberated from paper wrapped cigarettes "has a violent action in the nerve centers, producing degeneration of the cells of the brain, which is quite rapid among boys. Unlike most narcotics, this degeneration is permanent and uncontrollable. I employ no person who smokes cigarettes." Quoted from J. E. Brooks, *The Mighty Leaf* (Boston: Little, Brown, 1952), p. 274.

alcohol prohibitionists, by 1921 these zealots were successful in promoting the enactment of cigarette prohibition laws in 14 states, with an additional 92 anticigarette bills in various stages of the legislative process in 28 states. Tobacco prohibition laws were no more successful than those banning alcohol, and, by 1927, the last of the general statewide anticigarette laws was repealed.

The 1970s witnessed a renaissance in antismoking legislation, with the enactment of laws designed to protect the passive smoker from the potentially harmful effects of "second-hand"smoke. Lung associations and other proponents of laws limiting smoking in public places have argued that: (1) nonsmokers exposed to smoke in enclosed areas experience an increase in heart rate, a rise in blood pressure, and an elevation in carbon monoxide levels in the blood; (2) persons with respiratory and cardiovascular disorders are adversely affected by "second-hand" smoke; and (3) such smoke may affect the fetuses of pregnant women and infants during their first year of life. Recent evidence suggests that nonsmokers suffer lung damage from inhaling cigarette smoke, and have the same risk of respiratory impairment as do smokers who do not inhale and smokers who inhale the smoke of up to ten cigarettes daily.

Increasingly greater restrictions are being placed upon the social acceptability of smoking and ease with which an individual can smoke in the company of nonsmokers. The first state-wide antismoking law was passed in Arizona in 1973; by 1978, 33 states and the District of Columbia had enacted laws preventing smoking in public places.[15] "No smoking" is now the rule rather than the exception, with many laws stating that smoking is prohibited unless signs are posted that specifically permit this practice. Violation of the law is a misdemeanor and violators are subject to a fine. While the vigor with which these laws are enforced in various jurisdictions extends over a broad spectrum, the nonsmoker need no longer "choke and bear it."

TOBACCO DEPENDENCE

Tobacco smoking is a form of drug dependence and the modern cigarette is a highly efficient device for self-administering the drug nicotine. By inhaling, the smoker can get nicotine to his brain more rapidly than the heroin addict can get a "buzz" when he shoots heroin into a vein. . . . Furthermore, the smoker gets a "shot" of nicotine after each inhaled puff. At 10 puffs per cigarette, the pack-

---

[15] As might be anticipated, powerful interest groups are opposed to antismoking legislation. The tobacco producers and manufacturers are supported in their lobbying efforts by advertising interests who fear the loss of a primary and highly lucrative source of revenue. The enthusiasm of members of Congress to protect their constituents is tempered by the realization that the federal tax of 8 cents per pack of cigarettes added $2.5 billion to the credit side of the federal ledger in 1977 and a total of $3.5 billion in state and local taxes. The noneconomist should appreciate, however, that these tax revenues did not offset the estimated $27 billion expended for health costs associated with smoking.

a-day smoker gets more than 70,000 nicotine shots in his brain in a year. It is hardly surprising that nicotine smoking is so addictive.[16]

—Michael A. H. Russell (1977)

The curves [depicting the relapse rates for treated heroin users and smokers] are remarkably similar . . . but inferences concerning similar mechanisms need to be qualified. Relapse to heroin occurs against a steep gradient of immediate high risk and strong social disapproval, and merely obtaining the drug requires considerable effort. Relapse to smoking occurs in an environment that is almost neutral with respect to tobacco use, in which there is no immediate risk to health or social status, and in which the cigarettes are cheap and ubiquitous. While we may continue to wonder what drives the ex–opiate addict to relapse, given the multiple motives for smoking that have been postulated and the number of cigarettes a heavy smoker may have consumed over a 10-year period, we may find it remarkable that relapse is not universal.[17]

—Jerome H. Jaffe and Murray E. Jarvik (1978)

Reports of tobacco dependence by the native inhabitants of the Americas and the early European explorers appear in writings dating back to the sixteenth century. While 30 million Americans are former regular cigarette smokers, approximately 54 million are current regular smokers.

Tolerance and Physical Dependence

The neophyte smoker often experiences a drop in blood pressure, a slowing of the heart rate, nausea, salivation, cold sweat, pallor, and occasionally vomiting. With not strenuous effort, *tolerance* develops to these nicotine-induced effects. For example, while nonsmokers become nauseated after being administered 1 or 2 mg of nicotine, regular tobacco users can tolerate up to 8 mg.

A wide variety of psychological and physiological disturbances have been reported to occur after the cessation of the smoking habit; at this time, it is not clear whether all these effects can be solely attributed to a *nicotine withdrawal syndrome.* Among the symptoms commonly associated with the cessation of smoking include an intense craving for tobacco, tension, irritability, restlessness, depression, and impairment in the powers of concentration. Other symptoms may include a decrease in heart rate and blood pressure, weight gain, constipation, and sleep disturbances.

The smoking withdrawal syndrome generally appears within hours to several days after smoking cessation and may persist with varying degrees of in-

---

[16] "Smoking Problems: An Overview," in *Research on Smoking Behavior,* ed. M. E. Jarvik et al., NIDA Research Monograph 17, (Washington, D. C.: U.S. Government Printing Office, 1977), p. 15.

[17] *Psychopharmacology: A Generation of Progress,* ed. M. A. Lipton, A. DiMascio, and K. F. Killam, (New York: Raven Press, 1978), pp. 1674–75.

tensity for days to many months. Withdrawal irritability may be experienced even after relatively brief periods (90 minutes) of smoking deprivation.

Treatment

Since the initial dissemination of the health consequences of smoking to the public in the first Surgeon General's Report on Smoking and Health in 1964, a variety of methods have been introduced to assist the smoker to stop smoking. Such quitting methods are of two basic types: self-care and organized programs.

Self-care techniques may involve devising one's own way of quitting, receiving and following the advice of others, or using an instructional guide or filter device. While there are no long-term objective evaluations of the effectiveness of the numerous self-care techniques, it is estimated that 95 percent of the 30 million smokers who quit smoking since 1964 have done so on their own.

Most smokers accept the scientific evidence that smoking has an adverse effect on their health. While six of ten smokers have made a serious attempt to stop smoking, and another three of ten would try to quit if an easy way was available, most smokers need external aasistance in trying to break the smoking habit.

Organized smoking cessation methods are extremely diverse in nature and orientation and include individual counseling by physicians and other health professionals; educational programs conducted in the schools; group programs sponsored by voluntary public health (lung, heart, cancer) associations; hypnosis; aversive conditioning including electric shock, unpleasant tastes, breath holding, chain smoking until nauseated, or imagining that smoking is causing illness or other unpleasant effects; self-control involving the use of signal devices that interfere with environmental stimuli that normally lead to smoking; mass media activities combined with kits of antismoking materials; saturation antismoking campaigns involving entire communities or geographic areas; drugs;[18] and miscellaneous methods, usually employed in conjunction with another method, such as role playing, yoga, meditation, relaxation techniques, and reassuring telephone messages.

[18] Two general categories of **drugs** are employed by smokers seeking to quit: substitutes for smoking, and drugs that reduce the severity of the abstinence syndrome.

Lobeline, an alkaloid obtained from *Lobelia* (Indian tobacco), the most common smoking substitute, is reported to possess actions that are similar to those of nicotine. Lobeline is the active ingredient in a number of commercial products (Bantron, Lobidram, Nikoban, No-Kotin) promoted as smoking deterrents. Controlled studies suggest that lobeline is no more effective than a placebo in helping individuals stop smoking.

More recently, *nicotine-containing chewing gum* (Nicorette) has been developed which, in preliminary trials, appears to be effective in controlling the smoking abstinence syndrome. Each stick of gum, flavored with spice, contains 2 mg of nicotine; it is buffered to keep the saliva alkaline so that virtually all nicotine absorption will occur in the mouth. Each pack of gum is intended to replace a pack of cigarettes.

While it is far beyond the scope of this text to evaluate each of these treatment approaches, it should be noted that there has been a general lack of objective assessment of the success of these programs under carefully controlled conditions. No single treatment approach has been demonstrated to be clearly superior, and it now appears that the combined employment of multiple approaches may be most useful. While a very high percentage (60–80%) of participants completing many of the existing programs may have stopped smoking by the end of the formal treatment period, a mere 20 percent may be nonsmokers at the end of one year. Among the principal reasons commonly cited for relapse to smoking is the abstinence syndrome. It would appear that the severity of this abstinence syndrome is greater in women than men, and perhaps, to some measure, this accounts for the lower rate of achieving smoking cessation in women.

Youth-Oriented Programs

Despite a large number of educational programs directed at youths and adults, it is not known which approaches are most effective in preventing the initiation of smoking or terminating the habit once it has begun. Many youth-oriented programs have focused upon the long-term health hazards associated with smoking. While surveys indicate that 94 percent of teenagers know that smoking is harmful to their health, and 90 percent of teenage smokers are cognizant of the health threat that smoking poses, adolescents are interested in *now* and less moved by messages dwelling exclusively with the future.

A promising new approach seeks to fortify adolescents against the onslaught of various influences that lead to the initiation of smoking, including peer pressure, the mass media and advertising, and parent/older sibling smoking models. In these new programs, greater emphasis is placed on the *early* adverse effects to health caused by smoking. Since addictive smoking generally first appears during the high school years, the actual impact of smoking deterrent programs for adolescents cannot be accurately assessed until the youth has entered high school.

SUMMARY

The health hazards associated with the smoking of tobacco have now been ascertained with reasonable certitude. Of the more than 2000 compounds present in the gaseous and particulate phases of tobacco smoke, the alkaloid nicotine appears to be responsible for the behavioral effects and dependence associated with the regular use of cigarettes and other tobacco products. Depending upon the manner in which tobacco is smoked, nicotine may produce a state of arousal or relaxation. Smoking also causes transient increases in heart rate and blood pressure and suppression of appetite. Nicotine is among the most toxic chemicals commonly encountered; systemic absorption through the skin and after oral ingestion have resulted in many severe poisonings and even deaths in both children and adults.

Approximately one-third of the adult population (54 million) and 15 percent of teenagers in the United States smoke cigarettes. The prevalence of smoking among teenage females has been increasing at an alarming rate, and the average age at which smoking is initiated is declining.

Individuals continue to smoke for one or more of the following primary reasons: stimulation, sensorimotor manipulation (handling), pleasurable relaxation, to reduce negative feelings (antianxiety effects), to prevent or suppress tobacco craving, and through habit.

The mortality rate for all male adult cigarette smokers is 70 percent higher than for nonsmokers. Cigarette smoking is thought to be associated with more than an additional 340,000 deaths each year as well as severe illness resulting from cardiovascular diseases (heart attack, sudden cardiac death, atherosclerotic peripheral vascular disease); cancers of the lungs, oral cavity, larnyx, esophagus; respiratory diseases (emphysema, bronchitis); and peptic ulcer disease. The incidence of stillborns, neonatal deaths, and babies with lower birth weights is higher in smoking mothers. Smoking has been shown to reduce the magnitude of the pharmacological effects of some drugs. Cigarette smoke inhaled by nonsmokers ("second-hand" smoke) has been shown to have adverse effects on such individuals.

Tobacco dependence is characterized by psychological dependence (which may assume the extreme proportions of craving in some individuals), tolerance, and physical dependence. The incidence of relapse to smoking by persons seeking to quit is extremely high and may be related to the severity of the abstinence syndrome. Approximately 30 million persons have stopped cigarette smoking in the United States since 1964, 95 percent of whom have done so employing self-care techniques. Organized smoking cessation methods are extremely varied; none have been demonstrated to be clearly effective one year after the termination of treatment or even clearly superior to other existing methods. Lobeline is a drug used as a smoking deterrent, while nicotine-containing chewing gum is employed to reduce the severity of the abstinence syndrome. Vigorous attempts are currently underway to develop effective youth-oriented smoking deterrent programs.

SUPPLEMENTARY READINGS

Corti, A., *A History of Smoking*. London: George G. Harrap & Co., Ltd., 1931.

Jarvik, M. E., J. W. Cullen, E. R. Gritz, T. M. Vogt, and L. J. West, eds., *Research on Smoking Behavior*. NIDA Research Monograph No. 17. Washington, D.C.: U.S. Government Printing Office, 1977.

Jusko, W. J., "Role of Tobacco Smoking in Pharmacokinetics," *Journal of Pharmacokinetics and Biopharmaceutics* 6(1): 7–39 (1978).

Krasnegor, N. A., ed., *Cigarette Smoking as a Dependence Process.* NIDA Research Monograph No. 23. Washington, D.C.: U.S. Govenment Printing Office, 1979.

Krasnegor, N. A., ed., *The Behavioral Aspects of Smoking.* NIDA Research Monograph No. 26. Washington, D.C.: U.S. Government Printing Office, 1979.

Larson, P. S., and H. Silvette, *Tobacco: Experimental and Clinical Studies.* Supplement 3. Baltimore: Williams & Wilkins, 1975.

United States Public Health Service, *The Health Consequences of Smoking.* PHS Publication No. (CDC) 76-8704. Washington, D.C.: U.S. Government Printing Office, 1976.

United States Public Health Service, *Smoking and Health—A Report of the Surgeon General.* DHEW Publication No. (PHS) 79-50066. Washington, D.C.: U.S. Government Printing Office, 1979.

World Health Organization, *Smoking and Its Effect on Health: Report of a WHO Expert Committee.* WHO Technical Report Series No. 568. Geneva: World Health Organization, 1975.

Epilogue

Pharmacology as a science can aid us through its applications, if they are wisely made, to obtain those satisfactions in living which we all crave—satisfactions the drive for which is an inherent part of the built-in make-up of our integrating neurohumoral mechanisms for self-preservation and for the preservation of our human species, with its presumed humanity.

—Chauncey D. Leake (1961)

The earliest pharmacologist was doubtlessly a nameless inarticulate brute who, incapable of assuming an erect position and clad in an animal skin, was the first of this species to experience the biological effects of a plant ingested as a source of nourishment. History does not tell us whether this plant alleviated physical or mental suffering, altered behavior, or caused our ancestor to become violently ill and die. Moreover, we do not even know whether any fellow cave dwellers profited from this experience.

In the latter half of the last century, experimental pharmacology made its first appearance in Europe as an independent science. Among these early teachers was Oswald Schmiedeberg (1836-1921), whose pupils left his laboratory at Strassburg and established pharmacology departments throughout Europe and the United States. Today, tens of thousands of biomedical scientists housed in universities, research laboratories, and the multibillion-dollar pharmaceutical industry are actively studying the effects of drugs and their various influences on molecules and society. Scores of scholarly journals are reporting the results of these endeavors at an astronomical rate that can only be assimilated by large banks of computers fed by hordes of programmers.

Drugs have not only increased our life span, but have, more significantly, improved the quality of our lives. When your great-grandparents were about your age, a desolate and limited prognosis faced the patient afflicted with tuberculosis, meningitis, diabetes, high blood pressure, heart disease, schizophrenia, depression, severe allergic disorders, epilepsy, or arthritis. The few drugs that were then available possessed questionable therapeutic merit and were generally highly toxic to the patient. Today, all these diseases can be controlled with appropriate medication, thus enabling the patient to enjoy a more productive life.

What advances in pharmacology might we expect to witness during the course of our lifetimes or that of our children? Although disease will not cease to exist, drugs may be developed that are capable of preventing, more effectively treating, or even curing heart disease, mental illness, cancer, and illnesses of viral etiology. Drugs may be available to correct the genetic defects of the young, while others may postpone the mental and physical deterioration of the aged. Advances in pharmacology have not been uniformly distributed throughout the world. Although malaria and worm infestations have been largely eradicated in the Western world, today hundreds of millions of people in developing nations remain the prey of parasites. Diseases may, in the future, be managed by correcting their *underlying cause* and not by merely providing symptomatic relief. Optimal control of naturally occurring hormones and neurotransmitter substances may be achieved permitting disease to be managed in a "normal" physiological manner. Such control may result in some of the following therapeutic advances: enhancement of the rate of interferon synthesis to combat cancers and viral diseases; activation of endorphin release to alleviate pain and psychiatric disorders; selective elevation or reduction in specific members of the prostaglandin family of compounds to permit the management of inflammatory disorders, such as arthritis; and control of the immune system in a manner that permits a maintenance of its host defense capabilities to combat infectious disorders, while not rejecting tissues transplanted to replace worn-out or defective organs.

Humankind cannot achieve these goals until we more fully comprehend the nature of the biological processes occurring within our cells during health, disease, and aging, as well as the biochemical, physiological, and psychological mechanisms responsible for both normal and abnormal behavior. Such conquests of disease lie within the reaching fingertips of humankind and will be fully grasped only after the resolution of these enigmas. Drugs can play two fundamental roles in achieving these objectives. They may be utilized as experimental tools that will disclose the mysterious events that underlie the etiology of disease, and they may serve as instruments for achieving the prevention or cure of such disorders.

Index

A

Abortion, induced by:
  laxatives, 60–61
  prostaglandins, 39
Absences (petit mal seizures), 214, 216
Absorption of drugs, 47, 50 (*see also* specific
    drugs)
  definition, 47
  influenced by:
    disease, 67
    foods, 65, 223, 565–566
    physical-chemical drug properties, 47, 50
    routes of drug administration, 47, 48–49
    surface area, 50
  new drug development, 81
Abstinence syndrome (*see* Withdrawal
    syndrome)
Acetaldehyde, 224, 225, 241
Acetaminophen, 286, 517
  actions/effects, 287–288, 290
  chemistry, 287
  toxicity, 288

Acetanilid, 274
Acetazolamide, 216, 430, 432–433
Acetic acid, 276
Acetohexamide, 477
Acetone, 197
Acetophenazine, 328
Acetylcholine, 128–129 (*see also* Autonomic
    nervous system)
  acetylcholinesterase, 111, 129, 134
  actions/effects:
    cardiovascular system, 131
    central nervous system, 152, 175
    eye, 131, 133
    ganglionic transmission, 130, 160
    glandular secretions, 131, 490
    neuromuscular junction, 109, 130, 135, 160
    smooth muscles, 131, 531, 532
  antagonists, 112, 150–155, 160
  biosynthesis and breakdown, 129
  chemistry, 129
  choline acetyltransferase, 129
  drugs interacting with, 112, 175
  history, 106–107

Male sex hormones *(cont.)*
  representative drugs, table of, 468
  uses, 468, 588
Mandol (cefamandole), 564
Mandrax, 203
Mania, 340
  treatment, 331, 340–341
Mannitol, 428, 431, 435
Marax, 533
Marezine (cyclizine), 527
Marijuana, 368–385 *(see also Cannabis)*
Marijuana Tax Act, 371
Marine pharmacology, 77
Marplan (isocarboxazid), 339
Matulane (procarbazine), 589
Maximum effect, 34, 37
Mazindol, 315
MDA (methylenedioxyamphetamine), 352,
  354, 363
Mebaral (mephobarbital), 207, 216
Mecamylamine, 161, 420
Mechlorethamine, 584
Meclizine, 527, 529, 614
Median effective dose (ED50), 35, 36
Median lethal dose (LD50), 35, 36
Medicinal chemistry, 9
Medicine, use of drugs in, 11
Medihaler-Epi (epinephrine), 532
Medihaler-Iso (isoproterenol), 532
Medroxyprogesterone, 456, 465
Medulla oblongata:
  anatomy, 167
  functions, 172
  respiratory centers depressed by:
    barbiturates, 209
    general anesthetics, 196
    narcotics, 257, 258
    treatment, 209
Mefenamic acid, 290
Melanocyte-stimulating hormone, 451
Mellaril (thioridazine), 328
Melozets, 315
Melphalan, 584
Melsedin (methaqualone), 203
Membranes, cell, 26, 28–29
  drug passage across, 42–46
  inhibition of function, 550–551
  transport of chemicals, 446, 550
    hormonal influences, 447
Menopause, 456
Menstrual cycle, 454–455
  actions/effects of oral contraceptives on, 455
  treatment of disorders of, 456
Mental illness, 321–326
  causes, theories of, 324–326
    biochemical, 174, 250, 325–326, 329, 336,
    337
    genetic, 326
    psychological/sociocultural, 324–325

classifications and symptoms, 321–323
  affective disorders, 334
  depression, 334, 336
  mania, 340
  neuroses/psychoses, 322–323
general considerations, 321–322
hospital population statistics, 324
treatment with drugs:
  antianxiety, 341–346
  antidepressant, 337–340
  antimanic, 331, 340–341
  antipsychotic, 327–334, 335
  evolution of, 323–324, 326–327
Mental incapacitants, 16, 139, 140
Menthol, 275
Mepenzolate, 497
Meperidine, 252, 509
  actions/effects, 261
  chemistry, 251
Mephenesin carbamate, 342
Mephobarbital, 207, 216
Meprobamate, 202, 342, 343, 344
  abuse potential, 344
  actions/effects, 342, 344
  chemistry, 342
Mequin (methaqualone), 203
Merbaphen, 429
Merbromin, 27
Mercaptomerin, 430
Mercaptopurine, 586
Mercurial diuretics, 429, 430
Mercuric chloride, 429
Mercurochrome (merbromin), 27, 542, 604
Mercurous chloride, 429
Mercury, 604–605
  poisoning by, 85, 604–605
    treatment, 605, 624
  pollution, 604
  sources, 604
  therapeutic uses, 543, 604
Mercury bichloride, 429
Mering, J. von, 206, 471
Mersalyl with theophylline, 430
Mersalyn (mersalyl with theophylline), 430
Merthiolate (thimerosal), 27, 542, 604
Mescal buttons, 5
Mescaline, 354, 361–363
  actions/effects, 362–363
  adverse effects, 362
  chemistry, 352
  comparison with LSD, 356, 362
  derivatives, 352
  history, 5, 361–362
  peyote religion, 5, 361–362
Mesoridazine, 328
Mestinon (pyridostigmine), 135
Mestranol, 462
Metabolism (biotransformation) of drugs,
  54–56